AF668805

Pharmaceutical Biochemistry
- A Comprehensive Approach

Pharmaceutical Biochemistry
- A Comprehensive Approach

Dr. G. Saravanan
M. Pharm., Ph.D.
Professor
Department of Pharmaceutical Chemistry,
MNR College of Pharmacy,
Sangareddy, Hyderabad, TS, India.

Dr. V. Alagarsamy
M. Pharm, PhD, FIC, DOMH
Professor and Principal,
MNR College of Pharmacy,
Sangareddy - 502 294,
Hyderabad, TS, India.

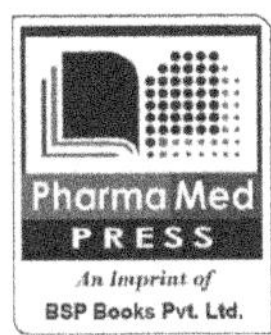

PharmaMed Press
An imprint of BSP Books Pvt. Ltd.,
4-4-309/316, Giriraj Lane,
Sultan Bazar, Hyderabad - 500 095.

Pharmaceutical Biochemistry - A Comprehensive Approach
by *G. Saravanan and V. Alagarsamy*

Published by:

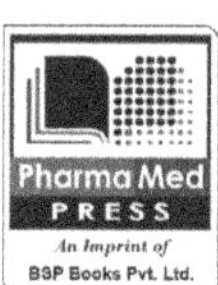

PharmaMed Press
An imprint of BSP Books Pvt. Ltd.,
A Unit of BSP Books Pvt. Ltd.
4-4-309/316, Giriraj Lane, Sultan Bazar, Hyderabad - 500 095.
Phone: 040-23445688; Fax: 91+40-23445611
E-mail: info@pharmamedpress.com
www.pharmamedpress.com/pharmamedpress.net

ISBN: 978-93-95039-13-0 (Hardback)

Dedication

Dr. G. Saravanan's Mother

Made to believe that anything is possible & for making everything possible

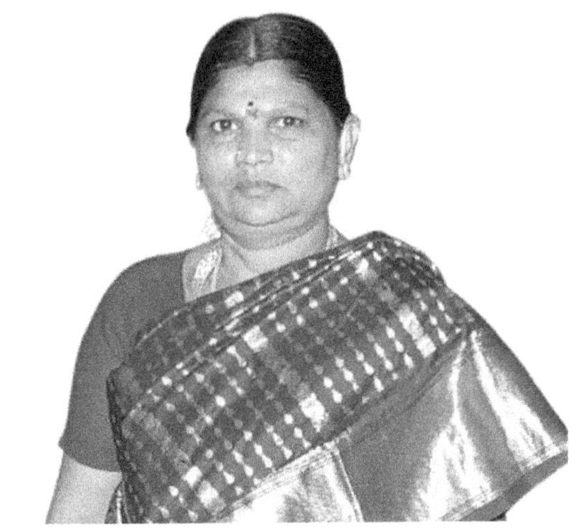

Shrimathi. G. NAGATHILAGAM

Preface

Biochemistry or biological chemistry is the branch of science that explores the chemical and physicochemical processes and substances that occur within and are related to living organisms. *The branch of science dealing with the study of all the life processes such as control and coordination within a living organism is called Biochemistry.* Biochemistry is a sub-discipline of both chemistry and biology. It may be divided into three fields: structural biology, enzymology, and metabolism. Over the last decades of the 20th century, biochemistry has become successful at explaining living processes through these three disciplines. Almost all areas of the life sciences are being covered and developed through biochemical methodology and research. Biochemistry focuses on understanding the chemical basis which allows biological molecules to give rise to the processes that occur within living cells and between cells, in turn relating greatly to the understanding of tissues and organs, as well as organism structure and function. Biochemistry is closely related to molecular biology, which is the study of the molecular mechanisms of biological phenomena.

Much of biochemistry deals with the structures, functions, and interactions of biological macromolecules, such as proteins, nucleic acids, carbohydrates, and lipids. They provide the structure of cells and perform many of the functions associated with life. The chemistry of the cell also depends upon the reactions of small molecules and ions. These can be inorganic (for example, water, and metal ions) or organic (for example, amino acids, which are used to synthesize proteins). The mechanisms used by cells to connect energy from their environment via chemical reactions are known as metabolism. The findings of biochemistry are applied primarily in medicine, nutrition, and agriculture. In medicine, biochemistry is used to investigate the causes and cures of diseases. In nutrition studies, biochemistry is used to maintain health and wellness and also the effects of nutritional deficiencies. In agriculture, biochemistry is used to investigate soil and fertilizers. Improving crop cultivation, crop storage, and pest control are also goals. Biochemistry covers a range of scientific disciplines, including genetics, microbiology, forensics, plant science, and medicine. Because of its breadth, biochemistry is very important and advances in this field of science over the past 100 years have been amazing.

Biochemistry is essential to understanding the following concepts. a) The chemical processes which transform diet into compounds that are characteristics of the cells of a particular species; b) The catalytic functions of enzymes; c) Utilizing the potential energy obtained from the oxidation of foodstuff consumed for the various energy-requiring processes of the living cell; d) The properties and structure of substances that constitute the framework of tissues and cells; e) To solve fundamental problems in medicine and biology.

The students often encounter various difficulties in grasping the fundamentals of biochemistry especially when they are supplied with inadequate information on basic biochemical reactions, enzymes, energetic metabolic pathways and principles, procedures, and the significance of the clinical biochemical test. Most of the books already published on this subject miss dealing with various aspects of biochemistry, particularly the clinical biochemistry part. For instance, a book gives the metabolism well but fails to explain the basic biomolecules and clinical biochemistry part; another book explains well about basic biomolecules and metabolic pathways but not the clinical biochemistry.

The vast academic experience helped us to realize the need of the students for a book that can help them to become masters in the subject. Many of our students were also inspired to learn biochemistry with the at most ease and simplified form of our clear and illustrative lecture notes. The main object of this book is to attract the B. Pharm., and Pharm. D graduate students, so that they feel an urge to explore and understand the basics of biochemistry including clinical biochemistry. This book thus aims at eliminating the inadequacy in teaching and learning biochemistry by providing enormous information about basic biochemical reactions, reasoning behind enzyme names, energetic aspects with clear representation, and regulation of metabolic pathways with inhibitors. In addition, the clinical biochemical test is well covered in this book with detailed principles, procedures, and clinical significance which will be beneficial for students, particularly Pharm. D., graduates. This book will add new encouragement to the study of the subject and will boost the spirit of research and provide new dimensions to the process of understanding biochemistry.

This book is an effect of our vision to discover the best biochemistry book, especially for pharmacy students, which consists of three parts. Part – I deals with the basic biochemistry including cell, biological membrane, transport of molecules, biological redox reactions, high energy compounds and various aspects of enzymes with well-labelled diagrams, illustrations and flow charts. Part – II deals with biomolecules and their metabolism. In this part, each biomolecule is discussed in a simplified manner with a clear definition, classification, properties and significance. For easy understanding and revision, classifications of biomolecules were schematically represented in colour and properties and biological significance was given point by point. One of the major highlights of this book is the metabolism of biomolecules which will clearly distinguish this book from the rest of the available books on the market.

Metabolic pathways were represented both in structural form and theoretical form along with the type of reaction, name of enzyme responsible and energetic aspects. The changes that take place in each biochemical reaction are highlighted in the structure for easy understanding of the type of reaction. Detailed explanation was given for each and every reaction of various metabolic pathways with the reasoning of enzyme name and energetic calculation. In the applicable places, regulation, inhibitors and metabolic disorders of biochemical reactions were also discussed. Part – III deals with clinical biochemistry including immunochemical techniques. In this part, the principle, reagents required, procedure, calculation and significance of various qualitative and quantitative biochemical tests were described in a student-friendly manner. Schematic representations of principle and procedure were given which is another highlight of this book. Probable questions including multiple-choice questions with keys, short answers and long answers given at end of each chapter add colours to this book. Swathing the entire features of biochemistry, a first of its kind, is the unique feature of this book. It facilitates the students to understand the subject more easily and interestingly. While writing this book, we felt that the book will bring about a re-orientation in the teaching and learning process of biochemistry.

The academic community in India is faced with a scarcity of books to cater to their needs. Numerous foreign writers' books deal well with basics and metabolic aspects related to biochemistry but lack clinical biochemistry aspects. Some Indian authors filled this lacuna to a certain extent by including the clinical biochemistry aspects but failed to give a clear explanation of metabolic pathways and clinical biochemistry tests. For this, the content of this book has been carefully tailored to cater for the needs of the academicians belonging to all Indian universities, pharmacologists, and clinical and industrial pharmacists by incorporating the missing links. We hope that this book will be a good source of information and reference for not only pharma graduates but also basic and applied researchers in this field. Moreover, it will also be of interest to a wide range of scientists, including organic chemists, medicinal chemists, pharmacologists and clinicians, who are interested in drug research. We welcome suggestions and constructive criticism from all corners of the scientific community.

Dr. G. Saravanan & Dr. V. Alagarsamy

Acknowledgement

A warm response to Prof. Alagarsamy's earlier books on the titles of "Text Book of Medicinal Chemistry", "Pharmaceutical Chemistry of Natural Products" (Published by Elsevier), Pharmaceutical Inorganic Chemistry, Pharmaceutical Organic Chemistry (Published by Pharma Book Syndicate) prompted us to write this Book on "Pharmaceutical Biochemistry - A Comprehensive Approach", covering all the topics suggested by the Pharmacy Council of India (PCI) for B. Pharm., and Pharm. D graduate students.

We wish to place on record our heartfelt thanks to everyone who has made this book possible, especially our beloved teachers from the first standard to the doctoral program. We dedicate this book to the many hundreds of budding graduates and pharmacy students, whom we have taught over the years, and our teachers who have encouraged us to convert our class notes into textbooks to reach a wide range of academic communities.

We are immensely grateful to Prof. K. Chinnaswamy and Dr. B. Suresh (**Pro-Chancellor, JSS University;** Ex-President, Pharmacy Council of India) for their constant support and inspiration extended to us to author this book.

We gratefully acknowledge the constant and continuous encouragement and moral support extended by Shri. M. N. Raju, Chairman, and Mr. M. Ravi Varma, Vice-Chairman, MNR Educational Trust, Hyderabad, for our entire academic and research pursuit, is a great motivation for us in taking up this new challenge.

We thank all the faculty members of the Faculty of Technology, Osmania University, Hyderabad for their constant support in all our academic activities.

We thank Mr. Anil Shah, Managing Director, PharmaMed Press for recognizing and inviting us to write this book. The friendly interaction experienced with the Pharma Book Syndicate, Mr. Naresh (Production Manager), and his team offered cordial support, which always made me furnish my input to make this Book one of the Best. Getting such a cooperative and energetic team encourages the authors to continue their writing always. We thank them wholeheartedly for accepting all views while designing the book and helping us reach this target.

Individually Dr. Saravanan expresses his sincere thanks to his father (Mr. V. Govindaraj), mother (Ms. G. Nagathilagam), father-in-law (Mr. T. R. Raja), mother-in-law (Ms. R. Rajathi), uncle (Mr. N. Manikandan & Mr. N. Thirupathi Vasagan), brother (Mr. G. Veeraputhiran), and cousin (Mr. R. Ramanarayanan & Mr. R. Lakshmana Kumar) for their kind encouragement and moral support throughout his career. The stimulation he got from his wife (Ms. R. Murugalakshmi) to reach this target is more than enzymes, and the patience and cooperation extended by his children (S. Veeraeshwaran and S. Veerakanishka), made him think of the goal without any diversion. He also expresses his sincere thanks to his friends especially Dr. T. Panneer Selvam, Dr. P. Dinesh Kumar, Dr. C. R. Prakash, Dr. K. Selvaraj, Dr. P. Parasuraman, and Dr. N. Kiruthiga for their support in his career.

Most of all, we thank The Almighty God for his endless blessings, knowledge, and strength to make this book possible.

G. Saravanan
sarachem1981@gmail.com
WhatsApp: +91-9963023257

V. Alagarsamy
drvalagarsamy@gmail.com
WhatsApp: +91-7674893936

Contents

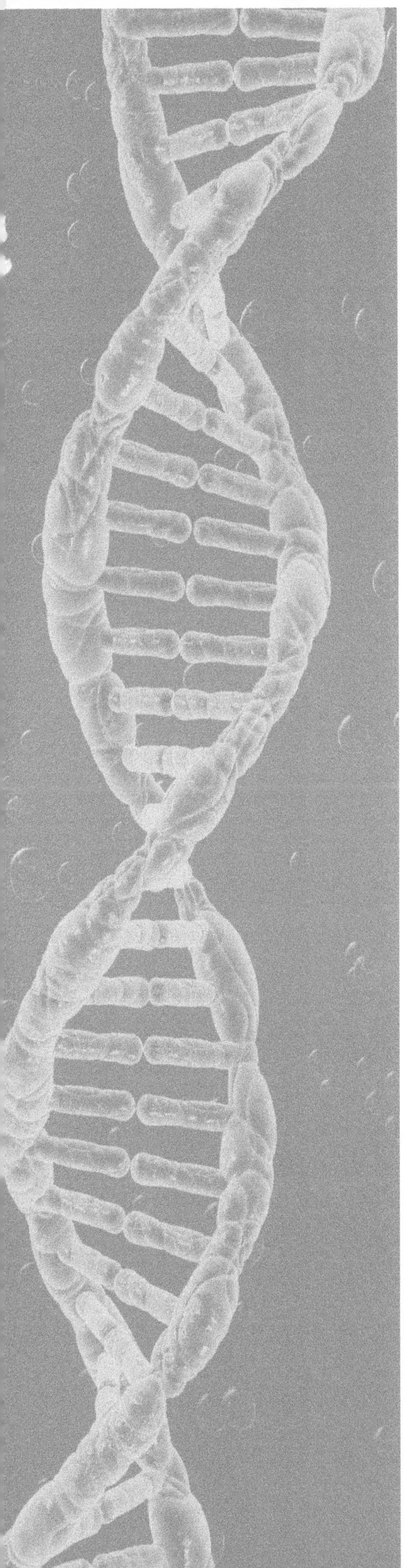

Part - I: Basic Biochemistry

1

Introduction to Biochemistry

The study of chemical processes within and relating to living organisms is called as **Biochemistry**. Sometimes it is also called as **biological chemistry**. The complexity of life is raised by biochemical processes. The chemical basis of biological molecules and its related process occur within living cells and between cells are focused and understand by biochemistry. This will help to study and understand tissues and organs, as well as organism structure and function. Structures, functions, and interactions of biological macromolecules, like proteins, nucleic acids, carbohydrates, and lipids are dealt by much of biochemistry. This biological macromolecule performs many of the functions associated with life and provides the structure of cells. The chemistry of the cell also depends on the reactions of smaller molecules and ions. These can be inorganic (**Example:** Water and metal ions) or organic (**Example:** The amino acids, which are used to synthesize proteins). Primarily in medicine, nutrition and agriculture the findings of biochemistry are applied. The causes and cures of diseases are investigated by biochemist in medicine. The effects of nutritional deficiencies and how to maintain health and wellness are studied in nutrition. Soil and fertilizers are investigated by biochemist in agriculture. They also try to discover ways to improve crop cultivation, crop storage, and pest control.

Cell

The structural and functional unit of life is cell. In all living organisms the basic unit of life is the cell. All organisms are made of cells or aggregates of cells. Unicellular organisms are organism composed of a single cell and multicellular organisms are organism composed of many cells. Independent existence and performing the essential functions of life are the capabilities of unicellular organisms. Live cell was first seen and described by Anton Von Leeuwenhoek and nucleus was later discovered Robert Brown. All the structural details of the cell were revealed by using electron microscope. Anything less than a complete structure of a cell does not ensure independent living.

Cells are the fundamental structural and functional unit of all living organisms or biological activity and are organized into subcellular organelles and each is assigned to specific function.

Composition of Cell

Elements: Living matter or cell is composed of many elements. Based on the quantities present in living matter elements are broadly classified into two major types.

1. **Major elements:** It constitutes about 90 % of dry body weight of human body. Carbon (C), hydrogen (H), oxygen (O), nitrogen (N), phosphorous (P) and sulfur (S) are the six major elements present in living matter.
2. **Minor elements:** Cell also contains several other elements in minute quantity which are functionally important. Sodium (Na), potassium (K), calcium (Ca), magnesium (Mg), fluorine (F), chlorine (Cl), iodine (I), zinc (Zn), iron (Fe), copper (Cu), cobalt (Co), molybdenum (Mo) and selenium (Se) are minor elements present in the cells.

The most predominant and versatile element of life is carbon because it is capable to form infinite number of compounds. The reason behind is ability of carbon to form stable covalent bonds and unlimited carbon–carbon (C-C) chain. In living system about 90% of compounds invariably contain carbon.

Macromolecules or Biomolecules: Life is composed of lifeless chemical molecules. About 6,000 and 1,00,00 different types of molecules are present in bacterium and man, respectively. Among these only few are characterized till now. Proteins, nucleic acid (such as DNA and RNA), polysaccharides and lipids are the important macromolecules or biomolecules composed of amino acids, nucleotides, monosaccharides and fatty acids, respectively. Strictly speaking lipids are not polymers but fatty acids are present in majority of lipids. The building blocks and functions of important biomolecules of cells are summarized in Table 1.1.

Table 1.1 Building blocks and functions of important biomolecules of cells.

S. No	Macromolecules or Biomolecules	Repeating Unit or Building Blocks	Important Functions
1	Protein	Amino acids	Static and dynamic functions of cell and fundamental basis of structure.
2	Deoxyribonucleic acid (DNA)	Deoxyribonucleotides	Storehouse of genetic information.
3	Ribonucleic acid (RNA)	Ribonucleotides	Essentially needed for biosynthesis of protein.
4	Glycogen or Polysaccharide	Glucose or monosaccharide	Storage form of energy to meet short term demands.
5	Lipid	Fatty acid, glycerol	Structural components of membrane and storage form of energy to meet long term demands.

Structural hierarchy of organism: Elements forms building blocks and macromolecules are formed from building blocks. Supramolecular assemblies like membranes are formed from macromolecules such as proteins, nucleic acid (such as DNA and RNA), polysaccharides and lipids. This supramolecular assembly organizes into organelles, cells, tissues, organs and finally the whole organism. The structural hierarchy of organism is depicted in Figure 1.1.

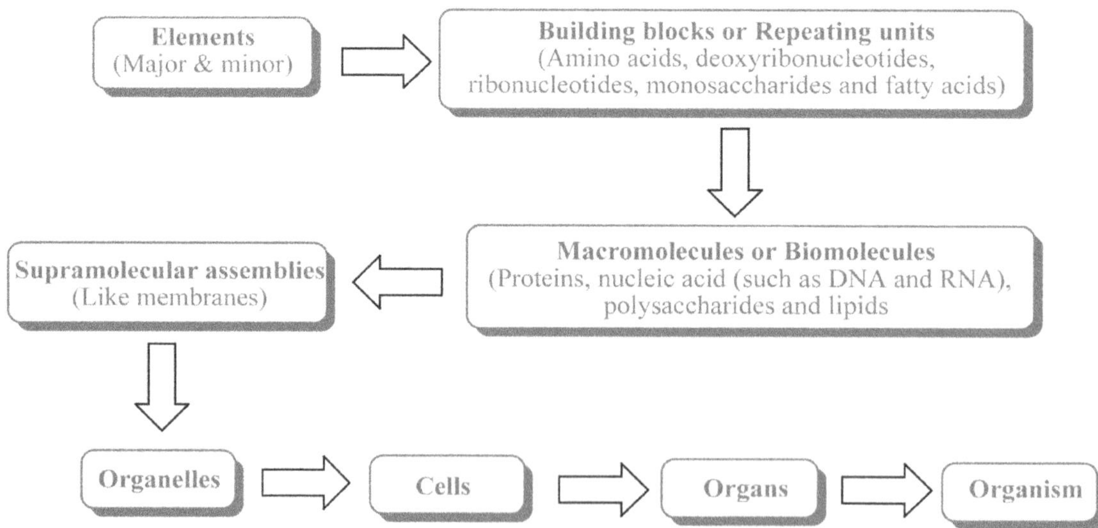

Figure 1.1 The structural hierarchy of organism.

Chemical composition of organism: The chemical composition of a normal healthy adult weighing 65 kg is summarized in Table 1.2. More than 60 % of the weight is contributed by the solvent of life i.e., water. Protein is mostly present in muscle and lipids are mostly present in adipose tissue contributes to weight followed by water. Minerals contributes about 6 % of body weight. Carbohydrate in the form of glycogen is present in low concentration and contributes less to weight.

Table 1.2 Chemical composition of a normal healthy adult weighing 65 kg.

S. No	Name of constituent	Composition (in percentage %)	Contribution to weight (in Kg)
1	Water	61.6	40
2	Protein	17.0	11
3	Lipid	13.8	9
4	Minerals	6.1	4
5	Carbohydrate	1.5	1
6	Total	100.0	65

Types of Cell

Based on the presence or absence of a membrane bound nucleus and other organelles, cells and hence organisms are broadly classified into two major types as,

1. Eukaryotic cell.
2. Prokaryotic cell.

A typical eukaryotic cell consists of a cell membrane, nucleus and cytoplasm and prokaryotic cell lacks membrane bound nucleus. Plant cells have a cell wall outside the cell membrane. **The volume of the cell is occupied by a semi-fluid matrix called cytoplasm in both prokaryotic and eukaryotic cells**.

Cells vary in their shape, size and activities/functions. **Example:** Only 0.3 μm is the length of smallest cell mycoplasmas, 3 to 5 μm is the length of bacteria and egg of an ostrich is the largest isolated single cell. 7.0 μm is the diameter of human red blood cells of multicellular organisms. Nerve cells are some of the longest cells. In addition to size, cells are also vary greatly in their shape. The shape of the cell may be columnar, polygonal, thread like, cuboid, disc-like, or even irregular. Based on the function they perform the shape of the cell may vary. Different shapes of cells are presented in Figure 1.2.

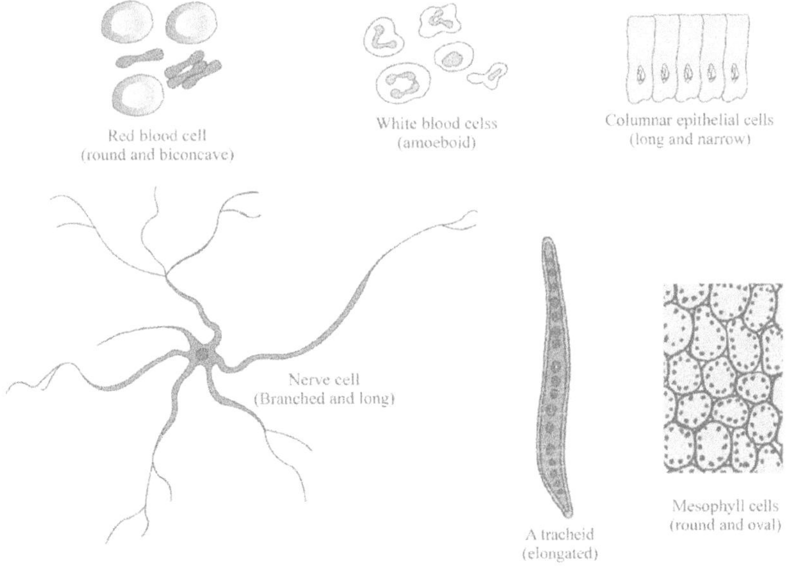

Figure 1.2 Different shapes of cells.

Prokaryotic Cells

In Greek "pro" means "before" and "karyon" means "nucleus". Prokaryotes lack nucleus and possess simple structure. In general, prokaryotic cells are smaller and multiply more rapidly as compared to eukaryotic cells. Bacteria, blue-green algae, mycoplasma and PPLO (pleuro pneumonia like organisms) are examples for prokaryotic cells. The size and shape of prokaryotic cells vary greatly. Rod like (*bacillus*), spherical (*coccus*), comma shaped (*vibrio*) and spiral (*spirillum*) are the four basic shapes of bacteria.

A wide variety of shapes and functions are exhibited by prokaryotic cell but the fundamental organizations are similar. Except in mycoplasma, cell wall surrounds the cell membrane in all prokaryotes. Cytoplasm is the fluid matrix filling the cell and there is no well-defined nucleus. Nuclear membrane do not envelop the genetic material and is basically naked. Outside the genomic DNA, small circular DNA known as plasmid is present in many bacteria in addition to the genomic DNA (the single chromosome/ circular DNA). Unique phenotypic characters like antibiotic resistance are conferred to such bacteria by this plasmid DNA. With foreign DNA, bacterial transformation is monitored by using this plasmid DNA in higher classes. In eukaryotes nuclear membrane is present. Except for ribosomes no organelles are found in prokaryotic cells like the ones in eukaryotic cells. The characteristic of prokaryotes is mesosome which is a specialized differentiated form of cell membrane. They are essentially in the folding of cell membrane. A typical eukaryotic cell and its comparison with other organism is presented in Figure 1.3.

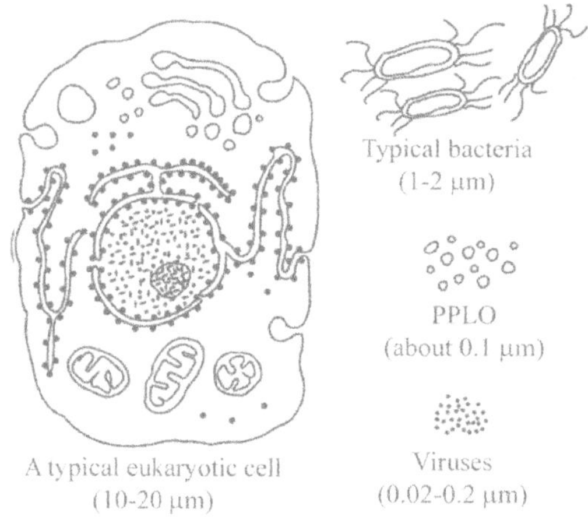

Figure 1.3 A typical eukaryotic cell and its comparison with other organism.

Cell envelope: Chemically complex cell envelope is present in many prokaryotic cells, mainly the bacterial cells. A tightly bound three layered structure is compose the cell envelope.

1. The outermost layer is glycocalyx
2. The centre layer cell wall
3. The inner layer plasma membrane.

Together these three layers perform single protective unit even though distinct functions are performed by each layer. Based on the cell envelope differences and response to Gram staining, bacteria are broadly classified into two major categories as Gram positive and Gram negative bacteria. Among different bacteria, composition and thickness of glycocalyx differs. In some bacteria the glycocalyx is slime layer (loose sheath) while in others it may be capsule (thick and tough). Apart from protection from bursting or collapsing, the cell wall prevents the bacterium by providing a strong structural support and the cell wall also determines the shape of the cell. In nature the plasma membrane is selectively permeable and interacts with the outside world. Structurally these membranes of prokaryotes are similar like eukaryotes.

In the cell extensions of plasma membrane, it forms a special membranous structure known as mesosome. Vesicles, tubules and lamellae are the different forms of extensions. Mesosomes help in cell wall formation, DNA replication and distribution to daughter cells. They also help in secretion processes, respiration, increasing the enzymatic content and surface area of the plasma membrane. Chromatophores which contain pigments are other membranous extensions into the cytoplasm which are present in some prokaryotes like cyanobacteria. Bacterial cells may be motile or non-motile. Flagella are the thin filamentous extensions from the bacterial cell wall present in motile bacterial cells. Bacteria show a range in the number and arrangement of flagella. Filament, hook and basal body are three parts of bacterial flagellum. The longest portion of flagellum is the filament and it extends from the cell surface to the outside. In bacteria pili and fimbriae are also the surface structures besides flagella but they don't have any role in motility. The pili made up of special protein are elongated tubular structures and the fimbriae sprouting out of the cell are small bristle like fibers. It helps to attach bacteria to rocks and also to the host tissues in some bacteria.

Ribosomes: With the plasma membrane ribosomes are associated in prokaryotic cell. They are made of two subunits namely 50S and 30S units which when present together form 70S prokaryotic ribosomes and the size is about 15 to 20 nm. Ribosomes are the site of protein synthesis. Polysome or polyribosomes are the chain formed by attachment of several ribosomes into a single mRNA. The ribosomes of a polysome translate the mRNA into proteins.

Inclusion bodies: Inclusion bodies are the storage form of reserve material present in cytoplasm of prokaryotic cells. In cytoplasm they lie free and are not bound by any membrane. **Example:** Phosphate granules, cyanophycean granules and glycogen granules. Green, purple and blue green photosynthetic bacteria contain gas vacuoles.

Eukaryotic Cells

In Greek "eu" means "true" and "karyon" means "nucleus". Eukaryotes possess well defined nucleus and are more complex in structure and functions. Protists, plants, animals and fungi are examples for eukaryotic cells. Presence of membrane bound organelles with an extensive compartmentalization of cytoplasm is present in eukaryotic cells. With a nuclear envelope, an organized nucleus is present in eukaryotic cells. In addition, various complex cytoskeletal and locomotory structures are also present in eukaryotic cells. Chromosomes are the organized genetic material of eukaryotic cells.

Cell walls, large central vacuole and plastids are present in plant cells and in animal cells these are absent; hence all eukaryotic cells are not identical. In other way, centrioles are present in animal cells whereas in plant cells these are absent. Structure of plant and animal cells are presented in Figure 1.4 and Figure 1.5, respectively.

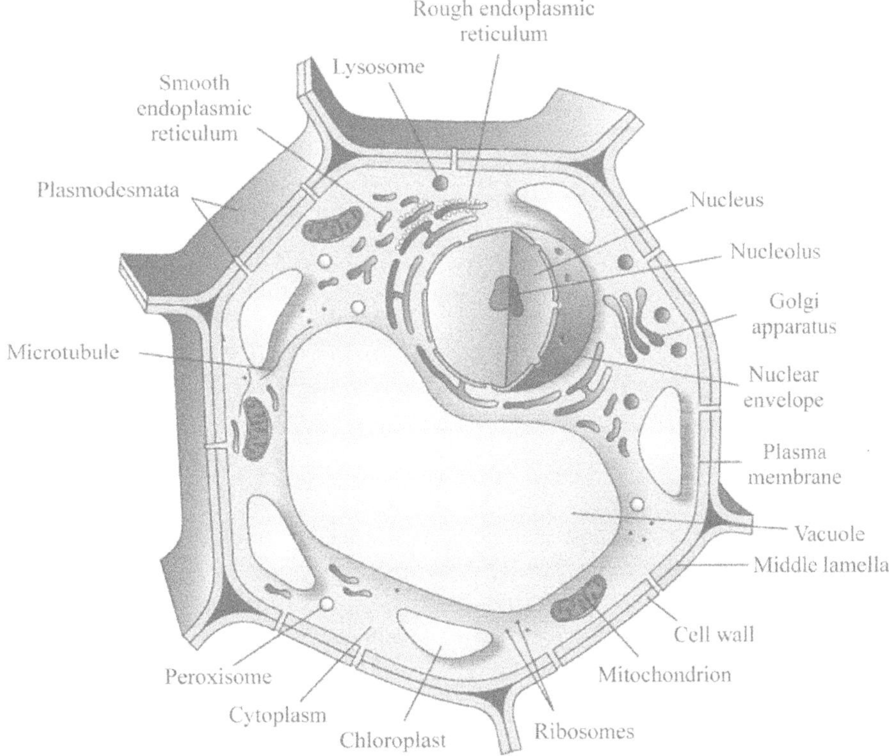

Figure 1.4 Structure of plant cell.

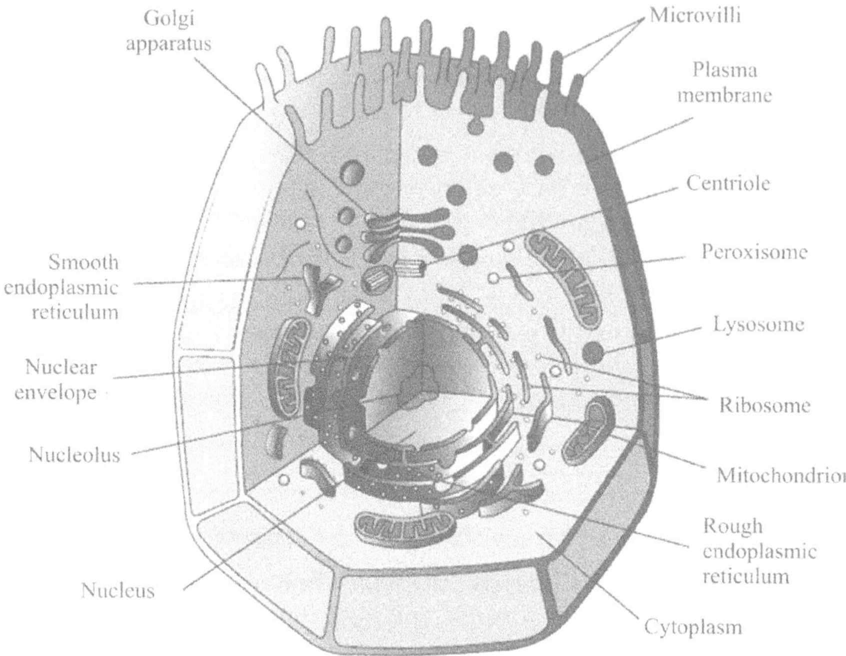

Figure 1.5 Structure of animal cell.

Human body possesses about 10^{14} cells with a size of 10 to 100 μm diameter. Plant cells possess rigid cell wall and chloroplasts which is the site of photosynthesis. Plasma membrane enveloped various subcellular organelles present in cells. Each subcellular organelles are isolated in pure form by differential centrifugation of tissue homogenate. Following are various organelles present in eukaryotic cells. They are,

1. Cell membrane
2. Nucleus
3. Mitochondria
4. Endoplasmic reticulum (ER)
5. Golgi complex
6. Lysosomes
7. Ribosomes
8. Microbodies or peroxisomes
9. Cytosol and cytoskeleton
10. Cilia and flagella
11. Centrosome and Centrioles
12. Cell wall
13. Vacuoles
14. Plastids

1. **Cell Membrane:**

   Lipids and proteins are the major components of cell membrane. Phospholipids are the major lipids which are arranged in a bilayer. Within the membrane polar heads and hydrophobic tails of the lipids are arranged towards the outer sides and the inner part of the cell membrane, respectively. This ensures that cells are protected from the aqueous environment by the non-polar tail of saturated hydrocarbons present in cell membrane.

2. **Nucleus:**

   It is the largest cellular organelle surrounded by the nuclear envelope, which consists of two parallel membranes with a perinuclear space between (10 to 50 nm). Between the materials present inside the nucleus and that of the cytoplasm, this perinuclear space forms a barrier. The outer membrane usually remains continuous with the endoplasmic reticulum and also bears ribosomes on it. Fusion of the two membranes forms the nuclear envelope, at a number of places which is interrupted by minute pores known as nuclear pores having diameter of about 90 nm. Between the nucleus and the cytoplasm RNA and protein molecules are moved in both directions through these nuclear pores only. In general, per cell only one nucleus is present but frequently it is observed variations in the number of nuclei. Even some mature cells lack nucleus. For example erythrocytes of many mammals and sieve tube cells of vascular plants. The ground material present in the nucleus is commonly known as nuclear matrix or the nucleoplasm. *DNA polymerase* and *RNA polymerase* are rich in nucleoplasm. In addition, enzymes involved in glycolysis, citric acid cycle and HMP shunt pathways are also present in nucleoplasm. Nucleolus and chromatin are the component of nucleoplasm. Nucleolus is the dense body present in nucleoplasm and possess spherical structures. RNA particularly rRNA is present in nucleolus and it enters the cytosol through nuclear pores. Protein syntheses are actively carried out in the cells through larger and more numerous nucleoli.

Chromatin is a loose and indistinct network of nucleoprotein fibers present in the nucleus. Chromatin contains DNA and some basic proteins called histones, some non-histone proteins and also RNA. Nucleosomes contain DNA and histones and the assembly of nucleosomes constitutes chromatin fibers of chromosome (In Greek "chromo" means "color" and "soma" means "body"). A single human cell has approximately two meter long thread of DNA distributed among its forty six (twenty three pairs) chromosomes. Kinetochores are disc shaped structures present on the sides of the primary constriction or the centromere which is essentially present in every chromosome. Two chromatids of a chromosome are held by centromere. The chromosomes are broadly classified into four types depending on the centromere position as follows.

(a) **Metacentric chromosome:** Centromere is present in middle and forms two equal arms of the chromosome.

(b) **Sub-metacentric chromosome:** Centromere is present slightly away from the middle leads to one longer and one shorter arm of the chromosomes.

(c) **Acrocentric chromosome:** Centromere is present close to its end leads to one very long and one extremely short arm of the chromosomes.

(d) **Telocentric chromosome:** Centromere is present in terminal or sometimes a few chromosomes have non-staining secondary constrictions at a constant location leads to the appearance of a small fragment called the satellite.

3. **Mitochondria:**

In Greek "mitos" means "thread" and "chondros" means "granule". Under the microscope, mitochondria are not easily visible unless specifically stained. Depends on the physiological activity of the cells the number of mitochondria present in each cell may vary. In addition, considerable degree of variability is observed in terms of size and shape also. In general, it is having 0.2-1.0 μm (average 0.5 μm) diameter and 1.0-4.1 μm length with cylindrical or sausage shape. Mitochondria is composed of,

(a) **Double membrane (inner membrane and outer membrane)**: This double membrane bound structure present in each mitochondrion divides its lumen distinctly into two aqueous compartments (inner compartment and outer compartment). Cristae are the number of infoldings formed in the inner membrane towards the matrix and these cristae increases the surface area. Own specific enzymes present in the two membranes are associated with the mitochondrial function.

(b) **Matrix:** It is a dense homogeneous substance filled in the inner compartment and the outer membrane forms the continuous limiting boundary of the organelle.

Mitochondria are the sites of aerobic cellular respiration and energy metabolism. Mitochondria are considered as 'power houses' of the cell because they produce cellular energy in the form of ATP. Single circular DNA molecule, a few RNA molecules, ribosomes (70S) and the components required for protein synthesis are also present in the matrix. Fission divides the mitochondria. About one fifth of cell volume is occupied by 2,000 mitochondria. About 10 % of mitochondrial proteins are synthesized in mitochondria itself from their own independent protein synthesizing machinery.

Endomembrane System: Some of the membranous organelles are considered together as their functions are coordinated and these membranous organelles are collectively known as endomembrane system. **Organelles such as endoplasmic reticulum (ER), Golgi complex, lysosomes and vacuoles come under this endomembrane system.** Whereas organelles such as mitochondria, chloroplast and peroxisomes do not come under this endomembrane system because their functions are not coordinated with the above components.

4. **The Endoplasmic Reticulum (ER):**

   Endoplasmic reticulum is a network or reticulum of tiny tubular structures scattered in the cytoplasm and it divides the intracellular space into two distinct compartments as,

   (a) Luminal (inside ER) compartment and

   (b) Extra luminal (cytoplasm) compartment

   There are two different types of ER depending on the presence of ribosomes attached to their outer surface as follows.

   (a) Rough endoplasmic reticulum (RER): This endoplasmic reticulum bearing ribosomes on their surface, hence they appeared rough. In the cells RER is frequently observed and it is involved actively in the synthesis of protein as it bears ribosomes. They are extensive and continuous with the outer membrane of the nucleus. As such microsomes do not occur in the cell. Microsomes are formed in small vesicles by disrupture of RER during the process of cell fractionation.

   (b) Smooth endoplasmic reticulum (SER): Ribosomes are not present in this type of ER; hence, they appear smooth. Synthesis of lipids such as phospholipids, triacylglycerol and sterols mainly takes place in the SER of the cell. It also supplies calcium for cellular function along with metabolism of drug

5. **Golgi apparatus or Golgi bodies:**

   Golgi bodies are the densely stained reticular structures present near the nucleus. Many disc-shaped, flat cisternae or sacs having diameter of 0.5 to 1.0 μm are present in Golgi apparatus. These are stacked parallel to each other. In a Golgi apparatus varied numbers of cisternae are present. Near the nucleus the Golgi cisternae are concentrically arranged with distinct the forming or convex cis face and the maturing or concave trans face. The forming and the maturing faces of the organelle are interconnected but entirely different. The principle function of the Golgi apparatus is acting as packaging materials, to be delivered either secreted outside the cell or to the intra-cellular targets. From the ER the materials in the form of vesicles to be packaged are fused with the *cis* face of the Golgi bodies and move towards the maturing face. For this reason, only Golgi bodies remain in close association with the ER. Before the number of proteins synthesized by ribosomes released from its *trans* face ER modifies in the cisternae of the Golgi bodies. Glycoproteins and glycolipids are mainly formed in the Golgi bodies because it is an important site for its formation.

6. **Lysosomes:**

   In the Golgi apparatus by the process of packaging these are formed as single membrane bound vesicular structures. All types of hydrolytic enzymes such as *hydrolases* are present very rich in the isolated lysosomal vesicles. These hydrolytic enzymes are optimally active at the acidic pH and are capable of digesting biomolecules such as carbohydrates, proteins, lipids and nucleic acids. Hence, **lysosomes are regarded as digestive tract of the cell. Example:** *Lipases* digest lipids; *proteases* digest proteins; *carbohydrases* digest carbohydrates; *nucleases* digest nucleic acid.

   Hydrolytic enzymes are responsible for maintaining the cellular compounds in a dynamic state through their degradation and recycling. The degraded product leaves the cell by diffusion for reutilization. Lipofuscin are the age pigments which are rich in lipids and proteins accumulate in the cells. When these hydrolytic enzymes are escaped into cytosol it results in destruction of functional biomolecules of the cells and leads to complication. **Example:** Arthritis, muscle disease and allergic disorder.

7. **Ribosomes:**

   Ribosomes are the dense particles possessing granular structures composed of ribonucleic acid (RNA) and proteins. They are not surrounded by any membrane. Larger and smaller subunits are the two subunits present in each ribosome. 60S and 40S are the two subunits of 80S ribosomes of eukaryotic cell; whereas 50S and 30S are the two subunits of 70S ribosomes of prokaryotic cell. 'S' denotes Svedberg's unit of sedimentation coefficient which is indirect measurement of density and size.

8. **Microbodies or Peroxisomes:**

   These are single membrane bound minute vesicles which are spherical or oval in shape. It is present in both plant and animal cells. It contains various enzymes particularly *catalases* which protect the cells from toxic effects of hydrogen peroxide (H_2O_2) into water and carbon dioxide. It is also involved in the synthesis of plasmogens and glycolipids and oxidation of long chain fatty acids containing more than eighteen carbons. Glyoxysomes are present in plants which are a special type of peroxisomes involved in the glyoxylate pathway.

9. **Cytosol and cytoskeleton:**

   Cytosol is a collective term representing cellular matrix. It is a compartment contains many enzymes, metabolites and salts in aqueous gel like medium.

   Cytoskeletons are collective term representing an elaborate network of filamentous proteinaceous structures present in the cytoplasm consisting of microfilaments, microtubules and intermediate filaments. Mechanical support, motility and maintenance of the shape of the cell are the major functions of cytoskeleton.

10. **Cilia and Flagella:**

    Hairs like outgrowth of the cell membrane covered with plasma membrane are known as cilia and flagella. Small structures which work like oars are cilia which cause the movement of either the surrounding fluid or the cell. When compared to cilia, flagella are longer and responsible for movement of cell. Flagella are also present in the prokaryotic bacteria but structurally differ from eukaryotic flagella. Axonemes are their core possesses a number of microtubules running parallel to the long axis. Nine doublets of radially arranged peripheral microtubules, and a pair of centrally located microtubules are present in the axoneme and this arrangement of axonemal microtubules is referred as the "9+2" array. Bridges connects the central tubules and central sheath also encloses it. Radial spoke connects to one of the tubules of each peripheral doublet; hence totally nine radial spokes are present. Linkers also interconnect the peripheral doublets. Basal bodies are the centriole-like structure from which both the cilium and flagellum are emerged.

11. **Centrosome and Centrioles:**

    Centrioles are cylindrical structures present in organelle centrosome. An amorphous pericentriolar material surrounds the two centrioles of centrosome. In a centrosome both the centrioles lie perpendicular to each other in which each has an organization like the cartwheel. Nine evenly spaced peripheral fibrils of tubulin protein are present in centrioles. Each of the peripheral fibril is a triplet and the adjacent triplets are also linked. Hub is the proteinaceous substance present in the proximal region central part of the centriole. Radial spokes made of protein connects hub with tubules of the peripheral triplets. In animal cells during cell division spindle apparatus are raised from spindle fibers and the centrioles form the basal body of cilia or flagella.

12. **Cell Wall:**

    In fungi and plants, cell wall forms an outer covering for the plasma membrane and the cell wall is a non-living rigid structure. The major functions of the cell wall are giving shape to the cell and protecting the cell from mechanical damage and infection. In addition, it also provides barrier to undesirable macromolecules and helps in cell-to-cell interaction. Cellulose, galactans, mannans and minerals like calcium carbonate are the components of cell wall of algae. Cellulose, hemicellulose, pectin and protein are the components of cell wall of other plants. The primary wall is the cell wall of a young plant cell, which is capable of growth. When the cell matures primary wall gradually diminishes with formation of the secondary wall on the inner (towards membrane) side of the cell. The different neighboring cells are holed or glued together by the middle lamella composed of calcium pectate. The cytoplasms of neighboring cells are connected by plasmodesmata which traversed the cell wall and middle lamellae.

13. Vacuoles:

In the cytoplasm the membrane bound space found is known as vacuole. Excretory product sap, water and other not useful materials are present in vacuoles. Tonoplasts are the single membrane which bounds the vacuole. 90 % volume of the plant cell is occupied by vacuoles. In plants, compared to cytoplasm in vacuole the concentration of tonoplast is significantly higher. Hence, transport of a number of ions and other materials into the vacuole is facilitated by the tonoplast against concentration gradients. For osmoregulation and excretion, the contractile vacuole present in *amoeba* is important. Food particles engulfment forms food vacuoles in many cells as in protists.

14. Plastids:

All plant cells and euglenoids contains plastids. They are large and bear some specific pigments which provide specific colors to the plants. Plastids are broadly classified into three types based on the type of pigments present in it as follows,

1. **Chloroplasts:** Chlorophyll and carotenoid pigments are present in chloroplast. Essential light energy necessary for photosynthesis is trapped by chloroplasts. In the mesophyll cells of the leaves, majority of the chloroplasts of the green plants are found. The space limited by the inner membrane of the chloroplast is called the stroma. A number of organized flattened membranous sacs called the thylakoids, are present in the stroma. The membrane of the thylakoids encloses a space called a lumen. The stroma of the chloroplast contains enzymes required for the synthesis of carbohydrates and proteins. It also contains small, double stranded circular DNA molecules and ribosomes. Chlorophyll pigments are present in the thylakoids.
2. **Chromoplasts:** Fat soluble carotenoid pigments like xanthophylls, carotene and others are present in chromoplast. Yellow, orange or red color was imparted to the plant by chromoplast.
3. **Leucoplasts:** These are colorless plastids of varied shapes and sizes with stored nutrients. **Example:** Amyloplasts of potato store carbohydrates (starch); elaioplasts store oils and fats whereas the aleuroplasts store proteins.

Comparison between Prokaryotes and Eukaryotes

The various characteristics of prokaryotic cells are compared with eukaryotic cell in the Table 1.3.

Table 1.3 Comparison between prokaryotes and eukaryotes.

S. No	Characteristic	Prokaryotic cell	Eukaryotic cell
1	Size	1 to 10 nm (Smaller than eukaryotes).	10 to 100 nm (Larger than prokaryotes).
2	Nucleus	No well-defined nucleus present, histones are absent and DNA is found in nucleoid.	Well defined nucleus surrounded by membrane is present and DNA associated with histone is present.
3	Cell membrane	Rigid cell wall envelopes the cell.	Flexible plasma membrane envelopes the cell.
4	Subcellular organelles	Not present.	Mitochondria, nucleus, lysosomes, etc are present.
5	Cytoplasm	Cytoskeleton and organelles are absent.	Cytoskeleton and organelles are present with a network of tubules and filaments.
6	Energy metabolism	Enzymes of energy metabolism are bound to membrane as mitochondria are absent.	Enzymes of energy metabolism are present in mitochondria.
7	Cell division	Cell division takes place by fission and not by mitosis.	Cell division takes place by mitosis.

Biochemical Organization of Cell Membrane

The cell membrane is an envelope which surrounds the cell. From the external environment cells are separated and protected by plasma membrane. In addition to that cell is connected to its environment by this plasma membrane only. Moreover, plasma membrane also surrounds the subcellular organelles such as mitochondria, nucleus and lysosomes.

Composition of Membrane

From tissue to tissue the actual composition of membrane varies. In general, the followings are the three substances which are the major components of cell membrane.

1. **Lipids:** In animal cell membrane amphipathic lipids (Lipids possessing both hydrophilic and hydrophobic groups) such as glycolipids, phospholipids and cholesterol are found.
2. **Proteins:** The proteins present in the membrane are broadly classified into two major types as extrinsic protein and intrinsic protein.
3. **Carbohydrates:** Glycocalyx are the thick coating of complex polysaccharides present in many animal cell membranes. In the tissue the oligosaccharides of glycocalyx interacts with collagen of intracellular matrix (Body substance which consists of ground substance and connective tissue fibers).

Structure of Membrane

In the year 1935, Davson proposed the lipid bilayer model for membrane structure and it was modified by Danielle. For membrane structure the most acceptable model and more recent model is "**Fluid mosaic model**" proposed by Singer and Niclolson. 5 to 8 nm is the usual thickness of the biological membrane. Lipid bilayer is the essential component of a membrane. At the core of the bilayer, non-polar (hydrophobic) region of the lipids face each other and the polar (hydrophilic) region face out ward. In this lipid bilayer globular proteins are embedded irregularly. These globular proteins are broadly classified into two major categories based on their position and type of attachment.

1. **Peripheral or extrinsic membrane protein:** These proteins lie on the surface of membrane and loosely bound to the surface membrane. Hence it can be easily separated from the membrane. **Example:** Cytochrome c of mitochondria.
2. **Integral or intrinsic membrane protein:** These integral proteins are partially or totally buried in the membrane and tightly bound to the lipid bilayer. Hence it cannot be easily separated from the membrane and it can be separated using detergents or organic solvents. **Example:** Cytochrome P_{450} and receptors of hormones.

According to this, the quasi-fluid nature of lipid enables lateral movement of proteins within the overall bilayer. This ability to move within the membrane is measured as its fluidity. The fluid nature of the membrane is also important from the point of view of functions like cell growth, formation of intercellular junctions, secretion, endocytosis, cell division etc. The proteins are distributed irregularly in membrane; hence, the membrane is asymmetric in nature. Like mosaic or ceramic tile, the membranes appeared due to arrangement of lipid bilayer and protein subunits. The membrane freely changes unlike a fixed ceramic tile. That's why the structure of the membranes is considered as fluid mosaic model. The fluid mosaic model of membrane structure is presented in Figure 1.6.

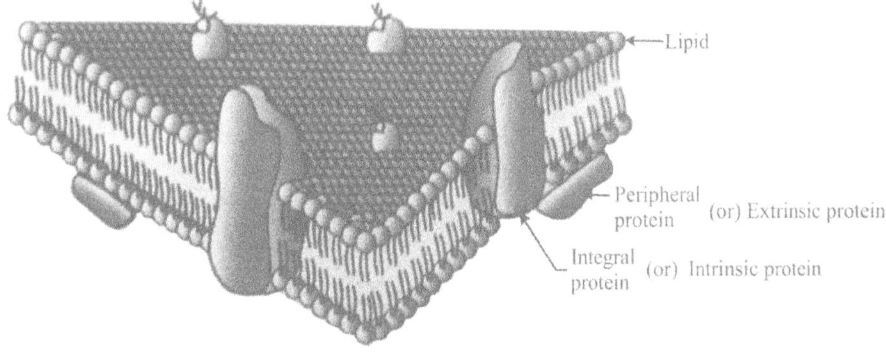

Figure 1.6 The membrane structure (Fluid mosaic model).

Transport of the Molecules Across Membranes

One of the most important functions of the plasma membrane is the transport of the molecules across it. Different types of transport of molecules across membranes are presented in Figure 1.7. The membrane is selectively permeable to some molecules present on either side of it. Depending on the size of molecules the transport processes across membranes are classified into two categories as,

1. Transport of metabolites or solutes
2. Transport of macromolecules

Transport of Metabolites or Solutes

In general, membrane forms a barrier for the free passage of compounds across the membrane.

Mechanism of transport system: Different mechanism involved in transport of metabolites or solutes is presented in Figure 1.8. Through membrane, metabolites or solutes are transported by two different mechanisms. They are,

(a) Passive transport
(b) Active transport

(a) Passive transport: It occurs along a concentration gradient (Solute moves from higher concentration to lower concentration) and this process is not dependent on the supply of metabolic energy (ATP is not necessary for passive transport). It was further subdivided into two types based on the requirements of carrier molecule as follows,

(i) Passive diffusion or Simple diffusion
(ii) Facilitated diffusion

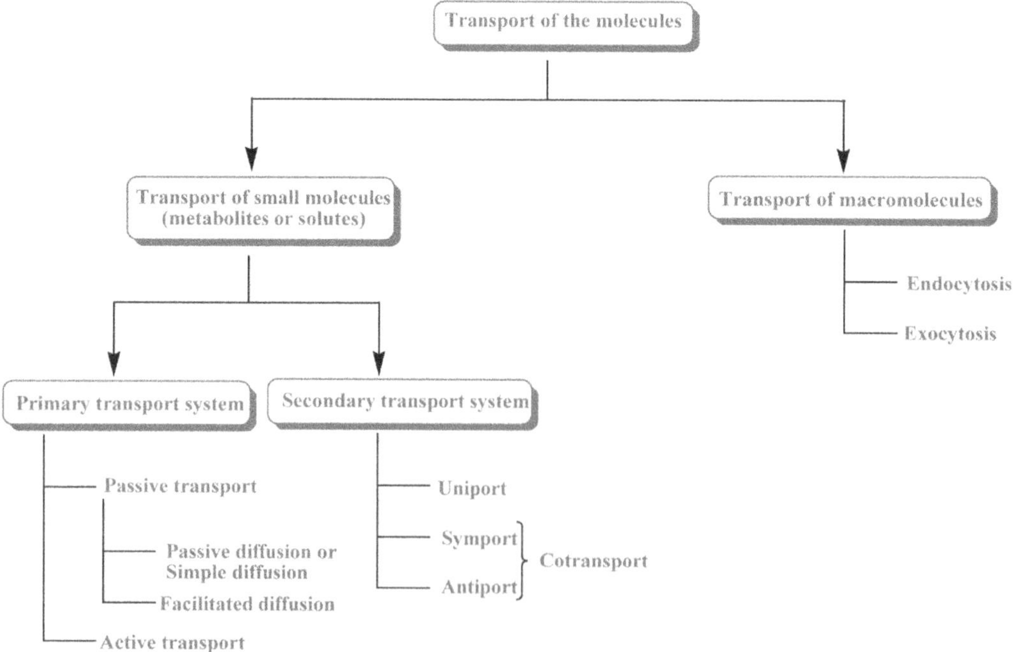

Figure 1.7 Types of transport of molecules across membranes.

(i) Passive diffusion or Simple diffusion: This process is a very simple process in which solutes move across the membrane along the concentration gradient. Presence of carrier or transport protein and supply of metabolic energy is not needed for this transport process. **Example:** Passage of water and gases.

Passive transport of water - Osmosis: The phenomenon of movement of water from dilute solution (Low osmotic pressure) to concentrated solution (High osmotic pressure) across the biological membrane is known as osmosis. In the body, movement of water occurs through osmosis which does not require any energy. Edema, diarrhea, cholera and inflammation are certain medical and health complications due to the disturbances in osmosis.

(ii) Facilitated diffusion: This process is also somewhat similar to passive diffusion. Like passive diffusion, solutes or metabolites move across the membrane along the concentration gradient and the supply of metabolic energy is not needed for this transport process also. The most important difference between passive and facilitated diffusion is presence of carrier or transport protein. Facilitated diffusion occurs through the mediation of carrier or transport protein; whereas passive diffusion occurs without mediation of carrier or transport protein. **Example:** Transport of active form of fatty acid i.e., acyl CoA (Carrier molecule: Carnitine); transport of glucose (Carrier molecule: Glucose transporter); transport of galactose, leucine and phenylalanine.

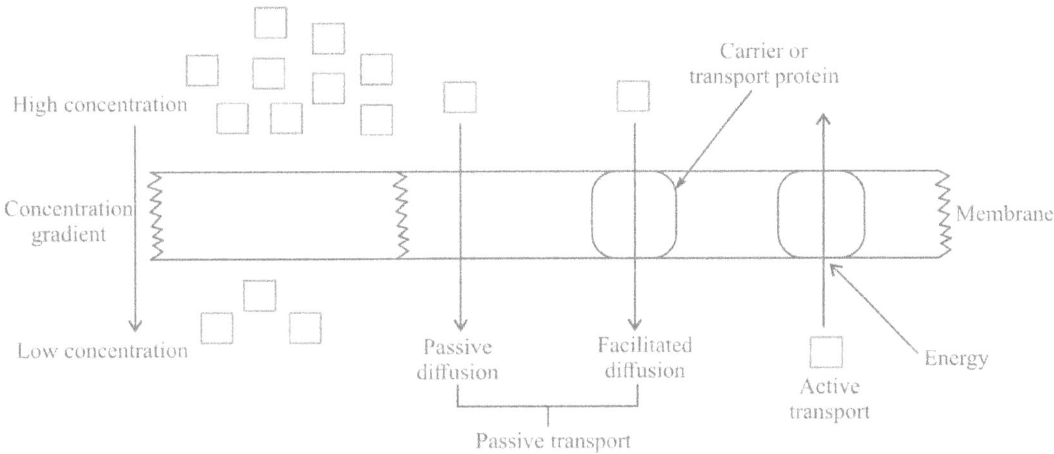

Figure 1.8 Transport of molecules across biological membrane.

Ping-Pong model: The occurrence of facilitated diffusion is explained by Ping-Pong model. Two conformations namely Ping conformation and Pong conformation exists for carrier or transport protein according to this mechanism. The carrier or transport protein exposed to the high solute concentration side in the "pong" conformation. This leads to attachment or binding of solute to specific sites of the carrier protein. Latter, carrier or transport protein undergoes conformational changes and exposed to the low solute concentration side in the "ping" conformation and releases solute molecule. Facilitated diffusion is generally regulated by hormones. This model is schematically represented in Figure 1.9. **Example:** Insulin increases transport of glucose in muscle and adipose tissue; transport of amino acid in liver and other tissue.

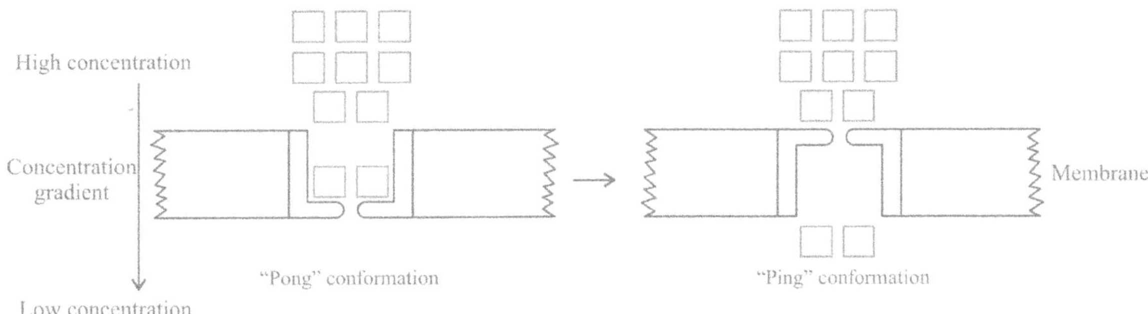

Figure 1.9 Facilitated diffusion – Ping Pong model.

(b) Active transport: It occurs against a concentration gradient (solute moves from lower concentration to higher concentration) and this process is dependent on the supply of metabolic energy (ATP is necessary for active transport). Like facilitated diffusion this process is also a carrier mediated process. Ion pumps particularly sodium-potassium (Na^+-K^+) pumps through the involvement of Na^+-K^+ *ATPase* or ion transporting *ATPase* are good examples for active transport process.

Sodium-potassium (Na^+-K^+) pump: Cells essentially need high intracellular potassium (K^+) concentration and low sodium (Na^+) concentration for their survival. Optimal glycolysis (*Pyruvate kinase* is dependent on potassium (K^+) concentration) and biosynthesis of proteins need high intracellular potassium (K^+) concentration. In addition, for nerve impulse transmission across plasma membrane sodium (Na^+) and potassium (K^+) gradients are needed. Sodium-potassium (Na^+-K^+) pump is diagrammatically represented in Figure 1.10.

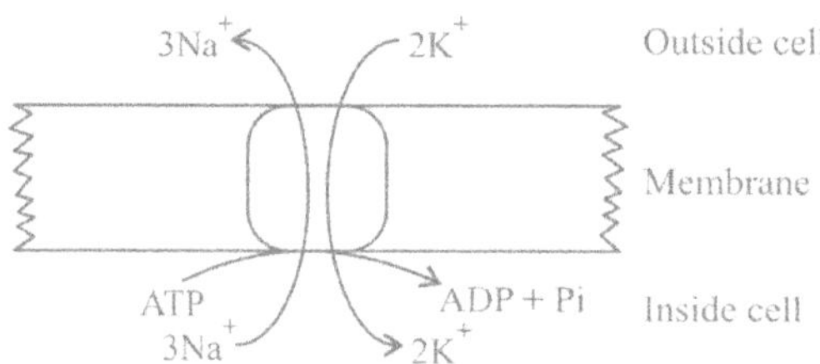

Figure 1.10 Sodium-potassium (Na^+-K^+) pump – An active transport.

In the cell, high potassium (K^+) concentration and low sodium (Na^+) concentration is maintained by the sodium-potassium (Na^+-K^+) pump. The *Na^+-K^+ ATPase* are the enzyme which is an integral plasma membrane protein having 2,50,000 molecular weight brought the above Na^+-K^+ concentration in the cells. Two α and two β subunits are present in *Na^+-K^+ ATPase*, hence it is represented as $(\alpha\beta)_2$. *Sodium-potassium (Na^+-K^+) ATPase* pumps three sodium (Na^+) to outside the cell from inside and brings two potassium (K^+) to inside the cell from outside. This requisite cytosolic sodium (Na^+) and potassium (K^+) levels are maintained using sodium-potassium (Na^+-K^+) pump by utilizing major portion of the cellular ATP (In nerve cells up to 70 %).

$$3\ Na^+\ (in) + 2\ K^+\ (out) + ATP \longrightarrow 3\ Na^+\ (out) + 2\ K^+\ (in) + ADP + Pi$$

Inhibitors of *Na^+-K^+ ATPase*: The followings are the two important inhibitors of the *Na^+-K^+ ATPase*.

1. **Ouabain:** It is a steroid derivative extracted from the seeds of an African shrub which inhibits *Na^+-K^+ ATPase*. Tribals in Africa use ouabain as poison to tip the hunting arrows (Arrow poison).
2. **Digoxin:** It is another *Na^+-K^+ ATPase* inhibitor and chemically it is steroid glycoside. In general digoxin improves cardiac contractility, hence used in the treatment of CHF (Congestive heart failure).

Types of Transport System

Based on the movement of molecules, transport systems are broadly classified into three major types as follows.

1. **Uniport system:** In this transport system, single molecules are transported through the membranes. **Example:** Transport of glucose to erythrocytes.
2. **Symport system:** In this transport system two different molecules are simultaneously transported in the same direction through the membrane. **Example:** From the gut sodium (Na^+) and glucose are transported to the intestinal mucosal cells.

3. **Antiport system:** In this transport system through the membrane two different molecules are simultaneously transported in the opposite direction. **Example:** Transport of chloride (Cl^-) and bicarbonate (HCO_3^-) in erythrocytes. Proton pump in the stomach is another example for antiport system of gastric parietal cells. In the lumen of stomach high acidic (pH ~ 1) condition is brought by the enzyme *H^+-K^+ ATPase*. For hydrolysis of one molecule of ATP, proton pump antiport two cytoplasmic protons ($2H^+$) and two extracellular potassium (K^+). The proton (H^+) combines with the chloride ion (Cl^-) secreted by the chloride ion (Cl^-) channel to form gastric HCl. Peptic ulcer is treated using omeprazole which is a drug that inhibits *H^+-K^+ ATPase* and results in decreased secretion of HCl.

   All the above-mentioned transport systems such as uniport systems, symport systems and antiport systems are considered as secondary active transport systems and are represented in Figure 1.11.

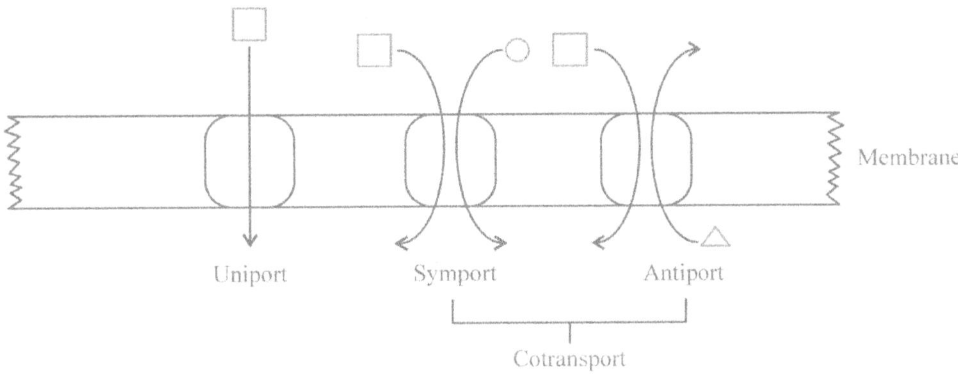

Figure 1.11 Different types of transport systems based on the movement of molecules.

Cotransport system: Through the membrane, transport of a substance coupled to the spontaneous movement of another substance is termed as cotransport system. Symport systems and antiport systems are very good examples for cotransport systems. Sodium (Na^+) cotransport system is another example. By this system amino acids and sugars are transported into the cells. Glucose (or amino acids) is passed into the cells with simultaneous movement of sodium (Na^+). Later sodium (Na^+) is pumped out from inside through *Na^+-K^+ ATPase* with the involvement of ATP.

Transport of Macromolecules

Across the membrane the transport of macromolecules such as proteins, polysaccharides and polynucleotides are also equally important. Two independent mechanisms are involved in the transport of macromolecules & are presented in Figure 1.12. They are,

1. **Endocytosis:** The processes of intake of macromolecules by the cells from the outside are termed as endocytosis. **Example:** Uptake of LDL by cells.
2. **Exocytosis:** The processes of release of macromolecules from the cells to the outside is termed as exocytosis. **Example:** Secretion of hormones such as insulin, parathyroid hormones from the cell.

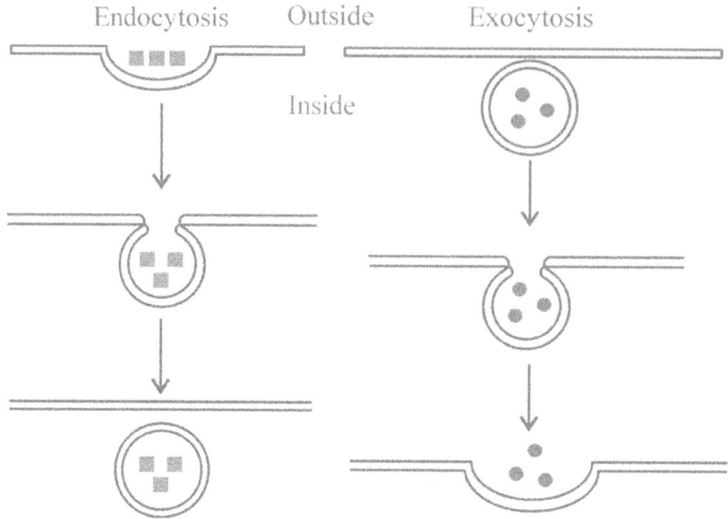

Figure 1.12 Transport of macromolecules.

Disorders of Membrane Transport System

Number of pathological conditions occur due to alterations in the membrane transport systems. The followings are some important diseases due to loss of membrane transport systems.

1. **Hartnup's disease:** In intestinal cells and renal tubules transport of neutral amino acids are decreased.
2. **Cystinuria:** It is the clinical condition in which excretion of cysteine, lysine, arginine and ornithine in urine is increased and leads to formation of renal cystine stones.
3. **Decreased glucose uptake:** Lack of specific sodium-glucose transporter decreases glucose uptake in some individuals.
4. **Decreased renal reabsorption of phosphate:** In vitamin D resistant rickets renal reabsorption of phosphate is decreased.

Bioenergetics (or) Biochemical Thermodynamics

Role of high energy compounds in biological process and basic knowledge of bioenergetics is very useful for better understanding of biological oxidation.

Study of energy changes (utilization and transfer) in biochemical reaction is termed as bioenergetics or biochemical thermodynamics. In bioenergetics mechanism of chemical reaction is not concerned but it concerned about the initial and final states of energy components of reactants. Based on energy released or consumed in biochemical reaction it was broadly classified into two types. They are,

1. **Exergonic reaction:** In this type biochemical reaction energy is released. ΔG^o value of this reaction is negative and the reactions will take place spontaneously. Almost all catabolic reactions are exergonic reactions. **Example:** Breakdown of ATP into ADP and inorganic phosphate liberates 7.3 Cal/mol energy.

$$ATP + H_2O \longrightarrow ADP + Pi \qquad (\Delta G^o = -7.3\ Cal/mol)$$

2. **Endergonic reaction:** In this biochemical reaction energy is consumed or utilized by the reactants. It needs energy; hence, energy must be supplied. ΔG° value of this reaction is positive and the reactions will not take place spontaneously. Almost all anabolic reactions, muscle contraction, nervous excitation, etc. are good examples for endergonic reactions. **Example:** Synthesis of ATP from ADP and inorganic phosphate. This reaction occurs only when 7.3 Cal/mol energy is supplied at least.

$$ADP + Pi \longrightarrow ATP + H_2O \quad (\Delta G^O = +7.3 \text{ Cal/mol})$$

Terms used in Bioenergetics:

To understand the bioenergetics reactions, it is necessary to know about the following terms

1. Free energy
2. Enthalpy
3. Entropy

1. **Free energy:** It is defined as the energy actually available for utilization or to do work. The feasibility of chemical reaction is predicted valuably using changes in free energy and is represented by the symbol "ΔG". If the reaction is accompanied by decrease in free energy then the reaction can occur spontaneously.

   Standard free energy change: It is defined as the free energy change when the reactants or products are at a concentration of 1 mol/*l* at pH 7.0. This standard free energy is denoted by the symbol "ΔG°".

   The free energy change (ΔG) may be either,

   (a) **Negative free energy change:** In a chemical reaction if there is a loss of free energy then ΔG is represented by negative sign and the reaction is called as exergonic reaction and the reaction proceeds spontaneously. Free energy changes of almost all catabolic reactions possess negative sign only. **Example:** Breakdown of ATP into ADP and inorganic phosphate liberates 7.3 Cal/mol energy.

$$ATP + H_2O \longrightarrow ADP + Pi \quad (\Delta G^\circ = -7.3 \text{ Cal/mol})$$

   (b) **Positive free energy change:** In a chemical reaction if free energy is supplied then the ΔG is represented by positive sign and the reaction is called as endergonic reaction and the reaction does not proceed spontaneously. Free energy changes of almost all anabolic reactions possess positive sign only. **Example:** Synthesis of ATP from ADP and inorganic phosphate and the reaction occurs only when 7.3 Cal/mol energy is supplied at least.

$$ADP + Pi \longrightarrow ATP + H_2O \quad (\Delta G^O = +7.3 \text{ Cal/mol})$$

   (c) **Zero free energy change:** In a chemical reaction ΔG becomes zero when it is at equilibrium.

$$A \rightleftharpoons B \quad (\Delta G^\circ = 0)$$

The free energy change (ΔG) is generally dependent on the actual concentrations of reactants and products at a constant temperature and pressure. Consider the below reaction in which reactant "A" is converted to product "B".

$$\underset{\text{(Reactant)}}{A} \longrightarrow \underset{\text{(Product)}}{B}$$

The following mathematical relationship can be derived when the reactant "A" is converted to product "B".

$$\Delta G = \Delta G^{o} + RT\, ln \frac{[B]}{[A]}$$

Where,

ΔG = Free energy change

ΔG° = Standard free energy change

R = 1.987 Cal / mol (Gas constant)

T = Absolute temperature in Kelvin (273 + °C)

ln = Natural logarithm

[B] = Concentration of product

[A] = Concentration of reactant

When reaction is at equilibrium then the free energy change is zero i.e., $\Delta G = 0$. Substitute the value of ΔG in above equation.

$$0 = \Delta G^{o} + RT\, ln \frac{[B]_{eq}}{[A]_{eq}}$$

Therefore, $$\Delta G^{o} = -RT\, ln \frac{[B]_{eq}}{[A]_{eq}}$$

Where, K_{eq} = Equilibrium constant

The free energy change (ΔG) is an additive value for pathways. A series of reactions are often involved in biochemical pathways. In such reaction the free energy change (ΔG) is an additive value. Whether the particular pathway will proceed or not is crucially determined by the sum of the free energy change (ΔG). The pathway can operate when the sum of the free energy change (ΔG) is negative even though some of the individual reactions may have positive free energy change (ΔG).

2. **Enthalpy:** It is a measure of the change in the heat content of the reactants compared to products. It is denoted by the symbol "ΔH". During the thermodynamic reaction either the heat may be released or absorbed. Based on this the chemical reactions are broadly classified into two major types as,
   (a) **Exothermic reaction:** During a chemical reaction if the heat is released then the reaction is said to be exothermic reaction. **Example:** Sodium hydroxide dissolved in water.
   (b) **Endothermic reaction:** During a chemical reaction if the heat is absorbed then the reaction is said to be endothermic reaction. **Example:** Benedict's test, Fehling's test, etc.
3. **Entropy:** It is the change in the randomness or disorder of reactants and products. It is usually represented by "ΔS". When the reaction attains equilibrium, entropy attains a maximum. In general, temporary decrease in entropy was observed in the reactions of biological systems.

Relationship between the change of free energy, enthalpy and entropy:

The relationship between the change of free energy, enthalpy and entropy is expressed in the below mentioned equation.

$$\Delta G = \Delta H - T\Delta S$$

Where,

ΔG = Free energy change

ΔH = Enthalpy

T = Absolute temperature in Kelvin (273 + °C)

ΔS = Entropy

Biological Oxidation

Oxidation is defined as addition of oxygen (or) loss of hydrogen (or) loss of electrons and reduction is defined as loss of oxygen (or) gain of hydrogen (or) gain of electron. The electron lost in the oxidation is accepted by acceptor which is said to be reduced. Both oxidation and reduction are coupled with each other. Hence oxidation-reduction reactions are commonly known as redox reaction (If one compound is getting oxidized the other one must reduce). **Example:** Inter conversion of Fe^{2+} (ferrous ion) to Fe^{3+} (ferric ion).

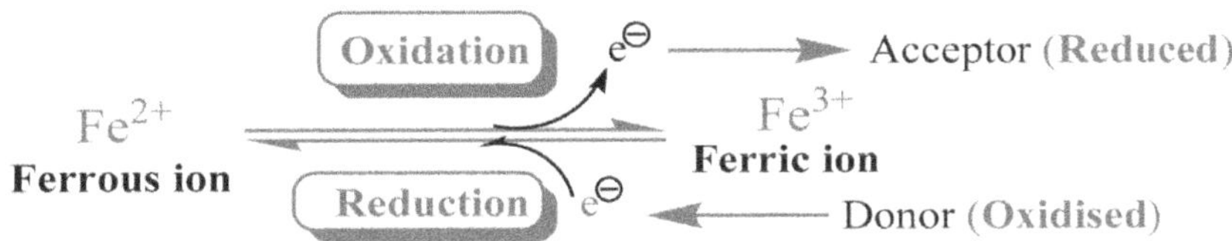

If the oxidation reduction reaction takes place in biological system then it is known as biological redox reaction (or) simply biological oxidation. The general oxidation-reduction principle is applicable to biological systems also. **Example:** The oxidation of NADH + H^+ to NAD^+ is coupled with simultaneous reduction of FMN to $FMNH_2$. In this example NADH + H^+ / NAD^+ and FMN / $FMNH_2$ are called as redox pair which differ in their tendency to lose or gain electrons.

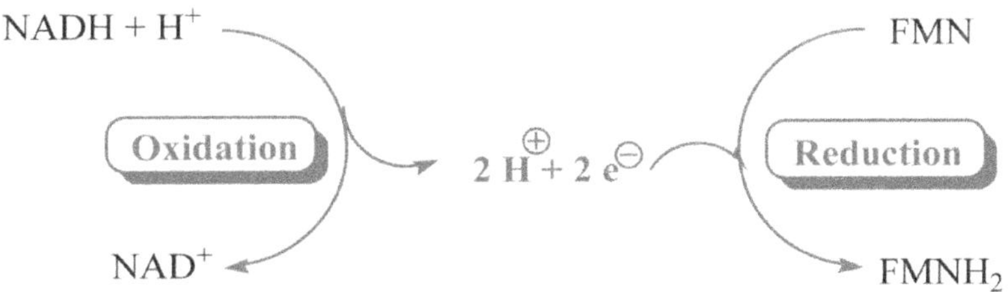

Redox Potential

Redox potential is otherwise known as oxidation-reduction potential. A quantitative measure of the tendency of a redox pair to lose or gain electrons is known as redox potential. Specific standard redox potential (E_o Volts) is assigned to each redox pair based on their tendency to lose or gain electrons at 25 °C and pH 7.0. The redox potential (E_o) is directly related to the change in the free energy ($\Delta G°$).

The specific standard redox potential (E_o) may be either positive or negative. More negative redox potential (E_o Volts) indicates greater tendency of reductant to lose electrons and a more positive redox potential (E_o Volts) indicates greater tendency of oxidant to accept electrons. Generally, the electrons flow from a redox pair with more negative redox potential (E_o Volts) to another redox pair with more positive redox potential (E_o Volts). Specific standard redox potential (E_o volts) of various redox pair system is summarized in Table 1.4.

Table 1.4 Specific standard redox potential (E_o Volts) of various redox pair system.

S. No	Redox pair	E_o in Volts
1	Succinate / α-ketoglutarate	- 0.67
2	$2H^+ / H_2$	- 0.42
3	NADH + H^+ / NAD^+	- 0.32
4	$NADP^+$ / NADP + H^+	- 0.32
5	FMN / $FMNH_2$ (Enzyme bound)	- 0.30
6	Lipoate (ox / red)	- 0.29
7	FAD / $FADH_2$	- 0.22
8	Pyruvate / Lactate	- 0.19
9	Fumarate / succinate	+ 0.03
10	Cytochrome b (Fe^{3+} / Fe^{2+})	+ 0.07
11	Coenzyme Q (ox / red)	+ 0.10
12	Cytochrome c_1 (Fe^{3+} / Fe^{2+})	+ 0.23
13	Cytochrome c (Fe^{3+} / Fe^{2+})	+ 0.25
14	Cytochrome a (Fe^{3+} / Fe^{2+})	+ 0.29
15	½ O_2 / H_2O	+ 0.82

Co-Enzyme System Involved in Biological Oxidation

Co-enzymes are defined as the non-protein, organic, low molecular weight and easily dialyzable substances associated with the functions of enzymes.

Holoenzyme (Active enzyme) ⟶ Apoenzyme (Protein part) + Co-enzyme (Non-protein part)

The followings are the various co-enzymes which are involved in biological oxidation. They are,

1. Flavin mononucleotide (FMN)
2. Flavin adenine dinucleotide (FAD)
3. Nicotinamide adenine dinucleotide (NAD^+)
4. Nicotinamide adenine dinucleotide phosphate ($NADP^+$)
5. Lipoic acid

Details of these co-enzymes along with its chemical structure is explained in enzyme topic.

Energy Rich Compounds

It is otherwise known as high energy compounds or high energy phosphates. In the biological systems certain compounds on hydrolysis yield energy. Energy rich compounds or high energy compounds are substances which possess sufficient free energy to liberate at least 7 Cal/mol at pH 7.0. Energy rich compounds are otherwise known as high energy compounds. Compared to hydrolysis of ATP into ADP and inorganic phosphates, all the high energy compounds liberate more energy when undergo hydrolysis. High energy compounds except acetyl CoA generally contains phosphate group in their structure, hence it is also known as high energy phosphates. **Example:** Phosphoenol pyruvate, carbamoyl phosphate, cAMP, 1,3-bisphosphoglycerate, phosphocreatine, acetyl phosphate, S-adenosylmethionine (SAM), pyrophosphate (PPi), acetyl CoA and ATP.

Compounds which liberate less than 7.0 Cal/mol (which is lower than hydrolysis of ATP into ADP and inorganic phosphate) are referred as low energy phosphates or low energy compounds. **Example:** ADP, glucose-1-phosphate, fructose-1-phosphate, glucose-6-phosphate and glycerol-3-phosphate. The standard free energy liberated during hydrolysis of some important compounds is summarized in Table 1.5.

Table 1.5 The standard free energy (ΔG°) liberated during hydrolysis of some important compounds.

S. No	Compounds Name	ΔG° (in Cal / mol)
High energy phosphates or High energy compounds		
1	Phosphoenol pyruvate	- 14.8
2	Carbamoyl phosphate	- 12.3
3	cAMP	- 12.0
4	1,3-Bisphosphoglycerate	- 11.8
5	Phosphocreatine	- 10.3
6	Acetyl phosphate	- 10.3
7	S-Adenosylmethionine (SAM; Sulfonium compound)	- 10.0
8	Pyrophosphate (PPi)	- 8.0
9	Acetyl CoA (Thioester)	- 7.7
10	ATP (Breakdown into ADP & inorganic phosphate)	- 7.3
Low energy phosphates or Low energy compounds		
11	ADP (Breakdown into AMP & inorganic phosphate)	- 6.6
12	Glucose-1-phosphate	- 5.0
13	Fructose-1-phosphate	- 3.8
14	Glucose-6-phosphate	- 3.3
15	Glycerol-3-phosphate	- 2.2

Classification of high energy compounds

High energy compounds are broadly classified into five major types according to type of bonds present in their structure. They are,

1. Pyrophosphate
2. Acyl phosphate
3. Enol phosphate
4. Thioester or thiol ester
5. Phosphagens or guanidino phosphate

Acid anhydride bonds particularly phospho anhydride bonds are high energy bonds which are usually present in all high energy compounds. Condensation of two acidic groups or related compounds generally produces this acid anhydride bonds. These bonds liberate free energy when it undergoes hydrolysis; hence it is known as high energy bonds. The symbol '~' is used by Lipmann to represent high energy bonds. ATP is instantly written as AMP-P-P. The various examples and bonds present in different classes of high energy compounds are summarized in Table 1.6.

Table 1.6 High energy compounds.

S. No	Class	Type of bond present	Example
1	Pyrophosphate	—C—(P)~(P)	Pyrophosphate, ATP
2	Acyl phosphate	O ‖ —C—O~(P)	Carbamoyl phosphate, 1,3-bisphosphoglycerate, acetyl phosphate
3	Enol phosphate	—CH ‖ —C—O~(P)	Phosphoenol pyruvate

Table 1.6 *Contd...*

S. No	Class	Type of bond present	Example
4	Thioester or thiol ester	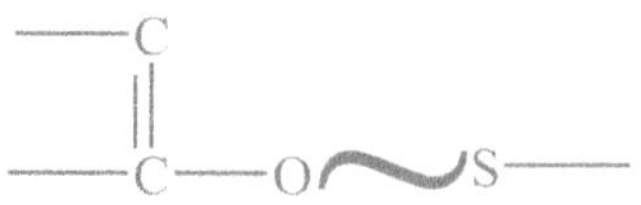 —C(=O)—O∼S—	Acetyl CoA, acyl CoA
5	Phosphagens or guanidino phosphate	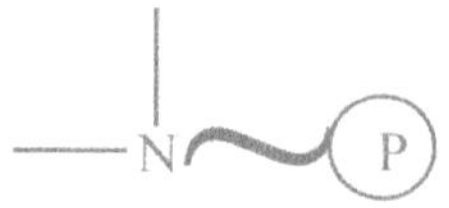 —N∼(P)	Phosphocreatine, phosphoarginine

Adenosine Triphosphate (ATP)

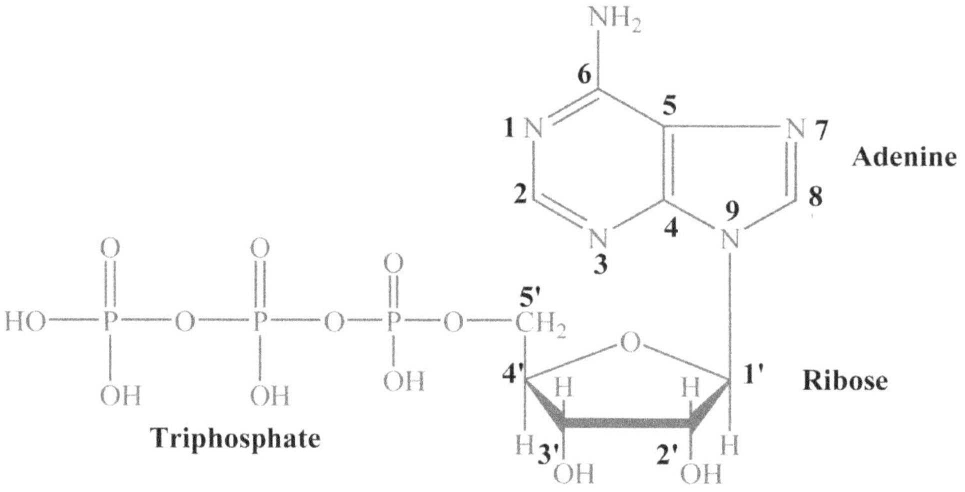

Adenosine triphosphate (ATP)

In living cells, the most important high energy molecule present is adenosine triphosphate (ATP). It is a nucleotide and composed of

1. Adenine (nitrogen base)
2. Ribose (sugar) and
3. A triphosphate groups.

In the triphosphate moiety of ATP, it contains two phospho anhydride bonds, hence ATP is a high energy compounds. ATP-ADP cycle evidences that ATP is the energy currency of the cell.

ATP-ADP Cycle

Large amount of energy (7.3 Cal/mol) is released when ATP is hydrolyzed to ADP and inorganic phosphate.

$$ATP + H_2O \longrightarrow ADP + Pi \qquad (\Delta G^\circ = -7.3\ Cal/mol)$$

Several processes in the biological systems such as muscle contraction, active transport, biosynthesis, etc. utilizes the energy liberated from the ATP when it breaks. In addition, energy rich compounds are biosynthesized from low energy compounds by reacting with high energy phosphates which is donated by ATP. Whilst, the compounds possessing higher free energy content donates high energy phosphates to ADP in order to produce ATP. ATP-ADP cycle is represented in Figure 1.13.

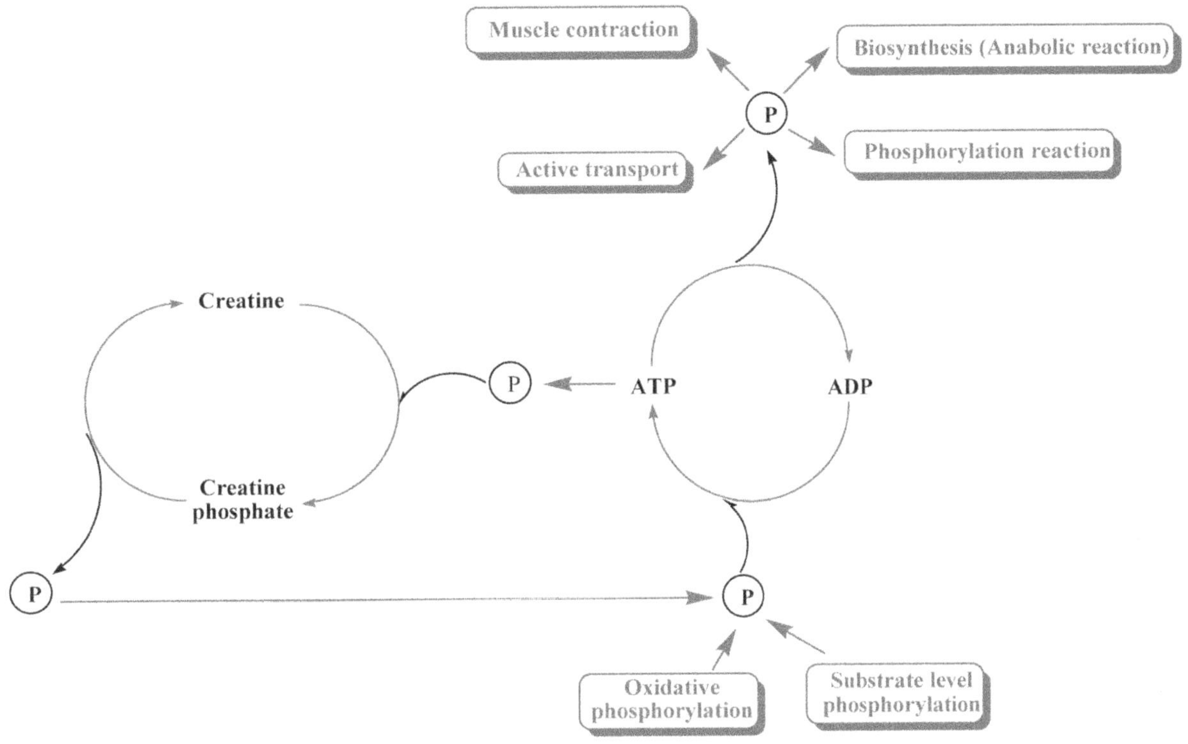

Figure 1.13 ATP-ADP cycle along with formation and breakdown of ATP (Phosphate will not exist free in biological system. It is only transferred).

Biological Significance of ATP

Biological importance of ATP is as follows

1. ATP is the short-term energy store of the cell.
2. Universally for all living things ATP is the energy currency of cell.
3. ATP is the source of phosphate moiety for phosphorylation reaction.
4. In addition, ATP can also donate pyrophosphate (PPi) and adenosine monophosphate (AMP) to other suitable acceptor for the formation of important biological compounds.
5. It easily participates in many biological reactions.
6. ATP is necessary for muscle contraction.
7. ATP is useful for nerve impulse transmission.
8. ATP is important for normal growth and development.
9. ATP is necessary for active transport.
10. ATP is also useful for homeostasis.
11. ATP is needed for all anabolic reactions.
12. ATP is helpful for intracellular signaling.
13. ATP is useful for the synthesis of nucleic acid.
14. ATP also plays a role in synthesis of proteins for the activation of amino acids.

Cyclic Adenosine Monophosphate (cAMP)

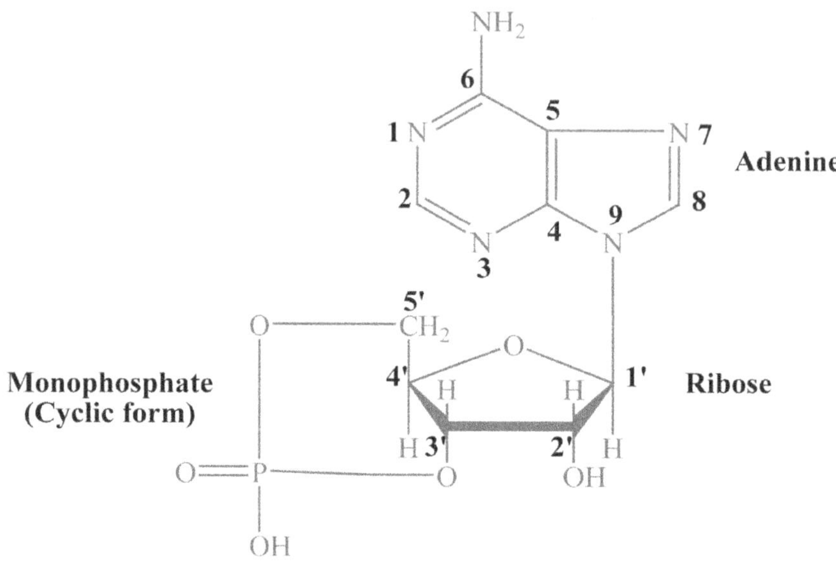

Cyclic adenosine monophosphate (*c*AMP)

In living cells, another important high energy molecule present is cyclic adenosine monophosphate (cAMP). The prefix 'cyclic' indicates the cyclic structure formed between phosphate moiety present at C-5 of ribose and hydroxyl group present at C-3 of ribose molecule.

It is a nucleotide and composed of

1. Adenine (nitrogen base)
2. Ribose (sugar) and
3. A monophosphate group.

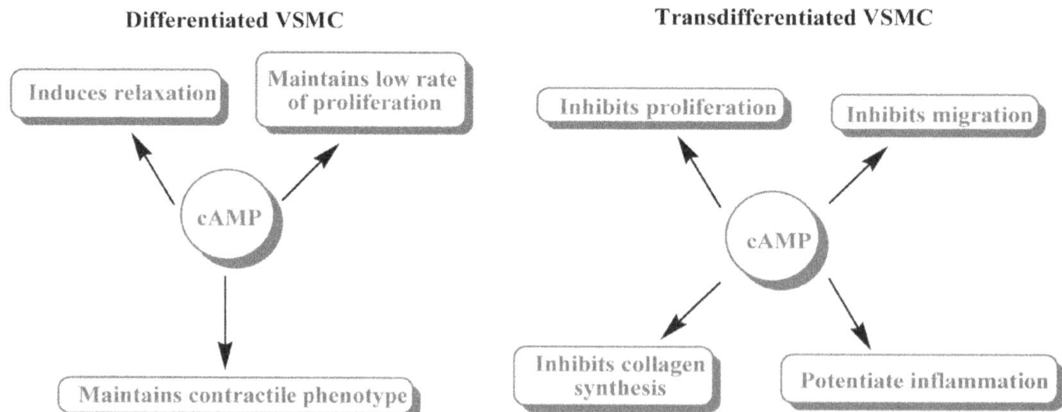

Biological Significance of cAMP

Biological responses of cAMP are,

1. It is the intracellular secondary messenger present in many biological processes.
2. It is used for signal transduction intracellularly.
3. cAMP plays an important key regulatory role in most type of cells.
4. *Adenyl cyclase* particularly alters cAMP and this cAMP regulates the enzyme called *phosphodiesteraeses*.

5. cAMP mediates some short-term aspects of synaptic transmission. In addition, some rapid actions of certain neurotransmitter on ion channels that do not involve ligand gated channels are mediated through cAMP.
6. Along with other intracellular messenger, cAMP plays a central role in mediating other aspects of synaptic transmission.
7. Virtually all other effects of neurotransmitter on target neuron functioning both short and long term are achieved through intracellular messengers.

Synthesis of ATP

ATP is generally synthesized by phosphorylation reaction from ADP and inorganic phosphate. Generally, the phosphorylation reaction used to synthesize ATP is broadly classified into two different types.

1. Substrate level phosphorylation
2. Oxidative phosphorylation

Substrate Level Phosphorylation

In this type of phosphorylation, ATP is directly synthesized in the metabolism during oxidation of substrate without involvement of ETC (Electron Transport Chain). To produce ATP, high energy phosphates are transferred usually from high energy compounds such as 1,3-bisphosphoglycerate, phosphoenol pyruvate (intermediates of glycolysis) and succinyl CoA (intermediates of citric acid cycle).

Example 1: 1,3-Bisphospho glycerate (1,3-BPG) produced 3-phospho glycerate (3-PG) by dephosphorylation reaction in presence of *phospho glycero kinase* (PGK) (In ATP / GTP involved reactions the enzymes acted are "*kinase*" and the substrate is "1,3-bisphospho glycerate").

COO—(P)
H—C—OH
CH_2O—(P)
1,3-Bisphospho glycerate (1,3-BPG)

Dephosphorylation
ADP ATP +1
1,3-Bisphospho glycerokinase ***(1,3-BPGK)***
$Mg^{2\oplus}$

$COO^{\ominus}$
H—C—OH
CH_2O—(P)
3-Phospho glycerate (3-PG)

Example 2: Phosphoenolpyruvate undergoes dephosphorylation and produce pyruvate in enol form in presence of *pyruvate kinase* (PK) (PEP) (In ATP / GTP involved reactions, the enzymes acted are "*kinase*" and the product formed is "pyruvate").

$COO^{\ominus}$
C—O—(P)
‖
CH_2
Phosphoenol pyruvate (PEP)

Dephosphorylation
ADP ATP +1
Pyruvate kinase ***(PK)***
$Mg^{2\oplus}$ (or) $Mn^{2\oplus}$

$COO^{\ominus}$
C—**OH**
‖
CH_2
Pyruvate (Enol form)

Example 3: Succinyl CoA is hydrolyzed into succinate with loss of co-enzyme A. The reaction is catalyzed by *succinate thiokinase* (STK) enzyme (In ATP / GTP involved reactions, the enzymes acted are "*kinase*", sulphur atom of CoA is involved and the product formed is "succinate"). One GDP is converted into GTP in this step by reacting with inorganic phosphate.

$$\underset{\text{Succinyl CoA}}{\begin{matrix} CH_2-COO^{\ominus} \\ | \\ CH_2-\underset{\underset{O}{\|}}{C}-SCoA \end{matrix}} \xrightarrow[\text{Succinate thiokinase (STK)}]{\text{Hydrolysis} \quad GDP,\ Pi \rightarrow GTP;\ H_2O \rightarrow CoASH} \underset{\text{Succinate}}{\begin{matrix} CH_2-COO^{\ominus} \\ | \\ CH_2-COO^{\ominus} \end{matrix}}$$

Oxidative Phosphorylation

In aerobic organism, oxidative phosphorylation is the major source of ATP. Oxidative phosphorylation is defined as the process of synthesizing ATP from ADP and Pi (inorganic phosphate) with the involvement ETC (electron transport chain). In general, the transport of electrons through the ETC is linked with the release of free energy. Oxidative phosphorylation is taking place in complex-V of inner mitochondrial membrane.

Phosphorous oxygen ratio (P:O): The phosphorous oxygen ratio i.e., P:O is defined as the number of inorganic phosphate molecules utilized for ATP generation for every atom of oxygen consumed. Otherwise it represents the number of molecules of ATP synthesized per pair of electrons carried through ETC. In general, the phosphorous oxygen ratio (P:O) for mitochondrial oxidation of NADH is three.

$$NADH + H^+ + \frac{1}{2}O_2 + 3\ ADP + 3\ Pi \longrightarrow NAD^+ + 3\ ATP + H_2O$$

The phosphorous oxygen ratio (P:O) for mitochondrial oxidation of $FADH_2$ is two.

$$FADH_2 + \frac{1}{2}O_2 + 2\ ADP + 2\ Pi \longrightarrow FAD + 2\ ATP + H_2O$$

Ten and six protons are pumped across the mitochondrial membrane by NADH + H^+ and $FADH_2$, respectively. Four protons are required for the synthesis of one ATP. Hence, there is a strong evidence that the phosphorous oxygen ratio (P:O) for mitochondrial oxidation of NADH + H^+ and $FADH_2$, is 2.5 and 1.5, respectively.

Site of oxidative phosphorylation in ETC: In ETC, there are three exergonic site which results in the synthesis of 3 ATP molecules.

1. Oxidation of $FMNH_2$ by Co-enzyme Q
2. Oxidation of cytochrome b by cytochrome c_1.
3. *Cytochrome oxidase* reaction.

Each one of the above sites represents the coupling site for the synthesis of one ATP. NADH + H^+ pass through all three coupling sites that results in production of three ATP. Whereas, $FADH_2$ by passing the first coupling site and pass through only last two coupling sites results in production of two ATP.

Energetic of oxidative phosphorylation: The simplified reactions involved in the transport of electrons to redox pair $\frac{1}{2}O_2$ / H_2O (E_0: + 0.82 V) from redox pair NAD^+ / NADH + H^+ (E_0: - 0.32 V) is represented as follows,

$$\frac{1}{2}O_2 + NADH + H^+ \longrightarrow H_2O + NAD^+$$

Between these two redox pairs the redox potential difference is 1.14 V [$\Delta E_0 = E_0$ of accepted redox pair - E_0 of donated redox pair i.e., 0.82 – (-0.32) which is 0.82 + 0.32)]. This 1.14 V redox potential equals to 52 Cal/mol of energy. In ETC, from the above electron transfers three ATPs are generated. Hence, the total energy of these three ATPs is 21.9 Cal/mol (One ATP energy is 7.3 Cal/mol. Hence, for three ATPs it is 7.3 X 3 = 21.9). From this, the energy conservation efficiency is calculated as follows,

$$\text{Energy conservation efficiency} = \frac{\text{Energy of 3 ATPS}}{\text{Total energy}} \times 100 = \frac{21.9}{52} \times 100 = 42\%$$

Thus, only 42 % of energy is trapped in the form of three ATPs when NADH + H^+ are oxidized and the remaining energy is lost as heat. This lost heat is not a waste one because it is necessary to maintain body temperature and it allows continuous generation of ATP in ETC.

Mechanism of Oxidative Phosphorylation

The mechanism involved in oxidative phosphorylation is tried to explain by several hypothesis. Out of several mechanisms proposed for oxidative phosphorylation the following three are most important.

1. Chemical coupling mechanism
2. Chemiosmotic mechanism
3. Conformational coupling mechanism

1. **Chemical coupling mechanism:** In the year 1953, Edward Slater proposed this hypothesis. According to this mechanism, in ETC during the course of electron transfer, ADP reacts with inorganic phosphate and produces a series of phosphorylated high energy intermediates which are utilized for synthesis of ATP. This reaction is believed to be analogous to the substrate level phosphorylation reactions occurring in glycolysis and TCA cycle. In addition, till date no evidence could prove this hypothesis since all attempts made to isolate any one of the phosphorylated high energy intermediates are not successful.

ADP + Pi ⟶ Several phosphorylated high energy intermediates ⟶ ATP

2. **Chemiosmotic mechanism:** This mechanism is widely accepted and it was proposed in the year 1961 by Peter Mitchell. This mechanism clearly explains the utilization of electrons transport in ETC for the production of ATP from ADP and inorganic phosphate. The energy stored in battery separated by positive and negative charges is generally used for comparison of chemiosmotic mechanism and is represented in Figure 1.14.

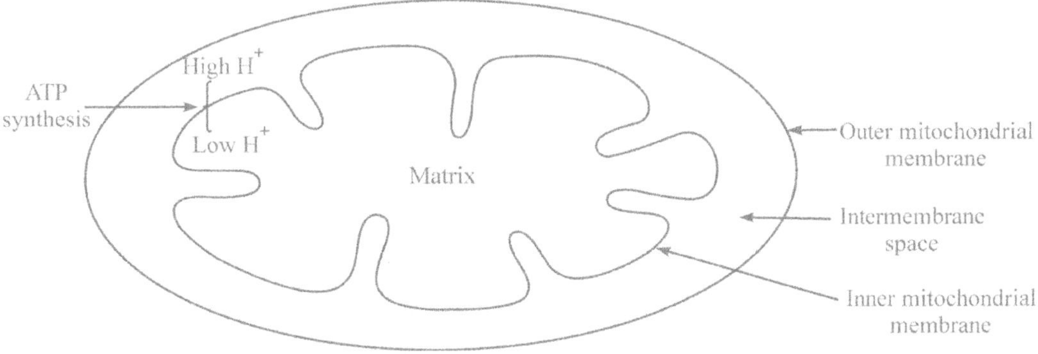

Figure 1.14 Outline of chemiosmotic mechanism for oxidative phosphorylation.

The inner mitochondrial membrane is impermeable to ions such as protons (H^+) and hydroxyl ions (OH^-). In ETC, across the coupling membrane (i.e., inner mitochondrial membrane) protons are translocated along with the transport of electrons to the inter membrane space from mitochondrial matrix. Electrochemical gradient or proton gradient takes place as a result of pumping of protons. The reason behind is accumulation of more protons (H^+) on the outer side of the inner mitochondrial membrane than the inner side. This formed electrochemical gradient or proton gradient due to flow of electrons in ETC is sufficient enough for the synthesis of ATP from ADP and inorganic phosphate.

The electrochemical gradient or proton gradient is utilized by the enzyme known as *ATP synthase* present in complex–V of inner mitochondrial membrane and produces ATP. The enzyme is also known as *ATPase* as it hydrolyzes ATP into ADP and inorganic phosphate. *ATP synthase* is a complex enzyme and are made up of two functional subunits namely F_1 and F_0. The structure of *ATP synthase* is comparable with the structure of lollipops. ATP is synthesized when the protons accumulated on the inter membrane space re-enter into the mitochondrial matrix. Chemiosmotic mechanism for oxidative phosphorylation is schematically represented in Figure 1.15.

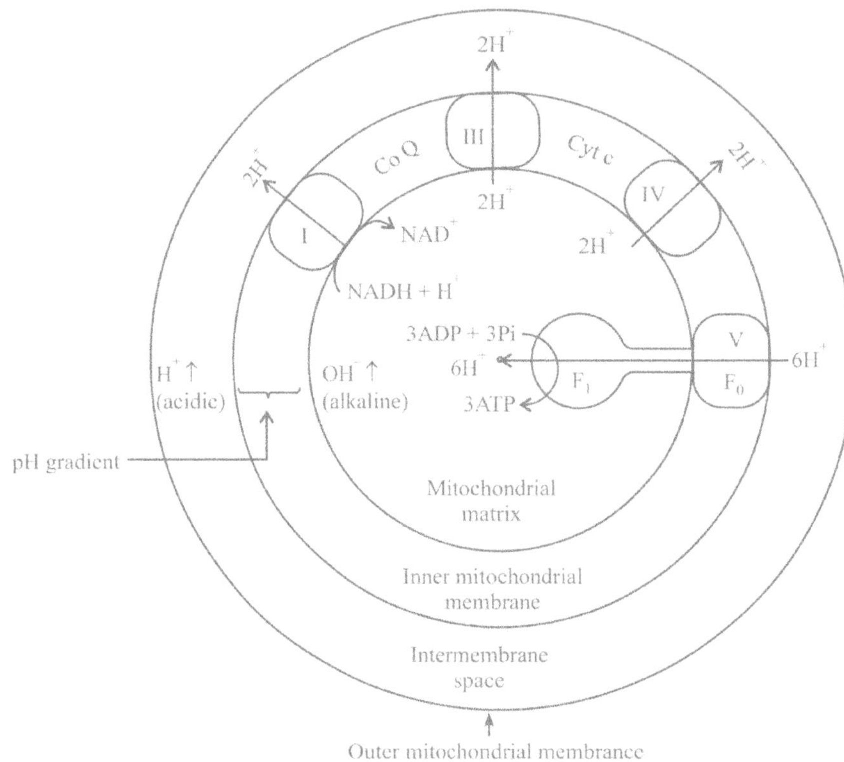

Figure 1.15 Schematic representation of chemiosmotic mechanism for oxidative phosphorylation.

Evidence for chemiosmotic mechanisms: There are several evidences available for supporting chemiosmotic mechanisms.

1. ATP synthesis takes place in inner mitochondrial membrane only.
2. Inner mitochondrial membrane is impermeable to various ions such as H^+, K^+ etc.
3. Additions of proton in inter membrane space of mitochondria results in increased ATP synthesis.
4. Any substances which increases the membrane permeability leads to decreased ATP synthesis. **Example:** 2, 4-Dinitrophenol (2,4-DNP).

3. **Conformational coupling mechanism:** According to this mechanism, inner mitochondrial membrane undergoes some conformational changes therefore ADP and Pi (inorganic phosphate) come close to each other during electron transfer in ETC which results in formation of ATP. There is an evidence for this mechanism as inner mitochondrial membrane undergoes conformational changes and it is explained by rotary motor model for ATP generation.

Rotary motor model for ATP generation: In 1964 Paul Boyer proposed that ATP is synthesized due to a conformational change in the mitochondrial membrane proteins. Now this hypothesis of Paul Boyer is considered as rotary motor or engine driving model or binding change model which is widely accepted. The enzyme *ATP synthase* is a complex one present in complex–V of inner mitochondrial membrane and it contains two major sub complexes namely F_0 and F_1. To the sub complex F_0 composed of channel protein C subunits, *F_1-ATP synthase* is attached. *F_1-ATP synthase* consist of three subunits namely α, β and γ. Generally, γ subunit is present centrally and is surrounded by alternative α and β subunits. Three α, three β and one γ subunit is present in *F_1-ATP synthase*. The γ subunit is rotated physically in response to proton flux leads to induction of conformational changes in $β_3$ subunit results in release of ATP. Different conformations were adapted by the three β subunits of *F_1-ATP synthase* according to the binding change mechanism. One subunit has O (open) conformation; the second one has L (loose) conformation; and the third one has T (tight) conformation. γ subunit rotation is induced by protons through unknown mechanism. This leads to conformational changes in β subunits. In L-conformation, ADP and inorganic phosphate binds to β subunits. When this L-site of β subunits changed to T-conformation, ATP is synthesized. The O-site is changed to L-conformation which binds to ADP and inorganic phosphate. The T-site is changed to O-conformation and releases ATP. This conformational change of β subunits is repeated and three ATPs are generated for each rotation. The release of ATP from O-conformation is energy dependent whereas synthesis of ATP is not dependent on energy. This is very crucial in synthesis of ATP by rotary motor model. This enzyme *ATP synthase* acting as a proton driving motor is a good example for rotary catalysis. Hence, in the world the smallest molecular motor is *ATP synthase*. Rotary motor model for ATP generation is represented in Figure 1.16.

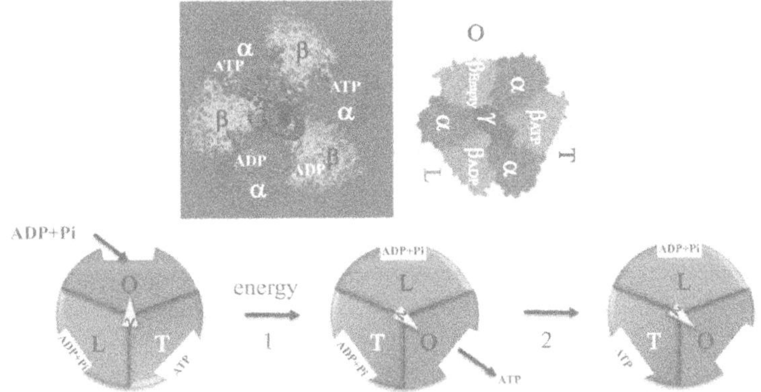

Figure 1.16 Rotary motor model for ATP generation.

Inhibitors of oxidative phosphorylation:

Oxidative phosphorylation can be inhibited by the following components.

1. Uncouplers
2. Ionophores
3. Inhibitors of *ATP synthase*
4. Inhibitors of adenine nucleotide carrier.

1. **Uncouplers:** These are the substances which uncouple or delink the transport of electrons in ETC during oxidative phosphorylation. Uncoupler oxidizes the reducing equivalents such as NADH + H^+ and $FADH_2$ without production of ATP. **Example:** 2,4-Dinitrophenol (2,4-DNP) and physiological uncouplers such as thyroxine, thermogenin and long chain fatty acids.
2. **Ionophores:** Ionophores is defined as lipophilic substances which increases the membrane permeability of various ions such as H^+, K^+, Cl^-, HCO_3^-, Na^+ etc. across the biological membrane. Even uncouplers are proton ionophores (uncouplers increase the membrane permeability of H^+ ions). **Example:** Valinomycin, gramicidin-A and nigericin are K^+ ionophores; 2,4-dinitophenol (2,4-DNP) is H^+ ionophores.
3. **Inhibitors of *ATP synthase*:** *ATP synthase* is an enzyme responsible for the synthesis of ATP. Hence, inhibition of *ATP synthase* may lead to decreased ATP synthesis. **Example:** Oligomycin
4. **Inhibitors of adenine nucleotide carrier:** ADP is an important component for the synthesis of ATP. Hence decreased supply of ADP may lead to decreased synthesis of ATP. This type of

inhibitors inhibits adenine nucleotide carrier which leads to block of adequate supply of ATP. **Example:** Atractyloside

Electron Transport Chain (ETC) or Respiratory Chain or Electron Transport System (ETS)

Through a series of biochemical reactions, energy rich biomolecules such as carbohydrates (specifically glucose), amino acids and fatty acids are oxidized in body into carbon dioxide and water. During these metabolic reactions from various metabolic intermediates the reducing equivalents are transferred into co-enzyme NAD^+ and FAD to produce NADH + H^+ and $FADH_2$ respectively. Through electron transport chain (ETC) these two reduced coenzymes finally reduce oxygen to water. Free energy loss is usually associated with ETC. From ADP and inorganic phosphate, ATP is synthesized by utilizing the part of this free energy . ETC is important for regeneration of oxidized form of reducing equivalent NAD^+ and FAD. Overview of biological oxidation and ETC are represented in Figure 1.17 and 1.18, respectively.

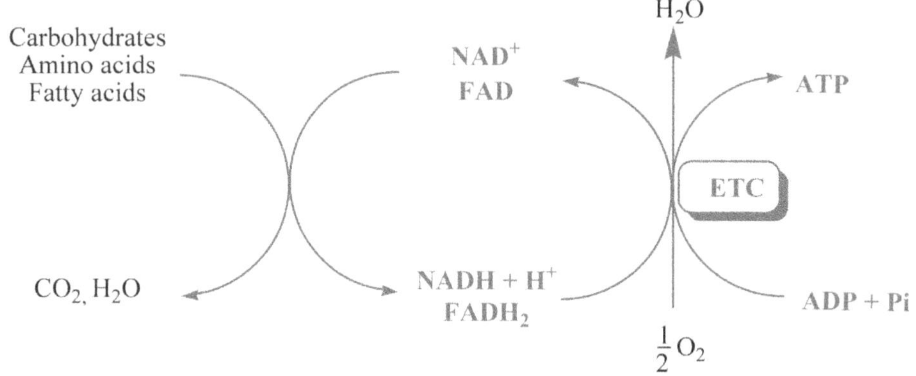

Figure 1.17 Overview of biological oxidation.

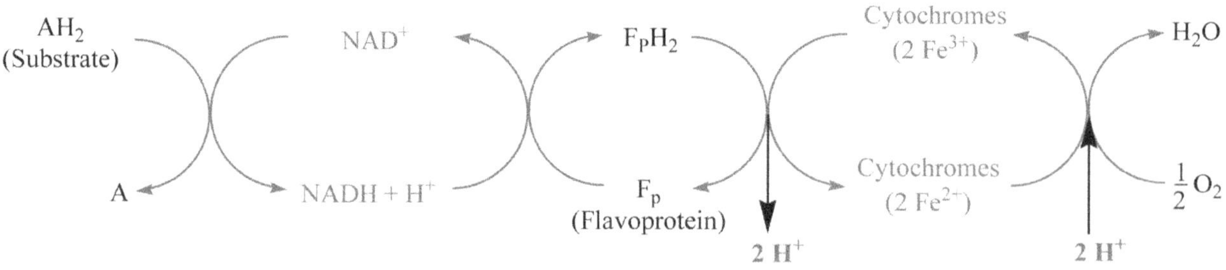

Figure 1.18 Overview of electron transport chain (ETC).

Mitochondria: Mitochondria are considered as the power house of the cell because mitochondria are the centre for metabolic oxidation reactions. The reduced coenzymes like NADH + H^+ and $FADH_2$ are oxidized to NAD^+ and FAD respectively in ETC of mitochondrion with energy liberation in the form of ATP. Five distinct parts are present in mitochondria. They are,

1. Outer mitochondrial membrane
2. Inner mitochondrial membrane
3. Inter membrane space
4. The cristae and
5. The mitochondrial matrix

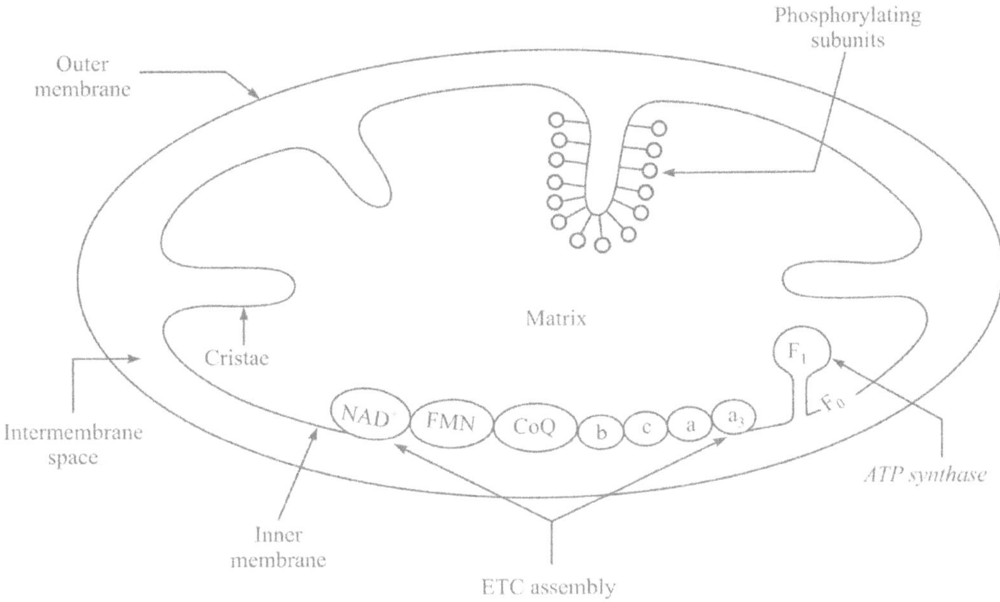

Figure 1.19 Structure of mitochondria depicting ETC.

In the inner mitochondrial membrane of the mitochondria, ETC and ATP synthesizing systems are located which is a specialized structure and rich in proteins. Inner mitochondrial membrane is impermeable to ions like sodium (Na^+), potassium (K^+), proton (H^+), etc. and small molecule like ADP, ATP, etc. The surface area of the inner mitochondrial membrane is greatly increased by forming cristae (highly folded membrane). The centre of ATP production i.e., a specialized particle phosphorylating subunits which look likes lollipops are present in the inner surface of the inner mitochondrial membrane. The mitochondrial matrix is the interior ground substance of the mitochondria. The enzymes involved in TCA cycle, oxidation of amino acids and β-oxidation of fatty acids are rich in the mitochondrial matrix. Structure of mitochondria depicting ETC is presented in Figure 1.19.

Mechanism of ETC

Five distinct enzyme or respiratory complexes are present in the inner mitochondrial membrane of the mitochondria. They are complex–I, complex–II, complex–III, complex–IV and complex–V. Electrons are carried by the first four complexes i.e., complex–I to complex–IV and the ATP is synthesized in complex–V. Certain mobile electron carriers such as, NADH, co-enzyme Q, cytochrome C and oxygen are present in ETC besides these five enzyme complexes. The electrons are transported collectively by the complex–I to complex–IV and the mobile electron carriers. Finally, the electrons react with oxygen and produced water. ETC of mitochondria utilizes the largest portion of oxygen consumed by the body. Mechanism of ETC with multiprotein complexes involved in ETC is represented schematically in Figure 1.20.

Components of ETC: There are the five major components which are distinct carriers that participate in the electron transport chain. These carriers are sequentially arranged and carry electrons from the substrate and finally combine with oxygen to produce water. The five major components of ETC are, 1) Nicotinamide nucleotides, 2) Flavoproteins, 3) Iron-sulphur proteins, 4) Co-enzyme Q and 5) Cytochromes.

1. **Nicotinamide nucleotide:** NAD^+ and $NADP^+$ are the two coenzymes of vitamin B_3 i.e., niacin. Out of these two, NAD^+ is actively involved in ETC. Generally, from the substrates (AH_2) such as glyceraldehyde-3-phosphate, pyruvate, isocitrate, α-ketoglutarate and malate, NAD^+ removes two hydrogen and reduced to NADH + H^+ in presence of *dehydrogenase* enzyme.

Redox reaction

$$\underset{\textbf{Substrate}}{AH_2} + NAD^+ \underset{\textit{Dehydrogenase}}{\rightleftharpoons} \underset{\textbf{Product}}{A} + NADH + H^+$$

Whereas $NADP^+$ is reduced to $NADPH + H^+$ in presence of $NADP^+$ dependent *dehydrogenase* enzyme which is not a substrate for ETC. $NADPH + H^+$ is mainly involved in fatty acid synthesis and cholesterol synthesis

2. **Flavoproteins:** *NADH-coenzyme Q reductase* or *NADH dehydrogenase* and *succinate-coenzyme Q reductase* or *succinate dehydrogenase* are the two important flavoproteins of the ETC. Prosthetic group present in flavoprotein *NADH dehydrogenase* is FMN. The co-enzyme FMN is converted to $FMNH_2$ by accepting two electrons and protons from $NADH + H^+$. *NADH dehydrogenase* is closely associated with iron-sulphur (Fe-S) proteins or non-heme iron (NHI) proteins.

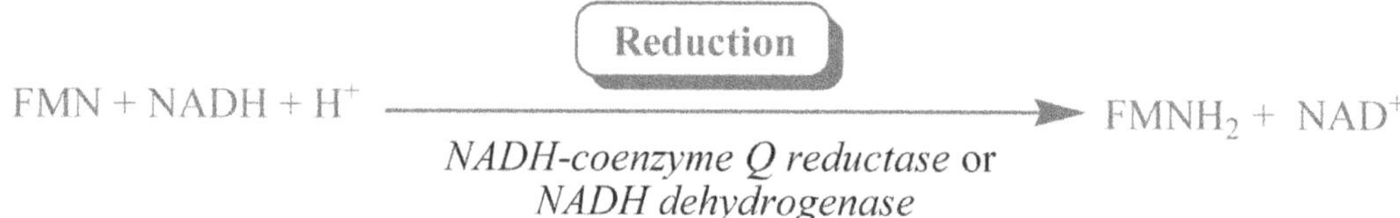

Prosthetic group present in flavoprotein *succinate dehydrogenase* is FAD. The coenzyme FAD is converted to $FADH_2$ by accepting two electrons and protons from succinate. *Succinate dehydrogenase* is also closely associated with iron-sulphur (Fe-S) proteins or non-heme iron (NHI) proteins.

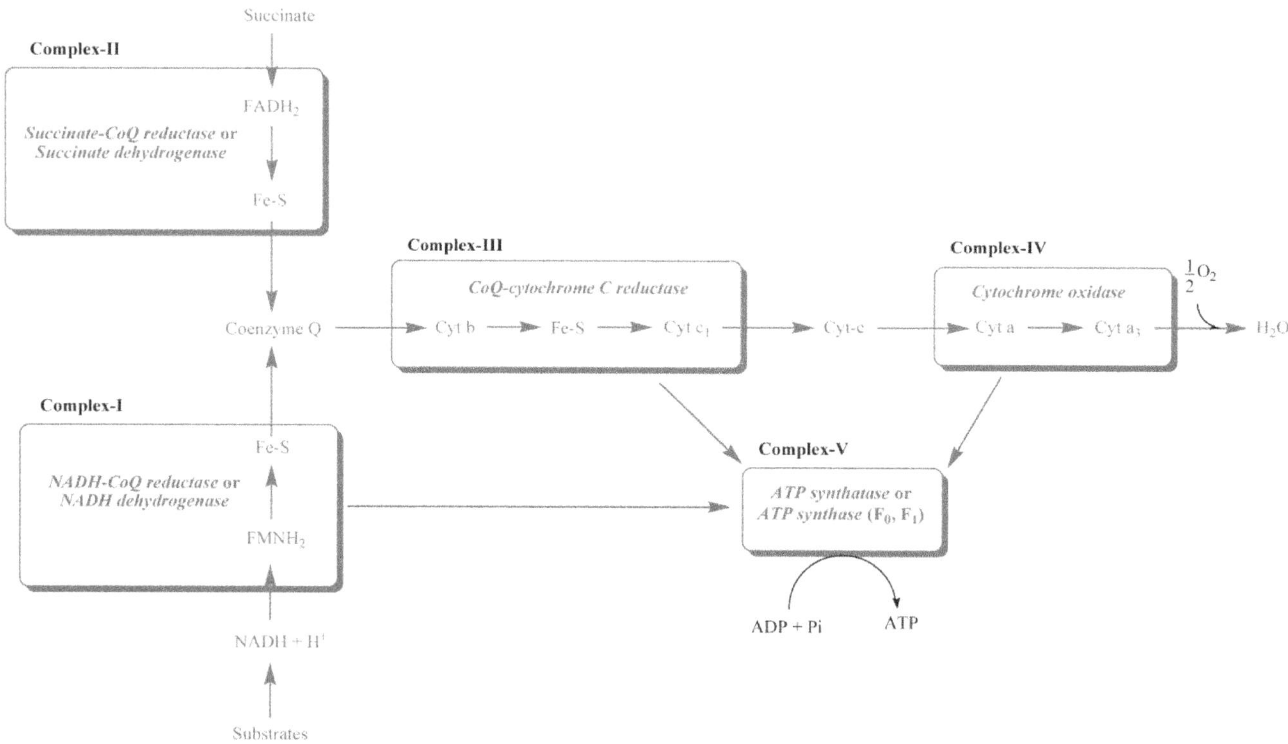

Figure 1.20 Mechanism of ETC with multiprotein complexes involved in ETC.

$$FAD + Succinate \xrightarrow[\textit{Succinate-coenzyme Q reductase or Succinate dehydrogenase}]{\text{Reduction}} FADH_2 + Fumarate$$

3. **Iron-sulphur (FeS) proteins:** There are about six iron-sulphur proteins which are involved in ETC and the exact mechanism involved in iron-sulphur protein is not clearly understood. In generals iron-sulphur proteins exist in two forms such as ferric i.e., Fe^{3+} (oxidized) and ferrous i.e., Fe^{2+} (reduced) which are inter convertible. Out of several iron-sulphur proteins, one is involved in the transfer of electron form $FMNH_2$ to coenzyme Q; the other one is involved in the transfer of electron form $FADH_2$ to coenzyme Q; the next one is the transfer of electron form cytochrome b to cytochrome c_1.
4. **Co-enzyme Q:** It is ubiquitous in living system; hence, it is also known as ubiquinone. Co-enzyme Q is a quinone derivative with a variable isoprenoid side chain. Quinone ring with ten isoprenoid unit side chain is present in mammalian tissues, hence it is commonly known as co-enzyme Q_{10} or CoQ_{10}. Co-enzyme Q is a lipophilic electron carrier. It accepts electron from both $FMNH_2$ produced in ETC and $FADH_2$ produced outside ETC (**Example:** *Succinate dehydrogenase, acyl CoA dehydrogenase,* etc.) In some organism like mycobacteria, co-enzyme Q is not present, hence, in these organism vitamin K performs the similar functions of co-enzyme Q. In body co-enzyme Q is directly synthesized because in animal there is no known vitamin precursors for co-enzyme Q .

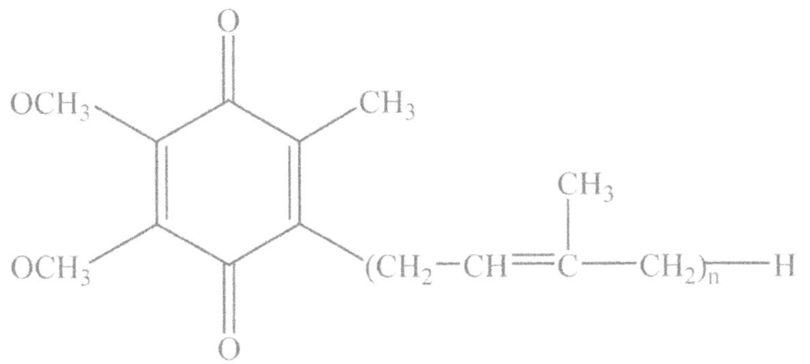

O
OCH_3 CH_3
CH_3
OCH_3 $(CH_2-CH=C-CH_2)_n-H$
O

5. **Cytochromes:** In general, cytochromes are hemoprotein containing heme as prosthetic group. Porphyrin ring with iron atom is present in heme. Compared to other hemoproteins such as hemoglobin, methemoglobin, heme present in cytochromes is different. In cytochromes, the iron is present in both reduced (ferrous i.e., Fe^{2+}) and oxidized (ferric i.e., Fe^{3+}) form alternatively which is essential for the transport of electrons in ETC. In case of other hemoproteins such as hemoglobin, methemoglobin, heme is present only in ferrous (Fe^{2+}) state.

   Depending upon the types of heme present and the respective absorption spectrum, initially three cytochromes are designated as cytochrome a, cytochrome b and cytochrome c. Latter, several additional cytochromes are discovered which are designated as cytochrome c_1, cytochrome b_1 and cytochrome a_3.

   Electrons are transported from co-enzyme Q into cytochromes in the following orders b, c_1, c, a and a_3. These cytochromes act as an effective electron carrier due to the presence of reversible oxidation–reduction property of heme iron present in it.

   Heme group and 104 amino acid containing small protein is cytochrome c (Molecular weight: 13,000). With an intermediate redox potential, cytochrome c acts as a central molecule in ETC. Cytochrome c can be easily extracted because it is loosely bounded in the inner mitochondrial membrane.

   In ETC, the terminal component is *cytochrome oxidase*. Cytochromes a and a_3 are collectively known as *cytochrome oxidase*. This is the only cytochrome which can directly react with molecular oxygen atom. Additionally, *cytochrome oxidase* also contains copper besides iron. Like iron, this copper also undergoes oxidation –reduction (cupric i.e., Cu^{2+} - curprous i.e., Cu^{+}) during the transport of electrons. Finally, water is produced in ETC from the transported electrons, free protons and the molecular oxygen atom.

Inhibitors of ETC

There are many site specific ETC inhibitors. Generally, inhibitors block the electron transport by binding with one component of ETC. This may lead to the accumulation of reduced components before the inhibitor

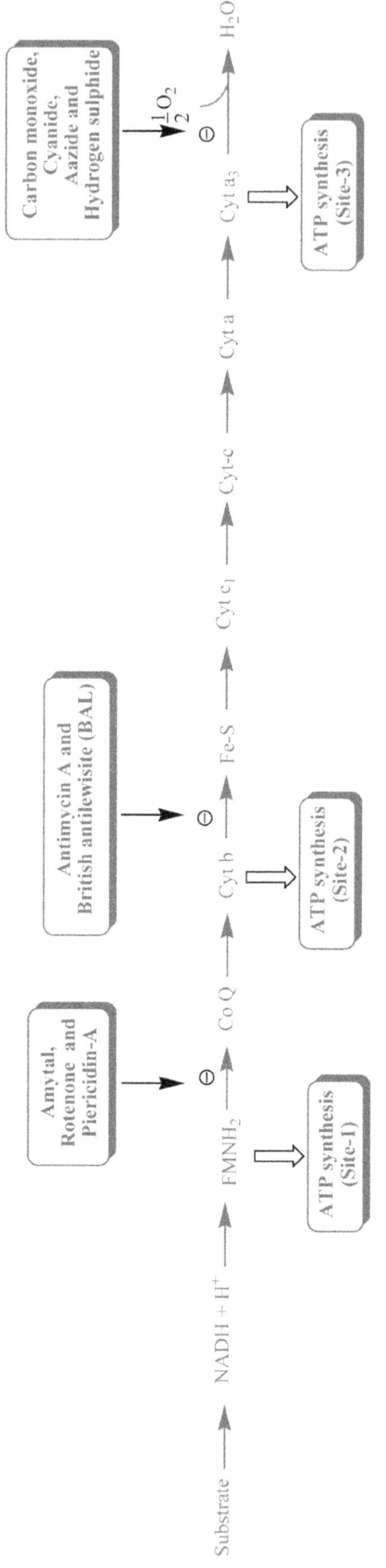

Figure 1.21 ETC with sites of ATP synthesis and inhibitors.

blockade step and oxidized components after the inhibitor blockade step. ATP synthesis i.e., phosphorylation mainly depends on ETC. Hence, ATP synthesis is also inhibited by the site specific ETC inhibitors. The inhibitors may act on three different sites of ATP synthesis as follows.

1. **Inhibitors at site-1:** The following chemical agents inhibits the synthesis of ATP in site-1 of ETC i.e., NADH and co-enzyme Q. **Example:** Amytal (barbiturate drug), rotenone (fish poison) and piericidin-A (antibiotic).
2. **Inhibitors at site-2:** The compounds inhibit the synthesis of ATP in site-2 of ETC i.e., cytochrome b and cytochrome c. **Example:** Antimycin-A (antibiotic) and British antilewisite i.e., BAL (Antidote used for war gas).
3. **Inhibition at site-3:** The compounds inhibit the synthesis of ATP in site-3 of ETC i.e., *cytochrome oxidase.* **Example:** Carbon monoxide (reacts with reduced form of cytochrome), cyanide and azide (reacts with oxidized form of cytochrome) and hydrogen sulphide (reacts with both oxidized and reduced form of cytochrome).

The most potent inhibitor of ETC is cyanide. It blocks the ETC by binding with the ferric ion of *cytochrome oxidase* which leads to death. Tissue asphyxia (mostly in CNS) is the reason behind the cyanide death. ETC with sites of ATP synthesis and inhibitors are presented in Figure 1.21.

PROBABLE QUESTIONS

PART – A: Multiple Choice Questions

1. __________ is the fundamental structural and functional unit of all living organisms.
   (a) Element (b) Macromolecule
   (c) Cell (d) Organ
2. Which of the following element is not a major element present in living matter?
   (a) Carbon (b) Sodium
   (c) Phosphorus (d) Sulphur
3. ____________ are the building blocks of lipids.
   (a) Fatty acid (b) Glycerol
   (c) Both a & b (d) None of the above
4. What is the percentage of water present in a normal healthy adult weighing 65 kg?
   (a) 52.4 (b) 61.6
   (c) 70.8 (d) 82.0
5. in both prokaryotic and eukaryotic cells, the volume of the cell occupied by a semi-fluid matrix called ________________.
   (a) Nucleus (b) Vacuole
   (c) Liposome (d) Cytoplasm
6. Which of the following is not a prokaryotic cell?
   (a) Fungi (b) Bacteria
   (c) PPLO (pleuro pneumonia like organisms) (d) Blue-green algae
7. __________ are the storage form of reserve material present in cytoplasm of prokaryotic cells.
   (a) Liposome (b) Mitochondria
   (c) Ribosome (d) Inclusion bodies
8. Which of the following are present in plant cells and absent in animal cells?
   (a) Cell walls (b) Large central vacuole
   (c) Plastids (d) All the above

9. In which chromosome, centromere is present in middle and forms two equal arms of the chromosome?
   (a) Metacentric chromosome (b) Sub-metacentric chromosome
   (c) Acrocentric chromosome (d) Telocentric chromosome
10. If enthalpy change for a reaction is zero, then $\Delta G°$ equals to ___________
   (a) $-T\Delta S°$ (b) $T\Delta S°$
   (c) $-\Delta H°$ (d) $\ln k_{eq}$
11. $\Delta G°$ is defined as the ___________
   (a) Residual energy present in the reactants at equilibrium
   (b) Residual energy present in the products at equilibrium
   (c) Difference in the residual energy of reactants and products at equilibrium
   (d) Energy required in converting one mole of reactants to one mole of products
12. For a reaction if $\Delta G°$ is positive, then ___________
   (a) The products will be favored
   (b) The reactants will be favored
   (c) The concentration of the reactants and products will be equal
   (d) All of the reactant will be converted to products
13. The study of energy relationships and conversions in biological systems is called as ___________
   (a) Biophysics (b) Biotechnology
   (c) Bioenergetics (d) Microbiology
14. Which of the following statement is false?
   (a) The reaction tends to go in the forward direction if ΔG is large and positive
   (b) The reaction tends to move in the backward direction if ΔG is large and negative
   (c) The system is at equilibrium if $\Delta G = 0$
   (d) The reaction tends to move in the backward direction if ΔG is large and positive
15. Anabolism and catabolism are chemically linked in the form of ___________
   (a) ADP (b) ATP
   (c) Phosphodiester linkage (d) ASP
16. Which of the following statements is false about ATP hydrolysis?
   (a) It is highly exergonic (b) Activation energy is relatively high
   (c) $\Delta G° = -30.5$ kJ/mol (d) $\Delta G° = 30.5$ kJ/mol
17. An endergonic reaction ___________
   (a) Proceeds spontaneously (b) Does not require activation energy
   (c) Releases energy (d) Requires energy
18. An exergonic reaction ___________
   (a) Proceeds spontaneously (b) Does not require activation energy
   (c) Releases energy (d) Requires energy
19. Phosphoryl groups are derivatives of ___________
   (a) Phosphorous acid (b) Phosphoric acid
   (c) Acetic acid (d) Citric acid
20. Water does a nucleophilic attack on phosphate monoester by producing ___________
   (a) Phosphorous chloride (b) Phosphorous sulfide
   (c) Inorganic phosphate (d) Organic phosphate

21. Which is an example of chemical to osmotic energy conversion that occurs in living organisms?
    (a) ATP-driven muscle contraction
    (b) ATP-dependent photon emission in fireflies
    (c) Light-induced electron flow in chloroplasts
    (d) ATP-driven active transport across a membrane
22. Which of the following statements about redox potential is false?
    (a) NADH/NAD^+ redox pair has the least redox potential
    (b) Oxygen/H_2O redox pair has the highest redox potential
    (c) The components of the electron transport chain are organized in terms of their redox potential
    (d) The redox potential of a system is usually compared with the potential of the hydrogen electrode
23. Which out of the following is not a flavoprotein?
    (a) *Succinate dehydrogenase* (b) Cytochrome c
    (c) *Xanthine oxidase* (d) *NADH dehydrogenase-Q reductase*
24. Which out of the following has the highest redox potential?
    (a) NAD^+ (b) FMN
    (c) FAD (d) O_2
25. Which one out of the following is not a NAD^+ requiring enzyme?
    (a) *Lactate dehydrogenase* (b) *Pyruvate dehydrogenase* complex
    (c) *Malate dehydrogenase* (d) *Acyl CoA dehydrogenase*
26. Which of the following enzyme catalyzes the direct transfer and incorporation of O_2 into a substrate molecule is
    (a) *Reductase* (b) *Oxidase*
    (c) *Oxygenase* (d) *Peroxidase*
27. Loss of electrons can be termed as ____________
    (a) Metabolism (b) Anabolism
    (c) Oxidation (d) Reduction
28. Gain of electrons can be termed as __________
    (a) Metabolism (b) Anabolism
    (c) Oxidation (d) Reduction
29. This is the major source of ATP in aerobic organism.
    (a) Substrate level phosphorylation (b) Oxidative phosphorylation
    (c) Glycolysis (d) TCA cycle
30. Name the compound with the greatest free energy
    (a) ATP (b) Phosphocreatine
    (c) Cyclic AMP (d) Phosphoenolpyruvate
31. 1,3-Bisphosphoglycerate is a example for which type of high energy compound?
    (a) Acyl phosphate (b) Enol phosphate
    (c) Pyrophosphate (d) Guanidino phosphate
32. In general, high energy compounds contain which type bond in its structure?
    (a) Peptide (b) Glycoside
    (c) Acid anhydride (d) Covalent

33. What happened to free energy changes when a reaction is at equilibrium?
    (a) Maximum (b) Minimum
    (c) Average (d) Zero
34. Standard redox potential of $NAD^+/NADH$ pair is ________ volts.
    (a) - 0.67 (b) - 0.22
    (c) +0.29 (d) - 0.32
35. The $FMNH_2$ is oxidized by __________
    (a) Cytochrome-c (b) Coenzyme Q
    (c) Cytochrome-a (d) Cytochrome-b
36. Which complex of inner mitochondrial membrane is the site of oxidative phosporylation?
    (a) III (b) IV
    (c) V (d) VI
37. Inner mitochondrial membrane is impermeable to which of the following ions?
    (a) H^+ (b) K^+
    (c) OH^- (d) All
38. Which of the following antibiotics act as ionophores for potassium ions.
    (a) Antimycin & Valinomycin (b) Piercidin-A & Valinomycin
    (c) Nigercin & Valinomycin (d) Antimycin & Piercidin-A
39. Protein that contains a nucleic acid derivative of riboflavin is called ________
    (a) Nucleic acid (b) Amino acid
    (c) Flavoprotein (d) None
40. NADP-linked *dehydrogenase* catalyzes ________
    (a) Glucose 6-phosphate+$NADP^+$ ↔ 6-phosphogluconate + NADPH + H^+
    (b) Lactate + NAD^+ ↔ pyruvate + NADH + H^+
    (c) Pyruvate + CoA + NAD^+ ↔ acetyl-CoA + CO_2 + NADH + H^+
    (d) L-Malate + NAD^+ ↔ oxaloacetate + NADH + H^+
41. A lipid-soluble benzoquinone with a long isoprenoid side chain is?
    (a) Ubiquinone (b) Cytochrome-b
    (c) Cytochrome-c (d) Cytochrome-a
42. The only membrane bound enzyme in the citric acid cycle is ________
    (a) *Succinate dehydrogenase* (b) *NADH dehydrogenase*
    (c) *ATP synthase* (d) *Acyl CoA dehydrogenase*
43. In ETC, complex-I is also called ________
    (a) *NADH dehydrogenase* (b) *Succinate dehydrogenase*
    (c) Cytochrome bc1 complex (d) *Cytochrome oxidase*
44. In ETC, complex-II is also called ________
    (a) *NADH dehydrogenase* (b) *Succinate dehydrogenase*
    (c) Cytochrome bc1 complex (d) *Cytochrome oxidase*
45. In ETC, complex-III is also called ________
    (a) *NADH dehydrogenase* (b) *Succinate dehydrogenase*
    (c) Cytochrome bc1 complex (d) *Cytochrome oxidase*

46. In ETC, complex-IV is also called ________
    (a) *NADH dehydrogenase* (b) *Succinate dehydrogenase*
    (c) Cytochrome bc1 complex (d) *Cytochrome oxidase*
47. In mitochondria, hydride ions are removed from substrates by ________
    (a) NAD-linked *dehydrogenases* (b) NADP-linked *dehydrogenases*
    (c) *ATP synthase* (d) *Succinate dehydrogenases*
48. Which of the following is the prosthetic group of *NADH dehydrogenase*?
    (a) NADH (b) FAD
    (c) NADPH (d) FMN
49. If mitochondria were blocked at the site of NADH oxidation and were treated with succinate as substrate, what would the P : O ratio is?
    (a) Same as that normally produced by succinate
    (b) One more than normally produced by succinate
    (c) One less than normally produced by succinate
    (d) Zero
50. ATP synthesis by chemiosmosis is by ___________
    (a) *ATP dehydrogenase* (b) *Gyrase*
    (c) *ATP synthase* (d) *Dehydrogenase*

Key for Multiple Choice Questions

1 (c)	2 (b)	3 (c)	4 (b)	5 (d)
6 (a)	7 (d)	8 (d)	9 (a)	10 (a)
11 (d)	12 (b)	13 (c)	14 (d)	15 (b)
16 (d)	17 (d)	18 (c)	19 (b)	20 (c)
21 (d)	22 (a)	23 (b)	24 (d)	25 (d)
26 (c)	27 (c)	28 (d)	29 (b)	30 (d)
31 (a)	32 (c)	33 (d)	34 (d)	35 (b)
36 (c)	37 (d)	38 (c)	39 (c)	40 (a)
41 (a)	42 (a)	43 (a)	44 (b)	45 (c)
46 (d)	47 (a)	48 (d)	49 (a)	50 (c)

PART – B: Short Answers

1. Explain the composition of cell.
2. Write a note on structural hierarchy of organism.
3. Define cell and list out different types of cell. Explain any one type of cell.
4. What are ribosomes and inclusion bodies?
5. How does an animal cell differs from plant cell.
6. Draw neat diagram of mitochondria and explain?
7. What is Golgi complex and endoplasmic reticulum?
8. Write the structural components of eukaryotic ribosomes.
9. Write a note on endomembrane system.
10. Compare prokaryotes and eukaryotes.
11. Write the characteristics of vesicular transport systems across cell membrane.
12. What is intrinsic and extrinsic protein?

13. What is free energy and free energy change?
14. Write the biochemical organization and functions of plasma membrane.
15. Write the characteristics of carrier mediated transport system.
16. Write the difference between passive transport and facilitated diffusion.
17. What is endocytosis and exocytosis?
18. Explain facilitated diffusion with the help of Ping-Pong model.
19. What is cotransport system?
20. Note on disorders of membrane transport system
21. What are the components present in the cell membranes?
22. What is energy rich compounds?
23. What are the main reasons for the ATP acts as universal energy currency molecule?
24. Write a brief account on ATP cycle.
25. Write about the biological significance of ATP & cAMP.
26. Explain redox potential & free energy constant.
27. Explain the biological significance of ATP.

PART – C: Long Answers

1. Write a detailed note on prokaryotic cells.
2. Explain eukaryotic cell with neat labelled diagram.
3. Write a detailed note on biochemical organization of cell membrane with neat labelled diagram.
4. How small molecules and macro molecules are transported in biological system. Explain with suitable diagram.
5. Write a detailed note on bioenergetics.
6. Define free energy, enthalpy and entropy. Explain the relationship between free energy, enthalpy and entropy.
7. List out various co-enzymes involved in biological oxidation and explain any two in detail with chemical structure.
8. Define and classify energy rich compounds. Explain any one compound in detail with chemical structure.
9. Explain about ETC & its mechanism.
10. Explain substrate level phosphorylation with suitable example.
11. Write an essay on electron transport chain & oxidative phosphorylation.
12. Write the biosynthesis and biological significance of ATP.
13. Write the biosynthesis and biological significance of cyclic AMP.
14. Explain the different mechanism or hypothesis proposed for oxidative phosphorylation.
15. Explain rotary motor model for ATP generation. Add a note on inhibitors of oxidative phosphorylation.
16. Outline how cyclic AMP is formed and destroyed. Comment on biological importance of cyclic AMP.
17. Difference between active and passive transport process.
18. Explain the components of respiratory chain in detail.
19. Explain the role of AMP in metabolism. Explain about active membrane transport.
20. Explain the terms: a) Passive diffusion; b) Active transport.
21. Write short notes on cyclic AMP.
22. Write briefly on: a) biological significance of ATP, b) Free energy, c) Energy rich compounds.
23. Write an account of high energy compounds metabolism.
24. Write a detailed note on inhibitors of ETC.
25. How does ATPs synthesized in biological system.

2

Enzymes

Enzymes are the bio-chemicals synthesized by living cells which increases the rate of the biochemical reaction without undergoing any changes itself. They are protein in nature (except RNA acting as *ribozyme*), colloidal (does not form true solution in water due to huge size), thermolabile (affected by heat) and specific in their action. They are huge in size with a small active site.

In biochemical lab, enzymes are highly used for diagnosis of various diseases. For example, in laboratory condition a couple of days are needed for hydrolysis of proteins even at 100 °C in presence of strong acid like hydrochloric acid, etc.; whereas the same reaction in a biological system is completed within 2 hours at body temperature itself in presence of GIT enzymes. This reaction shows the efficiency of enzymes.

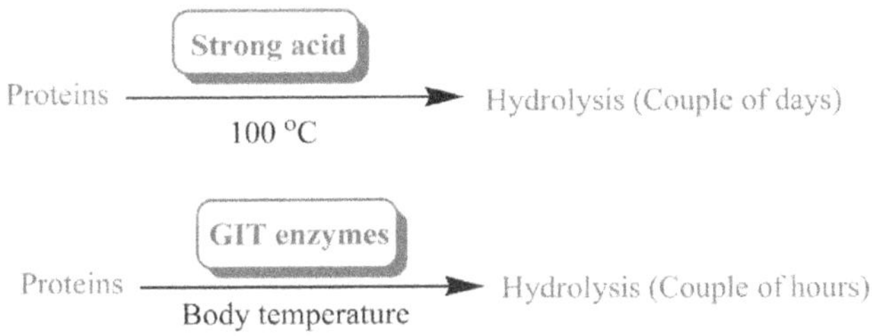

Properties

1. All enzymes are proteins except RNA as a *ribozyme.*
2. Holo-enzyme is the functional unit of enzyme and it is composed of two major parts namely apo-enzyme and co-enzyme. The Protein part of enzyme is called as apo-enzyme and the non-protein part of enzyme is called as co-enzyme.

Holoenzyme (Active enzyme) ⟶ **Apoenzyme** (Protein part) + **Co-enzyme** (Non-protein part)

3. Generally, co-enzymes are loosely bounded to apo-enzyme, hence can be easily separated by the process called dialysis. If the non-protein parts are tightly (covalently) bonded to the apo-enzyme then it is known as "prosthetic group" and it cannot be separated by dialysis.
4. Generally, enzymes are soluble in water but it does not form true solution instead it forms a colloidal solution. This property of an enzyme is due to its huge size.
5. The molecular weight of enzymes varies which depends upon the proteins present in enzymes.
6. Enzymes are varied in shape. It may be globular, oval, fibrous or elongated, etc.
7. Isoelectric pH (p^I) is defined as the pH at which proteins exists as zwitterion or dipolar ion. These dipolar or zwitterion are electrically neutral, hence in the electric field they do not migrate. Generally, at isoelectric pH the solubility is minimum, the precipitability is maximum and the buffering capacity is least.

8. Enzymes are big in size when compared to relatively smaller substrates. Only a smaller portion of the huge enzyme is directly involved in the substrate binding and catalysis. Active site or center of an enzyme represents the smaller region at which the substrate binds and participates in catalysis.
9. Enzymes contain a small active site and substrates bind with these active sites through weak non-covalent bonds.
10. The existence of an active site is due to the tertiary structure of protein resulting in three dimensional native confirmations. The amino acid present in the active site is responsible for the activity and specific action of the enzymes.
11. The active site is made up of amino acids which are far from each other in the linear sequences of amino acids (For example, the *lysozyme* is composed of 129 amino acids in which 35, 52, 62, 63 and 101 amino acids are present in the active site).
12. Active sites are not rigid in structure and are regarded as clefts or cervices or pockets occupying a small region in a big enzyme molecule. Serine is the most frequently found amino acid in active site.
13. Substrate binding site and catalytic binding sites are present in the active site of enzymes. The first one is for substrate and the second one is for catalyst for specific reactions. The co-enzymes or cofactors or prosthetic groups bind in the catalytic site only.
14. In general, enzyme binds with substrate and forms enzyme-substrate complex. This step is a reversible one. Later enzyme-substrate complex produces a product and regenerates enzymes for other fresh reaction.

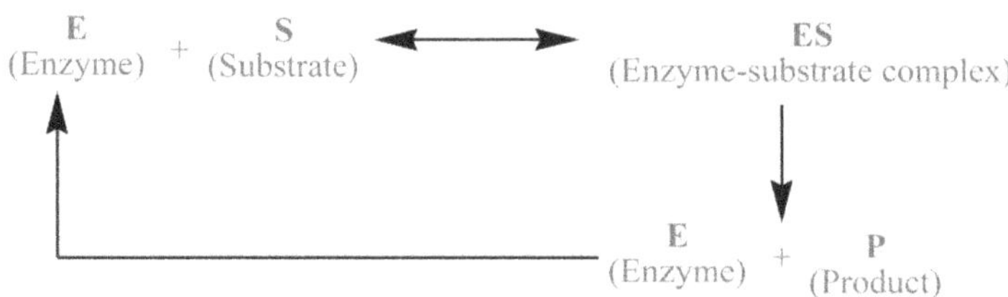

Nomenclature

Enzymes are named in three different ways a) Arbitrary manner, b) Tribal name, c) Enzyme commission name.

1. **Arbitrary Manner:** In olden days,the enzymes are named based on the discoveries. This system of naming doesn't convey any information like nature of the substrate on which it acts, the function of enzyme, etc. **Example:** *Pepsin, trypsin* and *chymotrypsin.*
2. **Tribal Name:** In this type of nomenclature the suffix "ase" is added to the substrate for giving a name to enzymes. This system also fails to provide complete information of enzyme catalyzed reaction such as type of reaction, cofactors required, etc. **Example:** *Lipase* acts on lipids, *nuclease* acts on nucleic acid, *protease* acts on protein, *lactase* acts on lactose. But this naming does not indicate about the type of reaction.
3. **IUB Name:** Enzyme commission allotted a four-digit enzyme commission (EC) number to every enzyme. This number is known as IUB (International union of biochemistry) name of enzymes. Each digit indicates certain information. The first digit of EC number indicates class of enzyme, the second digit indicates sub-class of enzyme, the third digit indicates sub-sub-class of enzyme and the fourth digit indicates individual enzyme name. This system provides all information related to biochemical reactions such as type of substrate, type of reaction catalyzed by the enzymes, co-enzyme required if any, etc. IUB names are not accepted for general use because they are complex and difficult to remember even though they are specific and unambiguous. Hence, usually tribal names along with EC numbers as and when needed are commonly used and are widely accepted.

Classification

Enzymes are classified in different ways as follows, a) IUB classification, b) Classification based on place or site of action, c) Classification based on the number of polypeptide chain, d) Classification based on the number of enzymes.

(a) IUB classification: In the year 1961, enzyme commission classified enzymes into six major categories according to the type of reactions catalyzed by enzyme. In general, the word **"OTHLIL"** may be memorized to remember six major categories of enzymes in correct order. All six classes of enzymes are summarized in Table 2.1 with type of reaction catalyzing, general reaction, example and biochemical reaction example.

Table 2.1 IUB classification of enzymes.

S. No.	Class of Enzyme	Type of reaction catalyzing	General Reaction	Example	Biochemical Reaction Example
1.	*Oxidoreductases*	It catalyzes oxidation reduction (redox) reaction	$AH_2 + B$ → (Oxidation-Reduction) → $A + BH_2$	*Alcohol dehydrogenase, cytochrome oxidase, L-amino acid oxidase, D-amino acid oxidase*	$CH_3CH_2OH + NAD^+$ (Ethanol) → *Alcohol dehydrogenase* (Oxidation-Reduction) → $CH_3CHO + NADH + H^+$ (Acetaldehyde)
2.	*Transferases*	It catalyzes the transfer of functional group other than hydrogen from one compound to another compound	$AX + B$ → (Functional group transfer other than hydrogen) → $A + BX$	*Choline acetyl transferase, transaminase, transmethylase, phoshorylase, hexokinase*	$CH_3COSCoA$ + Choline (Acetyl CoA) → *Choline acetyl transferase* (Transfer of acetyl group) → CH_3CO-Choline + CoASH (Acetyl choline)
3.	*Hydrolases*	It catalyzes hydrolysis reactions	$AB + H_2O$ → (Hydrolysis) → $AH + BOH$	*Cholinesterase, lipase, urease, pepsin, acid phosphatase, alkaline phosphatase*	CH_3CO-Choline + H_2O (Acetyl choline) → *Choline esterase* (Hydrolysis) → CH_3COOH + Choline (Acetic acid)
4.	*Lyases*	It catalyzes addition or removal of water, ammonia, carbon dioxide, etc. and results in the formation of double bond	A—X + B—Y → (Addition - Elimination) → AX—BY	*Aldolase, fumarase, Histidase*	Glyceraldehyde-3-phosphate + Dihydroxy acetone phosphate → *Aldolase* (Addition - Elimination) → Fructose-1,6-bisphosphate
5.	*Isomerases*	It catalyzes isomerization reaction	A ⇅ (Interconversion of isomers) A'	*Phospho triose isomerase, Phosphohexose isomerase, retinol isomerase*	Glyceraldehyde-3-phosphate ⇅ *Phospho triose isomerase* (Isomerization) Dihydroxy acetone phosphate
6.	*Ligases* or *synthetases* or *synthases*	It catalyzes synthetic reaction (In Greek "ligate" means to bind where two molecules joined together). It needs ATP	A + B → (Condensation usually depends on ATP; ATP → ADP + Pi) → A—B	*Glutamine synthase, succinate thiokinase, fatty acid synthase, acetyl CoA carboxylase*	Glutamic acid + NH_3 → *Glutamine synthase* (Condensation; ATP → ADP + Pi) → Glutamine

(b) **Classification based on place of action:** Enzymes are classified into 2 major types according to the place where it exhibits action.

1. **Intracellular enzyme:** In Greek "intra" means "within". These enzymes exhibit activity within the cell where they are synthesized. **Example:** *Hexokinase (HK), aldolase*, etc.
2. **Extracellular enzymes:** These enzymes exhibit activity outside the cell where they are not synthesized and not within the cell. **Example:** All digestive enzymes.

(c) **Classification based upon the number of polypeptide chains:** Based on the number of peptide chains present in enzyme it was classified into two major categories.

1. **Monomeric enzyme:** In Greek "mono" means "single". This enzyme is composed of single peptide chains. **Example:** *Trypsin.*
2. **Oligomeric enzyme:** In Greek "oligo" means "few". These enzymes are made up of a few peptide chains. **Example:** *Lactate dehydrogenase* **(LDH).**

(d) **Classification based upon the number of enzymes:** Enzymes are classified into two major categories according to the number of enzymes present in it.

1. **Mono-enzymes:** These enzymes are composed of single enzyme molecule only and are not depends on any enzyme for its activity. **Example:** Almost all enzymes like *hexokinase (HK), aldolase*, etc.
2. **Multi enzyme complex:** These are enzyme complexes made up of many enzyme molecules. The activity of enzymes depends on the activity of other enzymes present in complex. If any one enzyme is removed or inactivated the whole enzyme system becomes inactive. **Example:** *Lactate dehydrogenase (LDH), pyruvate dehydrogenase (PDH), fatty acid synthase (FAS)* complex.

Mechanism of Enzyme Action

Enzyme Decreases Activation Energy

Enzymes are powerful catalyst and catalysis is the prime functions of the enzyme. Similar to non-biological catalysis, it takes place in biological system also. The reactant must be changed to an activated state or transition state for any chemical reaction to take place. For this, the substances (reactants) needs some energy. The energy required by the reactants to undergo a chemical reaction is called activation energy. When heated the reactants attain this activation energy. The catalyst (enzyme in biological systems) brings down the activation energy hence the reactions takes place at lower temperature itself. Generally, equilibrium constants are not altered by enzymes and it only increases the velocity of reactions.

The role of enzyme or catalyst is usually compared with a tunnel made in the mountain to reduce the barrier as illustrated in Figure 2.1. Enzymes make the reaction go faster because it lowers the energy barriers of reactants. Enzyme made possible that all biochemical reaction occurs at body temperature itself (below 40 °C) by reducing activation energy of reactants as follows-.

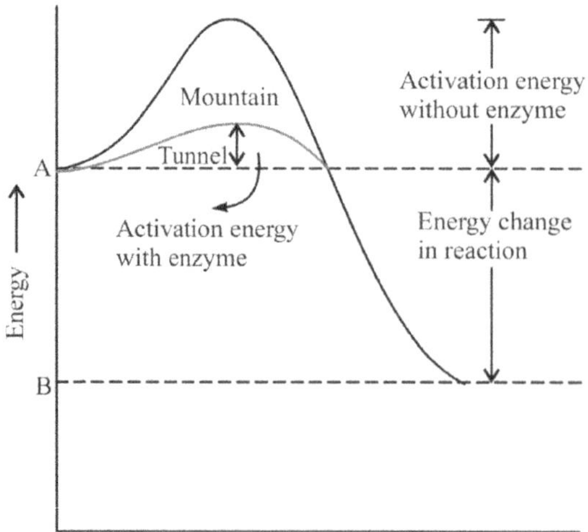

Figure 2.1 Effect of enzyme on activation energy of a reaction; A is substrate; B is product.

Formation of Enzyme-Substrate Complex

The primary basic in enzyme catalysis is binding of the substrate (S) with enzyme (E) on active site of enzyme and forms enzyme-substrate complex (ES). Finally, the product (P) is formed from enzyme-substrate complex (ES) with the regeneration of enzyme (E). This enzyme-substrate complex is otherwise called as a "Michaelis" complex.

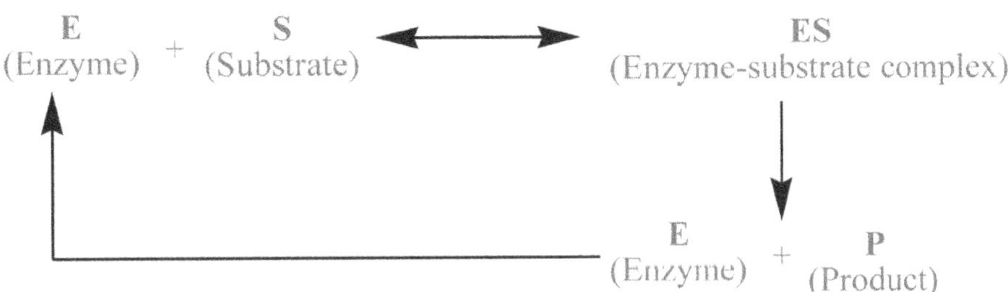

The above mechanism of enzyme-substrate complex formation is explained by the following theories like 1) Lock and key model or Fischer's template theory, 2) Induced fit theory or Koshland's model, 3) Substrate strain theory.

1. **Lock and key model or Fischer's template theory**

   The first theory to explain the mechanism of enzyme catalyzed reaction was proposed by German biochemist "Emil Fischer". According to this theory, the structure or conformation of enzymes is rigid in nature. Hence a particular substrate only fit into the enzymes just like a key fitted into a proper lock or hand in to the proper gloves. Hence the active site of an enzyme is pre-shaped and rigid where only specific substrate can bind and forms enzyme-substrate complex. But this theory not explains the flexible nature of enzymes, hence this theory fails to explain many facts of enzyme-catalyzed reactions particularly allosteric modulators. According to this theory, both enzyme and substrate are rigid in structure.

2. **Induced fit theory or Koshland's model**

   For enzyme-substrate complex formation, Koshland proposed more realistic and accepted model in 1958. According to this theory, the active sites of enzymes are not rigid and pre-shaped in structure. In nascent active site, the essential features of the substrate binding sites are present. When the enzyme is approached by a substrate, the enzyme undergoes some conformational changes which lead to the formation of strong substrate binding site. In addition, the active site is formed by the repositioning of appropriate amino acids due to induced fit and brings about the catalysis. As the substrate induces enzyme for binding it is known as induced fit theory. This theory explains the allosteric modulators and competitive enzyme inhibition on enzyme. There is enough evidence from X-ray diffraction studies for this model. According to this theory, enzyme is flexible in nature whereas substrate is rigid in structure.

3. **Substrate strain theory**

   This is another important theory which explains the mechanism of enzyme-substrate complex formation. In this model, the substrate is strained due to the induced conformation change in the enzyme. It is also possible that the enzyme induces a strain to the substrate when a substrate binds to the pre-formed active site. Product is formed from the strained substrate. According to this theory, both substrate and enzymes are flexible and not rigid in structure. In the enzymatic action, combination of induced fit theory or Koshland's model and substrate strain theory is operative. All three theories are represented in simple form in Figure 2.2 and Table 2.2

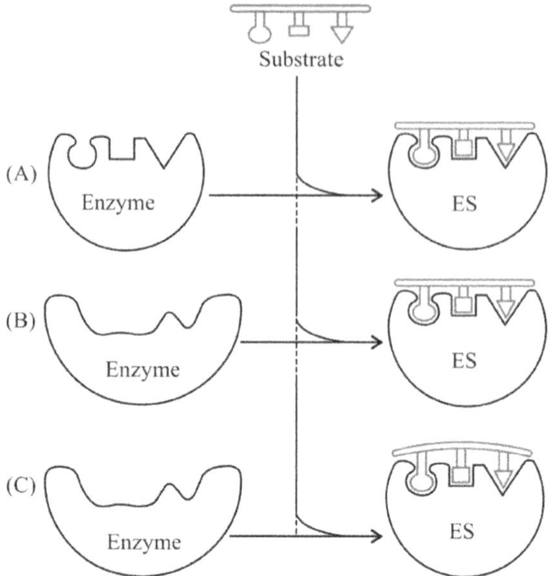

Figure 2.2 Theories of enzyme-substrate complex formation; A) Lock and key model or Fischer's template theory; B) Induced fit theory or Koshland's model; C) Substrate strain theory.

Table 2.2 Theories of enzyme substrate complex formation.

S. No.	Theory name	Structure or conformation	
		Enzyme	Substrate
1	Lock and key model or Fischer's template theory	Rigid	Rigid
2	Induced fit theory or Koshland's model	Flexible	Rigid
3	Substrate strain theory	Flexible	Flexible

Mechanism of Enzyme Catalysis

The product formation and the catalysis of an enzyme mainly depends on the formation of enzyme-substrate complex. Compared to non-catalyzed reaction the enzyme-catalyzed reactions are 10^6 to 10^{12} times faster. There are four processes behind this increased rate of reaction. They are 1) Acid-base catalysis, 2) Covalent catalysis, 3) Substrate strain catalysis, 4) Proximity catalysis or entropy effects.

1. **Acid-base catalysis:**
   In enzymology, the role of acids and bases are quite important. At physiological pH, histidine is the most important amino acid and the protonated form of histidine acts as an acid and its corresponding conjugate acts as base. The other acids of some amino acids are hydroxyl (OH) group of tyrosine, sulfhydryl (SH) group of cysteine and ε-amino (NH_2) group of lysine. The corresponding conjugates of these acids and carboxyl ions (COO^-) function as bases. At the active site of enzyme acidic group or basic group is present in the acid-base catalysis. This acidic or basic group is attacked by substrate results in acid-base catalysis of substrate with enzyme. **Example:** In RNA, pyrimidine loci and phosphodiester bonds are cleaved by *ribonuclease*.
2. **Covalent catalysis:**
   At the active site of enzyme, electrophilic (positive charge) group or nucleophilic (negative charge) group is present in the covalent catalysis. This electrophilic or nucleophilic group is attacked by substrate results in covalent binding of substrate with enzyme. **Example:** Covalent catalysis along with acid-base catalysis occurs in *serine proteases* (Serine is present in the active site).
3. **Substrate strain catalysis:**
   In substrate strain catalysis, substrate is strained due to the induced conformation change in the enzyme or the enzyme induces a strain to the substrate when a substrate binds to the pre-formed

active site. The energy level of substrate is increased during the induction of strain which may lead to transition state. **Example:** *Lysozyme* is an enzyme present in tear which cleaves 1,4-β-glycosidic linkage. The mechanism behind this enzyme is combination of substrate strain catalysis and acid-base catalysis.

4. **Proximity catalysis or entropy effects:**

   For appropriate catalysis to occur the substrate should come in close to the enzyme. The rate of reaction will be higher if the concentration of substrate is more. The catalysis will increase many folds (minimum thousand-fold) when the substrate binds with the active site of enzyme.

   More than one of the four processes such as acid-base catalysis, covalent catalysis, substrate strain catalysis and proximity catalysis or entropy effects are simultaneously taking place in the actual catalysis of the enzymes. This will help the substrate to form products through transition state.

Thermodynamics of Enzymatic Reactions

Based on the energy consideration (thermodynamics), the enzyme-catalyzed reactions are broadly classified into three groups as 1) Isothermic reaction, 2) Exothermic reaction, 3) Endothermic reaction.

1. **Isothermic reaction:** In this enzyme-catalyzed reactions the energy exchange between reactants and products are negligible. **Example:** *Glycogen phosphorylase*

$$\text{Glycogen} + \text{Pi} \xrightarrow[\textit{Glycogen phosphorylase}]{\text{Phosphorylation}} \text{Glucose-1-phosphate}$$

2. **Exothermic reaction:** This is otherwise known as exergonic reaction. Energy is liberated in these enzyme catalyzed reaction. **Example:** *Urease*

$$\underset{\text{Urea}}{NH_2CONH_2} + H_2O \xrightarrow[\textit{Urease}]{\text{Hydrolysis}} 2\ NH_3 + CO_2 + \text{Energy}$$

3. **Endothermic reaction:** This is otherwise known as endergonic reaction. In this enzyme catalyzed reactions, the energy is consumed. **Example:** *Glucokinase (GK)* or *Hexokinase (HK)*

$$\text{Glucose} + \text{ATP} \xrightarrow[\textit{Glucokinase} \text{ or } \textit{Hexokinase}]{\text{Phosphorylation}} \text{Glucose-6-phosphate} + \text{ADP}$$

Factors Affecting Enzyme Action

Contact between enzyme and substrate is pre-requisite or primary importance for enzyme activity. The velocity of enzyme-catalyzed reactions is affected by several important factors. They are as follows.

1. Contact between enzyme and substrate
2. Concentration of enzyme (Linear curve)
3. Enzyme kinetics or Concentration of substrate (Rectangular hyperbola curve)
4. Effect of temperature (Bell shape curve)
5. Effect of pH (Bell shape curve)
6. Effect of product concentration

7. Effect of enzyme activator
8. Effect of time
9. Effect of light and radiation
10. Effect of oxidizing substance

1. **Contact between enzyme and substrate:**

Contact between enzyme and substrate is the primary importance for the activity of enzyme. If enzymes are not contacted by substrate, it results in no activity. Enzymes are soluble in water but it does not form true solution instead of that it forms colloidal solution due to its huge size. Hence, the substrate must be water soluble substance. In case if the substrate is lipid soluble it must be emulsified then only it will come into contact with the enzyme. For example, *pancreatic lipase* is an enzyme which digests the lipids. *Pancreatic lipase* is water soluble whereas lipids are water insoluble. Hence, *pancreatic lipase* acts on lipids only when bile salts emulsify lipids. In this reaction, bile salts are act as emulsifying agent results in digestion of lipids. In case of obstructive jaundice where bile salts are absent in the intestinal tract, fats are not digested and hence fat is excreted in faeces undigested.

2. **Concentration of enzyme**

When concentration of enzyme increases the velocity of enzyme-catalyzed reaction also increases. While drawing a graph by taking enzyme concentration and velocity in X and Y axis, respectively it gives a linear curve (Figure 2.3). This property of enzyme is useful clinically to diagnose the diseases by keeping all other factors like substrate concentration, pH, temperature, etc. at the optimum level with the known volume of serum.

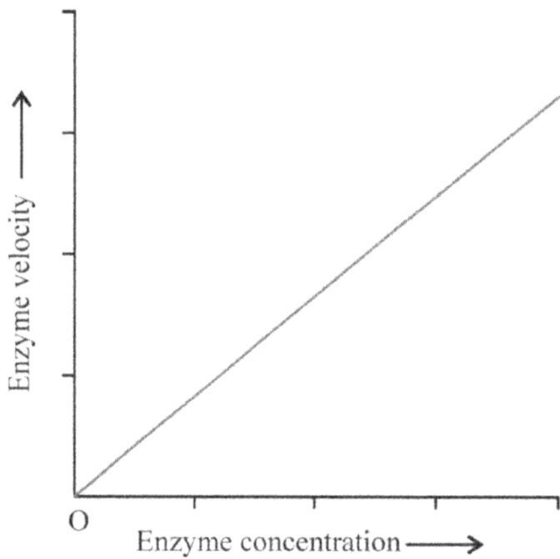

Figure 2.3 Effect of concentration of enzyme on velocity of enzyme.

3. **Enzyme kinetics or Concentration of substrate**

Initially, the increase in substrate concentration gradually increases the velocity of enzyme-catalyzed reactions within the limited range of substrate levels. After that concentration, a large change in substrate concentration produces a small change in velocity. Further increased concentration of substrate does not produce any change in velocity of reaction. The relationship between substrate concentration and velocity is explained by drawing a plot (graph) taking substrate concentration on X-axis and velocity on Y-axis. Generally, the graph for effect of concentration of substrate will be rectangular hyperbola (Figure 2.4).

In this graph three phases of reactions are observed. 1) Linear (A), 2) Curve (B), 3) Almost unchanged (C). Two different plots are used to explain the effect of substrate concentration in enzyme catalyzed reactions. They are a) Michaelis plot, and b) Lineweaver - Burk double reciprocal plot.

(a) **Michaelis plot**

K_m value or Michaelis-Menten constant is defined as the substrate concentration (in moles) required to produce half maximum velocity ($\frac{1}{2} V_{max}$) in an enzyme-catalyzed reactions. It is also known as **Brig's and Haldane's constant.** It indicates that when the substrate concentration is equal to K_m value, about 50 % of enzyme molecules are bonded with the substrate molecules. K_m value is not dependent on the concentration of enzymes. In K_m "K" stands for constant and "m" stands for Michaelis.

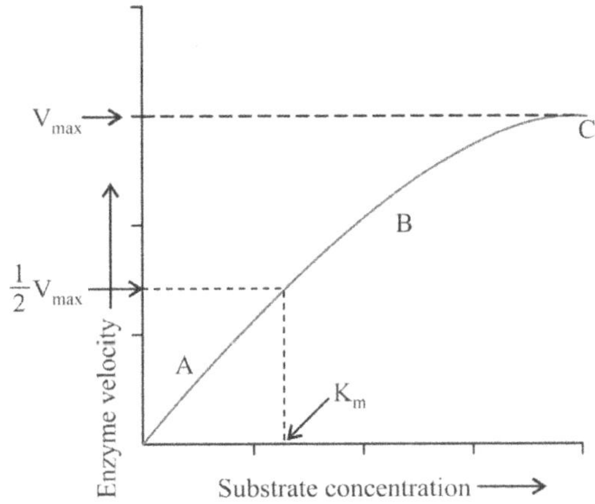

Figure 2.4 Effect of concentration of substrate on velocity of enzyme; A is linear; B is curve; C is almost unchanged.

In an enzyme catalyzed reaction, low K_m value indicates the strong affinity between enzyme and substrate; whereas high K_m value indicates the weak affinity between substrate and enzyme. Generally, the K_m value of most of the enzymes is in the ranges between 10^{-5} to 10^{-2} moles. When a substrate concentration is less than K_m value then the rate of reaction follows first order kinetics for substrate concentration; whereas when the substrate concentration is much greater than K_m value then it follows zero order kinetics in which the rate of reaction is independent of substrate concentration.

$$\underset{\text{(Enzyme)}}{E} + \underset{\text{(Substrate)}}{S} \underset{K_2}{\overset{K_1}{\rightleftharpoons}} \underset{\text{(Enzyme-substrate complex)}}{ES} \xrightarrow{K_3} \underset{\text{(Enzyme)}}{E} + \underset{\text{(Product)}}{P}$$

Where, K_1, K_2 and K_3 are velocity constants for respective reactions.

$$K_m = \frac{K_2 + K_3}{K_1}$$

After suitable modification of algebra,

$$V = \frac{V_{max}[s]}{K_m + [s]}$$

Where,
V = Measured velocity
V_{max} = Maximum velocity
[S] = Substrate concentration
K_m = Michaelis-Menten constant

If the measured velocity is equal to half maximum velocity *i.e.,* $(V = \frac{1}{2} V_{max})$ and substituting this in above equation results in,

$$\frac{1}{2} V_{max} = \frac{V_{max}[S]}{K_m + [S]}$$

$$K_m + [S] = \frac{2\,V_{max}[S]}{V_{max}}$$

$$K_m + [S] = 2\,[S]$$
$$K_m + 2\,[S] - [S]$$
$$K_m = [S]$$

(b) Lineweaver–Burk double reciprocal plot

Lineweaver–Burk double reciprocal plot is used to understand the effect of various inhibitors. For K_m value determination substrate saturation curve i.e., Michaelis plot is not very accurate. Lineweaver–Burk double reciprocal plot is very easier to calculate the K_m value.

$$V = \frac{V_{max}[S]}{k_m + [S]}$$

Therefore,

$$\frac{1}{V} = \frac{K_m + [S]}{V_{max}[S]}$$

$$\frac{1}{V} = \frac{K_m}{V_{max}} \times \frac{1}{[S]} + \frac{[S]}{V_{max}[S]}$$

$$\frac{1}{V} = \frac{K_m}{V_{max}} \times \frac{1}{[S]} + \frac{1}{V_{max}}$$

$$y = ax + b$$

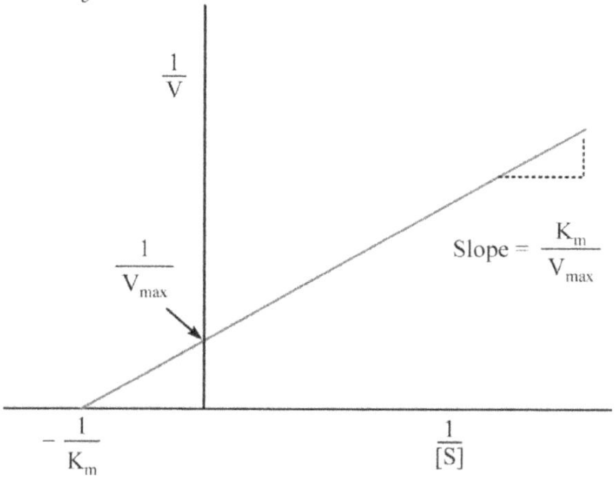

Figure 2.5 Lineweaver–Burk double reciprocal plot.

Where "a" is slope & "b" is the intercept. While drawing a graph by taking reciprocal of velocity ($\frac{1}{V}$) in "X" axis and reciprocal of substrate concentration ($\frac{1}{[S]}$) in "Y" axis, respectively it gives a straight line (Figure 2.5). Here the slope "a" is $\frac{K_m}{V_{max}}$ and the intercept "b" is $\frac{1}{V_{max}}$. It is very easy to calculate the K_m value from the intercept on "X" axis which is $\frac{-1}{K_m}$.

4. Effect of temperature

Initially, as the temperature increases velocity of enzyme reaction also increases up to a maximum. Further increase in temperature decreases the velocity of enzyme-catalyzed reaction. The initial increase in velocity of the enzyme reaction is due to higher activation energy and increased collision between molecules (enzyme & substrate) due to an increase in temperature. When enzymes are exposed to higher temperature leads to denaturation followed by derangement of protein structure which results in decreased activity. Usually while drawing a graph by taking temperature on X-axis and velocity on Y-axis will results in a bell-shaped curve (Figure 2.6). The temperature at which the maximum velocity is obtained is known as "optimum temperature". Temperature coefficient or Q_{10} is defined as the increases in velocity of enzyme reaction when the temperature is increased by 10 °C. For many enzymes, the Q_{10} value is 2 in between 0 to 40 °C. The ideal or optimum temperature for most of the enzyme is 40-45 °C. There are some exceptions such as *venom phosphokinase* and muscle *adenylate kinases* are active even at 100 °C. The optimum temperature for plant enzyme *urease* is 60 °C. The increased optimum temperatures of these enzymes are due to its very stable structure and conformation of enzymes.

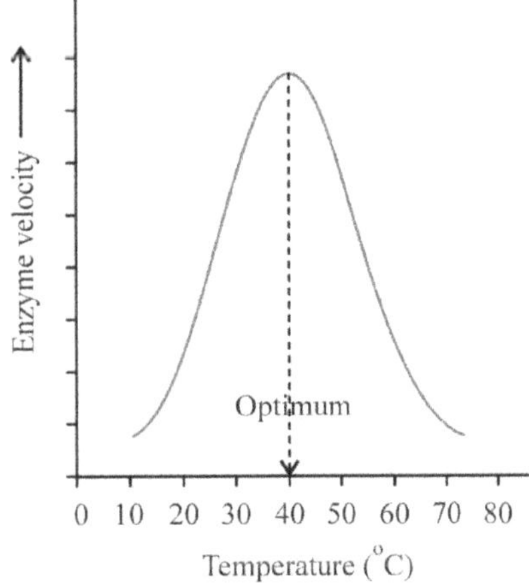

Figure 2.6 Effect of temperature on velocity of enzyme.

5. **Effect of pH**

The effect of pH is also similar to the effect of temperature. Effect of pH also produces bell-shaped curve (Figure 2.7) that means initially as the pH increases the velocity of enzyme reaction also increases up to a maximum. Further increase in pH decreases the velocity of enzyme-catalyzed reaction. The pH at which the maximum velocity is obtained is known as "optimum pH". Below and above this pH the enzyme activity is much lower and at extreme pH it becomes inactive. The ideal or optimum pH for most of the enzyme is around neutral pH i.e., 6 to 8. There are some exceptions such as *pepsin* (optimum pH: 1 to 2), *acid phosphatase* (optimum pH: 4 to 5), *alkaline phosphatase* (optimum pH: 10 to 11) and fungi and plant enzymes (optimum pH: 4 to 6).The concentration of the hydrogen ion influences the velocity of enzyme reactions by altering the ionic charges on the amino acids, substrate, enzyme-substrate complex, etc.

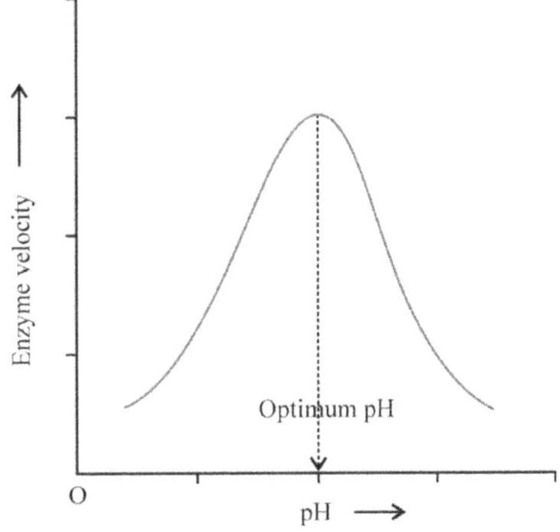

Figure 2.7 Effect of pH on velocity of enzyme.

6. **Effect of product concentration**

   Product concentration is indirectly proportional to the velocity of enzyme reaction. Generally, increased product concentration decreases the velocity of reaction because the product may bind with the active site of enzyme and forms a loose complex. Hence, it can be prevented by rapid removal of formed products.

7. **Effect of enzyme activators**

   Various metal substances may activate enzymes and increases the velocity of reactions. Some of the enzymes need metal cations such as Ca^{+2}, Mn^{+2}, Mg^{2+}, Co^{2+}, Cu^{2+}, Zn^{2+}, Na^{+}, K^{+}, etc. for their activity; whereas metal anions are rarely needed for activity of enzymes (Cl^{-} for *amylase*). The followings are the various mechanism of action of metals by which it activates the velocity of enzyme reactions.

   - Reaction with the substrate.
   - Formation of enzyme-substrate metal complex.
   - By modifying enzyme conformation.
   - Direct participation in the reaction.

   The enzymes are broadly classified into two major categories based on the metals required for their activity. They are a) Metal activated enzyme (The metal is loosely bonded with enzyme and can be easily exchanged by other ions). **Example:** Calcium and magnesium for *ATPase* and magnesium for *enolase*. b) Metallozymes (The metal is tightly bounded to the enzyme and cannot be easily exchanged). **Example:** Zinc in *alcohol dehydrogenase, carbonic anhydrase, alkaline phosphatase, carboxy peptidase* and *aldolase*; copper in *phenol oxidase*, manganese in *pyruvate oxidase*, Molybdenum in *xanthine oxidase*, iron and copper in *cytochrome oxidase*).

8. **Effect of time**

   If the enzyme catalyzed reaction is taking place in ideal conditions like optimum temperature, pH, etc. then the time required is less. If any parameter is not in ideal value than the time required is increased. Variation in the time of reaction is usually related to the alteration in temperature and pH.

9. **Effect of light and radiation**

   Generally, lights and radiations such as UV, IR, gamma radiations, X-rays may decrease the velocity of enzyme reaction due to the formation of peroxides which destructs structure of enzyme. **Example:** Salivary *amylase* activity is decreased by UV rays.

10. **Effect of oxidizing substances**

    Presence of oxidizing substances may decrease the velocity of enzyme reaction because activity of some enzymes depend on the sulfhydryl (-SH) group. These oxidizing substances oxidizes sulfhydryl (-SH) group into disulphide (S-S). **Example:** Reducing substances such as glutathione or cysteine may deactivate certain enzymes.

Enzyme Inhibition

Enzyme inhibitor is defined as the substance which binds with the enzyme and decreases the enzyme catalytic activity. The process by which the enzyme activity is decreased is known as enzyme inhibition. Enzyme inhibition is broadly classified into three major types.

1. Reversible enzyme inhibition
2. Irreversible enzyme inhibition
3. Allosteric enzyme inhibition

1. **Reversible enzyme inhibition (REI):**

   As the name indicates this type of enzyme inhibition is reversible in nature. In this type inhibitor binds with the enzyme by a weak non-covalent bond. Hence, the reactions can be reversed if the inhibitor is removed. Reversible enzyme inhibition is further sub-classified into two categories as a) Competitive enzyme inhibition (CEI), b) Non-competitive enzyme inhibition (NCEI).

(a) Competitive enzyme inhibition: There is a competition between substrate and inhibitor for binding to the active site of enzyme. The competition is due to structural similarities between real substrate (S) and the inhibitors (I). Hence, these inhibitors are regarded as analogue of substrate. Once the inhibitor (I) is bonded with enzyme (E) it forms enzyme inhibitor complex (EI) which leads to unavailability of enzyme for binding with substrate. During the reaction enzyme substrate complex (ES) are also formed.

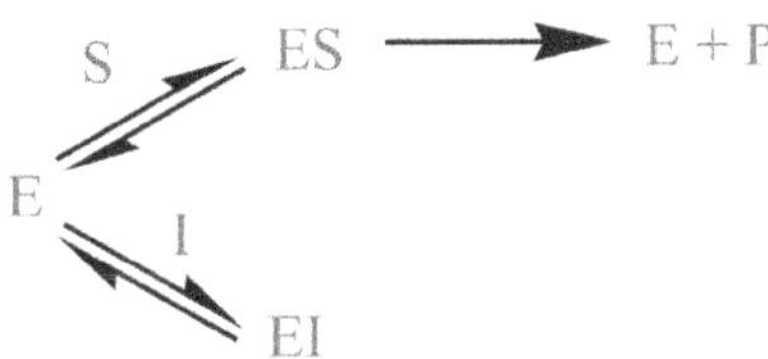

Followings are the two major factors which influence the competitive enzyme inhibition. They are i) Concentration of substrate and inhibitor, ii) Affinity of substrate and inhibitor with the enzyme. In general, high substrate concentration overcomes the competitive enzyme inhibition. K_m value is increasing and V_{max} is unchanged in competitive enzyme inhibition. A diagrammatic representation of competitive enzyme inhibition is presented in Figure 2.8 (A)and effect of competitive inhibitor on velocity of enzyme is presented in Figure 2.9.

Example 1: Enzyme: *Succinate dehydrogenase* (SDH), **Substrate:** Succinic acid, **Inhibitor:** Oxalic acid, malonic acid and glutaric acid. Here the structural similarities between substrate and inhibitors are presence of dicarboxylic group. Hence the inhibitors oxalic acid, malonic acid and glutaric acid competes with succinic acid for the active site of enzyme "*succinate dehydrogenase (SDH)*".

Succinic acid	Oxalic acid	Malonic acid	Glutaric acid
CH_2COOH – CH_2COOH	COOH – COOH	COOH – CH_2 – COOH	CH_2COOH – CH_2 – CH_2COOH

Example 2: Enzyme: *Alcohol dehydrogenase*(ADH), **Substrate:** Methanol (CH_3OH), **Inhibitor:** Ethanol (CH_3CH_2OH). In this example the structural similarities between substrate and inhibitors are presence of primary alcohol group. Hence the inhibitor ethanol competes with methanol for active site of enzyme "*alcohol dehydrogenase (ADH)*". For this reason, ethanol may be used in the treatment of methanol poisoning. Some more clinical and pharmacological significances of competitive enzyme inhibitors are listed in Table 2.3.

Example 3: Antimetabolites are the chemical substances which block the metabolic reaction due to its competitive enzyme inhibition with enzymes. Generally, they are used in the treatment of cancer. Examples are mentioned in Table. 2.3. The term antivitamins are used for the antimetabolites which block the biochemical actions of vitamins and leads to deficiencies of corresponding vitamins. **Example:** Sulphanilamide and dicoumarol.

Table 2.3 Clinical and pharmacological significances of competitive enzyme inhibitors.

S. No	Name of enzyme	Substrate name	Inhibitor name	Significance of inhibitors
1	*MAO (Monoamine oxidase)*	Nor-epinephrine, epinephrine	Ephedrine, amphetamine	Catecholamine elevators
2	*Xanthine oxidase*	Hypoxanthine, Xanthine	Allopurinol	Treatment of gout
3	*Dihydropteroate synthase*	PABA (*p*-Amino benzoic acid)	Sulfanilamide	Antibacterial agent
4	*Acetylcholine esterase*	Acetylcholine	Succinylcholine	In anesthetized patient used for muscle relaxation in surgery
5	*HMG CoA reductase*	HMG CoA	Lovastatin, Pravastatin	Antihyperlipidemic agent
6	*Dihydrofolate reductase*	Dihydrofolic acid	Methotrexate, Trimetrexate, Aminopterin	Treatment of leukemia and other cancers
7	*Vitamin K epoxide reductase*	Vitamin K	Dicoumarol	Anticoagulant

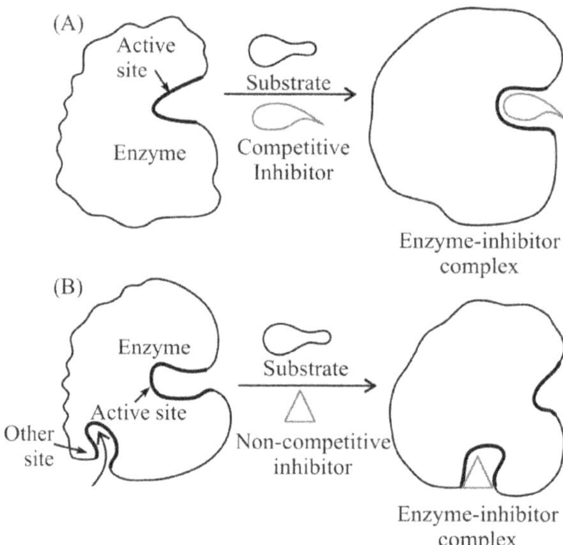

Figure 2.8 (A) Competitive enzyme inhibition; (B) Non-competitive enzyme inhibition.

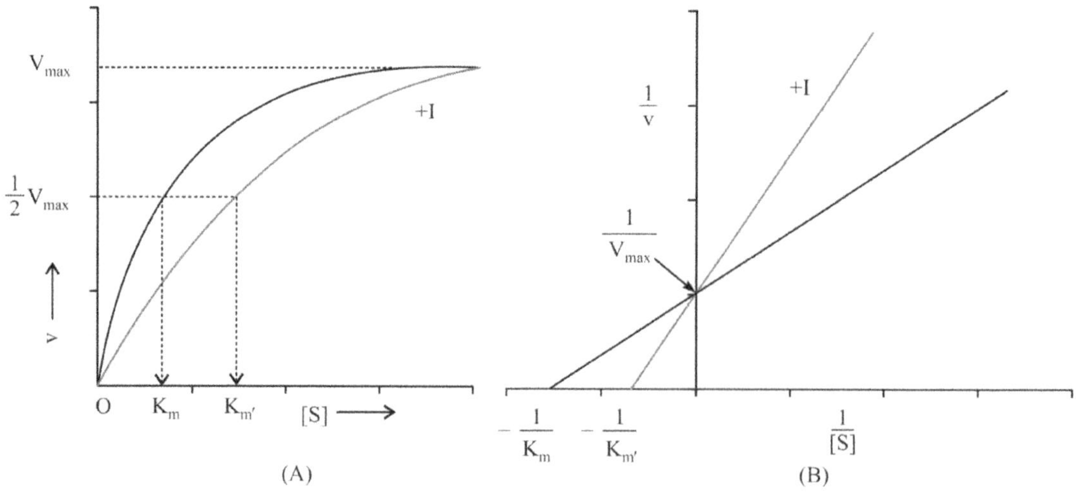

Figure 2.9 Effect of competitive inhibitor on velocity of enzyme; A) Velocity Vs Substrate; B) Lineweaver-Burk plot (Red line with inhibitor).

(b) **Non-competitive enzyme inhibition (NCEI):** In this type there is no competition between substrate and inhibitor for active site of enzyme because inhibitor bind with other sites on the enzyme surface and decreases the activity of enzyme. There are no structural similarities between substrate and inhibitors. Even though inhibitors exhibit strong affinities to bind in the second site of enzyme and it does not interfere with enzyme-substrate binding. The catalysis prevention may be due to enzyme conformation distortion. In this type, the inhibitor may bind with enzyme and enzyme-substrate complex as well . K_m value is unchanged and V_{max} is decreasing in non-competitive enzyme inhibition. A diagrammatic representation of non-competitive enzyme inhibition is presented in Figure 2.8 (B) and effect of non-competitive inhibitor on velocity of enzyme is presented in Figure 2.10.

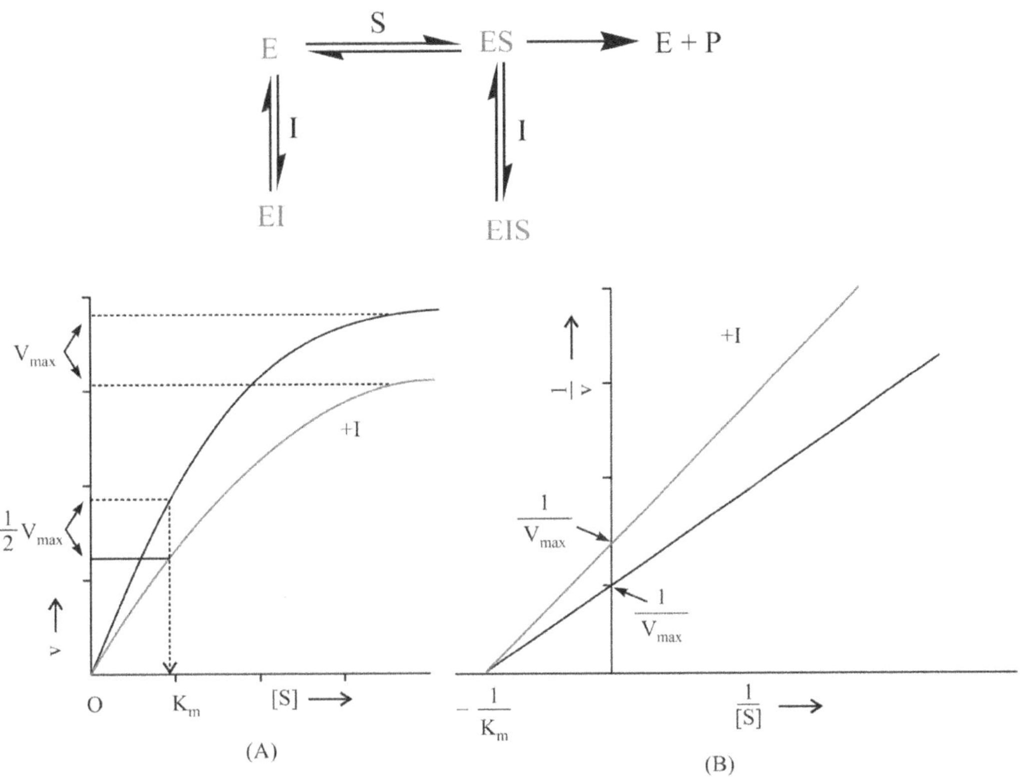

Figure 2.10 Effect of non-competitive inhibitor on velocity of enzyme; A) Velocity Vs Substrate; B) Lineweaver-Burk plot (Red line with inhibitor).

Example: Heavy metal ions like Hg^{2+}, Pb^{2+}, Ag^{+}, etc. binds with cysteinyl sulfhydryl group of enzymes non-competitively. Heavy metals also lead to formation of covalent bonds with carboxyl group and histidine often resulting in irreversible inhibition.

$$E{-}SH + Hg^{2+} \rightleftharpoons E{-}S{\cdots}Hg^{2+} + H^{+}$$

2. **Irreversible enzyme inhibition:**

In this type of enzyme inhibition substrate binds to the enzyme by a covalent bond which is very strong in nature. Hence, the bond cannot be broken easily. This leads to an irreversible reaction. Generally, these irreversible inhibitors are toxic substances which poisons the enzymes. The following reaction represents irreversible enzyme inhibition. The characteristics of various irreversible enzyme inhibitors are listed in Table 2.4.

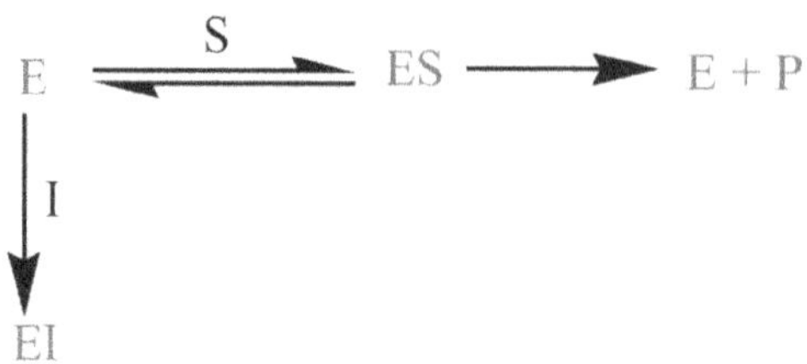

Table 2.4 Irreversible enzyme inhibitors.

S. No	Name of the enzyme	Inhibitor name	Characteristics
1	*Papain*, and *glyceraldehyde-3-phosphate*	Iodoacetate	Iodoacetate combine with –SH group of these enzyme and make them inactive
2	*Aldehyde dehydrogenase (ADH)*	Disulfiram	Treatment of alcoholism due to accumulation of acetaldehyde
3	Serine containing enzymes	Penicillin	Blocks the synthesis of bacterial cell wall.
4	*Serine protease, acetylcholine esterase (AchE)*	Diisopropyl fluorophosphates (DFP)	DFP is a nerve gas used in second world war by German.
5	*Acetylcholine esterase (AchE)*	Organophosphorus insecticides like parathion and malathion	Produces paralysis of vital body functions due to block of nerve conduction.

Suicide inhibition is a specialized form of irreversible inhibition. In this case, the actual or the original inhibitor is converted to a more potent form of inhibitor by the same enzyme itself. The actual or original inhibitor binds with enzyme reversibly (Mostly structural analogue or competitive inhibitor), whereas the newly formed inhibitor binds with enzyme irreversibly. Examples of various suicidal inhibitors and its uses are listed in Table 2.5.

Table 2.5 Suicide inhibitors.

S. No	Name of the enzyme	Original inhibitor name	Newly formed inhibitor	Uses
1	*Xanthine oxidase*	Allopurinol	Alloxanthine	Treatment of gout
2	*Thymidylate synthase*	5-Fluorouracil	Fluorodeoxy uridylate	Treatment of cancer

3. **Allosteric enzyme inhibition:**

   In Greek, "allo" means "other". Few of the enzymes possess additional sites known as allosteric site along with the active site. These enzymes are known as allosteric enzymes. In the enzyme molecules, these allosteric sites are unique places. Generally, allosteric enzymes exist in two conformation state in the concerted model as a) T-state (Tense or taut), b) R-state (Relaxed). The T and R states are in equilibrium. If enzymes are present in relaxed form the activity will be more whereas if the enzymes are present in tense form the activity will be less. In general, allosteric activators favors R-state of enzyme and allosteric inhibitors favor T-state. **Example:** Glucose-6-phosphate for *hexokinase(HK)*, ATP for *phosphofructokinase (PFK)* and *isocitrate dehydrogenase (ICDH)*, AMP for *fructose-1,6-bisphosphatase (F1,6BPase)*, and palmitate for *acetyl CoA carboxylase*. Various form of allosteric enzyme and its activator and inhibitor is diagrammatically represented in Figure 2.11.

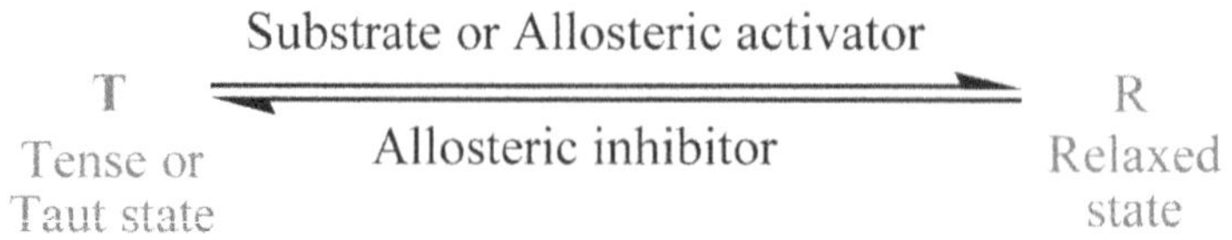

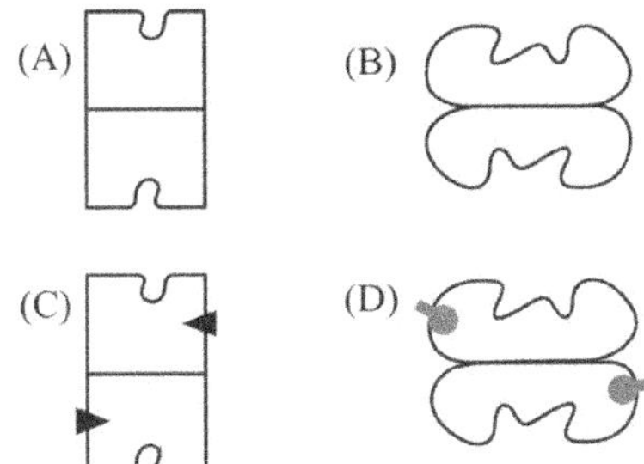

Figure 2.11 Allosteric enzyme; A) T-form; B) R-form; C) Effect of allosteric inhibitor; D) Effect of allosteric activator.

Enzyme Regulation

Enzyme regulation occurs in biological system in different stages in order to achieve cellular economy. Cellular metabolism is a molecular economy that is functionally organized into supply and demand blocks linked by metabolic products and co-factor cycles. The various ways of enzyme regulation are as follows.

1. Allosteric regulation
2. Latent enzyme activation
3. Metabolic pathways compartmentation
4. Enzyme synthesis control
5. Enzyme degradation
6. Iso-enzyme

1. **Allosteric regulation**

The unique places of allosteric enzymes are alloesteric site which is additional site beside active site of enzyme. In these allosteric sites the allosteric modulators (modifiers or effectors) binds and regulate the activity of enzyme. In the allosteric site, binding of a positive allosteric modifiers results in increased enzyme activity and the allosteric site is known as activator site. Similarly, Binding of a negative allosteric modifier results in decreased enzyme activity and the allosteric site is known as inhibitor site.

Allosteric enzymes are the enzymes which are regulated by allosteric mechanism. Based on the effect of allosteric modifiers or effectors on K_m and V_{max} the allosteric enzymes are broadly classified into two types.

(a) **K-class allosteric enzymes:** In this class, allosteric effectors change the K_m and not the V_{max} value. Similar to competitive enzyme inhibition double reciprocal plots are obtained for this class of allosteric enzymes. **Example:** *Phosphofructokinase (PFK).*

(b) **V-class allosteric enzymes:** In this class, allosteric effectors change the V_{max} and not the K_m value. Similar to non-competitive enzyme inhibition double reciprocal plots are obtained for this class of allosteric enzymes. **Example:** *Acetyl CoA carboxylase.*

The sub-units of the oligomeric allosteric enzyme may be different or identical. In the active site of the enzyme conformational changes are taking place due to the reversible non-covalent binding of allosteric effectors that results in increased or decreased catalytic activity of enzyme. Generally, allosteric enzymes exist in two conformation state in the concerted model as a) T-state (Tense or taut), b) R-state (Relaxed). Normally allosteric activators favors R-state of enzyme and allosteric inhibitors favors T-state. Substrate will bind only to the R-state of the enzyme, hence increased substrate concentration increases R-state of the enzyme molecule. Hence, allosteric enzyme and substrate binding is said to be co-operative. Sigmoidal curve is obtained instead of rectangular hyperbola for allosteric enzymes when the graph is plotted between velocity and substrate concentration.

If the effects of allosteric modulator promote the binding of substrate to the enzyme which results in positive effect always is known as homotrophic effect. Incase if the effects of allosteric modulator promote the binding of substrate to the enzyme which results in either positive or negative effect is known as heterotrophic effect. The various examples for allosteric enzymes are listed in Table 2.6.

Table 2.6 Allosteric enzyme & their effectors.

S. No	Metabolic pathway name	Enzyme name	Allosteric activator	Allosteric inhibitor
1	Glycolysis	*Hexokinase (HK)*	-------	Glucose-6-phosphate
2	Glycolysis	*Phosphofructokinase (PFK)*	AMP, ADP	ATP
3	TCA cycle	*Isocitrate dehydrogenase (ICDH)*	ADP, NAD^+	ATP
4	Gluconeogenesis	*Pyruvate carboxylase (PC)*	Acetyl CoA	-------
5	Gluconeogenesis	*Fructose-1,6-bisphosphatase (F1,6-BPase)*	-------	AMP
6	Urea cycle	*Carbamoyl phosphate synthase – I (CPS – I)*	N-Acetyl glutamate (NAG)	-------
7	Tryptophan metabolism	*Tryptophan oxygenase (TO)*	L-Tryptophan	-------
8	Fatty acid synthesis	*Acetyl CoA carboxylase (ACC)*	Isocitrate	Palmitate

Feedback regulation: Feedback regulation is defined as the process in which first step of the series of enzyme catalyzed reaction is inhibited by the final product of that reaction. For example, product "E" is synthesized from substrate "A" in the following series of reaction.

$$A \xrightarrow{e_1} B \xrightarrow{e_2} C \xrightarrow{e_3} D \xrightarrow{e_4} E$$

E

Where, A = Initial substrate

B, C and D = Intermediate compounds

E = End product

e_1, e_2, e_3 and e_4 = Enzymes

For regulating the pathway of above reactions, very first step (A to B by enzyme e_1) is the most effective by the final product E. This type of regulation is known as negative feedback regulation because increased final product concentration itself decreased its synthesis by inhibiting enzyme e_1. It will save the cellular economy by blocking the wasteful expenditure utilized for the synthesis of already existing compound. End product inhibition or feedback inhibition is the special type of allosteric enzyme inhibition used to control metabolic pathways for efficient cellular functions.

Example: *Aspartate transcarbamoylase (ATC)* is inhibited by CTP (cytidine triphosphate) in biosynthesis of pyrimidine.

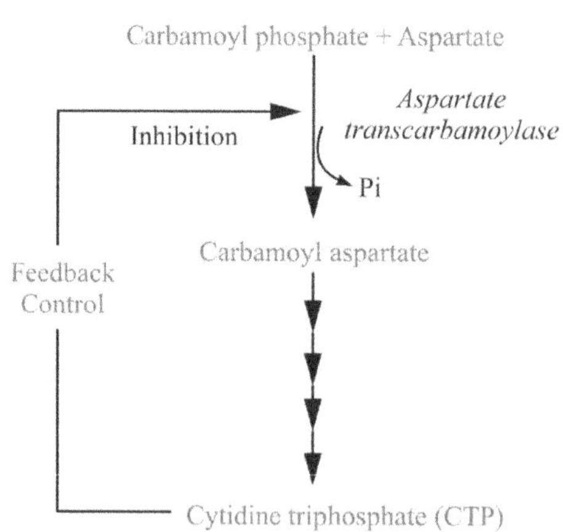

In general, feedback regulation represents a phenomenon while feedback inhibition involves the mechanism of regulation. For instance, through feedback regulation hepatic cholesterol synthesis is decreased by dietary cholesterol. Dietary cholesterol does not directly inhibit the regulatory enzyme *HMG CoA reductase*, hence feedback inhibition is not involved in this process. However, cholesterol reduces (repression) the activity of gene encoding this enzyme.

2. **Latent enzyme activation**

As such latent enzymes are inactive. Latent enzymes whose activity only becomes manifest when the conditions are changed. The term "latent enzyme" is used especially of a particulate enzyme that becomes active when the particles are disrupted. Some of the enzymes are synthesized as zymogens or pro-enzymes which undergoes irreversible covalent activation by breakdown of one or more peptide bonds. Conversion of pro-enzymes *chymotrypsinogen, pepsinogen* and *plasminogen* into active enzymes *chymotrypsin, pepsin* and *plasmin,* respectively are very good examples.

Depending on the needs of biological systems some of the enzymes exist in both active and inactive forms which are inter convertible. Reversible covalent modifications such as oxidation and reduction of disulfide bonds and phosphorylation and dephosphorylation brings the above inter conversion.

Example 1: To provide energy, the muscle enzyme *glycogen phosphorylase* breaks glycogen. This enzyme possesses two identical subunits (homodimer) and exists in two inter convertible forms. The inactive form of enzyme is *phosphorylase-b* (dephospho enzyme) which is phosphorylated at serine residues and converted into active form *phosphorylase-a*. The inactive form *phosphorylase-b* is produced from active form by dephosphorylation reaction.

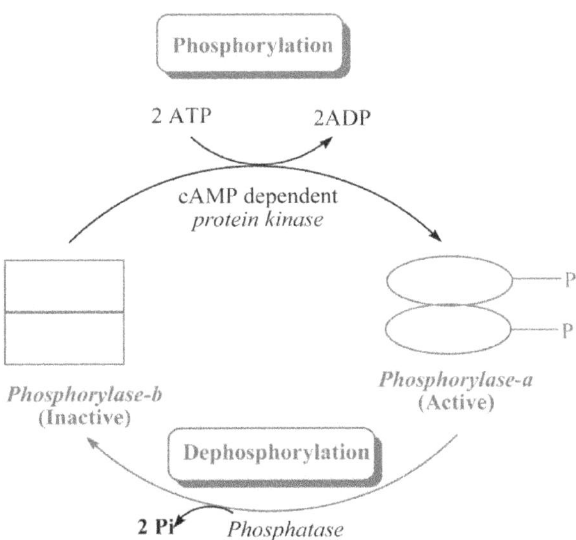

Citrate lyase and *fructose-2,6-bisphosphatase* are the other examples for phosphorylated active enzymes. Some enzymes are active in dephosphorylated form and converted into inactive form by phosphorylation. *Acetyl CoA carboxylase, glycogen synthase* and *HMG CoA reductase* are examples for dephosphorylated active enzymes.

Sulfhydryl (-SH) group is necessary for the activity of some enzymes. Stability of these enzymes is brought by reducing substances like glutathione.

E—S—S—E → E—SH + E—SH

Oxidized form of enzyme (Inactive)

2G—SH → GS—SG

Glutathione **(Reduced form)**

Glutathione **(Oxidized form)**

Reduced form of enzyme (Active)

3. **Metabolic pathways compartmentation**

In biological systems, both synthesis and degradations are occurring for some substances like fatty acid and glycogen. Simultaneous occurrences of both the pathways are not possible. To achieve maximum cellular economy anabolic (synthetic) and catabolic (breakdown) pathways are taking place in different cellular organelles. For example, fatty acid oxidation occurs in mitochondria whereas fatty acid synthesis occurs in cytosol. Intracellular locations of certain enzymes are presented in Table 2.7.

Table 2.7 Intracellular locations of certain enzymes.

S. No	Intracellular organelle	Enzymes or metabolic pathways
1	Nucleus	Replication and transcription
2	Mitochondria	Krebs cycle, amino acid oxidation, urea cycle, fatty acid oxidation, oxidative phosphorylation and ETC
3	Microsomes (Endoplasmic reticulum)	Protein synthesis, triacylglycerol and phospholipid synthesis, steroid synthesis and reduction, *esterase* and *cytochrome* P_{450}
4	Golgi apparatus	*Glucose-6-phosphatase*, *glucosyl* and *galactosyl transferases* and *5-nucleotidase*
5	Lysosomes	*Proteases, lipases, nucleases, phosphatases, phospholipases, hydrolases* and *lysozyme*
6	Peroxisomes	*D-Amino acid oxidase*, long chain fatty acid oxidation, *urate oxidase* and *catalase*
7	Cytoplasm	Glycolysis, HMP shunt pathway, fatty acid synthesis, purine and pyrimidine catabolism, and *aminotransferases*

4. **Enzyme synthesis control**

Many enzymes importantly regulating enzymes are present in very low concentration. The velocity of enzyme catalyzed reactions is directly controlled by number of enzymes. Enzyme levels are efficiently regulated because the half lives of many rate limiting enzymes are very short. Based on the level of enzymes present in biological systems, the enzymes are broadly classified into two classes namely a) Constitutive enzymes, b) Adaptive enzyme.

(a) **Constitutive enzymes:** The levels of these enzymes are fairly constant and are not controlled. It is otherwise known as housekeeping enzymes.

(b) **Adaptive enzymes:** The levels of these enzymes are not constant and are decreased or increased based on the body demands. Hence, these enzymes are well regulated by the genes. The enzyme levels may increase or decrease by increasing the synthesis of enzyme (Induction) or decreasing the synthesis of enzyme (Repression). At the gene level the enzyme concentrations are determined by induction or repression through the mediation of hormones or other substances.

Induction: Increased synthesis of enzyme is represented by the term "induction". **Example:** The synthesis of *glucokinase (GK), phosphofructokinase (PFK), pyruvate kinase (PK)* and *glycogen synthase (GS)* are induced by the hormone insulin. All these enzymes are involved in utilization of glucose. Similarly, the synthesis of *pyruvate carboxylase (PC), tryptophan oxygenase (TO)* and *tyrosine aminotransferase (TAT)* is induced by the hormone cortisol.

Repression: Decreased synthesis of enzyme is represented by the term "repression". Substrate can repress the enzyme synthesis in many instances. **Example:** The synthesis of *pyruvate carboxylase(PC)* is repressed by substrate glucose.

5. **Enzyme degradation:**

Generally, enzymes are not immortal because it creates many problems. Half-life of the individual enzymes varies a lot. Half-life of some enzymes are in days while for others in hours or in minutes (**Example:** LDH_4: 5 to 6 days, LDH_1: 8 to 12 hours, *Amylase*: 3 to 5 hours). The regulatory and key enzymes are most rapidly degraded. When there is no need it rapidly disappears and as when required it synthesized immediately. In majority cases long half-life possessing enzymes are sluggish in catalytic activity.

6. **Iso-enzymes:**

   Iso-enzymes are defined as the different form of the same enzyme [differ in amino acid sequence] exhibits similar activity. These iso-enzymes also help in regulation of enzyme activity. Many iso-enzymes are tissue specific. Iso-enzymes catalyze the same reaction of a given enzyme. But iso-enzymes differ in many properties such as K_m value, V_{max}, Isoelectric pH, electrophoretic mobility, optimum temperature, optimum pH, effect on heat, quantities present, etc.

Co-enzymes

Protein parts of the enzymes are not sufficient always to bring about the catalytic activity. Majority of the enzymes for its catalysis activity additionally need small non-protein factors collectively known as co-factors. In nature these co-factors may be either organic or inorganic.

Co-enzymes are defined as the non-protein, organic, low molecular weight and easily dialyzable substances associated with the functions of enzymes. If the organic non-protein substances are tightly bounded to protein part of enzyme then the term prosthetic group is used. Inorganic co-factors such as Ca^{2+}, Mg^{2+}, Mn^{2+}, etc. which are necessary to increase the activity of enzyme are called activators.. However, three terms such as co-enzyme, prosthetic group and activator are used interchangeably.

Holo-enzyme is the functional unit of enzyme and it is composed of two major parts namely apo-enzyme and co-enzyme. The protein part of enzyme is called as apo-enzyme and the non-protein part of enzyme is called as co-enzymes. Co-enzymes do not decide the specificity of enzyme. The specificity of enzyme is mostly depending on the apo-enzyme only.

Holoenzyme (Active enzyme) ⟶ Apo-enzyme (Protein part) + Co-enzyme (Non-protein part)

Usually co-enzymes are considered as co-substrate or second substrate because it also possess affinity with enzyme comparable with that of the substrates. During the enzymatic reactions co-enzymes undergoes modification but later regenerated, whereas substrate is converted to the product. Co-enzymes play a crucial role in functions of enzyme. In general co-enzymes are participated in several reactions involving transfer of atoms or groups like hydrogen, aldehydes, keto, amino, acyl, methyl, carbon dioxide, etc.

Types of co-enzymes:

There are four different types of co-enzymes as 1) Vitamin co-enzymes, 2) Non-vitamin co-enzymes, 3) Nucleotide co-enzymes, 4) Protein co-enzymes.

1. **Vitamin co-enzymes:** It is otherwise known as co-enzymes from vitamin B-complex because most of the co-enzymes are the derivatives of water-soluble B-complex vitamins. The B-complex vitamin exhibits its biological function through its respective co-enzymes only and the details are presented in Table 2.8.
2. **Non-vitamin co-enzymes:** Not all co-enzymes are vitamin derivatives. There are several other organic substances which have no relation with vitamins but act as co-enzymes. These organic substances are known as non-vitamin co-enzymes and various non-vitamin co-enzymes are listed in Table 2.9.

Table 2.8 Vitamin co-enzymes.

S. No	Vitamin name	Co-enzyme name	Chemical structure of co-enzyme	Important structural features of co-enzyme	Deficiency / Disorder	Atom or group transferred	Example of dependent enzyme
1	Vitamin-B_1 (Thiamine)	TPP (Thiamine pyrophosphate)	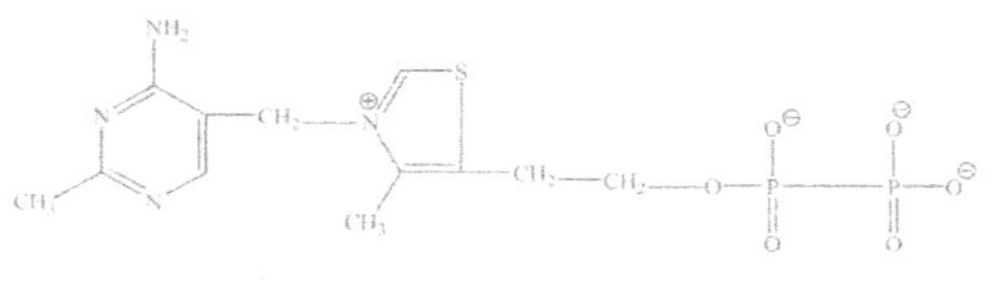	Pyrimidine, thiazole and methylene bridge	Beri-beri (dry or wet or mixed or infantile), peripheral neuropathy and Wernicke-Korsakoff syndrome	Aldehyde or keto	*Transketolase*
2	Vitamin B_2 (Riboflavin)	FMN (Flavin mono nucleotide)	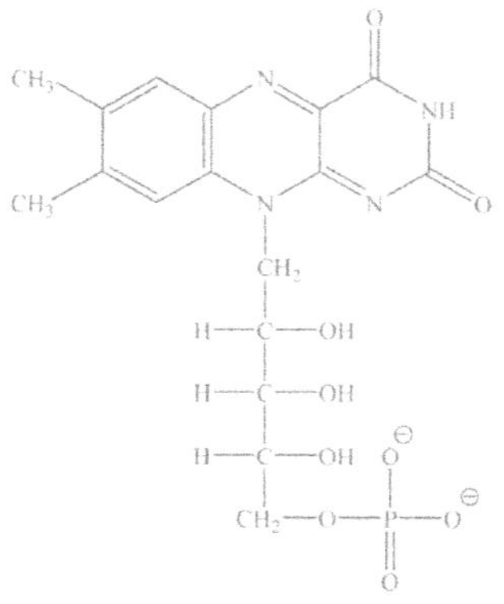	Isoalloxazine ring and ribitol	Cheilosis, glossitis and dermatitis	Hydrogen and electron	*L-Amino acid oxidase*
3		FAD (Flavin adenine dinucleotide)	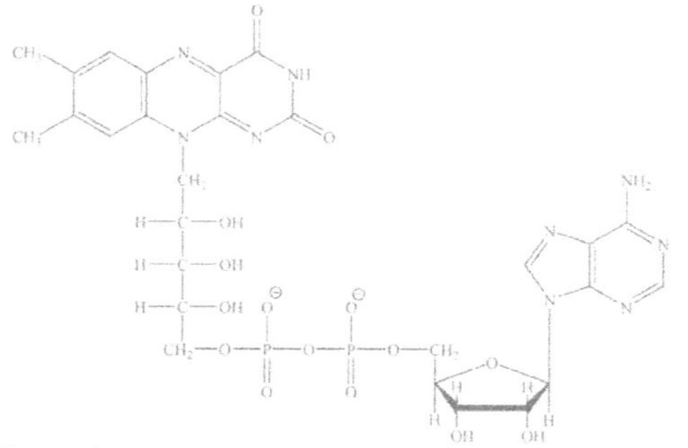	Isoalloxazine ring, ribitol, adenine and ribose	Cheilosis, glossitis and dermatitis	Hydrogen and electron	*D-Amino acid oxidase*

Table 2.8 Contd...

S. No	Vitamin name	Co-enzyme name	Chemical structure of co-enzyme	Important structural features of co-enzyme	Deficiency / Disorder	Atom or group transferred	Example of dependent enzyme
4	Vitamin-B_3 (Niacin)	NAD^+ (Nicotinamide adenine dinucleotide)	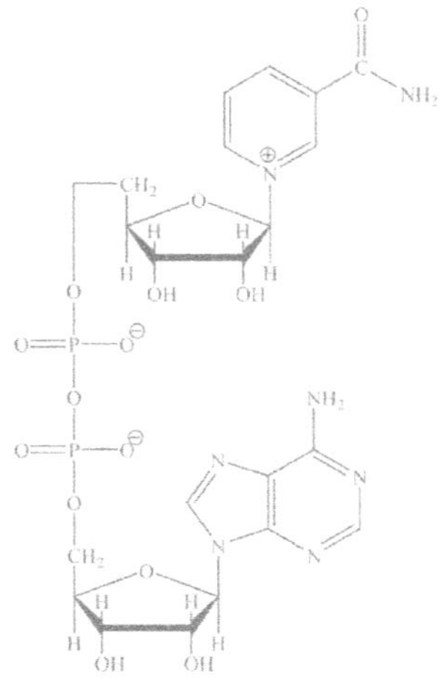	Pyridine, adenine and ribose	Pellagra (Dermatitis, diarrhea and dementia)	Hydrogen and electron	*Lactate dehydrogenase (LDH)*
5		$NADPH^+$ (Nicotinamide adenine dinucleotide phosphate)	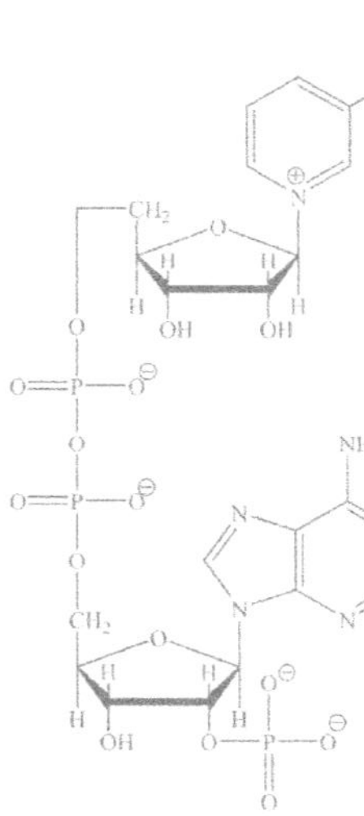	Pyridine, adenine and ribose	Pellagra (Dermatitis, diarrhea and dementia)	Hydrogen and electron	*Glucose-6-phosphate dehydrogenase (G6PD)*

Table 2.8 Contd...

S. No	Vitamin name	Co-enzyme name	Chemical structure of co-enzyme	Important structural features of co-enzyme	Deficiency / Disorder	Atom or group transferred	Example of dependent enzyme
6	Lipoic acid or Thioctic acid or 6,8-dithiooctanoic acid	Lipoic acid	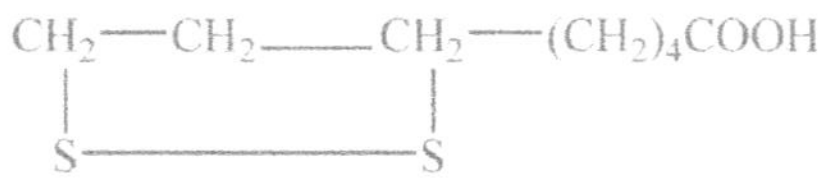 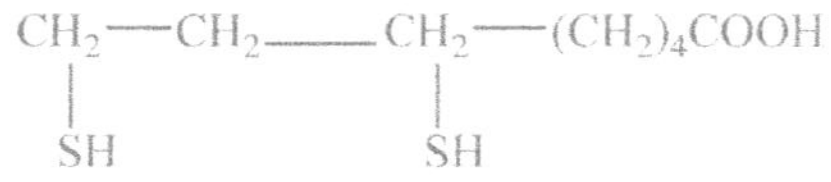 $CH_2—CH_2—CH_2—(CH_2)_4COOH$ (S—S bridge) **Oxidized form** $CH_2—CH_2—CH_2—(CH_2)_4COOH$ (SH, SH) **Reduced form**	Octanoic acid and thio group	Therapeutically used as antioxidant to prevent stroke, myocardial infarction, etc.	Hydrogen and electron	*Pyruvate dehydrogenase (PDH)*
7	Vitamin-B_5 (Pantothenic acid)	CoA (Co-enzyme-A)	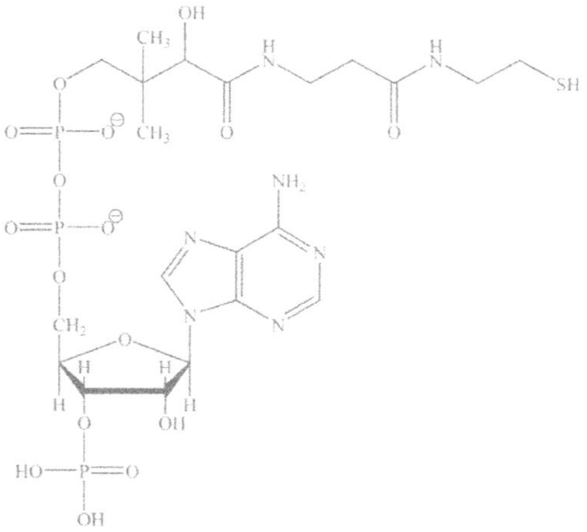	Pantoic acid, β-alanine, adenine and ribose	Burning feet syndrome (Pain and numbness in the toes, sleeplessness, fatigue, etc.). In animal (Anemia, fatty liver, decreased steroid synthesis)	Acyl group	*Thiokinase (TK)*
8	Vitamin-B_6 (Pyridoxine)	PLP (Pyridoxal phosphate)	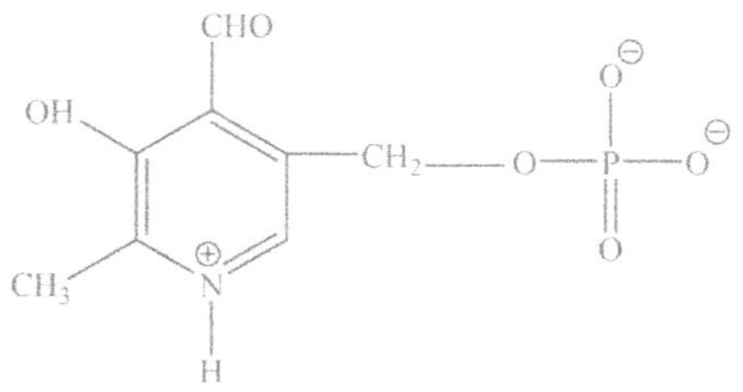	Pyridine	Neurological symptoms like depression, irritability, nervousness and mental confusion.	Amino or keto group	*Alanine transaminase (ATA)*

Table 2.8 Contd...

S. No	Vitamin name	Co-enzyme name	Chemical structure of co-enzyme	Important structural features of co-enzyme	Deficiency / Disorder	Atom or group transferred	Example of dependent enzyme
9	Vitamin-B_7 (Biotin)	Biocytin	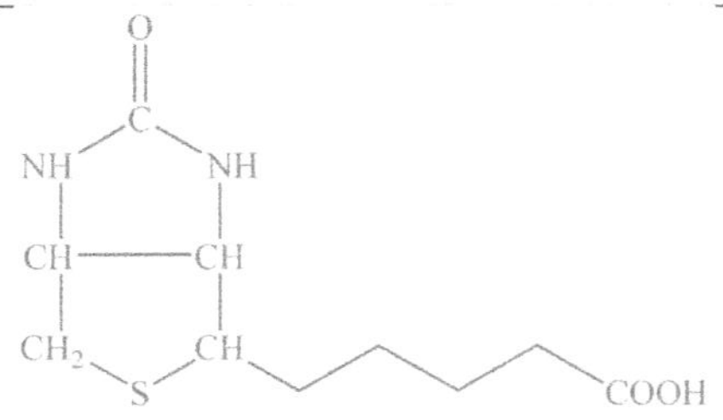	Imidazole and thiophene ring	Anemia, loss of appetite, nausea, dermatitis, glossitis, depression, hallucination and muscle pain.	Carbon dioxide	*Pyruvate carboxylase*
10	Vitamin-B_9 (Folic acid)	FH_4 or THF (Tetrahydro folic acid)	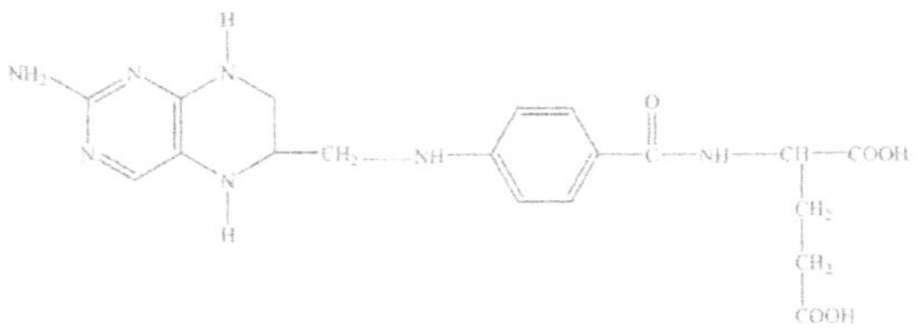	Pteridine, PABA (*p*-amino benzoic acid) and glutamate	Macrocytic anemia and neural defects in fetus. Formiminoglutamate (FIGLU) accumulates and excretes in urine	Formyl, methyl, etc. (One carbon)	*Formyl transferase*
11	Vitamin-B_{12} (Cyanocobalamin)	Methyl cobalamin, S-Deoxy adenosyl cobalamin	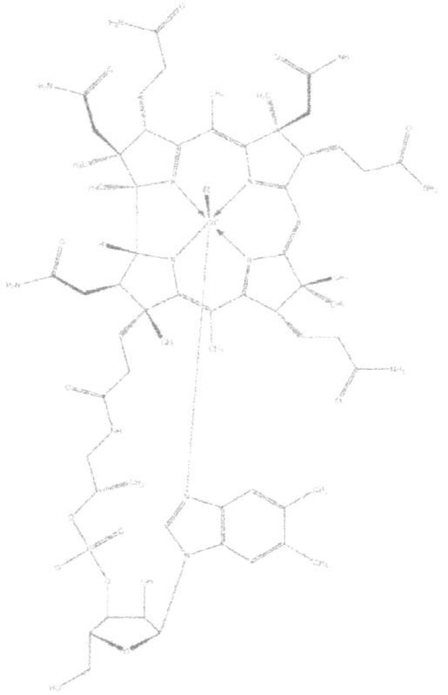 R = Methyl (Methyl cobalamin) R = 5'-Deoxy adenosyl cobalamin (S-Deoxy adenosyl cobalamin)	Porphyrin ring, pyrrole ring, amino isopropanol, dimethyl benzimidazole and cobalt atom	Pernicious anemia, neuronal degeneration and demyelination of nervous system	Methyl or isomerization	*Methyl malonyl CoA mutase*

Table 2.9 Non-vitamin co-enzymes.

S. No.	Name	Abbreviation	Structure	Biochemical functions
1	Adenosine triphosphate	ATP	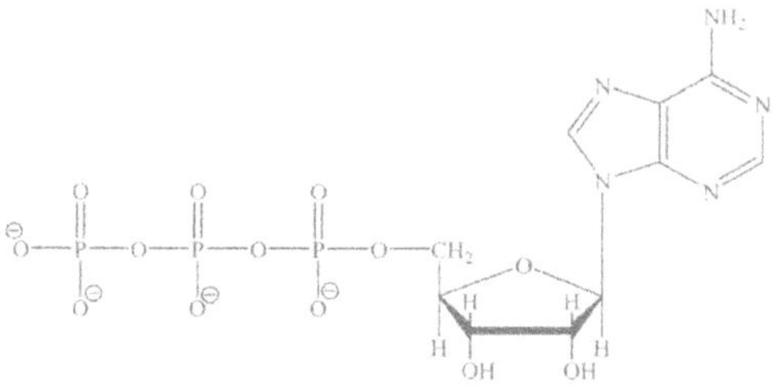	Donates phosphate, adenosine and AMP (adenosine monophosphate) moieties in biosynthetic reaction.
2	Uridine diphosphate	UDP	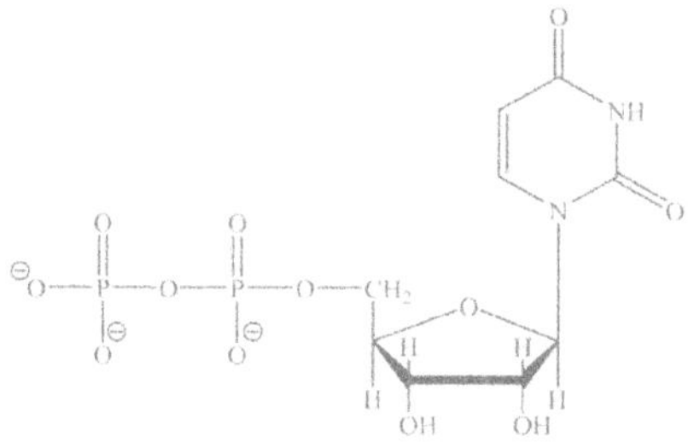	Carries molecule of mono saccharides like glucose and galactose for glycogen synthesis.
3	Cytidine diphosphate	CDP	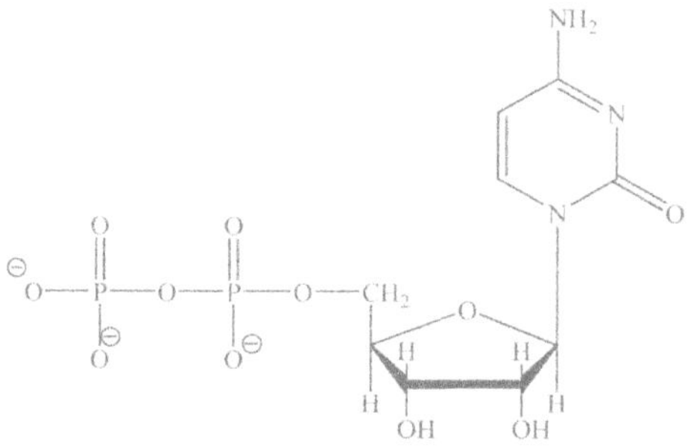	Carrier molecule of ethanolamine and choline for phospholipid synthesis.
4	S-Adenosyl methionine	SAM	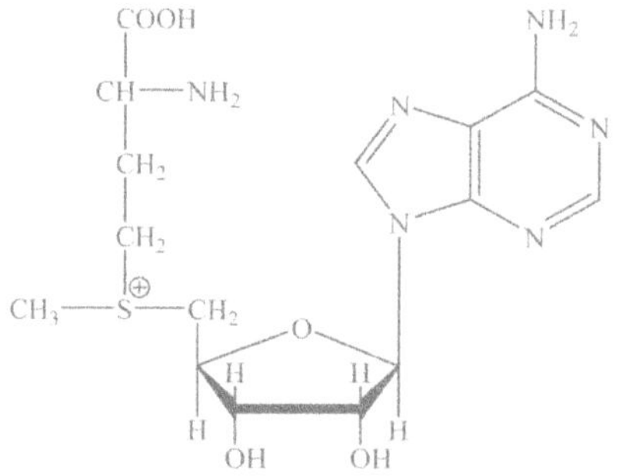	Donates methyl group in biosynthetic reaction.
5	Phosphoadenosine-phosphosulphate	PAPS	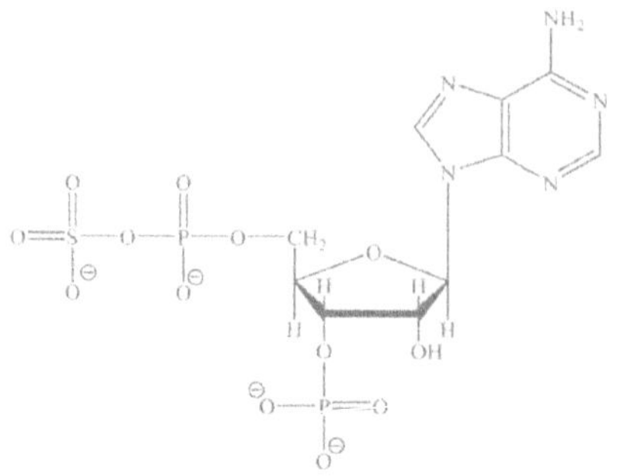	Donates sulphate groups for synthesis of muco ploy saccharides.

3. **Nucleotide co-enzyme:** The co-enzymes which are composed of nitrogen base, sugar and phosphate moieties are known as nucleotide co-enzymes. **Example:** FMN, FAD, NAD^+, $NADP^+$, Co-enzyme A, etc.
4. **Protein co-enzyme:** Some of the protein may serve as a co-enzyme for few enzymes. **Example:** Thioredoxin for *ribonucleotide reductase.*

Iso-enzymes

Iso-enzyme is defined as the multiple forms of an enzyme catalyzing the same reactions. They differ in their physical and chemical properties. The presences of iso-enzymes are confirmed from the following facts.

1. From the different genes iso-enzymes are synthesized. **Example:** *Malate dehydrogenase (MDH)* present in mitochondria is different from that found in cytosol.
2. Oligomeric enzymes are made up of more than one sub-units. **Example:** *Lactate dehydrogenase (LDH)* and *creatinine phosphokinase (CPK).*
3. As a monomer or oligomer, the enzymes may be active. **Example:** *Glutamate dehydrogenase (GDH).*
4. Difference in carbohydrate content in glycoprotein may be responsible for iso-enzymes. **Example:** *Alkaline phosphatase (AP).*

Therapeutic and Diagnostic Applications of Isoenzyme:

The following are the therapeutic and diagnostic applications of various iso-enzymes.

Example 1 (*Lactate dehydrogenase* or *LDH*)

$CH_3-CH(OH)-COOH$ (Lactic acid) ⇌ [Oxidation; NAD^+ → $NADH + H^+$; *Lactate dehydrogenase (LDH)*] $CH_3-C(=O)-COOH$ (Pyruvic acid)

Lactic acid **Pyruvic acid**

The enzyme commission number of *LDH* is 1.1.1.27. The systemic name of *LDH* is *L-lactate-NAD⁺ oxidoreductase* and it catalyzes the interconversion of lactate and pyruvate.

There are five different *LDH* iso-enzymes namely LDH_1, LDH_2, LDH_3, LDH_4 and LDH_5. It is an oligomeric (tetrameric) enzyme made up of four polypeptide sub units. Different genes produce two type of sub units namely "M" for muscle (Basic) and "H" for heart (Acidic). One or both the sub-units are present in the iso-enzymes LDH_1 to LDH_5. The characteristic features of *LDH* iso-enzymes are presented in Table 2.10.

Example 2 (*Creatinine phosphokinase* or *CPK*)

It is otherwise known as *creatine kinase* or *CK*. It catalyzes the interconversion of creatine phosphate or phosphocreatine into creatine.

Creatine phosphate or Phosphocreatine ⇌ [**Dephosphorylation**; ADP → ATP] Creatine

Creatine phosphokinase (CPK) or *Creatine kinase (CK)*

Table 2.10 Characteristic features of LDH iso-enzymes.

S. No.	Name of iso-enzyme	Composition	Tissues present	Electrophoretic mobility	Liability to heat at 60 °C	% present in normal serum	Significance of differential catalytic activity	Diagnostic importance
1	*LDH_1*	H H H H H_4	Heart and RBC	Fastest	Not affected	25 %	*LDH_1* is inhibited by pyruvate. Hence pyruvate is not converted into lactate in muscle. Pyruvate is converted to acetyl CoA which enters in TCA cycle. *LDH_1* has high K_m value for pyruvate.	In myocardial infarction *LDH_1* is much greater than *LDH_2*. It happens within 12 to 24 hours after infarction.
2	*LDH_2*	H H H M H_3M	Heart and RBC	Faster	Not affected	35 %	---------	In healthy individual *LDH_2* is higher than *LDH_1*. *LDH* activity in RBC is 80 to 100 times more than in serum. Hence, for estimation of serum or its iso-enzyme serum should be totally free from hemolysis.
3	*LDH_3*	H M H M H_2M_2	Brain and kidney	Fast	Partially affected	27 %	---------	---------
4	*LDH_4*	H M M M HM_3	Liver and skeletal muscle	Slow	Completely affected	8 %	---------	---------
5	*LDH*	M M M M M_4	Liver and skeletal muscle	Slowest	Completely affected	5 %	Inhibition of *LDH_5* by pyruvate is minimum. Hence pyruvate is converted into lactate. LDH_5 has low K_m value for pyruvate.	Increased activity of *LDH_5* in serum is an indicator of liver disease.

There are three different *CPK* iso-enzymes namely CPK_1, CPK_2 and CPK_3. It is an oligomeric (dimeric) enzyme made up of two polypeptide sub-units. Different genes produce two type of sub-units namely "M" for muscle and "B" for brain. The sub-unit of CPK_1, CPK_2 and CPK_3 are BB, MB and MM, respectively. CPK_1, CPK_2 and CPK_3 are mainly present in brain, heart and skeletal muscle, respectively. The normal serum level of CPK_2 is very less (less than 2 % of total *CPK*). Within first 6 to 18 hours after myocardial infarction serum level of CPK_2 increases to as high as 20 %. Hence, estimation of serum level of CPK_2 is the earliest reliable indication of myocardial infarction. In skeletal muscle disorder serum level of CPK_2 is not elevated.

Example 3 (*Alkaline phosphatase* or *ALP*)

It is otherwise known as *basic phosphatase*. It catalyzes the hydrolysis of phosphate monoesters at basic pH values.

There are six different *ALPs* iso-enzymes namely α_1*-ALP*, α_2*-heat labile ALP*, α_2*-heat stable ALP*, *pre-β-ALP*, *γ-ALP*, etc. It is a monomeric enzyme and the iso-enzymes are due to the difference in carbohydrate content (Sialic acid residues). Hepatitis is diagnosed by increased concentration of α_2*-heat labile ALP* and bone diseases are diagnosed from increased serum *pre-β-ALP*.

Example 4 (*Alcohol dehydrogenase* or *ADH*)

It catalyzes the interconversion of alcohol into aldehyde.

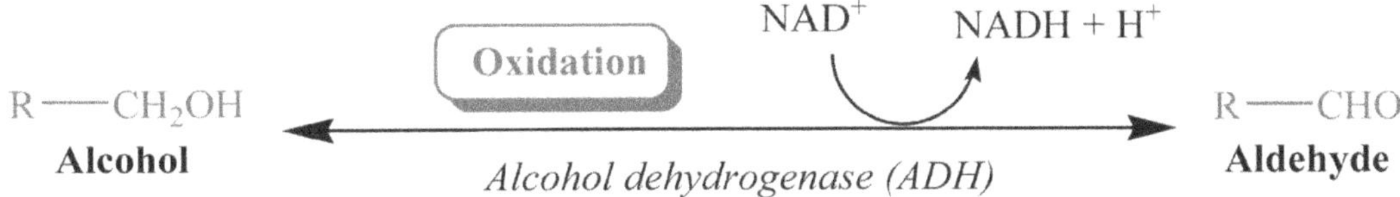

It is otherwise known as *creatine kinase* or *CK*. It catalyzes the interconversion of creatine phosphate or phosphocreatine into creatine.

There are two iso-enzymes available for *alcohol dehydrogenase*. $\alpha\beta_1$*-ADH* is present in white Americans and Europeans and $\alpha\beta_2$*-ADH* is present in Japanese and Chinese (Orientals). The $\alpha\beta_2$*-ADH* iso-enzymes more rapidly converts alcohol into aldehydes. Among oriental accumulation of acetaldehyde is associated with tachycardia and facial flushing. This is not common in whites. The increased sensitivity of Japanese and Chinese to alcohol is due to the presence of $\alpha\beta_2$*-ADH* iso-enzymes.

Applications of Enzymes

The applications of enzymes are broadly classified into five major categories 1) Therapeutic applications, 2) Analytical applications, 3) Applications in genetic manipulation, 4) Industrial applications, 5) Diagnostic applications.

1. **Therapeutic applications:**

   Various enzymes are therapeutically useful for the treatment of various diseases. They are,

   (a) From *streptococcus, streptokinase* was prepared and is used for clearing blood clots. *Streptokinase* is an enzyme which activates the conversion of plasma plasminogen into plasmin. This plasmin activates the conversion of fibrin clot into soluble products.

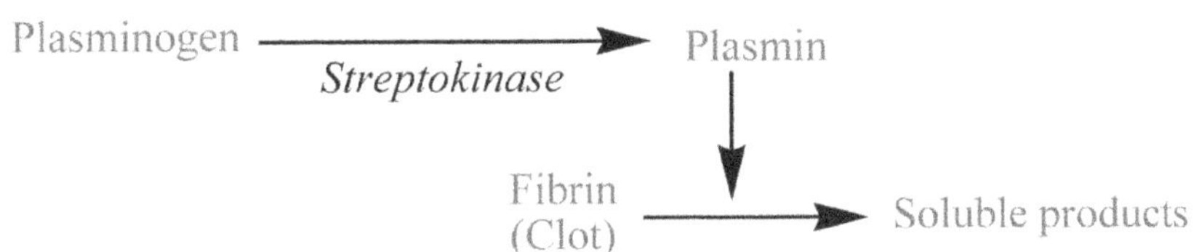

(b) Tumor cells are dependent on asparagine of the host's plasma for their multiplications. *Asparaginase* drastically decreases the host's plasma asparagine which may lead to decreased viability of the tumor cells. Hence, *asparaginase* enzyme is used in the treatment of leukemias.

(c) *Papain* is used as an anti-inflammatory agent.

(d) Enzyme α_1-*antitrypsin* is used for the treatment of emphysema.

(e) Pancreatic enzymes like *lipase* and *trypsin* are used for the digestion in pancreatic diseases.

2. **Analytical applications:**

In the clinical laboratories some of the enzymes are used for the measurements of drugs, substrates and even the activities of other enzymes also. Compared to the conventional chemical methods, enzymatic methods are more accurate and specific for the estimation of various biochemical compounds like glucose, urea, uric acid, cholesterol, etc.

(a) Plasma glucose is estimated by using *glucose oxidase* and *peroxidase* enzymes.

(b) Few of these enzymes are immobilized by binding with insoluble solid matrix. Stability and catalytic activity of enzymes are not affected by this solid matrix. The commonly used solid matrixes are beaded gels and cyanogen bromide activated sepharose. Without losing the activity the bound enzymes can be preserved for long periods. *Glucose oxidase* and *peroxidase*, immobilized and coated on a strip of paper is used clinically for the detection of glucose in urine. Based on the concentration of glucose, the intensity of blue color varies. Hence, strip method is useful for semi-quantitative estimation of glucose in urine.

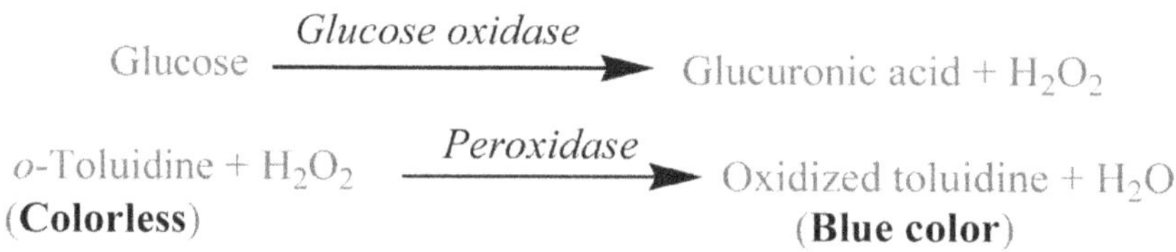

(c) *Urease* is used for the estimation of urea.

(d) Uric acid is estimated using *uricase* enzymes.

(e) *Lipase* is used for the estimation of triglycerides.

(f) Bacterial contamination of food substances is identified by *luciferase* enzymes.

(g) In the analytical technique ELISA, *horse radish peroxidase* or *alkaline phosphatase* are useful.

3. **Applications in genetic manipulation:**

Some of the enzymes also play a role in the genetic engineering.

(a) *Restriction endonucleases* are useful for gene transfer and DNA finger printing.

(b) *Taq DNA polymerase is* useful for the *polymerase* chain reactions.

4. **Industrial applications:**

In industries, enzymes can be used as catalytic agents.

(a) For preparation of cheese, enzyme *rennin* is used in industries.

(b) In food industries *α-amylase* is used.

(c) High fructose syrups are produced by using *glucose isomerase*.

(d) Washing powders are produced in industries with the help of enzyme *proteases*.

5. **Diagnostic applications:**

Clinically the enzyme activities in biological fluids are more important. There are two classes of enzymes present in the circulation. They are 1) Plasma functional or plasma specific enzymes, 2) Plasma non-functional or non-plasma specific enzymes.

Plasma functional or plasma specific enzymes: In general, the activities of these enzymes are high in plasma than in the tissues. It is mainly synthesized in liver and enters into the circulation to perform specific functions. **Example:** *Lipoprotein lipase, plasmin, thrombin, choline esterase, ceruloplasmin,* etc.

Plasma non-functional or non-plasma specific enzymes: In general concentration of these enzymes are high in tissues compared to plasma either low or absent. **Example:** Digestive enzymes like *amylase, pepsin, trypsin, lipase,* etc. and constitutive enzymes like *lactate dehydrogenase (LDH), transaminase, acid and alkaline phosphatase (ACP or ALP), creatine phosphokinase (CPK),* etc. For the diagnosis or prognosis of many diseases these plasmas non-functional or non-plasma specific enzymes are very useful. The balance between the enzyme synthesis and its release in the normal cell turnover is indicated by the normal serum level of enzymes.

Elevated serum level enzymes in diagnosis: The serum enzyme levels may increase due to cellular damage, proliferation of cells, increased synthesis of enzymes and increased rate of cell turnover. Generally, to detect the cellular damages serum enzymes are used conveniently as markers which help in the diagnosis of diseases. The followings are some important examples of elevated serum level enzymes used for the diagnosis purpose.

(a) Increased serum *amylase* is seen in acute pancreatitis, chronic pancreatitis, acute parotitis (mumps), severe diabetic ketoacidosis and obstruction of pancreatic duct.
(b) Increased serum *lipase* is seen in acute pancreatitis and moderate elevation seen in carcinoma of pancreas.
(c) In acute hepatitis of viral or toxic origin, cirrhosis of liver and jaundice serum *alanine transaminase (ALT)* or *serum glutamate pyruvate transaminase (SGPT)* is elevated. It is more specific for diagnosis of liver diseases because it is a cytosomal enzyme.
(d) Serum *aspartate transaminase (AST)* or *serum glutamate oxaloacetate transaminase (SGOT)* is elevated in liver diseases and myocardial infarction. It is more specific for diagnosis of heart diseases because it is found in both cytostome and mitochondria.
(e) In some liver and bone disease *serum alkaline phosphatase (ALP)* is elevated. Hence it is useful for the diagnosis of rickets, obstructive jaundice, carcinoma of bone and hyperparathyroidism.
(f) *Serum acid phosphatase (ACP)* is elevated in the prostate cancer. Hence, tartrate labile *ACP* is used for the prognosis and diagnosis of prostate cancer.
(g) *Creatine kinase (CK)* is elevated in myocardial infarction and hence, useful for the diagnosis of myocardial infarction.
(h) *Lactate dehydrogenase (LDH)* is useful for the diagnosis of myocardial infarction, infective hepatitis, leukemia and muscular dystrophy.
(i) Serum *aldolase* is elevated in muscular dystrophy.
(j) In hepatitis, serum *5-nucleotidase* level is elevated.
(k) Alcohol sensitively is detected by using *γ-glutamyl transpeptidase (GGT)*. It is also elevated in obstructive jaundice and infective hepatitis.

Decreased serum level enzymes in diagnosis: Sometimes due to congenital deficiency or decreased enzyme synthesis the plasma level of enzymes may decrease than normal. This is also useful for the diagnosis of certain diseases.

(a) In liver diseases *amylase* serum level is decreased.
(b) Serum *pseudocholinesterase (ChE II)* is decreased in cirrhosis of liver, liver cancer, viral hepatitis and malnutrition.
(c) Wilson disease is diagnosed from decreased serum *ceruloplasmin*.
(d) Decreased *glucose-6-phosphate dehydrogenase (G-6-PD)* in RBC is useful for the diagnosis of congenital deficiency with hemolytic anemia.

Estimation of enzymes in other body fluids and tissues: Estimation of enzymes in other body fluids and tissues other than serum or plasma is also used for diagnosis of several diseases.

(a) In acute pancreatitis urinary *amylase* is increased and in renal graft dysfunction urinary *β-N-acetylgalactosidase* is elevated. *B-Glucuronidase* is increased in the urinary bladder cancer and pancreatic cancer.
(b) Meningitis is diagnosed using *lactate dehydrogenase (LDH)* in cerebrospinal fluid (CSF).
(c) Gastric carcinoma is diagnosed from elevated *β-glucuronidase*.

(d) Cystic fibrosis is diagnosed from decreased fetal *trypsin* levels.
(e) Type – I glycogen storage disease is diagnosed from decreased *glucose-6-phosphatase* in liver.
(f) In McArdle's disease muscle *phosphorylase* activity is decreased.
(g) Thiamine deficiencies are diagnosed using decreased *transketolase* activity.
(h) For the diagnosis of in born error cultured fibroblasts and amniotic cells are frequently used. **Example:** In cultured amniotic cells deficiency of *phenylalanine hydroxylase* is observed in phenylketonuria.

Enzyme patterns in important diseases: It is better to estimate few (three or more) enzymes instead of single enzymes for the better diagnosis of a particular disease. The followings are the enzyme patterns in important diseases.

(a) Myocardial infarction is diagnosed from elevated serum levels of *creatine phosphokinase (CPK), aspartate transaminase (AST)* and *lactate dehydrogenase (LDH)*. For the early diagnosis of myocardial infarction, the protein *cardiac troponins* are highly useful. Similarly, the protein *myoglobin* is also an early marker for the diagnosis of myocardial infarction.
(b) The elevated serum level of *alanine transaminase (ALT), aspartate transaminase (AST)* and *lactate dehydrogenase (LDH)* are useful for the diagnosis of liver dysfunction due to jaundice, toxic hepatitis, cirrhosis and hepatic necrosis. Alcoholic liver diseases are diagnosed using serum *γ-glutamyl transpeptidase (GGT)*. *Alkaline phosphatase* and *5-nucleotidase* are elevated markedly in intrahepatic and extrahepatic cholestasis.
(c) Serum levels of *creatine phosphokinase (CPK), aldolase* and *aspartate transaminase (ATA)* are elevated in muscular dystrophies.
(d) Prostate cancer is diagnosed from elevated serum *acid phosphatase (ACP)*. For lung cancer, neuroblastoma, pheochromocytoma, etc. neuron specific *enolase* is serving as a marker.

PROBABLE QUESTIONS

PART – A: Multiple Choice Questions

1. Which one is the functional unit of the enzyme?
   (a) Apo-enzyme (b) Holo-enzyme
   (c) Co-enzyme (d) Iso-enzyme
2. Which of the following is example for oligomeric enzymes?
   (a) *Nuclease* (b) *Trypsin*
   (c) *Lactate dehydrogenase* (d) *Hexokinase*
3. The Michaelis-Menten constant or Brigs and Haldane constant (K_m), is given by which of the following formula?
   (a) $k_m=(k_1+k_2)/k_3$ (b) $k_m=(k_2+k_3)/k_1$
   (c) $k_m=(k_3+k_1)/k_2$ (d) $k_m=k_2/k_1$
4. At the active sites of enzymes which amino acid is most frequently found?
   (a) Aspartate (b) Cysteine
   (c) Serine (d) Arginine
5. Which class of enzyme does not exhibit stereo specificity?
   (a) *Isomerase* (b) *Lyase*
   (c) *Hydrolase* (d) *Ligase*
6. Which of the following is non-protein part of the enzyme?
   (a) Apo-enzyme (b) Co-enzyme
   (c) Holo-enzyme (d) Iso-zyme

7. Which part of enzyme is responsible for specificity of enzyme?
   (a) Co-enzyme (b) Holo-enzyme
   (c) Apo-enzyme (d) Iso-enzyme
8. Which enzyme is useful for clearing the blood clots?
   (a) *Asparaginase* (b) *Papain*
   (c) *α_1-antitrypsin* (d) *Streptokinase*
9. The digestive enzyme belongs to which category?
   (a) Secretary enzyme (b) Constitutive enzyme
   (c) Serum enzyme (d) Iso-enzyme
10. Which of the following co-enzyme is not involved in hydrogen transfer?
    (a) FMN (b) FAD
    (c) NAD^+ (d) FH_4
11. Which word may be memorized to remember the six classes of enzymes in correct order.
    (a) OLLITH (b) OHLITL
    (c) OLTHIL (d) OTHLIL
12. Which of the following statement is incorrect?
    (a) Enzymes increases the activation energy (b) Enzymes decreases the activation energy
    (c) Enzymes are colloidal in nature (d) Enzymes are thermo liable in nature
13. What indicates low Km value?
    (a) Strong affinity between enzyme & co-enzyme
    (b) Weak affinity between enzyme & co-enzyme
    (c) Strong affinity between enzyme & substrate
    (d) Weak affinity between enzyme & substrate
14. Disulfiram is a very good example for which type of enzyme inhibition?
    (a) Irreversible (b) Reversible
    (c) Competitive (d) Non-competitive
15. Which enzyme is useful for the diagnosis of obstructive jaundice?
    (a) *Acid phosphatase* (b) *Alkaline phosphatase*
    (c) *SGOT* (d) *SGPT*
16. Which of the following is true about Michaelis-Menten kinetics?
    (a) K_m, the Michaelis constant, is defined as that concentration of substrate at which enzyme is working at maximum velocity
    (b) It describes single substrate enzymes
    (c) K_m, the Michaelis constant is defined as the dissociation constant of the enzyme-substrate complex
    (d) It assumes covalent binding occurs between enzyme and substrate
17. When the velocity of enzyme activity is plotted against substrate concentration, which of the following is obtained?
    (a) Hyperbolic curve (b) Parabola
    (c) Straight line with positive slope (d) Straight line with negative slope

18. The rate determining step of Michaelis-Menten kinetics is __________
    (a) The complex dissociation step to produce products
    (b) The complex formation step
    (c) The product formation step
    (d) None of the mentioned
19. The molecule which acts directly on an enzyme to lower its catalytic rate is __________
    (a) Repressor (b) Inhibitor
    (c) Modulator (d) Regulator
20. Which of the following is an example for irreversible inhibitor?
    (a) Disulfiram (b) Oseltamivir
    (c) Protease inhibitors (d) DIPF
21. Which of the following is an example of reversible inhibitor?
    (a) DIPF (b) Penicillin
    (c) Iodoacetamide (d) Protease inhibitors
22. Where does inhibitor binds on enzyme in mixed inhibition?
    (a) At active site (b) Allosteric site
    (c) Does not bind on enzyme (d) Binds on substrate
23. The catalytic efficiency of two distinct enzymes can be compared based on which of the following factor?
    (a) K_m (b) Product formation
    (c) Size of the enzymes (d) pH of optimum value
24. What is the general mechanism of an enzyme?
    (a) It acts by reducing the activation energy (b) It acts by increasing the activation energy
    (c) It acts by decreasing the pH (d) It acts by increasing the pH
25. The allosteric inhibitor of an enzyme __________
    (a) Causes the enzyme to work faster (b) Binds to the active site
    (c) Participates in feedback regulation (d) Denatures the enzyme
26. Which of the following is false about allosteric feedback inhibition?
    (a) Bacterial enzyme system is the first known example
    (b) Conversion of L-leucine to L-isoleucine
    (c) *Threonine dehydratase* is inhibited by isoleucine
    (d) If the isoleucine concentration decreases, the rate of threonine dehydration increases
27. Which of the following is false?
    (a) Methyl, phosphoryl, adenyl, uridylyl and adenosine diphosphate ribosyl groups are the modifying groups
    (b) An example of an enzyme regulated by methylation is the methyl-donating chemo taxis protein of bacteria
    (c) The protein is a part of the system that permits a bacterium to swim towards attractant
    (d) The methylating agent is S-adenosylmethionine
28. Which of the following is false?
    (a) Allosteric modulators may be inhibitory or stimulatory
    (b) Based on the nature of modulator, allosteric enzymes are of two types

(c) Homotropic allosteric enzymes have the substrate and modulator same
(d) Heterotropic allosteric enzymes have the substrate and modulator same

29. In the case of allosteric enzymes what is the graphical representation when initial velocity is plotted against substrate concentration?
(a) Straight line with negative slope
(b) Hyperbola
(c) Sigmoid curve
(d) Parabola

30. Which is the enzyme that acts as a regulatory enzyme in a four-step metabolic pathway?
(a) First enzyme
(b) Fourth enzyme
(c) Second enzyme
(d) Third enzyme

31. A Holo-enzyme is
(a) Functional unit
(b) Apo-enzyme
(c) Co-enzyme
(d) All of these

32. Example of an extracellular enzyme is
(a) *Lactate dehydrogenase*
(b) *Cytochrome oxidase*
(c) *Pancreatic lipase*
(d) *Hexokinase*

33. Enzymes, which are produced in inactive form in the living cells, are called
(a) Co-enzyme
(b) Lysozymes
(c) Apoenzymes
(d) Proenzymes

34. The enzyme which can add water to a carbon-carbon double bond or remove water to create a double bond without breaking the bond is
(a) *Hydratase*
(b) *Hydroxylase*
(c) *Hydrolase*
(d) *Esterase*

35. Fischer's "lock and key" model of the enzyme action implies that
(a) The active site is complementary in shape to that of substance only after interaction
(b) The active site is complementary in shape to that of substance
(c) Substrates change conformation prior to active site interaction
(d) The active site is flexible and adjusts to substrate

36. A sigmoidal plot of substrate concentration ([S]) verses reaction velocity (V) may indicate
(a) Michaelis-Menten kinetics
(b) Co-operative binding
(c) Competitive inhibition
(d) Non-competitive inhibition

37. An inducer is absent in the type of enzyme
(a) Allosteric enzyme
(b) Constitutive enzyme
(c) Co-operative enzyme
(d) Isoenzymic enzyme

38. In reversible non-competitive enzyme activity inhibition
(a) V_{max} is increased
(b) K_m is increased
(c) K_m is decreased
(d) Concentration of active enzyme is reduced

39. The pH optima of most of the enzymes is
(a) Between 2 and 4
(b) Between 5 and 9
(c) Between 8 and 12
(d) Above 12

40. Co-enzymes are
(a) Heat stable, dialyzable, non-protein organic molecules
(b) Soluble, colloidal, protein molecules

(c) Structural analogue of enzymes
(d) Different forms of enzymes

41. An example of hydrogen transferring co-enzyme is
(a) CoA (b) NAD^+
(c) Biotin (d) TPP

42. An example of group transferring co-enzyme is
(a) NAD^+ (b) $NADP^+$
(c) FAD (d) CoA

43. *Co-carboxylase* is
(a) Thiamine pyrophosphate (b) Pyridoxal phosphate
(c) Biotin (d) CoA

44. A co-enzyme containing non aromatic hetero ring is
(a) ATP (b) NAD
(c) FMN (d) Biotin

45. A co-enzyme containing aromatic hetero ring is
(a) TPP (b) Lipoic acid
(c) Co-enzyme Q (d) Biotin

46. Iso-enzymes are
(a) Chemically, immunologically and electrophoretically different forms of an enzyme
(b) Different forms of an enzyme similar in all properties
(c) Catalyzing different reactions
(d) Having the same quaternary structures like the enzymes

47. Iso-enzymes can be characterized by
(a) Proteins lacking enzymatic activity that are necessary for the activation of enzymes
(b) Proteolytic enzymes activated by hydrolysis
(c) Enzymes with identical primary structure
(d) Similar enzymes that catalyze different reaction

48. Which of the following are factors affecting enzyme activity?
(a) Concentration (b) pH
(c) Temperature (d) All of these

49. The iso-enzymes LDH_5 is elevated in
(a) Myocardial infarction (b) Peptic ulcer
(c) Liver disease (d) Infectious disease

50. Lineweaver – Burk double reciprocal plot is related to
(a) Substrate concentration (b) Enzyme activity
(c) Temperature (d) Both (a) and (b)

51. The co-enzyme not involved in the formation of acetyl-CoA from pyruvate is
(a) TPP (b) Biotin
(c) NAD^+ (d) FAD

52. Characteristic features of active site are
(a) Flexible in nature (b) Site of binding
(c) Acidic (d) Both (a) and (b)

53. Which of the following is an example of enzyme inhibition?
(a) Reversible inhibition (b) Irreversible inhibition
(c) Allosteric inhibition (d) All of these

54. Which of the following co-enzyme takes part in hydrogen transfer reactions?
(a) Tetrahydrofolate (b) Co-enzyme A
(c) Co-enzyme Q (d) Biotin

55. Which of the following co-enzyme takes part in oxidation-reduction reactions?
(a) Pyridoxal phosphate (b) Lipoic acid
(c) Thiamin diphosphate (d) None of these

56. A co-enzyme required in transamination reactions is
(a) Co-enzyme A (b) Co-enzyme Q
(c) Biotin (d) Pyridoxal phosphate

57. Co-enzyme A contains a vitamin which is
(a) Thiamin (b) Ascorbic acid
(c) Pantothenic acid (d) Niacinamide

58. Cobamides contain a vitamin which is
(a) Folic acid (b) Ascorbic acid
(c) Pantothenic acid (d) Vitamin B_{12}

59. A co-enzyme required in carboxylation reactions is
(a) Lipoic acid (b) Co-enzyme A
(c) Biotin (d) All of these

60. Which of the following co-enzyme takes part in tissue respiration?
(a) Co-enzyme Q (b) Co-enzyme A
(c) $NADP^+$ (d) Cobamide

Key for Multiple Choice Questions

1. (b)	2. (c)	3. (b)	4. (c)	5. (a)
6. (b)	7. (c)	8. (d)	9. (a)	10. (d)
11. (d)	12. (b)	13. (c)	14. (a)	15. (b)
16. (b)	17. (a)	18. (a)	19. (b)	20. (d)
21. (d)	22. (b)	23. (a)	24. (a)	25. (c)
26. (b)	27. (b)	28. (d)	29. (c)	30. (a)
31. (d)	32. (c)	33. (d)	34. (a)	35. (b)
36. (b)	37. (b)	38. (d)	39. (b)	40. (a)
41. (b)	42. (d)	43. (c)	44. (d)	45. (a)
46. (a)	47. (b)	48. (d)	49. (c)	50. (d)
51. (b)	52. (d)	53. (d)	54. (c)	55. (b)
56. (d)	57. (c)	58. (d)	59. (c)	60. (a)

PART – B: Short Answers

1. What is intra-cellular enzyme & extra-cellular enzyme?
2. What is monomeric & oligomeric enzyme?
3. Explain multi enzyme complex with suitable examples.
4. How enzyme-substrate complex are formed?
5. Write a short note on Fischer's template theory.
6. What is substrate strain theory?
7. Define exothermic and endothermic reaction.
8. Explain the term "enzyme kinetics".
9. What are co-enzymes? Write the biochemical role of nicotinamide co-enzymes.
10. Define Michaelis-Menten constant and write its significance.
11. Note on Lineweaver–Burk double reciprocal plot.
12. How temperature and pH influence the enzyme velocity.
13. What is competitive enzyme inhibition?
14. Write a note on suicide inhibition.
15. Explain allosteric enzyme inhibition.
16. Define constitutive enzyme and adaptive enzyme.
17. Define enzyme induction and repression.
18. What is iso-enzyme? Write clinical applications of iso-enzymes.
19. Write a short note on non-vitamin co-enzyme.
20. With suitable example explain about co-enzymes and co-factors.
21. How many classes of enzymes are there according to the IUB?
22. Explain the effect of substrate concentration on enzyme activity.
23. Give a brief account of co-enzymes and iso-enzymes.
24. Explain enzyme inhibition.
25. List out various therapeutic applications of enzy**mes.**

PART – C: Long Answers

1. Explain the characteristics of reversible enzyme inhibition with their kinetics.
2. Explain the nomenclature and classification of enzymes.
3. Describe different types of enzyme inhibitors. How do you distinguish a competitive inhibitor from non-competitive inhibitor?
4. Describe various factors effecting enzyme activity. Comment on enzyme inhibition.
5. Briefly explain the effect of substrate concentration on enzyme activity. Write about the different types of enzyme inhibition process. Define enzyme induction.
6. Explain about diagnostic & therapeutic applications of enzymes & isoenzymes.
7. Define & classify enzymes.
8. Write the clinical applications of enzymes.
9. Define & explain the following: a) Enzymes, b) Isoenzymes, c) Co-enzymes.
10. Explain kinetics, mechanism of action & inhibition of enzymes.
11. What are enzymes? Classify enzymes with examples. Explain the mechanism of enzyme action.
12. Write briefly on activators & deactivators of enzymes.
13. Explain the clinical significance of enzymes, isoenzymes & co-enzymes.
14. Explain the mechanism of action of enzyme & its inhibition.
15. What are co-enzymes? Give the example & explain their significance.
16. What is regression, induction & control of enzyme synthesis.

17. Sketch the clinical applications of enzymes & isozymes.
18. Explain the role of cAMP in enzyme activation, repression & induction with suitable examples.
19. Discuss briefly the specificity & mechanism of action of enzymes.
20. Discuss briefly on the mechanism of enzyme repression & induction.
21. Explain the various properties of enzymes.
22. Write a detailed note on nomenclature of enzymes.
23. Explain various theories associated with enzyme-substrate complex formation.
24. Explain the mechanism of enzyme catalysis in detail.
25. How are enzymes regulated in biological systems?

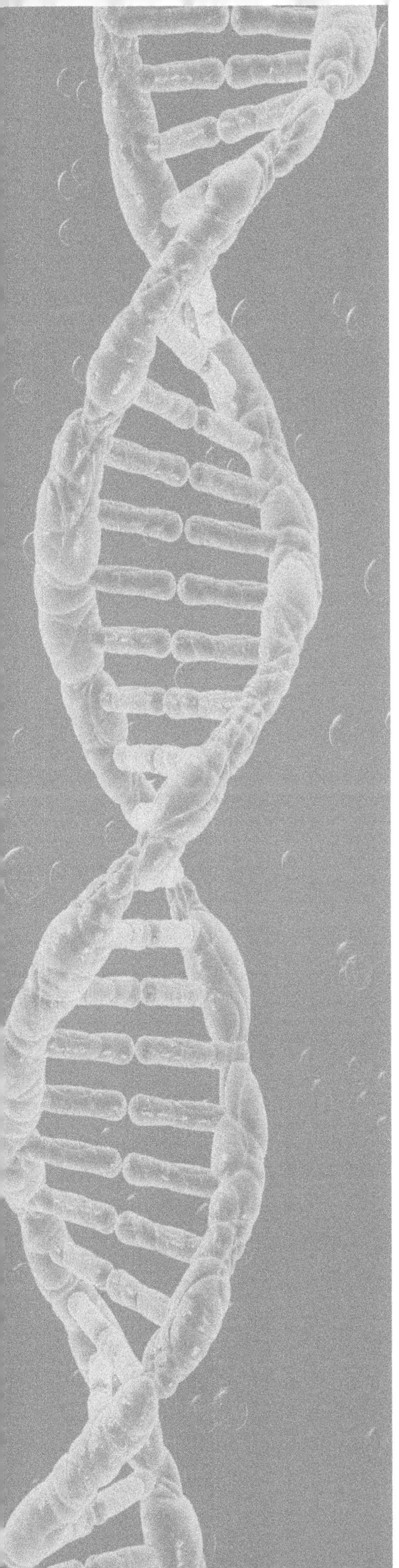

PART - II

Biomolecules & Its Metabolism

3

Carbohydrates & Its Metabolism

In nature carbohydrates are the most abundant organic molecules and widely distributed in plants and animals. They are synthesized in plants by photosynthesis and serves as storage of energy (e.g. starch and glycogen) and source of energy (e.g. sugars). Earlier, carbohydrates were regarded as the **hydrates of carbon i.e., C(H_2O)** (carbo indicates "carbon"; hydrates indicates "water"), hence they are named as carbohydrates. The hydrogen and oxygen are present in the same ratio as in water, hence the term hydrates is added. They are primarily composed of carbon, hydrogen and oxygen. **$(CH_2O)_n$ or $C_nH_{2n}O_n$ (where n > 3)** is the empirical formula of most of the carbohydrates. **Example:** Glucose ($C_6H_{12}O_6$), ribose ($C_5H_{10}O_5$), etc. But some non-carbohydrates also appear as hydrates of carbon. **Example:** Formaldehyde (CH_2O; HCHO), acetic acid ($C_2H_4O_2$; CH_3COOH), lactic acid ($C_3H_6O_3$; $CH_3CH(OH)COOH$) and inositol ($C_6H_{12}O_6$). In addition, some genuine carbohydrates do not satisfy this empirical formula. **Example:** Rhamnose, ($C_6H_{12}O_5$), digitoxose ($C_6H_{12}O_4$), rhamnohexose ($C_7H_{14}O_6$). Therefore, carbohydrates are not always considered as hydrates of carbon. The general formula for polysaccharides is **$(C_6H_{10}O_5)_n$**.

Carbohydrates are defined as optically active polyhydroxy aldehydes or ketones or compounds which produce them on hydrolysis. Nitrogen, phosphorus, or sulfur is also present in some of the carbohydrates apart from the carbon, hydrogen and oxygen. Because of their sweet taste, the simpler members of carbohydrate family are also known as saccharides (In Latin, **saccharum means "sugar"**).

Classification

Based on solubility, crystal structure and taste, carbohydrates are broadly classified into two major types as,

1. Sugars
2. Non-sugars or polysaccharides or glycans

1. Sugars: Sugars are soluble in water, crystalline in structure and are sweet in taste. Further based on the number of sugar molecules present sugars are classified into two categories

A. Monosaccharides
B. Oligosaccharides

A. Monosaccharides: In Greek, mono means "single" and in Latin, saccharum means "sugar", hence monosaccharides are composed of single sugar molecules. Monosaccharides are defined as polyhydroxy aldehydes or ketones which cannot be hydrolysed to simpler sugars. Monosaccharides having more than four carbon atoms possess cyclic structures. In nature the most commonly found monosaccharides are D-glucose (aldohexose) and D-fructose (ketohexose). In nucleic acids, nucleotides and nucleosides, aldopentoses such as D-ribose and 2-deoxy-D-ribose are present.

Based on the nature of carbonyl group, present monosaccharides are further sub divided into two types.

(i) **Aldoses or Aldose sugar:** Carbonyl group present is aldehyde, hence aldoses are monosaccharides composed of polyhydroxy aldehydes.

(ii) **Ketoses or Ketose sugar:** Carbonyl group present is ketone, hence ketoses are monosaccharides composed of polyhydroxy ketones.

These aldose and ketose sugars are further divided into several types based on the number of carbon atoms in the molecules as follows.

(a) **Trioses:** Tri means "three", hence trioses are monosaccharides made up of three carbon atoms. **Example:** Glyceraldehyde (Aldotriose) and dihydroxy acetone (Ketotriose).

(b) **Tetroses:** Tetra means "four", hence tetroses are monosaccharides made up of four carbon atoms. **Example:** Erythrose, threose (Aldotetrose) and erythrulose (Ketotetrose).

(c) **Pentoses:** Penta means "five", hence pentoses are monosaccharides made up of five carbon atoms. **Example:** Ribose, arabinose, xylose, lyxose (Aldopentose) and ribulose, xylulose (Ketopentose).

(d) **Hexoses:** Hexa means "six", hence hexoses are monosaccharides made up of six carbon atoms. **Example:** Allose, altrose, glucose, mannose, gulose, idose, galactose, talose (Aldohexose) and allulose, fructose, sorbose, tagatose (Ketohexose).

(e) **Heptoses:** Hepta means "seven", hence heptoses are monosaccharides made up of seven carbon atoms. **Example:** Glycero mannoheptose (Aldoheptose) and sedoheptulose (Ketoheptose).

(f) **Nanoses:** Nano means "nine", hence nanoses are monosaccharides made up of nine carbon atoms. **Example:** Neuraminic acid (Ketonanose).

B. **Oligosaccharides:** In Greek, oligo means "few" and in Latin, saccharum means "sugar", hence oligosaccharides are composed of few (two to ten) sugar molecules. In oligosaccharides short chain of monosaccharide units or residues are present and are linked by characteristic linkages known as glycosidic linkage. On hydrolysis these carbohydrates yield two to ten monosaccharide molecules. Hence, further based on the number of monosaccharide units formed on hydrolysis they are divided into various classes as follows.

(i) **Diasaccharides:** In Greek, di means "two" and in Latin, saccharum means "sugar", hence disaccharides are composed of two sugar molecules i.e, two monosaccharide residues. These two monosaccharide residues are attached covalently by an O-glycosidic bond, which is formed when a hydroxyl group of one monosaccharide reacts with the anomeric carbon of the other monosaccharide. These sugars on hydrolysis give two moles of the monosaccharides. **Example:** Maltose on hydrolysis yields two molecules of α-D-glucose (α-1,4-glycosidic linkage); Lactose on hydrolysis yields one molecules each of β-D-glucose and β-D-galactose (β-1,4-glycosidic linkage); Sucrose on hydrolysis yields one molecules each of α-D-glucose and β-D-fructose (1,2-glycosidic linkage); Isomaltose on hydrolysis yields two molecules of α-D-glucose (α-1,6-glycosidic linkage); Cellobiose on hydrolysis yields two molecules of β-D-glucose (β-1,4-glycosidic linkage).

(ii) **Trisaccharides:** In Greek, tri means "three" and in Latin, saccharum means "sugar", hence trisaccharides are composed of three sugar molecules i.e, three monosaccharide residues. These sugars on hydrolysis give three moles of the monosaccharides. Most oligosaccharides consisting of three or more units do not occur as free entities but are linked to non-sugar molecules (lipids or proteins) in glycoconjugates. **Example:** Raffinose on hydrolysis yields one molecule each of α-D-glucose, β-D-fructose and α-D-galactose or sucrose and α-D-galactose

(iii) Tetrasaccharides: In Greek, tetra means "four" and in Latin, saccharum means "sugar", hence tetrasaccharides are composed of four sugar molecules i.e, four monosaccharide residues. These sugars on hydrolysis give four moles of the monosaccharides. **Example:** Stachyose on hydrolysis yields one molecule each of α-D-glucose and β-D-fructose and two molecules of α-D-galactose.

(iv) Pentasaccharides: In Greek, penta means "five" and in Latin, saccharum means "sugar", hence pentasaccharides are composed of five sugar molecules i.e, five monosaccharide residues. These sugars on hydrolysis give five moles of the monosaccharides. **Example:** Verbascose on hydrolysis yields one molecule each of α-D-glucose and β-D-fructose and three molecules of α-D-galactose.

2. **Non-sugars or Polysaccharides or glycans:** (Non-sugars are insoluble in water and forms colloids, non-crystalline in structure and are tasteless (not sweet in taste). In Greek, poly "means" many and in Latin, saccharum means "sugar", hence polysaccharides are composed of many sugar molecules i.e, many monosaccharide residues. These sugars on hydrolysis give many moles of the monosaccharides. Chemically they are long chain or polymers of monosaccharides. Some polysaccharides, such as cellulose, are linear chains; others, such as starch, glycogen, are branched. Glycosidic linkage can be formed at any one of the hydroxyl group of monosaccharides that's why branches are occurring in polysaccharides. Further based on composition i.e., repeating units, polysaccharides are further classified into two categories as,

   A. Homopolysaccharides or homoglycans

   B. Heteropolysaccharides or heteroglycans

   A. Homopolysaccharides or homoglycans: (In Greek homo means "same", poly means "many" and in Latin, saccharum means "sugar", hence homopolysaccharides are composed of same sugar molecules i.e, same monosaccharide residues. Only a single type of monosaccharide is obtained on hydrolysis of homopolysaccharides. They are further classified into two types based on monosaccharide present as

   (i) Glucosan: They are polymers of glucose i.e., repeating unit is glucose. **Example:** Starch, glycogen, cellulose, dextrans, dextrins, chitin, etc.

   (ii) Fructosan: They are polymers of fructose i.e., repeating unit is fructose. **Example:** Inulin, etc.

   B. Heteropolysaccharides or heteroglycans: (In Greek hetero means "different", poly means "many" and in Latin, saccharum means "sugar", hence heteropolysaccharides are composed of different sugar molecules i.e, different monosaccharide residues. Mixture of few monosaccharide or its derivatives is obtained on hydrolysis of heteropolysaccharides. Mucopolysaccharides are heteroglycans made up of repeating units of sugar derivatives namely amino sugars and uronic acids. Mucopolysaccharides are commonly known as glycosaminoglycans (GAG). Some of mucopolysaccharides are found in combination with proteins to form proteoglycans or mucoids or mucoproteins. In proteoglycans 5 % protein and 95 % carbohydrates are present. Various examples of mucopolysaccharides are, keratan sulphate, heparin, dermatan sulphate, chondroitin sulphate, hyaluronic acid, etc.

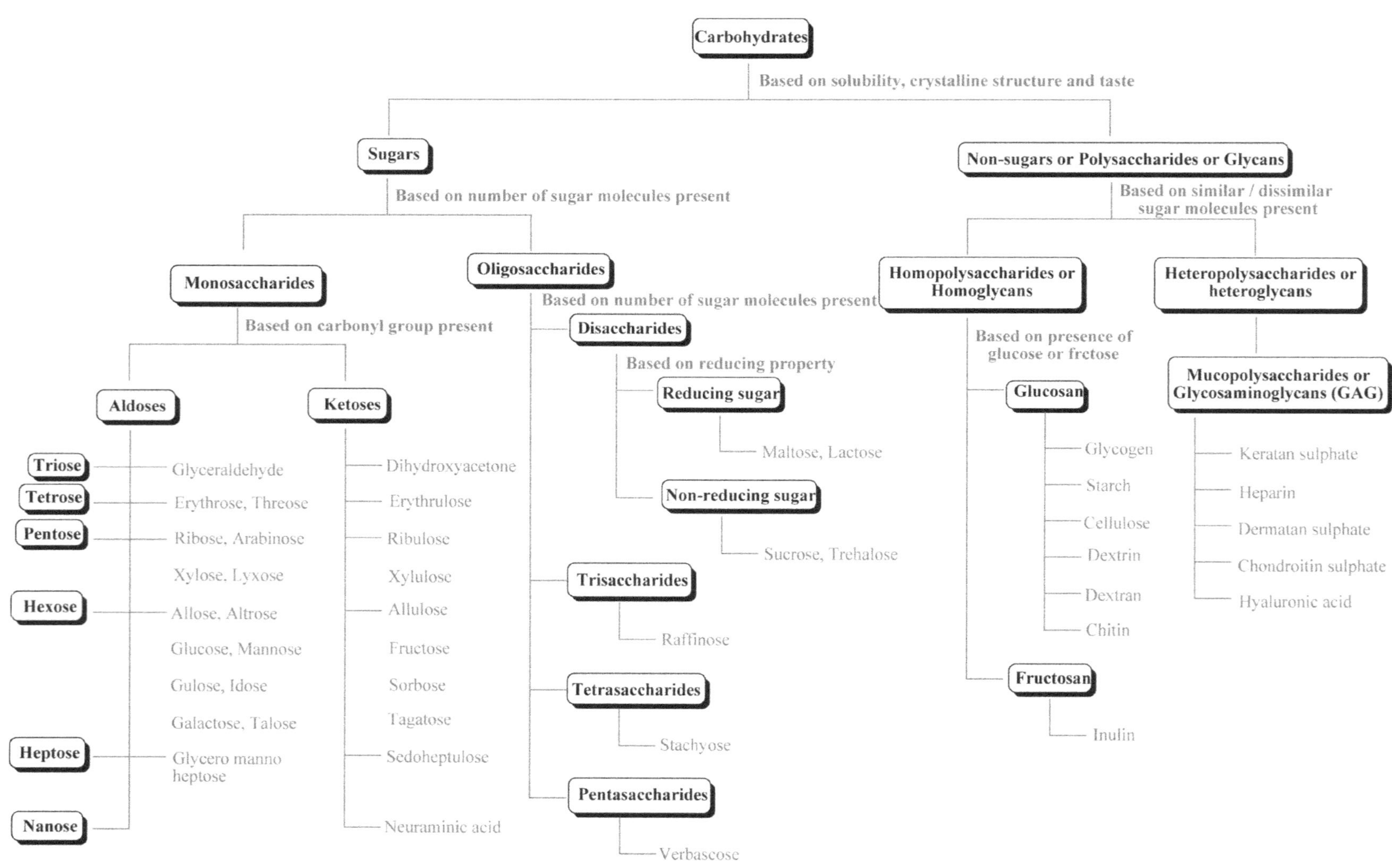

Carbohydrates
Based on solubility, crystalline structure and taste
Sugars
Based on number of sugar molecules present
Monosaccharides
Based on carbonyl group present
Aldoses
Triose
Tetrose
Pentose
Hexose
Heptose
Nanose
Glyceraldehyde
Erythrose, Threose
Ribose, Arabinose
Xylose, Lyxose
Allose, Altrose
Glucose, Mannose
Gulose, Idose
Galactose, Talose
Glycero manno heptose
Ketoses
Dihydroxyacetone
Erythrulose
Ribulose
Xylulose
Allulose
Fructose
Sorbose
Tagatose
Sedoheptulose
Neuraminic acid
Oligosaccharides
Based on number of sugar molecules present
Disaccharides
Based on reducing property
Reducing sugar
Maltose, Lactose
Non-reducing sugar
Sucrose, Trehalose
Trisaccharides
Raffinose
Tetrasaccharides
Stachyose
Pentasaccharides
Verbascose
Non-sugars or Polysaccharides or Glycans
Based on similar / dissimilar sugar molecules present
Homopolysaccharides or Homoglycans
Based on presence of glucose or frctose
Glucosan
Glycogen
Starch
Cellulose
Dextrin
Dextran
Chitin
Fructosan
Inulin
Heteropolysaccharides or heteroglycans
Mucopolysaccharides or Glycosaminoglycans (GAG)
Keratan sulphate
Heparin
Dermatan sulphate
Chondroitin sulphate
Hyaluronic acid

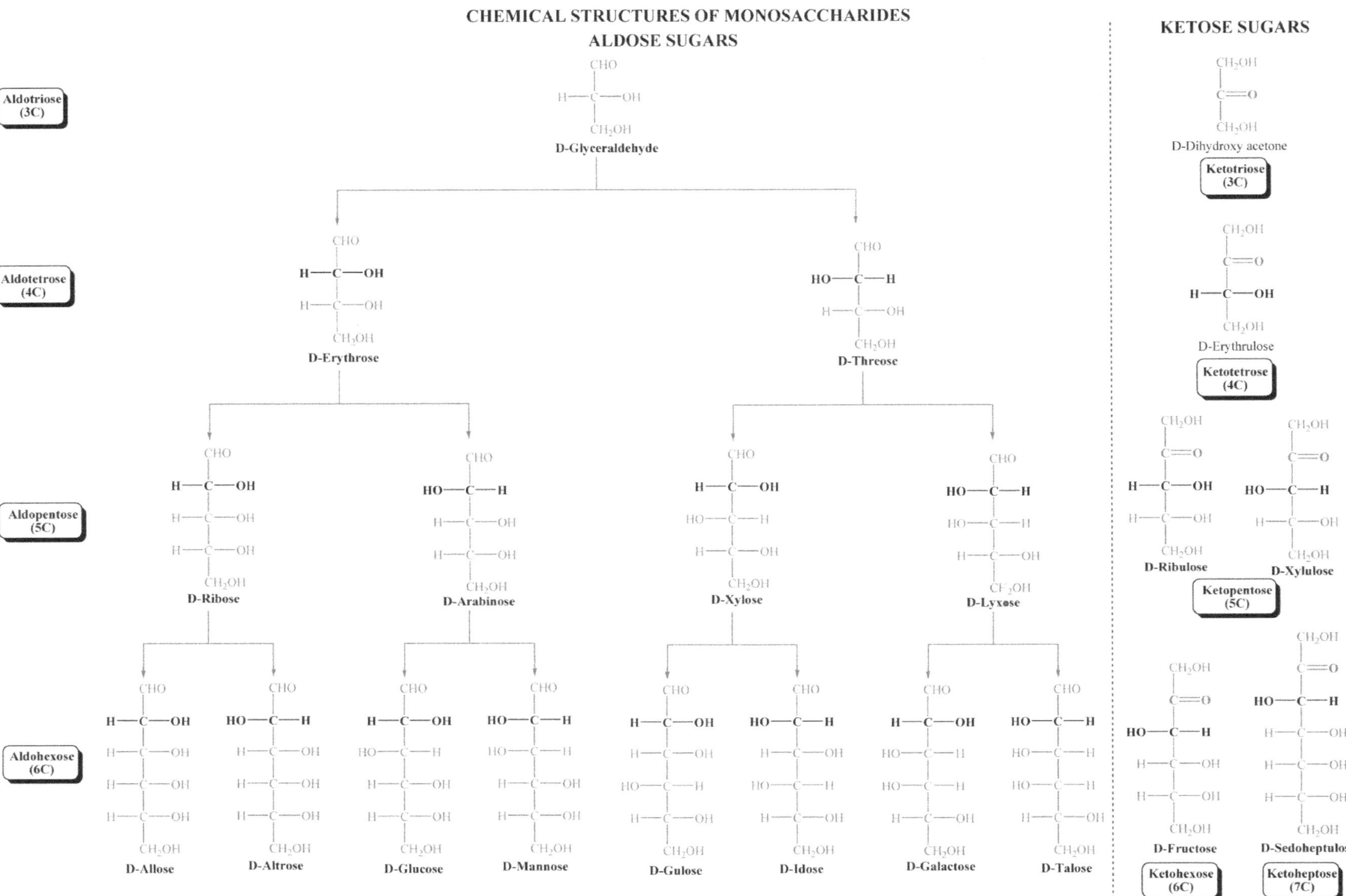
CHEMICAL STRUCTURES OF MONOSACCHARIDES
ALDOSE SUGARS
Aldotriose (3C)
D-Glyceraldehyde
Aldotetrose (4C)
D-Erythrose
D-Threose
Aldopentose (5C)
D-Ribose
D-Arabinose
D-Xylose
D-Lyxose
Aldohexose (6C)
D-Allose
D-Altrose
D-Glucose
D-Mannose
D-Gulose
D-Idose
D-Galactose
D-Talose
KETOSE SUGARS
D-Dihydroxy acetone
Ketotriose (3C)
D-Erythrulose
Ketotetrose (4C)
D-Ribulose
D-Xylulose
Ketopentose (5C)
D-Fructose
Ketohexose (6C)
D-Sedoheptulose
Ketoheptose (7C)

CHEMICAL STRUCTURES OF DISACCHARIDES

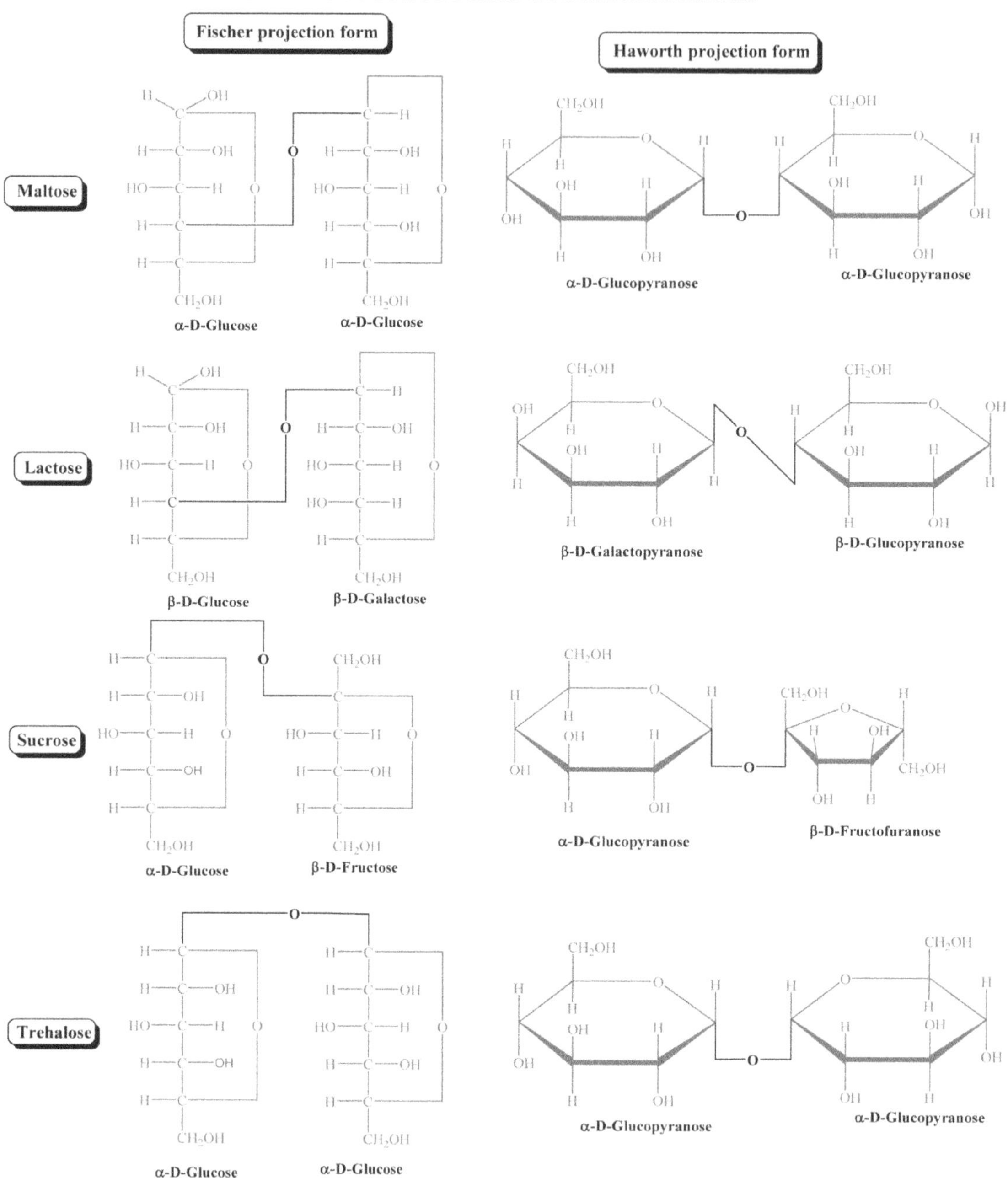

Chemical Nature

The followings are some important structural aspects of carbohydrates particularly monosaccharides. They are,

1. Stereoisomerism (D- & L-isomers)
2. Optical activity
3. Configuration of D-aldoses and D-Ketoses
4. Epimers
5. Enantiomers & Diastereomers
6. Anomers
7. Mutarotation

1. **Stereoisomerism:**

The important characteristic of monosaccharides is stereoisomerism. Compounds possessing same molecular formula, but different structural formula are termed as stereoisomer. Asymmetric or chiral carbon is defined as carbon attached to four different atoms or groups. The number of possible isomers (2^n) of given compound is determined from the number of chiral carbon (n) present. Four asymmetric carbons are present in glucose, hence 16 isomers are possible.

D- & L-isomers: The spatial arrangement of hydrogen (-H) and hydroxyl (-OH) group on the carbon atom that is adjacent to the terminal primary alcohol carbon (penultimate carbon or in glucose it is C-5 or in glyceraldehyde it is C-2) will determine whether the monosaccharide is D- or L-isomer. In D-isomer the hydroxyl (-OH) group is present in right side whereas in L-isomer the hydroxyl (-OH) group is present in left side. The simplest asymmetric carbon possessing monosaccharide is glyceraldehyde. Hence, it is chosen as reference monosaccharide to represent all other monosaccharides structure. The D- and L-isomers are mirror images of each other. In mammalian tissue, the naturally occurring monosaccharide are mostly D-isomers only. In addition, D-series of monosaccharide is specifically metabolized by the enzyme machinery of the cell.

```
H—C=O
H—C—OH
  CH2OH
```
D-Glyceraldehyde

```
H—C=O
OH—C—H
   CH2OH
```
L-Glyceraldehyde

```
H—C=O
H—C—OH
HO—C—H
H—C—OH
H—C—OH
  CH2OH
```
D-Glucose

```
H—C=O
HO—C—H
H—C—OH
HO—C—H
HO—C—H
   CH2OH
```
L-Glucose

2. **Optical activity:**

The characteristic feature of the asymmetric carbon is optical activity. The optical isomers rotate the plane polarized light into either right side or left side. When normal light (disperse in all direction) is passed into nickel prism it will be converted in to plane polarized light (disperse in only one direction). If optical isomers rotate the plane polarized light into right side, it is known as dextrorotatory compound and is denoted by the symbol "d or +", whereas if optical isomers rotate the plane polarized light into left side, it is known as levorotatory compound and is denoted by the symbol "l or -". Generally, based on the structural relationship with glyceraldehyde optical isomers are denoted as D(+), D(-), L(+) and L(-). Racemic mixture contains equal amount of d- and l-isomers and does not exhibit any optical activity because dextrorotatory and levorotatory activities cancel each other. The term dextrose is used for glucose solution in medical practice because of dextrorotatory nature of glucose.

3. **Configuration of D-aldoses and D-ketoses:**

The configurations of various D-aldoses are mentioned by increasing the chain length by one carbon atom at a time in Kiliani Fischer synthesis. Among various aldoses, the most predominant which occurs in nature is glucose.

There are five D-ketoses which are physiologically important are D-erythrulose, D-ribulose, D-xylulose, D-fructose and D-sedoheptulose. The configuration of various D-aldoses and D-ketoses are mentioned under chemical structures of monosaccharides.

4. **Epimers:**

Epimers are defined as two compounds differing from each other around a single specific carbon (other than anomeric carbon) in their configuration. The reaction involving interconversions of epimers is known as epimerization and the enzyme involved is *epimerase*. **Example:** Glucose and mannose (C-2 epimer because they differ in their configuration around C-2); Glucose and galactose (C-4 epimer because they differ in their configuration around C-4).

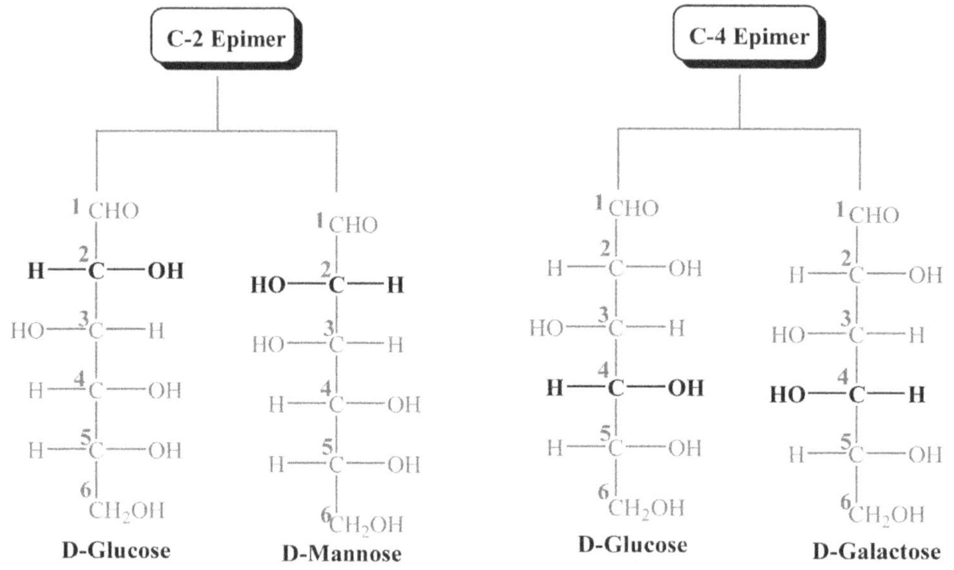

C-2 Epimer: D-Glucose, D-Mannose

C-4 Epimer: D-Glucose, D-Galactose

5. **Enantiomers & Diastereomers:**

Enantiomers: The stereoisomers which are mirror images of each other are known as enantiomers. The D- and L-isomers are mirror images of each other, hence they are enantiomers. **Example:** D-Glucose and L-glucose.

Diastereomers: The stereoisomers which are not mirror images of each other are known as diastereomers. **Example:** D-Glucose and D-mannose.

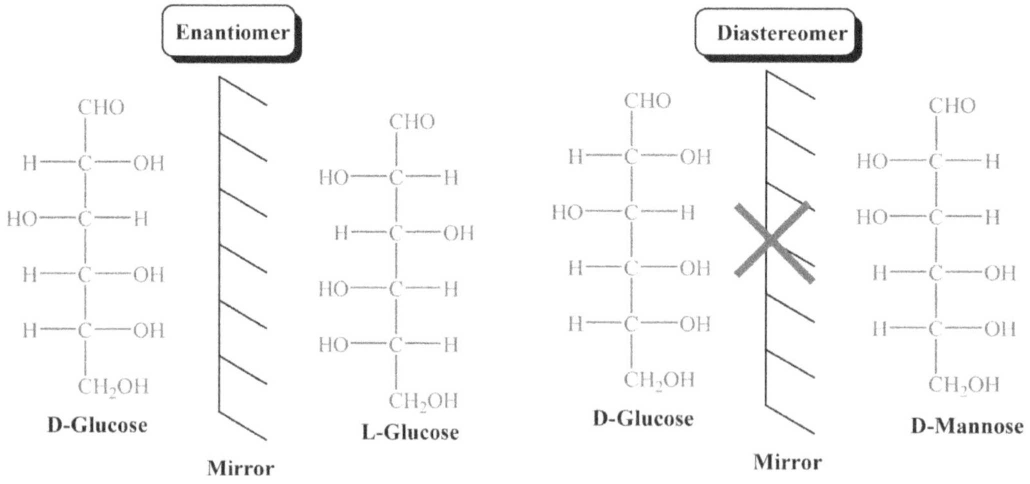

Enantiomer: D-Glucose, Mirror, L-Glucose

Diastereomer: D-Glucose, Mirror, D-Mannose

6. **Anomers:**

Two isomers differ from each other around a single specific carbon i.e., anomeric carbon in their configuration is known as anomers. Anomeric carbon is the functional group carbon atom which is involved in the formation of hemiacetal or hemiketal. Simply the two isomers differing only in the configuration of C-1 (in aldoses) or C-2 (in ketoses) are known as anomers, while such a carbon atom is known as anomeric carbon atom. **Example:** The α-and β-cyclic forms of D-glucose. In Haworth ring structure of D-glucose if the hydroxyl (-OH) group of anomeric carbon is present on the opposite side to the terminal primary alcoholic (-CH_2OH) group then it is known as α-D-glucose. Similarly, if the hydroxyl (-OH) group of anomeric carbon is present on the same side to the terminal primary alcoholic (-CH_2OH) group then it is known as β-D-glucose.

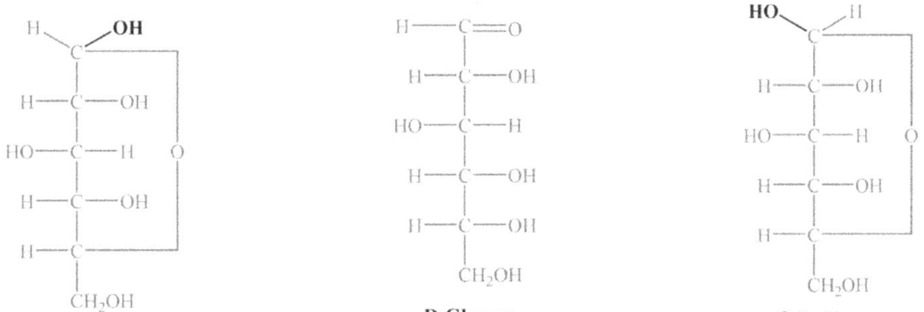

α-D-Glucose

D-Glucose
(Open chain form)

β-D-Glucose

Fischer projection: Anomeric form of D-glucose

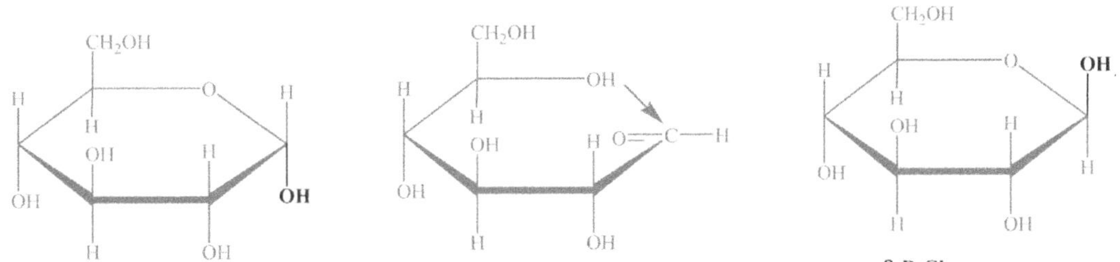

α-D-Glucopyranose

D-Glucose
(Acyclic form)

β-D-Glucopyranose

Haworth projection: Anomeric forms of D-glucose

7. **Mutarotation:**

Two distinct configurations (α and β) of the hemiacetals and hemiketals can occur when the cyclic structure open and re-closes due to the rotation of carbon atom bearing the reactive carbonyl group. The carbon atom which is involved in this rotation is known as anomeric carbon and the obtained two forms are termed as anomers. Mutarotation is defined as the change in specific optical rotation representing the interconversion of α- and β-forms to an equilibrium mixture.

Example: The specific optical rotation of freshly prepared solution of α-D-glucose and β-D-glucose in water is + 112.2 ° and + 18.7 ° respectively. But the specific optical rotation of both α-D-glucose and β-D-glucose gradually changes and attains equilibrium with a constant value of + 52.7 ° due to mutarotation of glucose. The equilibrium mixture contains 36 % of α-D-glucose, 63 % of 7-D-glucose and 1 % of open chain form.

	α-D-Glucose	⇌	Equilibrium mixture	⇌	β-D-Glucose
Specific optical rotation	+ 112.2 °		+ 52.7 °		+ 18.7 °

Chemical Reactions of Monosaccharides

The monosaccharide contains two or more hydroxyl groups with either aldehyde or ketone functional group. Hence, they give most of the reactions but not all the reactions of the carbonyl group as well as of the alcoholic group. In addition, in the same molecule as it contains alcoholic and carbonyl group, they may give typical reactions. The various chemical reactions of monosaccharide are,

1. Enolization or tautomerization
2. Reducing properties
3. Dehydration
4. Epimerization
5. Reduction

6. Oxidation
7. Osazone formation
8. Ester formation
9. Glycoside formation

1. **Enolization or tautomerization:**

   Tautomerization is defined as the shifting of hydrogen from one carbon to adjacent carbon oxygen to form enediol. Generally, carbohydrates undergo enolization in presence of strong alkali such as sodium hydroxide and the anomeric carbon atom is involved in this reaction. The enediols are highly reactive, hence monosaccharide in alkaline solution are powerful reducing agent. In presence of dilute alkali or amines, sugars undergo rearrangement to form a mixture of more than one sugar. **Example:** In the presence of very dilute alkali (0.02 N sodium hydroxide), glucose is converted into a mixture of glucose, mannose and fructose. This is due to the formation of common enediol for all three sugars. This reaction is known as Lobry de Bruyn-van Ekenstein rearrangement.

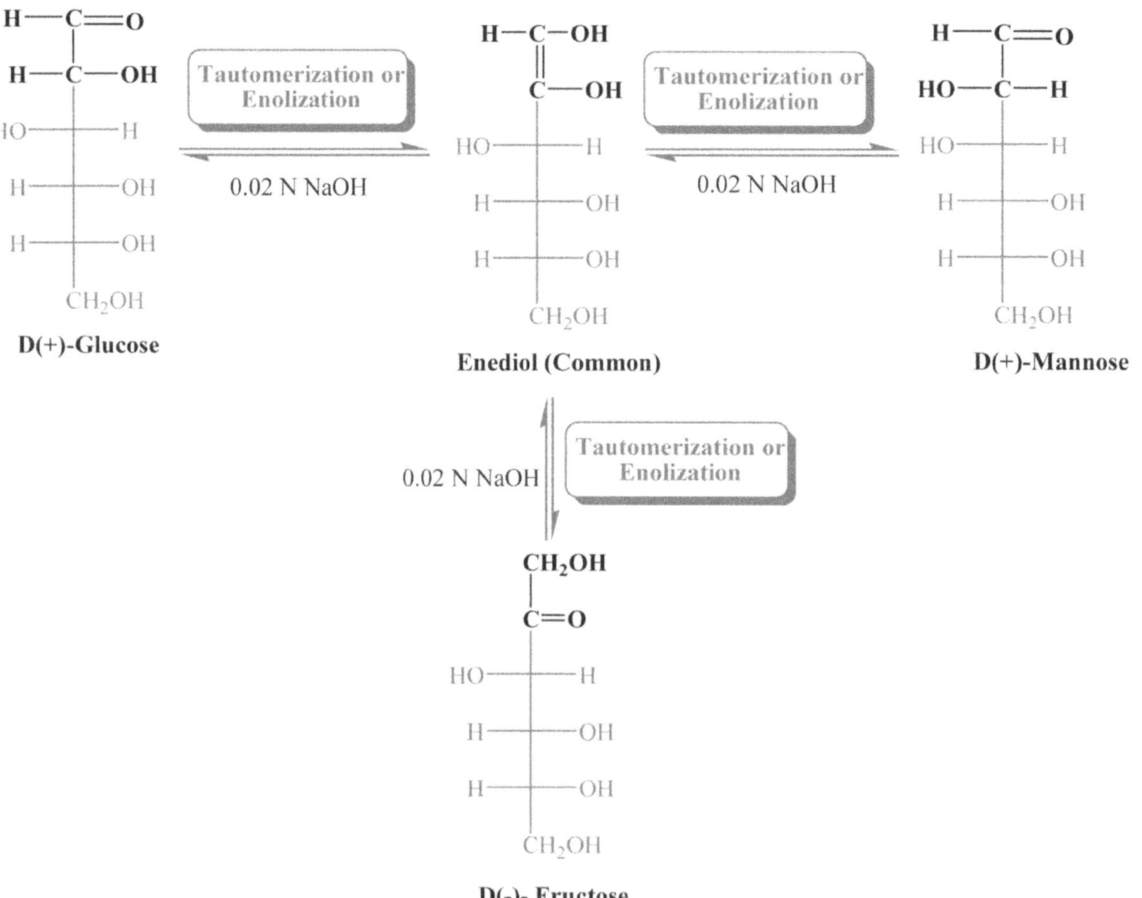

2. **Reducing properties:**

   The reducing properties of sugar is due to formation of enediol in the presence alkali. Free carbonyl group like aldehyde or ketone is necessary for the formation of enediol. Hence, sugars possessing free aldehyde or ketone group reduces cupric ion (Cu^{+2}) of copper sulphate into cuprous ion (Cu^{+}). These sugars are called as reducing sugars. This is the basic principle involved in reducing sugar tests such as Benedict's test, Fehling's test, Barfoed's test, etc. A non-reducing sugar lacks free carbonyl group like aldehyde or ketone and hence, it cannot reduces cupric ion (Cu^{+2}) of copper sulphate into cuprous ion (Cu^{+}).

Reducing sugar

Alkali

Enediol Sugar acid

$CuSO_4$ **Copper sulphate** → Cu^{2+} **Cupric ion** → Cu^{+} **Cuprous ion** → (H_2O) 2 CuOH **Cupric hydroxide (Yellow colour)** → ($- H_2O$) Cu_2O **Cuprous oxide (Red colour)**

3. Dehydration:

Monosaccharide undergoes dehydration and loses three molecules of water when it is treated with dehydrating agents like concentrated sulphuric acid. In general, on dehydration hexose sugars form hydroxymethyl furfural and pentoses form furfural. Thus the formed hydroxymethyl furfural or furfural forms complex with phenolic compounds like α-naphthol and produces colored complex. This is the principle behind most popular Molisch test. Oligosaccharides and polysaccharides initially produce monosaccharide by hydrolysis in the presence of concentrated sulphuric acid and then it undergoes dehydration.

D-Glucose → Dehydration, Conc. H_2SO_4, $- 3\ H_2O$ → **Hydroxymethyl furfural** → Phenolic compound (α-Naphthol), Complexation → **Violet or purple colour complex**

D-Ribose → Dehydration, Conc. H_2SO_4, $- 3\ H_2O$ → **Furfural** → Phenolic compound (α-Naphthol), Complexation → **Violet or purple colour complex**

4. Epimerization:

In a molecule containing several asymmetric centers, conversion of one epimer into other epimer or the process of inversion of configuration at one asymmetric centre is known as epimerization. Epimers are defined as two compounds differing from each other around a single specific carbon (other than anomeric carbon) in their configuration. In general aldose is converted into its epimer via aldonic acid (**Example:** Gluconic acid and mannaonic acid) in presence of bromine water and pyridine at 150 °C.

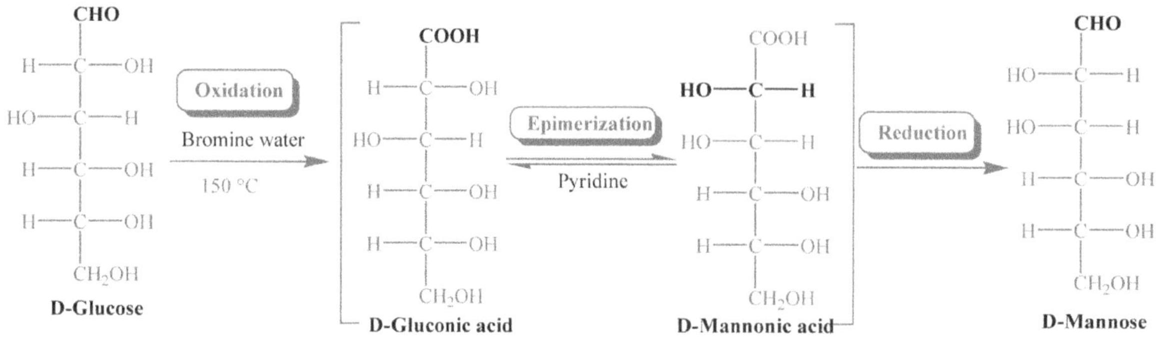

D-Glucose → Oxidation (Bromine water, 150 °C) → [D-Gluconic acid ⇌ Epimerization (Pyridine) ⇌ D-Mannonic acid] → Reduction → D-Mannose

5. **Reduction:**

Monosaccharides are reduced to corresponding alditols by electrolytic reduction, high pressure hydrogenation over a nickel or copper chromite catalyst, or sodium borohydride. In these type of reductions an aldose gives only one type of alcohol (**Example:** Glucose gives sorbitol and mannose gives mannitol), whereas due to the introduction of a new asymmetric carbon atom (shown by asterisk) a ketose gives a mixture of two alcohols (**Example:** Fructose gives a mixture of sorbitol and mannitol). The reason behind is two different configurations of a new asymmetric carbon.

If monosaccharides undergo reduction in presence of hydroiodic acid and red phosphorus it converts hydroxyl groups into methylene group.

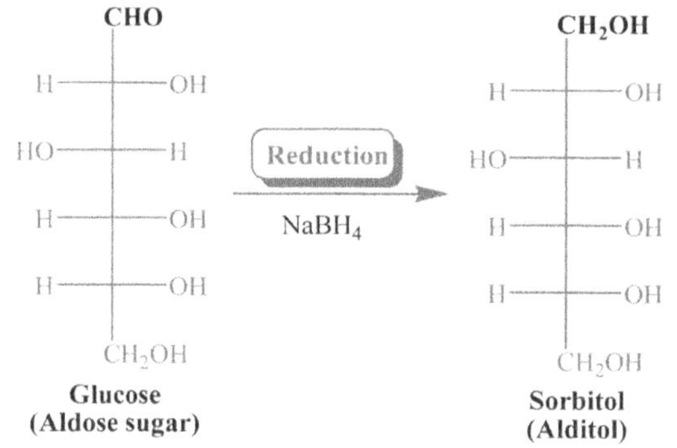

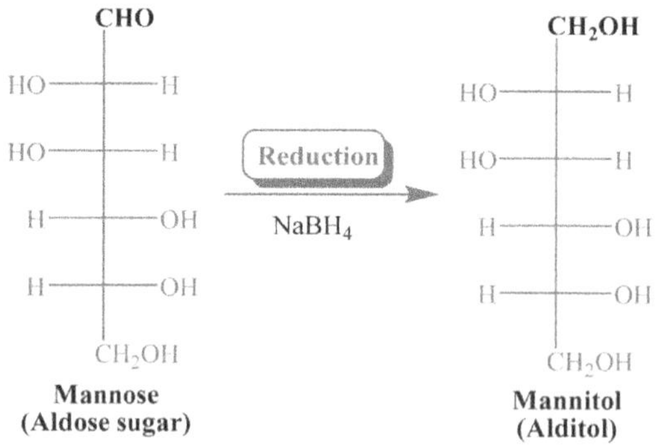

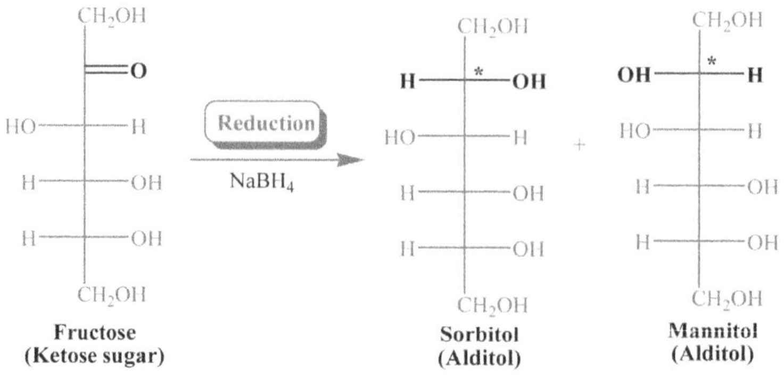

Glucose (Aldose sugar) → Reduction ($NaBH_4$) → Sorbitol (Alditol)

Mannose (Aldose sugar) → Reduction ($NaBH_4$) → Mannitol (Alditol)

Fructose (Ketose sugar) → Reduction ($NaBH_4$) → Sorbitol (Alditol) + Mannitol (Alditol)

6. **Oxidation:**
Monosaccharide undergoes oxidation and produce variety of products depending on the nature of oxidizing agents used. Various important oxidizing agents used and their corresponding oxidized products are listed in Table 3.1.

Table 3.1 List of oxidizing agents and their corresponding oxidized products.

S. No.	Oxidizing agents used	Products formed
1	Benedict's, Fehling's and Tollen's reagent (Mild oxidizing agents)	Aldoses are oxidized to corresponding aldonic acid (aldehyde group oxidized to acid group) and α-hydroxy ketoses are oxidized to corresponding α-hydroxy ketonic acid (Primary alcohol oxidized to acid group).
2	Bromine water (Mild oxidizing agent)	Aldoses are oxidized to corresponding aldonic acid (aldehyde group oxidized to acid group) and ketoses are not oxidized. Stable δ-lactone is obtained on evaporation of aldonic acid. Original aldose can be obtained when lactone is reduced with sodium-amalgam (Na/Hg) in the presence of a trace of acid. The lactone may also be reduced to alcohol by adding aqueous lactone to aqueous sodium borohydride whereas ketoses are not oxidized by bromine water.
3	Nitric acid (Strong oxidizing agent)	Aldoses are oxidized to corresponding dicarboxylic acid known as aldaric acid (both aldehyde and primary alcohol group oxidized to acid group). Ketoses are oxidized to mixture of acids having fewer carbon atoms.
4	Lead tetraacetate and periodic acid (Strong oxidizing agent)	It oxidizes the 1,2-glycolic portions of the monosaccharide molecules with the cleavage of the C-C bond. Between every two 1,2-glycolic groups, one molecule of the reagent is consumed. For convenient handling, periodic acid is more preferred than lead tetraacetate.

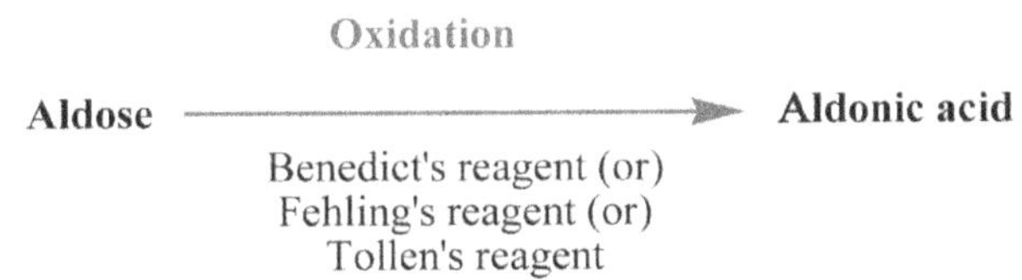

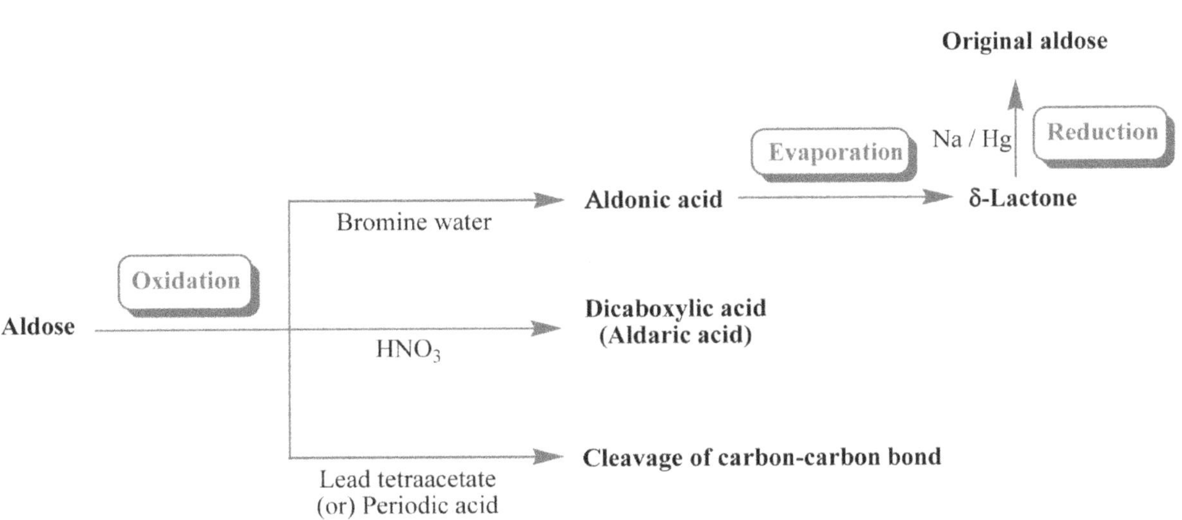

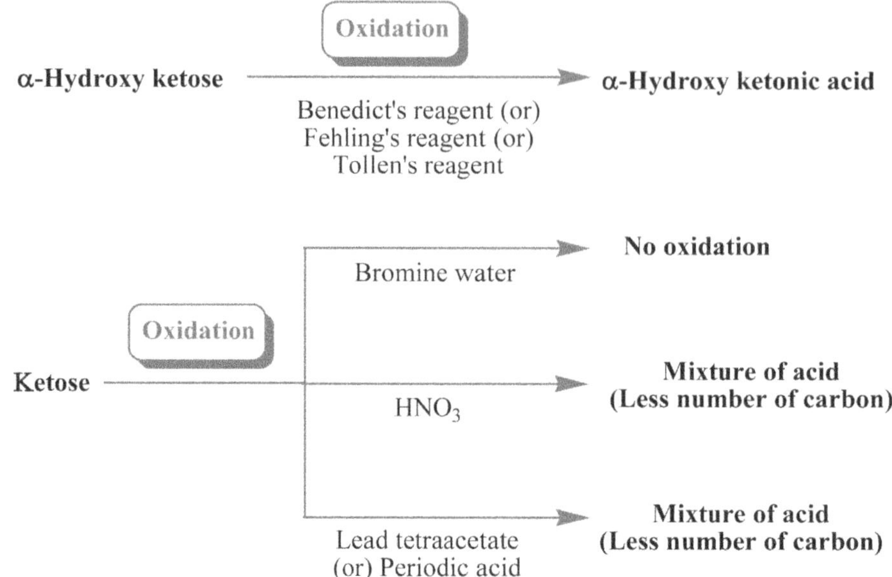

7. **Osazone formation:**

In general carbonyl group reacts with one molecule of hydroxylamine and forms corresponding aldoxime or ketoxime. But aldoses and ketoses react with three molecules of phenylhydrazine in acetic acid to yield osazones, through phenylhydrazones. Generally, all reducing monosaccharides and disaccharides form osazones (**Example:** Maltose produce sunflower shaped crystals and lactose produce powder puff shaped crystals). The first two carbons are involved in the formation of osazone. Hence, sugars differ in these carbons form same osazone. **Example:** Glucose, fructose and mannose produce needle shaped crystals.

Glucose $\xrightarrow[-H_2O]{\text{Dehydration},\ C_6H_5NHNH_2}$ Glucose phenylhydrazone $\xrightarrow[-C_6H_5NH_2,\ -NH_3]{\text{Oxidation},\ C_6H_5NHNH_2}$ Phenylhydrazone of glucosone $\xrightarrow[-H_2O]{\text{Dehydration},\ C_6H_5NHNH_2}$ Glucosazone

Fructose $\xrightarrow[-H_2O]{\text{Dehydration},\ C_6H_5NHNH_2}$ Fructose phenylhydrazone $\xrightarrow[-C_6H_5NH_2,\ -NH_3]{\text{Oxidation},\ C_6H_5NHNH_2}$ Phenylhydrazone of fructosone $\xrightarrow[-H_2O]{\text{Dehydration},\ C_6H_5NHNH_2}$ Fructosazone

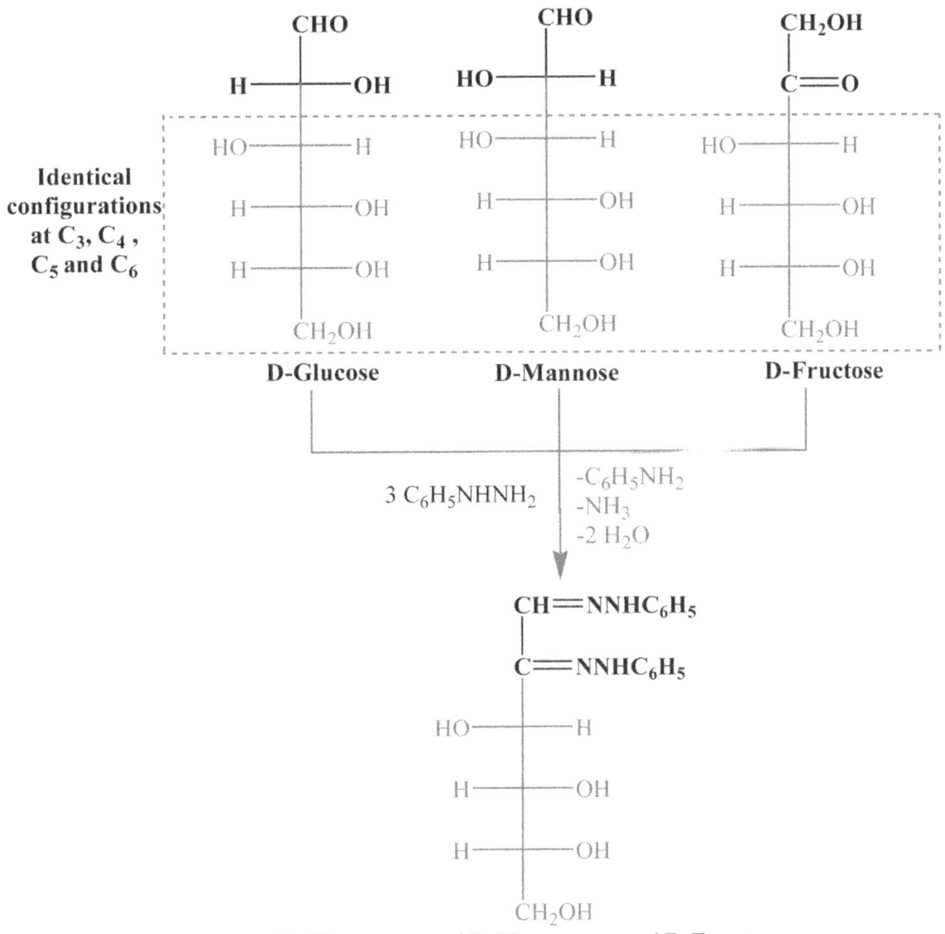

D-Glucosazone / D-Mannosazone / D-Fructosazone
(Needle shaped crystals)

8. **Ester formation:**
The alcoholic group of monosaccharides undergoes esterification either enzymatically or non-enzymatically. The common reaction in metabolism is esterification of carbohydrates with phosphoric acid. In general ATP donates the phosphate moiety for esterification. **Example:** Formation of glucose-6-phosphate form glucose and ATP in presence of *glucokinase* or *hexokinase*.

Esterification
ATP → ADP
Glucokinase (GK) or *Hexokinase (HK)*
Mg^{2+}

Glucose → $CH_2—O—PO_3^{2-}$ (or) $CH_2—O—PO(OH)_2$ (or) $CH_2—O—Ⓟ$

Glucose
Glucose-6-phosphate

9. **Glycoside formation:**
Hemiacetal or hemiketal hydroxyl group of one carbohydrate reacts with a hydroxyl group of other carbohydrates or a non-carbohydrate (**Example:** Methyl alcohol, phenol and glycerol) and forms glycosides. Thus the formed bond is known as glycosidic bond, the non-carbohydrate moiety is referred as aglycone and the carbohydrate moiety is referred as gly**cone. Disaccharides, oligosaccharides and polysaccharides are formed from monosaccharides held together by glycosidic bonds.**

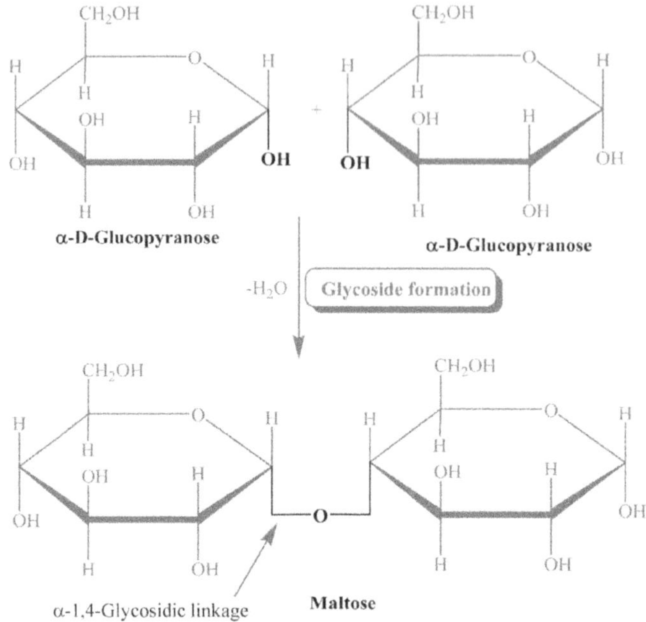

Biological Significance of Carbohydrates

1. For all organism carbohydrates are the principal dietary source of energy (4 Cal/g).
2. Carbohydrates are used as a precursor for the synthesis of many organic compounds like fats and amino acids. Degradation products of carbohydrates act as "promoters" or "catalysts".
3. In the form of glycoprotein and glycolipids carbohydrates participate in the cell membrane structure and important cellular functions like cell growth, adhesion and fertilization.
4. For many organism carbohydrates are the structural components including cellulose fiber of plants, exoskeleton of some insects and the cell wall of microorganisms.
5. The immediate energy demands of the biological systems are satisfied by carbohydrates as glycogen (storage form of energy).
6. To the mammals except ruminant, glucose is the most important energy source of carbohydrates.
7. In medicinal practice dextrose is frequently used.
8. Erythrocytes and brain cells utilize glucose solely for energy purposes.
9. Glucose can be converted to glycogen (storage form of energy), galactose (component of lactose) and ribose (nucleic acid component).
10. High concentration of fructose is present in the semen which produces energy for motility of sperms. Sperms utilize fructose for energy. Fructose is formed in the seminiferous tubular epithelial cells from glucose.
11. Large amount of maltose present in several food preparations particularly baby foods are produced by hydrolysis of grains. Disaccharides are easily digestible from the nutritional point of view.
12. The lactose is synthesized from glucose in lactating mammary gland by the duct epithelium. For the newborn baby good source of energy is lactose present in breast milk.
13. A non-pathogenic *Coliform bacillus (E. coli)* usually ferments lactose, whereas pathogenic *Typhoid bacillus* does not ferment lactose generally. This test is used to distinguish two microorganisms.
14. *E. coli* and *A. aerogenes* present in milk converts milk to lactic acid in many organisms.
15. Osmotic condition of the blood is changed when sucrose is administered parentrally which causes flow of water from the tissues into blood.
16. Inulin a homoglycans composed of fructose is used in estimation of GFR (Glomerular filtration rate) to assess the renal function. It is also used for the estimation of body water i.e., ECF (extra cellular fluid).

17. Heparin is a mucopolysaccharide used as anticoagulant.
18. Cellulose is non-digestible carbohydrates which decrease the intestinal absorption of glucose and cholesterol thereby increases bulk of faeces. Hence, cellulose is used to avoid constipation.
19. In joints the mucopolysaccharide hyaluronic acid act as shock absorbent and lubricant.
20. Hyaluronidase is an enzyme present in semen that degrades the gel (contains hyaluronic acid) present around ovum. Hence, it may lead to effective penetration of sperm into the ovum.
21. The solutions of dextrin are used as "mucilages".
22. The solution of dextran having molecular weight approximately 75,000 has been used as plasma expander.
23. In constipation, agar is used as laxative and agar is used in agar plate for culture medium preparation.
24. Certain derivatives of carbohydrates are used as drugs. **Example:** Cardiac glycosides like digoxin and digitoxin and antibiotics like aminoglycosides and streptomycin.
25. Antifreeze glycoprotein present in antarctic fish is responsible for their survival below -2 °C.
26. Derangement of glucose metabolism is seen in diabetes mellitus, glycogen storage diseases and galactosemia.
27. Certain pathological conditions such as cataract, nephropathy is due to the accumulation of sorbitol and dulcitol in the tissues.

Metabolism of Carbohydrates

All major pathways of carbohydrate metabolism relate to glucose. Hence, glucose is the central molecule of carbohydrate metabolism. The various other important monosaccharides involved in carbohydrate metabolism are fructose, galactose and mannose. Overview of carbohydrate metabolism is presented in Figure 3.1 & Table 3.2.

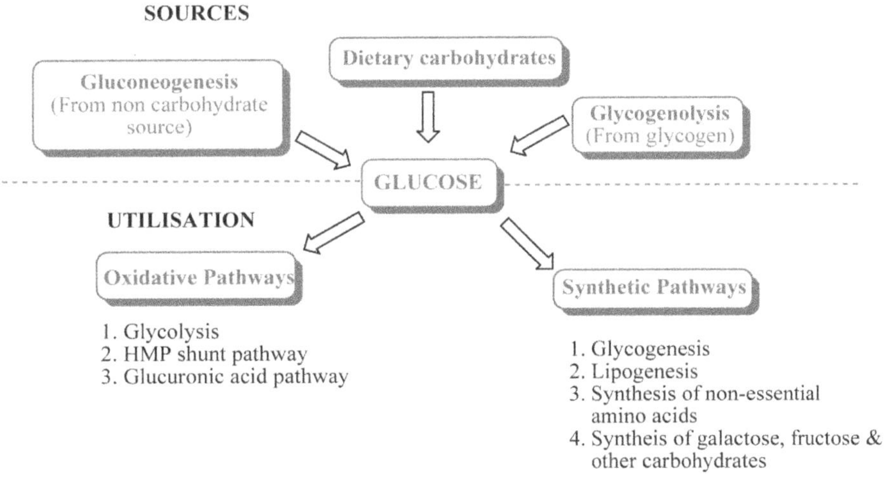

Figure 3.1 Overview of carbohydrate metabolism.

Transport of Glucose

Compared to blood glucose concentration (< 100 mg/dl), cell glucose concentration is very low. Even though, glucose is not entered the cell by simple diffusion (Movement from high concentrated area to low concentrated area without energy and carrier molecule). Glucose is transported into the cell by the following two specific transport system.

1. **Insulin independent transport system:** This transport system of glucose is not dependent on hormone insulin. This transport system comes under the category of facilitated diffusion (Movement from high concentrated area to low concentrated area without energy using specific carrier molecule i.e., glucose transporters or GLUT). There are five different glucose transporters (GLUT-1, GLUT-2, GLUT-

3, GLUT-4 and GLUT-5) identified in cell membranes. In hepatocytes, brain and erythrocytes, glucose is transported by this transport system. In erythrocytes, GLUT-1 is abundantly present.

2. **Insulin dependent transport system:** This transport system of glucose is dependent on hormone insulin. This transport system also comes under the category of facilitated diffusion like insulin independent transport system. In muscles and adipose tissue, glucose is transported by this transport system. In skeletal muscle and adipose tissue, GLUT-4 is abundantly present. In skeletal muscle and adipose tissue, insulin increases and promotes the activity of GLUT-4. Transport of glucose in cell by facilitated diffusion is presented in Figure 3.2.

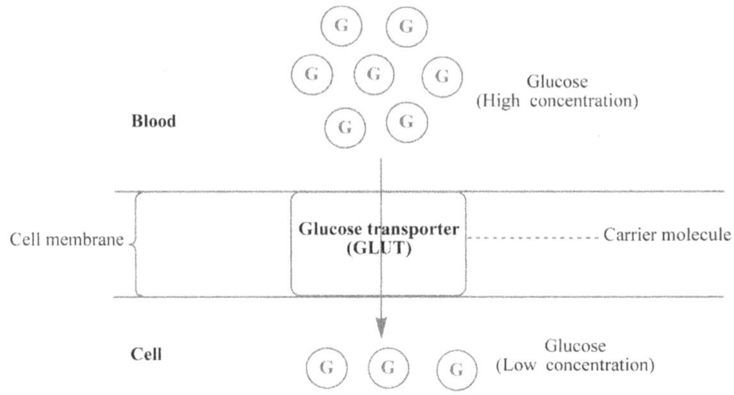

Figure 3.2 Transport of glucose in cell by facilitated diffusion.

Table 3.2 Overview of carbohydrate metabolism.

S. No.	Name of the pathway	Definition	Schematic representation
1.	Glycolysis or Embden Meyerhof pathway or EM pathway	Oxidation of glucose or glycogen into pyruvate or lactate with the production of ATP	Glucose / Glycogen → (Oxidation) → Pyruvate / Lactate + n ATP
2.	Kreb's cycle or Citric acid cycle or Tri carboxylic acid cycle or TCA cycle	Oxidation of acetyl CoA to carbon dioxide with the production of ATP	Acetyl CoA → (Oxidation) → CO_2 + n ATP
3.	Glycogenesis	Formation of glycogen from glucose	Glucose + n ATP → (Synthesis) → Glycogen

Table 3.2 Contd...

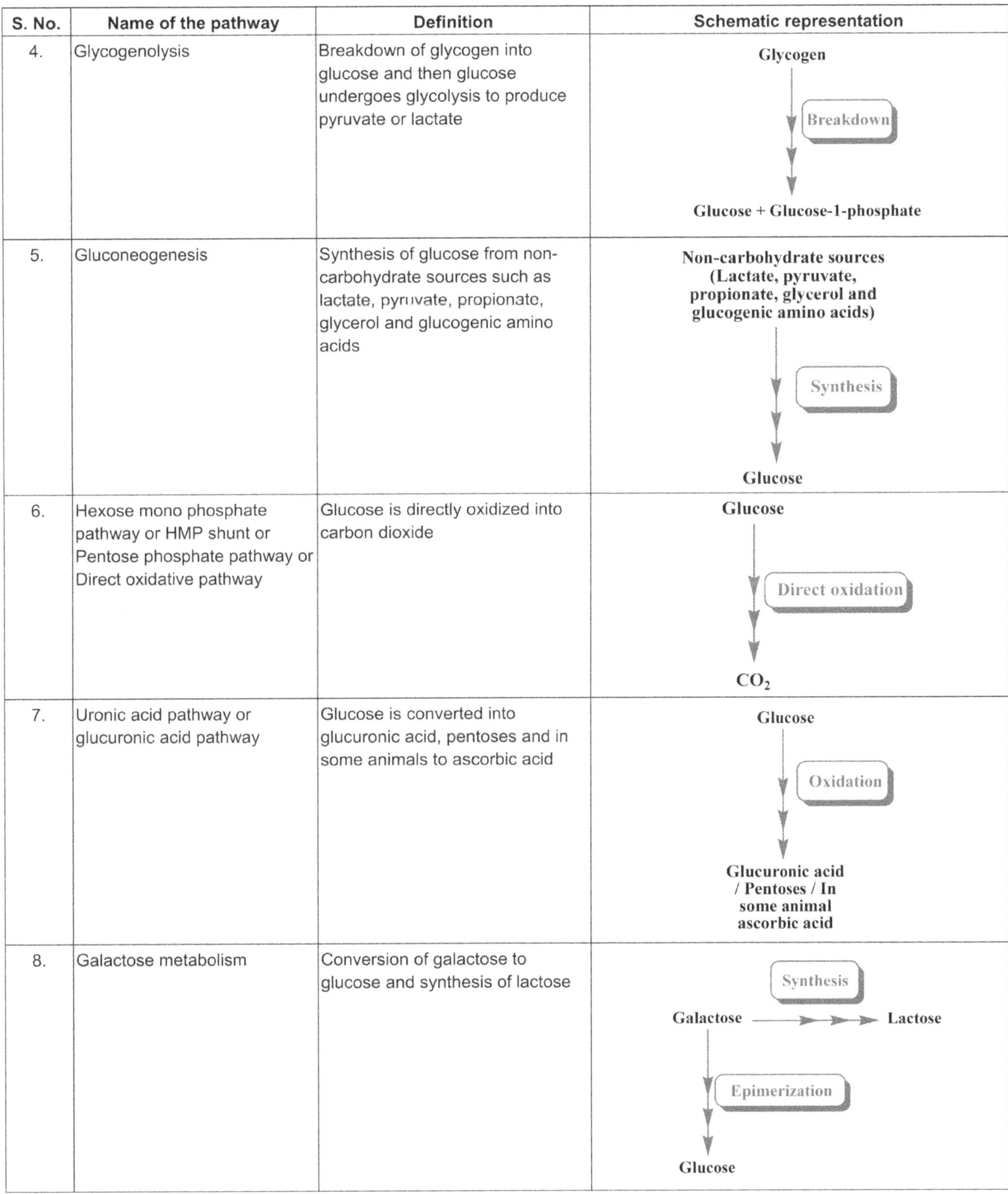

S. No.	Name of the pathway	Definition	Schematic representation
4.	Glycogenolysis	Breakdown of glycogen into glucose and then glucose undergoes glycolysis to produce pyruvate or lactate	Glycogen → (Breakdown) → Glucose + Glucose-1-phosphate
5.	Gluconeogenesis	Synthesis of glucose from non-carbohydrate sources such as lactate, pyruvate, propionate, glycerol and glucogenic amino acids	Non-carbohydrate sources (Lactate, pyruvate, propionate, glycerol and glucogenic amino acids) → (Synthesis) → Glucose
6.	Hexose mono phosphate pathway or HMP shunt or Pentose phosphate pathway or Direct oxidative pathway	Glucose is directly oxidized into carbon dioxide	Glucose → (Direct oxidation) → CO_2
7.	Uronic acid pathway or glucuronic acid pathway	Glucose is converted into glucuronic acid, pentoses and in some animals to ascorbic acid	Glucose → (Oxidation) → Glucuronic acid / Pentoses / In some animal ascorbic acid
8.	Galactose metabolism	Conversion of galactose to glucose and synthesis of lactose	Galactose → (Synthesis) → Lactose; Galactose → (Epimerization) → Glucose

Table 3.2 Contd...

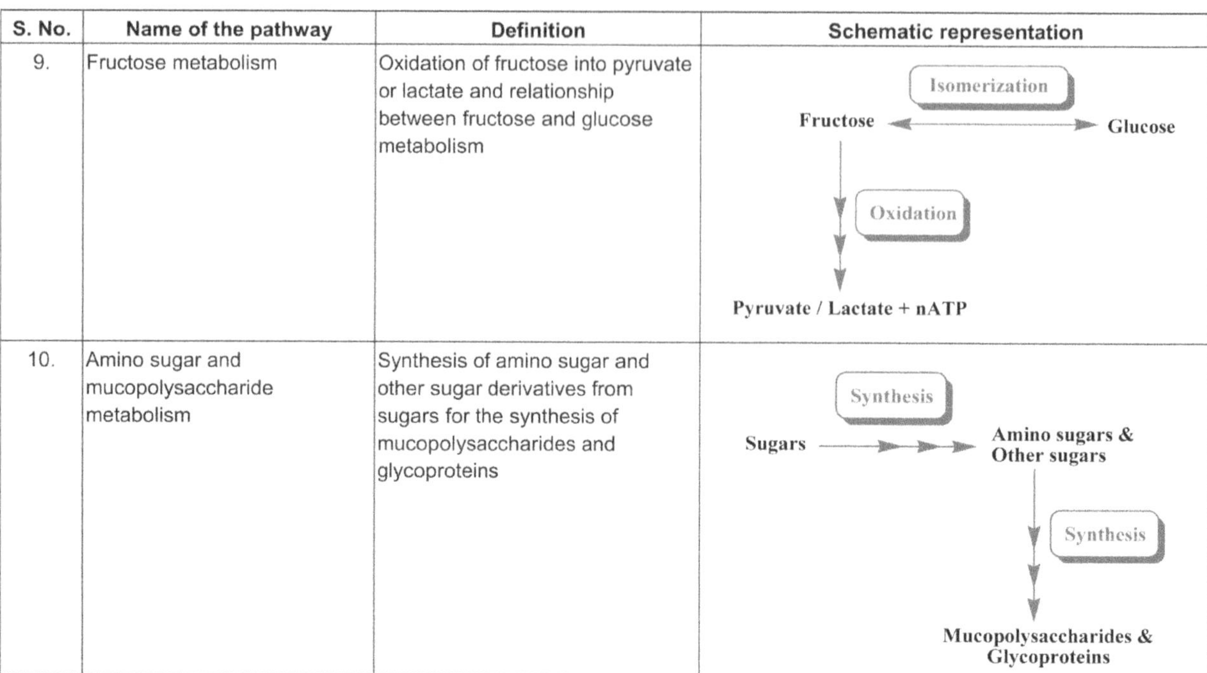

S. No.	Name of the pathway	Definition	Schematic representation
9.	Fructose metabolism	Oxidation of fructose into pyruvate or lactate and relationship between fructose and glucose metabolism	Fructose ⟷ Glucose (Isomerization); Fructose → Pyruvate / Lactate + nATP (Oxidation)
10.	Amino sugar and mucopolysaccharide metabolism	Synthesis of amino sugar and other sugar derivatives from sugars for the synthesis of mucopolysaccharides and glycoproteins	Sugars → Amino sugars & Other sugars (Synthesis); Amino sugars & Other sugars → Mucopolysaccharides & Glycoproteins (Synthesis)

GLYCOLYSIS

Definition: In Greek glycose means "sugar or sweet" and lysis means "dissolution or breakdown". Hence glycolysis means "breakdown or dissolution of sugar or sweet". It is also known as *Embden-Meyerhof pathway* or EM pathway. **Glycolysis is defined as "A series of chemical reactions taking place in biological system which converts glucose or glycogen into pyruvate or lactate with the production of energy".**

$$\text{Glucose or Glycogen} \xrightarrow{\text{Biological System}} \text{Pyruvate or Lactate} + \text{n ATP}$$

Glycolysis takes place in all the cells of the body and the necessary enzymes are present in cytosol fraction of the cell. Various intermediates produced in glycolysis are useful for the synthesis of several non-essential amino acids and glycerol (which is useful for formation of fat). Glucose can be synthesized from lactate or pyruvate (Reverse of glycolysis) by making alternate arrangements at three irreversible steps of glycolysis and the process is known as gluconeogenesis.

Types: Glycolysis can take place either in the presence or in the absence of oxygen. Based on this there are two different types of glycolysis.

1. **Aerobic glycolysis:** It takes place in presence of oxygen and the end product is pyruvate. The aerobic glycolysis can be summarized as follows.

$$\textbf{Glucose} + 2\ NAD^+ + 2\ ADP + 2\ Pi \longrightarrow \textbf{2 Pyruvate} + 2\ NADH + 2\ H^+ + 2\ ATP$$

2. **Anaerobic glycolysis:** It takes place in absence of oxygen and the end product is lactate. The anaerobic glycolysis can be summarized as follows.

$$\textbf{Glucose} + 2\ ADP + 2\ Pi \longrightarrow \textbf{2 Lactate} + 2\ ATP$$

Pathway

There are three important stages in glycolysis as a) Priming stage or Energy investment stage, b) Splitting stage c) Energy generation stage.

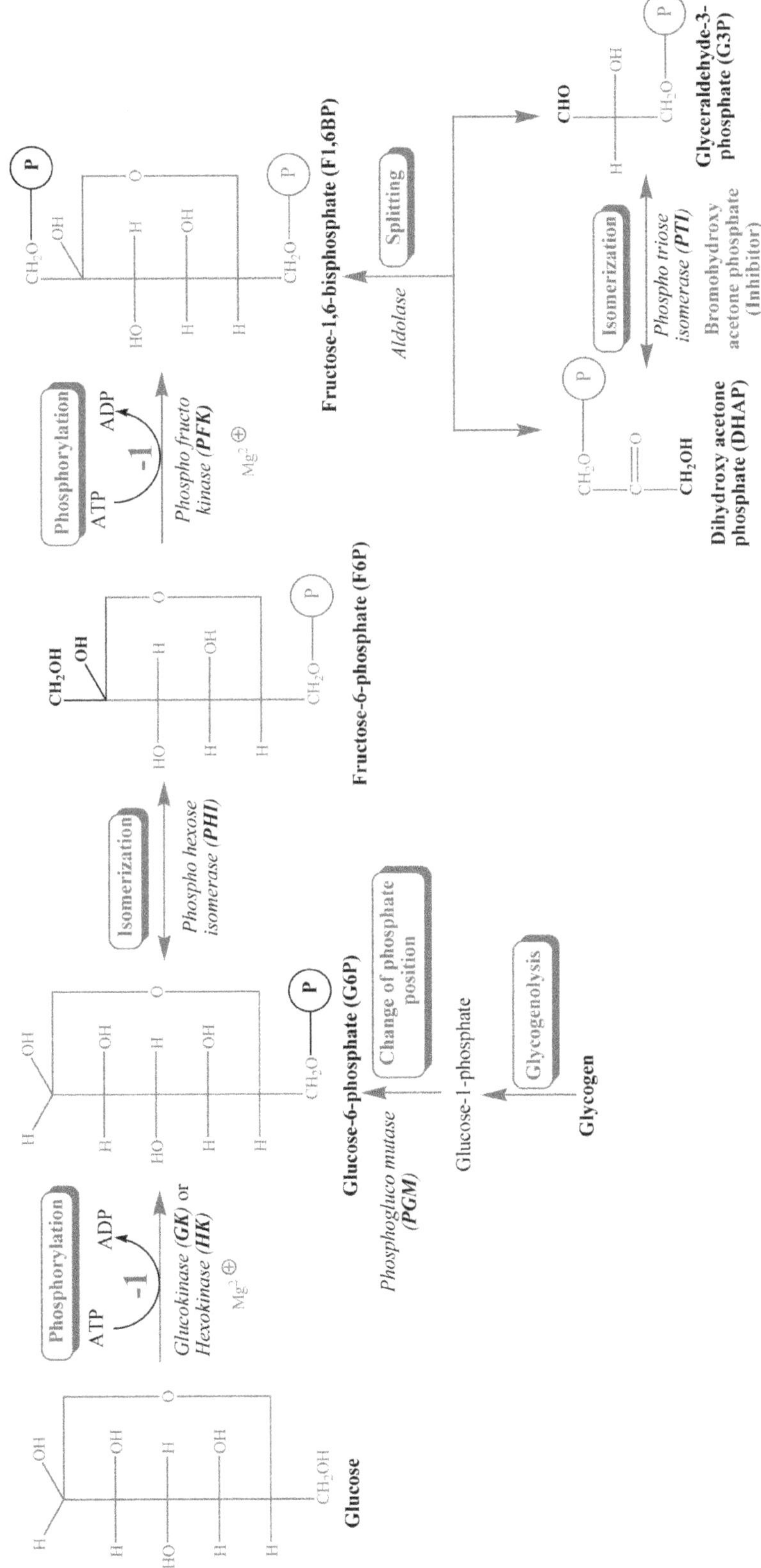
Glucose
Phosphorylation
ATP
ADP
-1
Glucokinase (GK) or Hexokinase (HK)
Mg2+ ⊕
Glucose-6-phosphate (G6P)
Phosphogluco mutase (PGM)
Change of phosphate position
Glucose-1-phosphate
Glycogenolysis
Glycogen
Isomerization
Phospho hexose isomerase (PHI)
Fructose-6-phosphate (F6P)
Phosphorylation
ATP
ADP
-1
Phospho fructo kinase (PFK)
Mg2+ ⊕
Fructose-1,6-bisphosphate (F1,6BP)
Splitting
Aldolase
Dihydroxy acetone phosphate (DHAP)
Isomerization
Phospho triose isomerase (PTI)
Bromohydroxy acetone phosphate (Inhibitor)
Glyceraldehyde-3-phosphate (G3P)

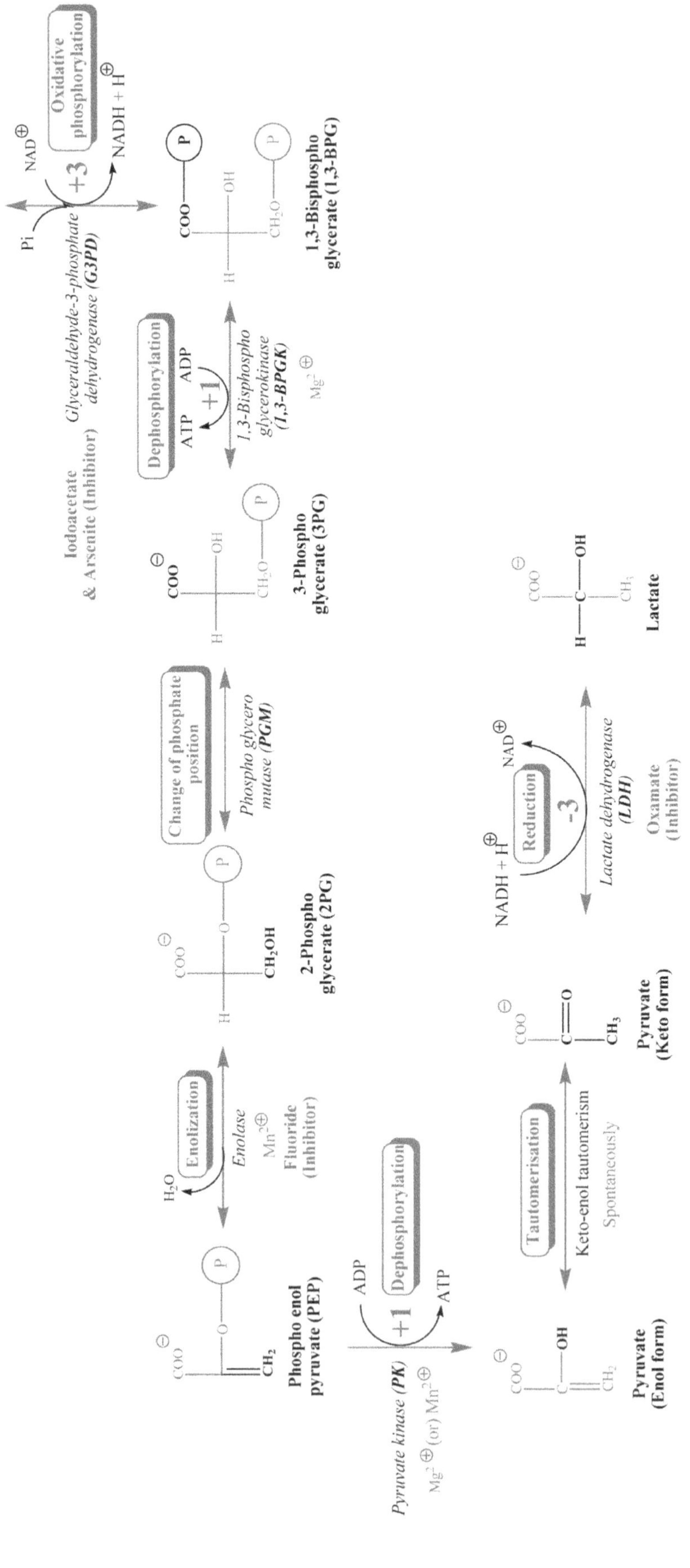

Pi
NAD⊕
Iodoacetate
& Arsenite (Inhibitor)
*Glyceraldehyde-3-phosphate dehydrogenase (**G3PD**)*
+3
Oxidative phosphorylation
NADH + H⊕

1,3-Bisphospho glycerate (1,3-BPG)

Dephosphorylation
ATP ADP
+1
*1,3-Bisphospho glycerokinase (**1,3-BPGK**)*
Mg^{2}⊕

3-Phospho glycerate (3PG)

Change of phosphate position
*Phospho glycero mutase (**PGM**)*

2-Phospho glycerate (2PG)

H_2O
Enolization
Enolase
Mn^{2}⊕
Fluoride (Inhibitor)

Phospho enol pyruvate (PEP)

ADP
*Pyruvate kinase (**PK**)*
Mg^{2}⊕(or) Mn^{2}⊕
+1
Dephosphorylation
ATP

Pyruvate (Enol form)

Tautomerisation
Keto-enol tautomerism
Spontaneously

Pyruvate (Keto form)

NADH + H⊕
Reduction
NAD⊕
-3
*Lactate dehydrogenase (**LDH**)*
Oxamate (Inhibitor)

Lactate

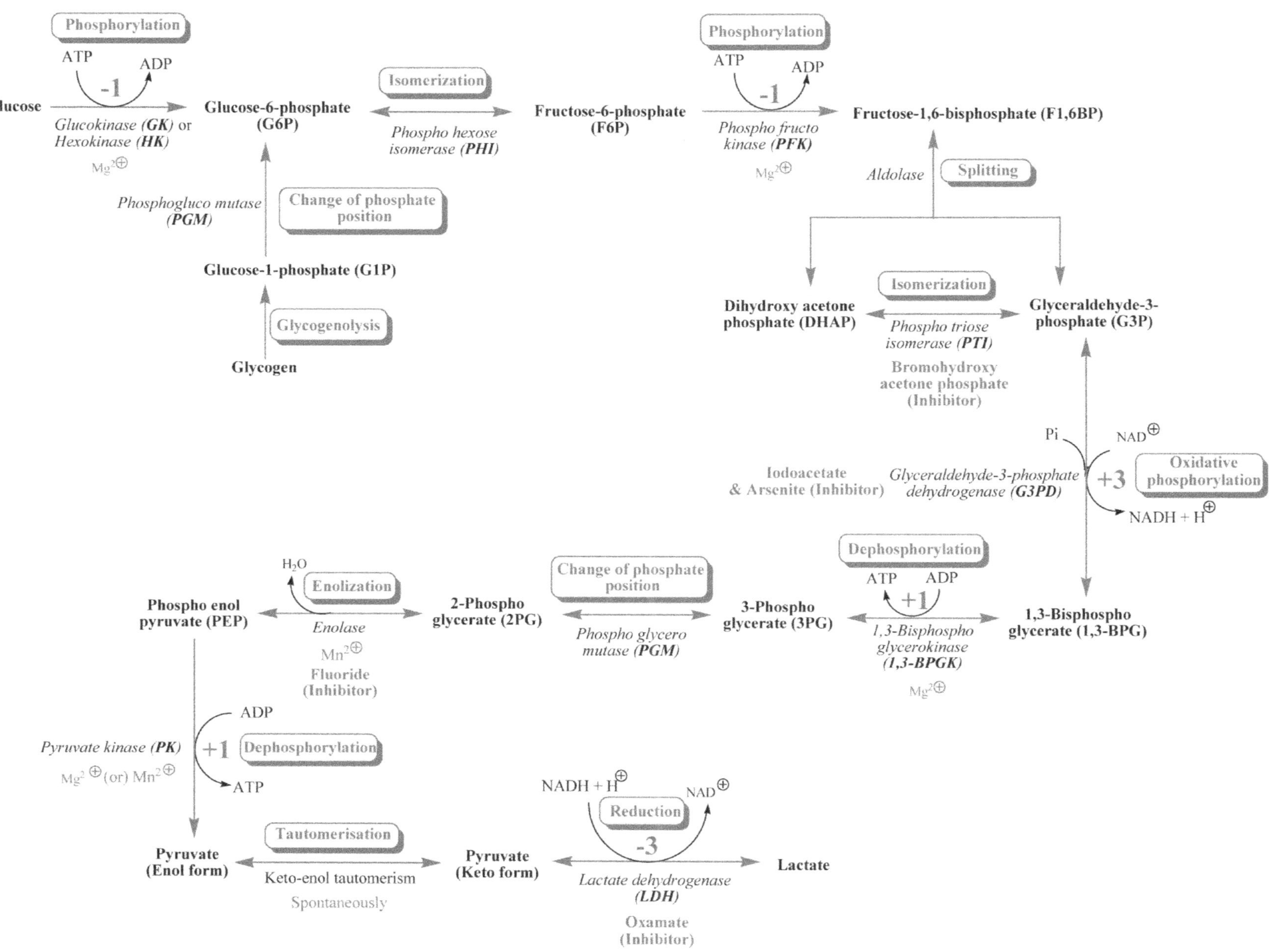
Phosphorylation
ATP
ADP
-1
Glucose
Glucokinase (GK) or Hexokinase (HK)
Mg2⊕
Glucose-6-phosphate (G6P)
Isomerization
Phospho hexose isomerase (PHI)
Fructose-6-phosphate (F6P)
Phosphorylation
ATP
ADP
-1
Phospho fructo kinase (PFK)
Mg2⊕
Fructose-1,6-bisphosphate (F1,6BP)
Aldolase
Splitting
Phosphogluco mutase (PGM)
Change of phosphate position
Glucose-1-phosphate (G1P)
Glycogenolysis
Glycogen
Isomerization
Dihydroxy acetone phosphate (DHAP)
Phospho triose isomerase (PTI)
Bromohydroxy acetone phosphate (Inhibitor)
Glyceraldehyde-3-phosphate (G3P)
Pi
NAD⊕
Iodoacetate & Arsenite (Inhibitor)
Glyceraldehyde-3-phosphate dehydrogenase (G3PD)
+3
Oxidative phosphorylation
NADH + H⊕
Dephosphorylation
ATP
ADP
+1
1,3-Bisphospho glycerokinase (1,3-BPGK)
Mg2⊕
1,3-Bisphospho glycerate (1,3-BPG)
3-Phospho glycerate (3PG)
Change of phosphate position
Phospho glycero mutase (PGM)
2-Phospho glycerate (2PG)
H2O
Enolization
Enolase
Mn2⊕
Fluoride (Inhibitor)
Phospho enol pyruvate (PEP)
ADP
+1
Dephosphorylation
ATP
Pyruvate kinase (PK)
Mg2⊕ (or) Mn2⊕
Pyruvate (Enol form)
Tautomerisation
Keto-enol tautomerism
Spontaneously
Pyruvate (Keto form)
NADH + H⊕
NAD⊕
Reduction
-3
Lactate dehydrogenase (LDH)
Oxamate (Inhibitor)
Lactate

(a) Priming stage or Energy investment stage

1. The first step in glycolysis is a simple phosphorylation reaction. In this step glucose is phosphorylated at 6th position in the presence of enzyme called "*hexokinase* (*HK*) or *glucokinase* (*GK*)" (In ATP / GTP involved reactions, the enzymes acted are "*kinase*" and the substrate is "glucose" which is a "hexose" sugar) and produces glucose-6-phosphate (G6P). *Kinase* enzyme needs magnesium ion (Mg^{2+}) as co-factor for its activity. **This step is the first irreversible step of glycolysis.** In this step one ATP is converted into ADP **(1 ATP is utilized)**.
2. Glucose-1-phosphate (G1P) is the product of glycogenolysis obtained from glycogen. Further, phosphate group present in 1st position of glucose-1-phosphate is shifted to 6th position and produces glucose-6-phosphate (G6P). The enzyme responsible is *phospho gluco mutase* (*PGM*) (In change of position of phosphate group involved reactions, the enzymes acted are "*mutase*" and the substrate is "glucose-1-phosphate").
3. In the next step glucose-6-phosphate (G6P) is isomerized into fructose-6-phosphate (F6P) by "*phospho hexose isomerase* (*PHI*)" (glucose-6-phosphate and fructose-6-phosphate are "phospho hexose sugar" and the reaction involved is "isomerization").
4. **This is the second irreversible step of glycolysis.** Like first step, fructose-6-phosphate (F6P) undergoes phosphorylation at 1st position and produces fructose-1,6-bisphosphate (F1,6BP) in the presence of "*phospho fructo kinase* (*PFK*)" (In ATP / GTP involved reactions, the enzymes acted are "*kinase*" and the substrate is "fructose-6-phospha**te").** One ATP is converted into ADP in this step **(1 ATP utilized).**

(b) Splitting stage

5. Dihydroxy acetone phosphate (DHAP) and glyceraldehyde-3-phosphate (G3P) are formed from fructose-1,6-bisphosphate (F1,6BP) by splitting reaction using "*aldolase*" enzyme. In this step 6 carbon fructose-1,6-bisphosphate is broken into two 3 carbon containing compounds (Dihydroxy acetone phosphate (DHAP) and glyceraldehyde-3-phosphate (G3P)). DHAP and G3P are functional isomers like glucose and fructose. These two are interconvertible by "*phospho triose isomerase* (*PTI*)" enzyme (Dihydroxy acetone phosphate (DHAP) and glyceraldehyde-3-phosphate (G3P) are "phospho triose sugar" and the reaction involved is "isomerization") There is no role for dihydroxy acetone phosphate (DHAP) except its conversion into glyceraldehyde-3-phosphate (G3P).

(c) Energy generation stage

6. Glyceraldehyde-3-phosphate (G3P) undergoes oxidative phosphorylation by reacting with inorganic phosphate and produces 1,3-bisphospho glycerate (1,3BPG). *Glyceraldehyde-3-phosphate dehydrogenase* (*G3PD*) enzyme (In NAD^+ / $NADP^+$ / FAD involved reactions, the enzymes acted are "*dehydrogenase*" and the substrate is "glyceraldehyde-3-phosphate") catalyzes this step. During this reaction one molecule of NAD^+ is reduced to NADH + H^+ **(3 ATP generated)**.
7. In the next step 1,3-bisphospho glycerate (1,3BPG) produced 3-phospho glycerate (3PG) by dephosphorylation reaction in presence of *phospho glycero kinase* (*PGK*) (In ATP / GTP involved reactions, the enzymes acted are "*kinase*" and the substrate is "1,3-bisphospho glycerate"). One ADP is converted into ATP in this step **(1 ATP generated)**.
8. Further, phosphate group present in 3rd position of 3-phospho glycerate (3PG) is shifted to 2nd position and produces 2-phospho glycerate (2PG). The enzyme responsible is *phospho glycero mutase* (*PGM*) (In change of position of phosphate group involved reactions, the enzymes acted are "*mutase*" and the substrate is "3-phospho glycerate").
9. In the succeeding step, 2-phospho glycerate (2PG) produces phospho enol pyruvate (PEP) by enolization reaction in the presence of *enolase* (In reverse reaction, "enol" is the substrate and type of reaction is "hydrolysis"). *Enolase* needs magnesium ion (Mg^{2+}) as co-factor for its activity.
10. In the next step phospho enol pyruvate (PEP) undergoes dephosphorylation and produces pyruvate in enol form in the presence of *pyruvate kinase* (*PK*) (In ATP / GTP involved reactions,

the enzymes acted are "*kinase*" and the product formed is "pyruvate"). One ADP is converted into ATP in this step **(1 ATP generated). This step is the third irreversible step of glycolysis.**

11. Spontaneously pyruvate is converted into its keto form by keto-enol tautomerism from enol form. Pyruvate is the end product of aerobic glycolysis.
12. In absence of oxygen, pyruvate is converted into lactate with the help of *lactate dehydrogenase (LDH)* (In NAD^+ / $NADP^+$ / FAD involved reactions, the enzymes acted are "*dehydrogenase*" and the product is "lactate"). During this reaction one molecule of NADH + H^+ is oxidized to NAD^+ **(3 ATP utilized)**. Lactate is the end product of anaerobic glycolysis.

Regulation:

The three irreversible steps regulate glycolysis i.e., *hexokinase* (*HK*) or *glucokinase* (*GK*), *phospho fructo kinase* (*PFK*) and *pyruvate kinase* (*PK*). These three enzymes are rate limiting enzymes of glycolysis. Bromohydroxy acetone phosphate inhibits *phospho triose isomerase* (*PTI*); iodo acetate and arsenite inhibits *glyceraldehyde-3-phosphate dehydrogenase* (*G3PD*); fluoride inhibits *enolase* and oxamate inhibits *lactate dehydrogenase* (*LDH*).

Importance / Significance:

1. In the absence of oxygen, glycolysis is an emergency energy yielding pathway to the cells.
2. It is an important pathway which synthesizes ATP in the tissue lacking mitochondria (**Example:** Erythrocyte, cornea and lens).
3. Glycolysis is also significant for ATP synthesis in some other tissues having a smaller number of mitochondria (**Example:** Kidneys, testes and leucocytes).
4. Glycolysis occurrence is pre-requisite for the aerobic oxidation of carbohydrates which later takes place in the cells having mitochondria.
5. Glycolysis is very essential for brain because it is dependent on glucose for its energy demand. Glucose present in the brain must undergo glycolysis before it is oxidized into carbon dioxide.

Energetics

Energetic of aerobic and aerobic glycolysis are summarized in Table 3.3.

Table 3.3 Energetic of glycolysis.

S. No	Enzyme responsible	Conversion takes place	No. of moles involved	No. of ATP generated or utilized
1	*Hexokinase (HK)* or *glucokinase (GK)*	One ATP is converted into ADP	1	- 1
2	*Phospho fructo kinase (PFK)*	One ATP is converted into ADP	1	- 1
3	*Glyceraldehyde-3-phosphate dehydrogenase (G3PD)*	One NAD^+ is reduced to NADH + H^+ (One NADH + H^+ is equals to 3 ATP)	2	+ 6
4	*Phospho glycero kinase (PGK)*	One ADP is converted into ATP	2	+ 2
5	*Pyruvate kinase (PK)*	One ADP is converted into ATP	2	+ 2
	Net ATP generated in aerobic glycolysis (-1 -1 + 6 + 2 + 2)			**8**
6	*Lactate dehydrogenase (LDH)*	One NADH + H^+ is oxidized to NAD^+ (One NADH + H^+ is equals to 3 ATP)	2	- 6
	Net ATP generated in anaerobic glycolysis (8-6)			**2**

Metabolic disorders:

1. **Pasteur effect:** It is defined as the process of inhibition of glycolysis by oxygen (aerobic condition). It is due to the inhibition of *phospho fructo kinase* (*PFK*) enzyme.
2. **Crabtree effect:** Crabtree effect is basically opposite to Pasteur effect. It is defined as the phenomenon of inhibition of oxygen consumption by the addition of glucose to tissues having high aerobic glycolysis. This effect is due to increased competition of glycolysis for inorganic phosphate and NAD^+ which limits the availability for phosphorylation and oxidation.

CONVERSION OF PYRUVATE TO ACETYL CoA

Pyruvate dehydrogenase (*PDH*) (In NAD^+ / $NADP^+$ / FAD involved reactions, the enzymes acted are "*dehydrogenase*" and the substrate is "pyruvate") is an enzyme which converts pyruvate in to acetyl CoA by oxidative decarboxylation (Both oxidation and decarboxylation takes place). Decarboxylation of pyruvate produces acetaldehyde which on further oxidation produces acetic acid. Finally, acetic acid reacts with coenzyme A and produced acetyl CoA by esterification. One molecule of NAD^+ is reduced to $NADH + H^+$ during this reaction (**3 ATP generated**).

$CH_3—C(=O)—COO^{\ominus}$
Pyruvate

CoASH; $NAD^{\oplus}$
Pyruvate dehydrogenase (***PDH***)
+3 Oxidative decarboxylation
CO_2, H_2O; $NADH + H^{\oplus}$

$CH_3—C(=O)—SCoA$
Acetyl CoA

Cardiac muscle and kidney contain high concentration of *PDH*. It is found only in mitochondria. It is a very good example for multi enzyme complex which requires the following five co-factors for its activity. 1) TPP (Thiamine pyrophosphate); 2) Lipoamide; 3) FAD; 4) Co-enzyme A and 5) NAD^+. Lactic acidosis is observed in patients with inherited deficiency of *PDH* usually after glucose load. Arsenic and mercuric ion binds with sulfhydryl (–SH) groups of lipoic acid; hence it inhibits *PDH* activity.

CITRIC ACID CYCLE

Other Names: 1) TCA (tricarboxylic acid) cycle (First few compounds formed are tricarboxylic acid derivatives like citrate, cis-aconitate, isocitrate and oxalosuccinate), 2) Krebs cycle (In 1937, Hans Adolf Krebs proposed this cycle based on studies of oxygen consumption in pigeon breast muscle. He got noble prize in 1953 in physiology and medicine for this discovery).

Definition: Citric acid cycle is defined as a process of oxidation of acetyl CoA into carbon dioxide with the production of 12 ATPs in a cyclic manner. The first product formed in this cycle is citrate; hence this cycle is known as citric acid cycle.

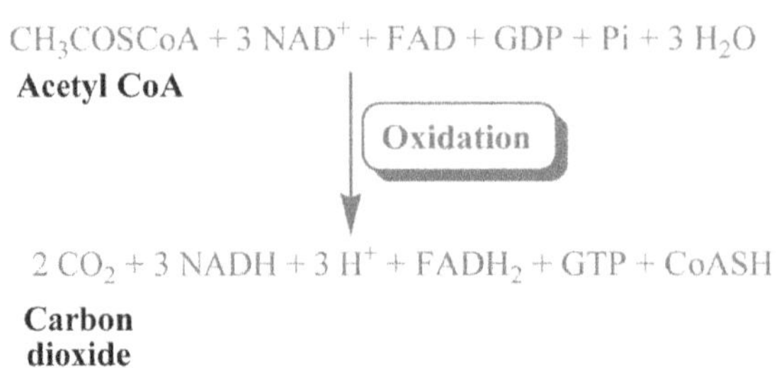

Pathway:

Glycolysis and TCA cycle are linked by oxidative decarboxylation of pyruvate to acetyl CoA. The enzymes necessary for citric acid cycle are present very near to ETC in mitochondrial part of cell. In this pathway a two-carbon acetyl CoA reacts with four-carbon oxaloacetate and produced six-carbon citrate. During pathways, two carbons are oxidized into carbon dioxide and oxaloacetate is regenerated and utilized again. Hence, **oxaloacetate is considered to play catalytic role in TCA cycle**.

1. In the first step, acetyl CoA reacts with oxaloacetate by aldol condensation like reaction and produced tricarboxylic acid citrate with the removal of co-enzyme A. *Citrate synthase* (*CS*) enzyme (The product formed is "citrate" and the type of reaction is "synthesis") catalyzed this step.
2. In the next step, citrate loses one molecule of water (-OH from C-2 and -H from C-1) and produced cis-aconitate by dehydration in presence of *cis-aconitase* (*CA*) (It is reversible reaction. In reverse reaction, substrate is "cis-aconitate" and the type of reaction is "hydrolysis").
3. Further, the cis-aconitate undergoes hydrolysis in the presence of same *cis-aconitase* (*CA*) enzyme and forms isocitrate (In citrate the position of -OH group is C-2; whereas in isocitrate it is C-1. Hence, it is good example for positional isomer).
4. Oxalosuccinate is produced when isocitrate (IC) reacts with reducing equivalent NAD^+ by dehydration reaction. *Isocitrate dehydrogenase* (*ICDH*) (In NAD^+ / $NADP^+$ / FAD involved reactions, the enzymes acted are "*dehydrogenase*" and the substrate is "isocitrate") catalyzes this reaction. During this reaction one molecule of NAD^+ is reduced to NADH + H^+ **(3 ATP generated)**.
5. This step is also catalyzed by *isocitrate dehydrogenase* only. It is a decarboxylation reaction in which C-2 carboxylic (-COOH) group of oxalosuccinate is removed as carbon dioxide and results in formation of α-ketoglutarate **(First carbon dioxide is produced)**.
6. α-Ketoglutarate (α-KG) undergoes oxidative decarboxylation reaction and produces succinyl CoA in presence of *α-ketoglutarate dehydrogenase* (*α-KGDH*) (In NAD^+ / $NADP^+$ / FAD involved reactions, the enzymes acted are "*dehydrogenase*" and the substrate is "α-ketoglutarate"). This reaction is similar to pyruvate to acetyl CoA catalyzed by *pyruvate dehydrogenase* (*PDH*). Like *pyruvate dehydrogenase* (PDH), *α-ketoglutarate dehydrogenase* (*α-KGDH*) also needs five co-factors such as 1) TPP (Thiamine pyrophosphate); 2) Lipoamide; 3) FAD; 4) Co-enzyme A and 5) NAD^+ for its activity. During this reaction one molecule of NAD^+ is reduced to NADH + H^+ **(3 ATP generated and second carbon dioxide is produced)**.
7. In the next step succinyl CoA is hydrolyzed into succinate with loss of co-enzyme A. The reaction is catalyzed by *succinate thiokinase* (*STK*) enzyme (In ATP / GTP involved reactions, the enzymes acted are "*kinase*", sulphur atom of CoA is involved and the product formed is "succinate"). One GDP is converted into GTP in this step by reacting with inorganic phosphate **(1 ATP generated)**.
8. Succinate is reduced to fumarate in the succeeding step by *succinate dehydrogenase* (*SDH*) (In NAD^+ / $NADP^+$ / FAD involved reactions, the enzymes acted are "*dehydrogenase*" and the substrate is "succinate"). During this reaction one molecule of FAD is reduced to $FADH_2$ **(2 ATP generated)**.
9. In presence of *fumarase* (Substrate is "fumarate" and the type of reaction is "hydrolysis"), maleate is produced from fumarate by hydrolysis reaction with one mole of water.
10. In the last step, oxaloacetate is regenerated from maleate by simple reduction with the involvement of NAD^+. *Maleate dehydrogenases* (*MDH*) enzyme (In NAD^+ / $NADP^+$ / FAD involved reactions, the enzymes acted are "*dehydrogenase*" and the substrate is "maleate") catalyze this reaction. During this reaction one molecule of NAD^+ is reduced to $NADH^+$ H^+ **(3 ATP generated)**.

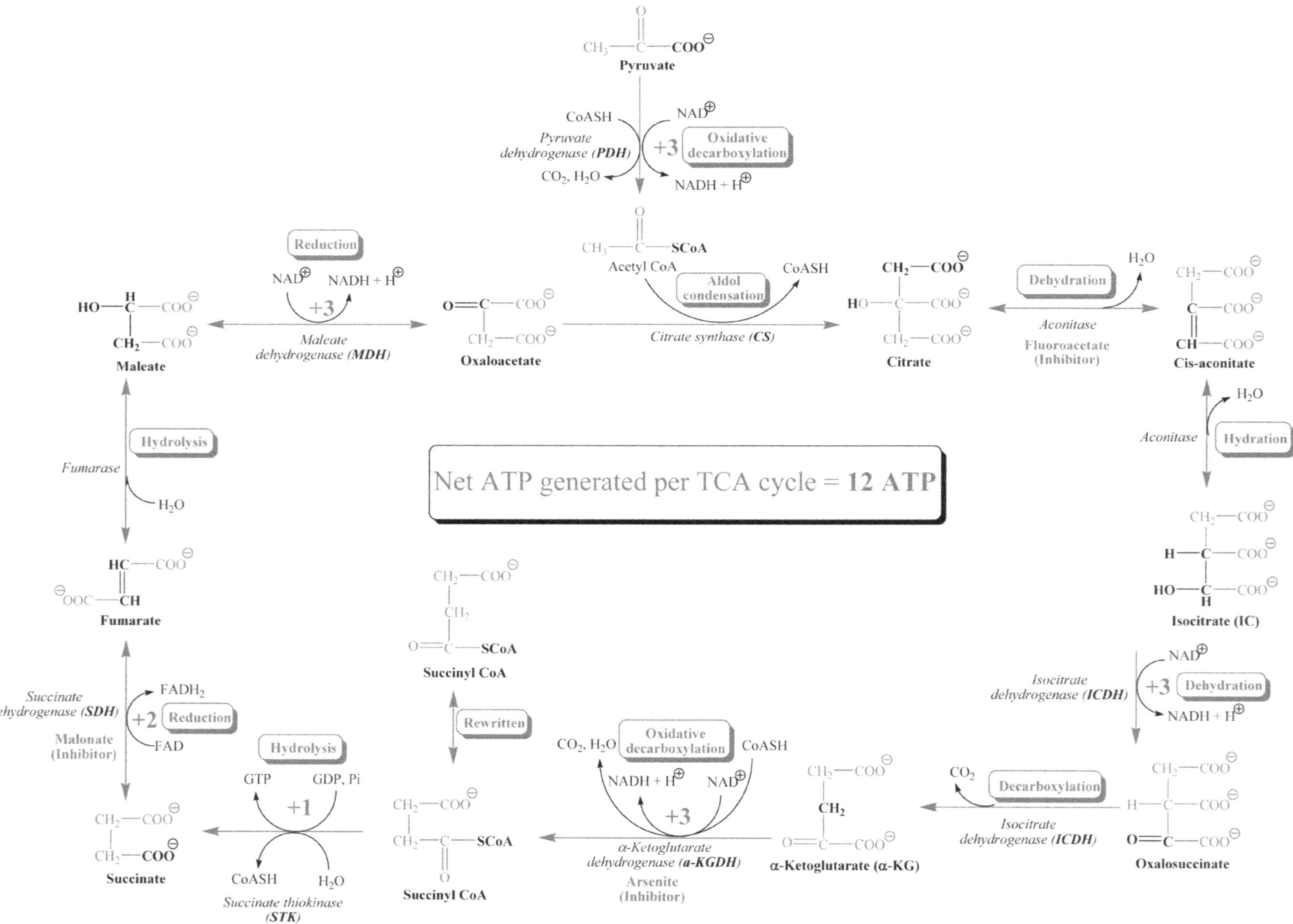
Pyruvate
CoASH
NAD⊕
Pyruvate dehydrogenase (PDH)
+3
Oxidative decarboxylation
CO_2, H_2O
NADH + H⊕
Acetyl CoA
Reduction
NAD⊕
NADH + H⊕
+3
Maleate dehydrogenase (MDH)
Maleate
Oxaloacetate
Aldol condensation
CoASH
Citrate synthase (CS)
Citrate
Dehydration
H_2O
Aconitase
Fluoroacetate (Inhibitor)
Cis-aconitate
H_2O
Aconitase
Hydration
Hydrolysis
Fumarase
H_2O
Net ATP generated per TCA cycle = 12 ATP
Fumarate
Succinyl CoA
Isocitrate (IC)
NAD⊕
Isocitrate dehydrogenase (ICDH)
+3
Dehydration
NADH + H⊕
Succinate dehydrogenase (SDH)
$FADH_2$
+2
Reduction
FAD
Malonate (Inhibitor)
Rewritten
Oxidative decarboxylation
CO_2, H_2O
CoASH
NADH + H⊕
NAD⊕
+3
α-Ketoglutarate dehydrogenase (α-KGDH)
Arsenite (Inhibitor)
α-Ketoglutarate (α-KG)
CO_2
Decarboxylation
Isocitrate dehydrogenase (ICDH)
Oxalosuccinate
Hydrolysis
GTP
GDP, Pi
+1
CoASH
H_2O
Succinate thiokinase (STK)
Succinate
Succinyl CoA

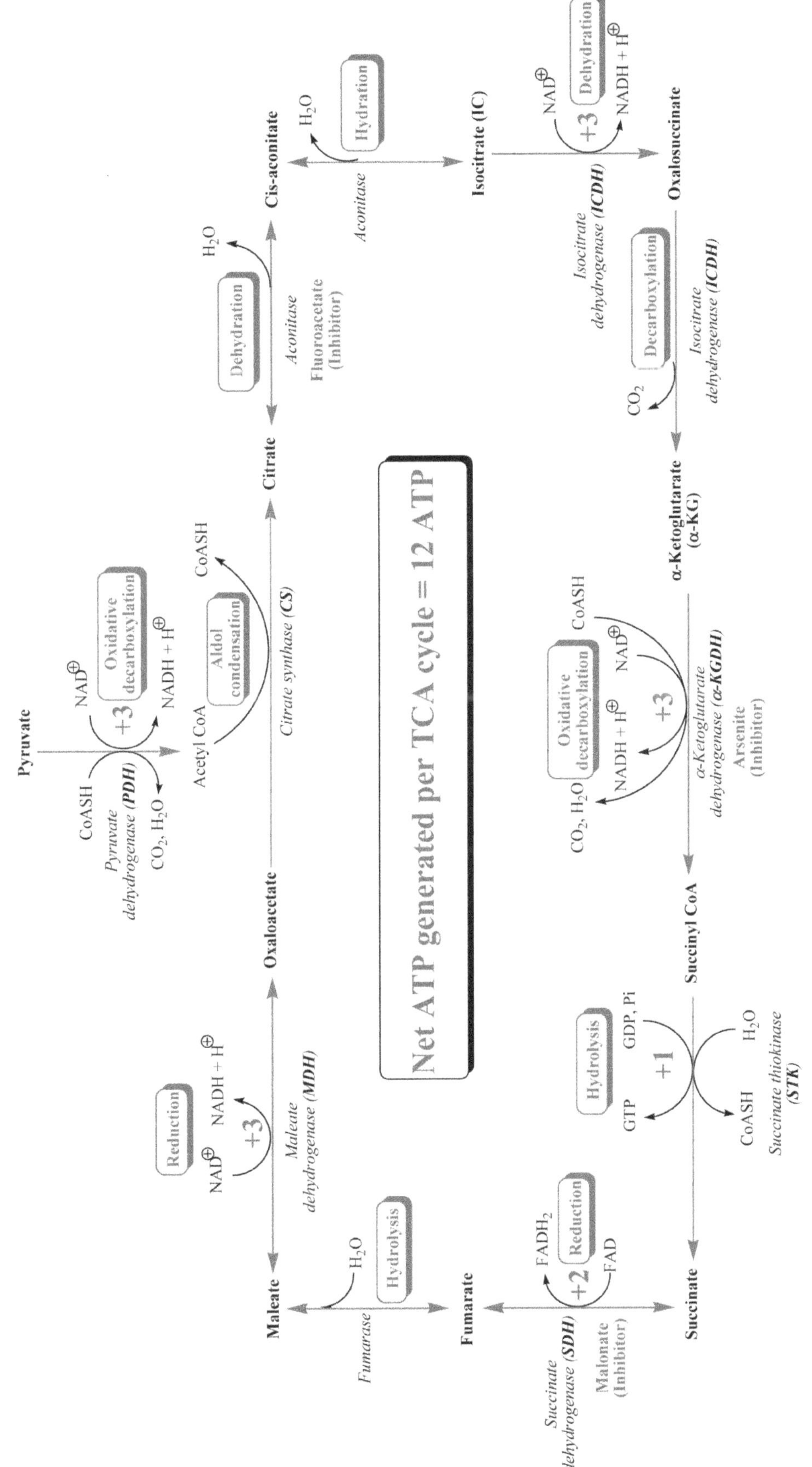
Pyruvate
CoASH
Pyruvate dehydrogenase (PDH)
CO_2, H_2O
$NAD^{\oplus}$
+3
Oxidative decarboxylation
$NADH + H^{\oplus}$
Acetyl CoA
Aldol condensation
CoASH
Citrate synthase (CS)
Oxaloacetate
Citrate
Dehydration
H_2O
Aconitase
Fluoroacetate (Inhibitor)
Cis-aconitate
H_2O
Aconitase
Hydration
Isocitrate (IC)
$NAD^{\oplus}$
+3
Dehydration
$NADH + H^{\oplus}$
Isocitrate dehydrogenase (ICDH)
Oxalosuccinate
CO_2
Decarboxylation
Isocitrate dehydrogenase (ICDH)
α-Ketoglutarate (α-KG)
CO_2, H_2O
Oxidative decarboxylation
CoASH
$NADH + H^{\oplus}$
$NAD^{\oplus}$
+3
α-Ketoglutarate dehydrogenase (α-KGDH)
Arsenite (Inhibitor)
Succinyl CoA
Hydrolysis
GTP
GDP, Pi
+1
CoASH
H_2O
Succinate thiokinase (STK)
Succinate
Succinate dehydrogenase (SDH)
$FADH_2$
+2
Reduction
FAD
Malonate (Inhibitor)
Fumarate
Fumarase
H_2O
Hydrolysis
Maleate
Reduction
$NAD^{\oplus}$
$NADH + H^{\oplus}$
+3
Maleate dehydrogenase (MDH)
Net ATP generated per TCA cycle = 12 ATP

Importance / Significance:

1. It is the final common oxidative pathway for carbohydrates, proteins and lipids.
2. About 65-70 % of total ATPs are synthesized in citric acid cycle. Hence, it is important metabolic pathway for the supply of energy.
3. About 2/3 of the oxygen consumed by the biological system is utilized by this cycle.
4. It is the most important central pathway because it connects either directly or indirectly almost all other individual metabolic pathway.
5. In addition to energy supply, TCA cycle also produces many intermediates necessary for the synthesis of glucose, amino acids, heme, etc.
6. Krebs cycle is amphibolic because it is both catabolic (breakdown of acetyl CoA to carbon dioxide) and anabolic (produces many intermediates necessary for the synthesis of glucose, amino acids, heme, etc.) in nature.
7. It is a cyclic process but not the closed one. It is open chain cycle i.e., several compounds may enter and leave the cycle at different stages.
8. Presence of oxygen is necessary for TCA cycle, even though oxygen is not directly participated. Because for the regeneration of reducing equivalent NAD^+ and FAD from NADH+ H^+ and $FADH_2$ in ETC needs oxygen.
9. Citric acid cycle will not take place in the absence of oxygen (anaerobic condition).

Regulation:

Citric acid cycle is regulated by the following three enzymes such as 1) *Citrate synthase* (*CS*), 2) *Isocitrate dehydrogenase* (*ICDH*) and 3) α-*Ketoglutarate dehydrogenase* (α-*KGDH*). ADP availability is the most important one because accumulation of NADH and $FADH_2$ inhibits the above rate limiting enzymes of TCA cycle. Fluoroacetate and arsenite non-competitively inhibits *aconitase* and α-*ketoglutarate dehydrogenase* (α-*KGDH*), respectively; whereas malonate competitively inhibits *succinate dehydrogenase* (*SDH*).

Energetic

Energetic of citric acid cycle are summarized in Table 3.4.

Table 3.4 Energetic of citric acid cycle.

S. No.	Enzyme responsible	Conversion takes place	No. of moles involved	No. of ATP generated or utilized
1	*Isocitrate dehydrogenase (ICDH)*	One NAD^+ is reduced to NADH + H^+ (One NADH + H^+ is equals to 3 ATP)	1	+ 3
2	*α-Ketoglutarate dehydrogenase (α-KGDH)*	One NAD^+ is reduced to NADH + H^+ (One NADH + H^+ is equals to 3 ATP)	1	+ 3
3	*Succinate thiokinase (STK)*	One GDP is converted into GTP	1	+ 1
4	*Succinate dehydrogenase (SDH)*	One FAD is reduced into $FADH_2$	1	+ 2
5	*Maleate dehydrogenase (MDH)*	One NAD^+ is reduced to NADH + H^+ (One NADH + H^+ is equals to 3 ATP)	1	+ 3
6	**Net ATP generated in TCA cycle for one acetyl CoA**			**12**

Energetic of glucose oxidation

(a) Aerobic condition

Energetic of complete oxidation of one glucose molecule in presence of oxygen is summarized in Table 3.5.

(b) Anaerobic condition

Energetic of complete oxidation of one glucose molecule in absence of oxygen is summarized in Table 3.6.

Table 3.5 Energetic of aerobic glucose oxidation.

S. No.	Pathway name	Conversion takes place	No. of ATP generated or utilized
1	Aerobic glycolysis	One glucose into 2 pyruvate	+ 8
2	Connecting link	2 Pyruvate to 2 acetyl CoA (For one mole of pyruvate 3 ATP generated. Hence for 2 pyruvate it is 6)	+ 6
3	TCA cycle	2 Acetyl CoA to 4 CO_2 (For one acetyl CoA 12 ATP generated. Hence for 2 acetyl CoA it is 24)	+ 24
4	**Net ATP generated for complete oxidation of one glucose molecule in aerobic condition**		**+ 38**

Table 3.6 Energetic of anaerobic glucose oxidation.

S. No.	Pathway name	Conversion takes place	No. of ATP generated or utilized
1	Anaerobic glycolysis	One glucose into 2 lactate (Lactate is not undergoing any further oxidative pathways and it is excreted in urine)	+ 2
2	**Net ATP generated for complete oxidation of one glucose molecule in anaerobic condition**		**+ 2**

GLUCONEOGENESIS

Definition: Gluco means "glucose / glycogen", in Greek neo means "new (other than carbohydrates)" and genesis means "synthesis". **Gluconeogenesis is defined as the process of synthesising glucose or glycogen from non-carbohydrate sources such as lactate, pyruvate, propionate, glycerol and glucogenic amino acids.**

Pathway:

Gluconeogenesis is the reverse of glycolysis. The three irreversible steps of glycolysis are modified / reversed by specific alternate enzymes. The enzymes are mainly present in cytosol even though few precursors are synthesized in mitochondria. Mostly gluconeogenesis takes place in liver and to small extent in kidney also,. The enzymes involved in three irreversible steps of glycolysis are "1) *Gluco kinase* (*GK*) or *hexo kinase* (*HK*), 2) *Phospho fructo kinase* (*PFK*) and 3) *Pyruvate kinase* (*PK*)". The alternative for these enzymes in gluconeogenesis are "1) *Glucose-6-phosphatase* (*G6Pase*), 2) *Fructose-1,6-bisphosphatase* (*F1,6BPase*), and 3) *Phospho enol pyruvate carboxy kinase* (*PEPCK*)".

1. ***Glucose-6-phosphatase* (*G6Pase*):** This step is the final step of gluconeogenesis. This enzyme directly reverses the reaction catalyzed by *gluco kinase* (*GK*) or *hexo kinase* (*HK*). *Glucose-6-phosphatase* (Substrate is "glucose-6-phosphate" and the type of reaction is "hydrolysis") hydrolyses glucose-6-phosphate (G6P) into glucose with removal of one molecule of inorganic phosphate. *Glucose-6-phosphatase* (*G6Pase*) is mainly present in liver and kidney but not present in muscle, brain and adipose tissue.

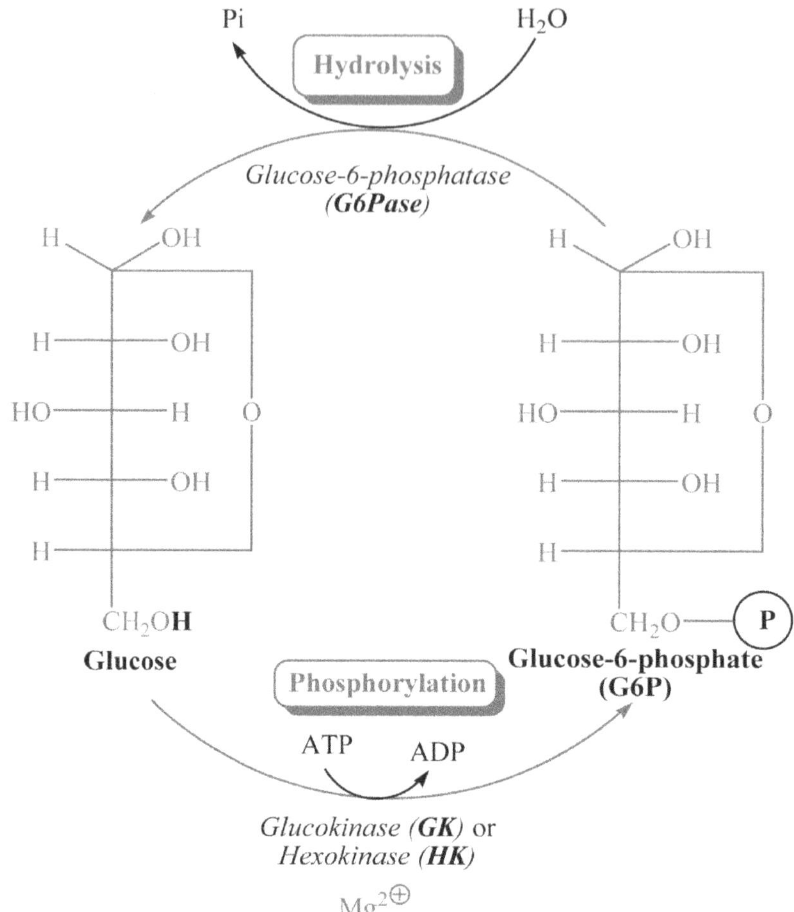

2. ***Fructose-1,6-bisphosphatase (F1,6BPase):*** This enzyme directly reverses the reaction catalyzed by *phospho fructo kinase* (PFK). *Fructose-1,6-bisphosphatase* (Substrate is "fructose-1,6-bisphosphate" and the type of reaction is "hydrolysis") hydrolyses fructose-1,6-bisphosphate (F1,6BP) into fructose-6-phosphate (F6P) with removal of one molecule of inorganic phosphate. *Fructose-1,6-bisphosphatase (F1,6BPase)* is not present in smooth muscle and heart muscle.
3. ***Phospho enol pyruvate carboxy kinase* (PEPCK):** This enzyme reverses the reaction catalyzed by *pyruvate kinase* (*PK*) but not directly. Pyruvate from cytosol enters into mitochondria where it reacts with carbon dioxide and get converted to oxaloacetate by carboxylation reaction in the presence of *pyruvate carboxylase* (*PC*) ("Pyruvate" is the substrate and the type of reaction is "carboxylation"). The energy for this anabolic reaction is obtained from the breakdown of ATP into ADP and inorganic phosphate **(1 ATP utilized)**. Later, oxaloacetate undergoes oxidation with the involvement of NADH and produces maleate. *Maleate dehydrogenase* (*MDH*) (In NAD^+ / $NADP^+$ / FAD involved reactions, the enzymes acted are "*dehydrogenase*" and the product is "maleate") catalyze this reaction. During this reaction one molecule of NADH + H^+ is oxidized to NAD^+ **(3 ATP utilized)**. Later maleate is transported from mitochondria to cytosol. In cytosol maleate produces oxaloacetate in the presence of *maleate dehydrogenase* (*MDH*) (Same reaction but in reverse manner i.e. reversible reaction) **(Hence, 3 ATP generated)**. Finally, oxaloacetate undergoes decarboxylated phosphorylation and produces phospho enol pyruvate (PEP). The enzyme responsible is *phospho enol pyruvate carboxy kinase* (*PEPCK*) (Product is "phospho enol pyruvate", the type of reaction is "carboxylation" (reverse reaction) and in ATP / GTP involved reactions, the enzymes acted are "*kinase*"). One GTP is converted into GDP in this step by donating one inorganic phosphate to substrate **(1 ATP utilized)**. Totally 2 ATP are utilized for the conversion of pyruvate to phospho enol pyruvate (PEP). But only one ATP is generated when phospho enol pyruvate (PEP) is converted into pyruvate.

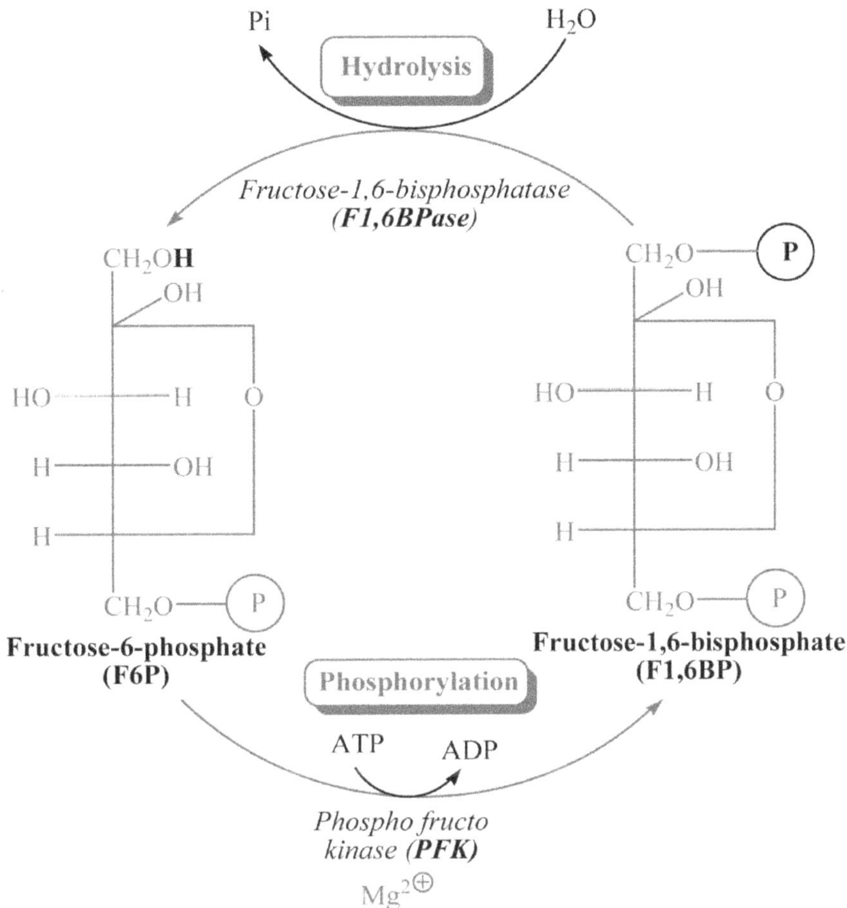

The overall reaction of pyruvate to glucose are summarized as follows,

$$2\text{ Pyruvate} + 4\text{ ATP} + 2\text{ GTP} + 2\text{ NADH} + 2\text{ H}^+ + 6\text{ H}_2\text{O}$$

$$\downarrow$$

$$\textbf{Glucose} + 4\text{ ADP} + 2\text{ GDP} + 6\text{ Pi} + 2\text{ NAD}^+$$

Due to lack of *glucose-6-phosphatase* (*G6Pase*) and *fructose-1,6-bisphosphatase* (*F1,6BPase*) in muscle, it can't utilize lactate or pyruvate to produce glucose. But through "Cori cycle" lactate present in muscle is transported to liver where glucose is synthesized by gluconeogenesis followed by transport of glucose into muscle.

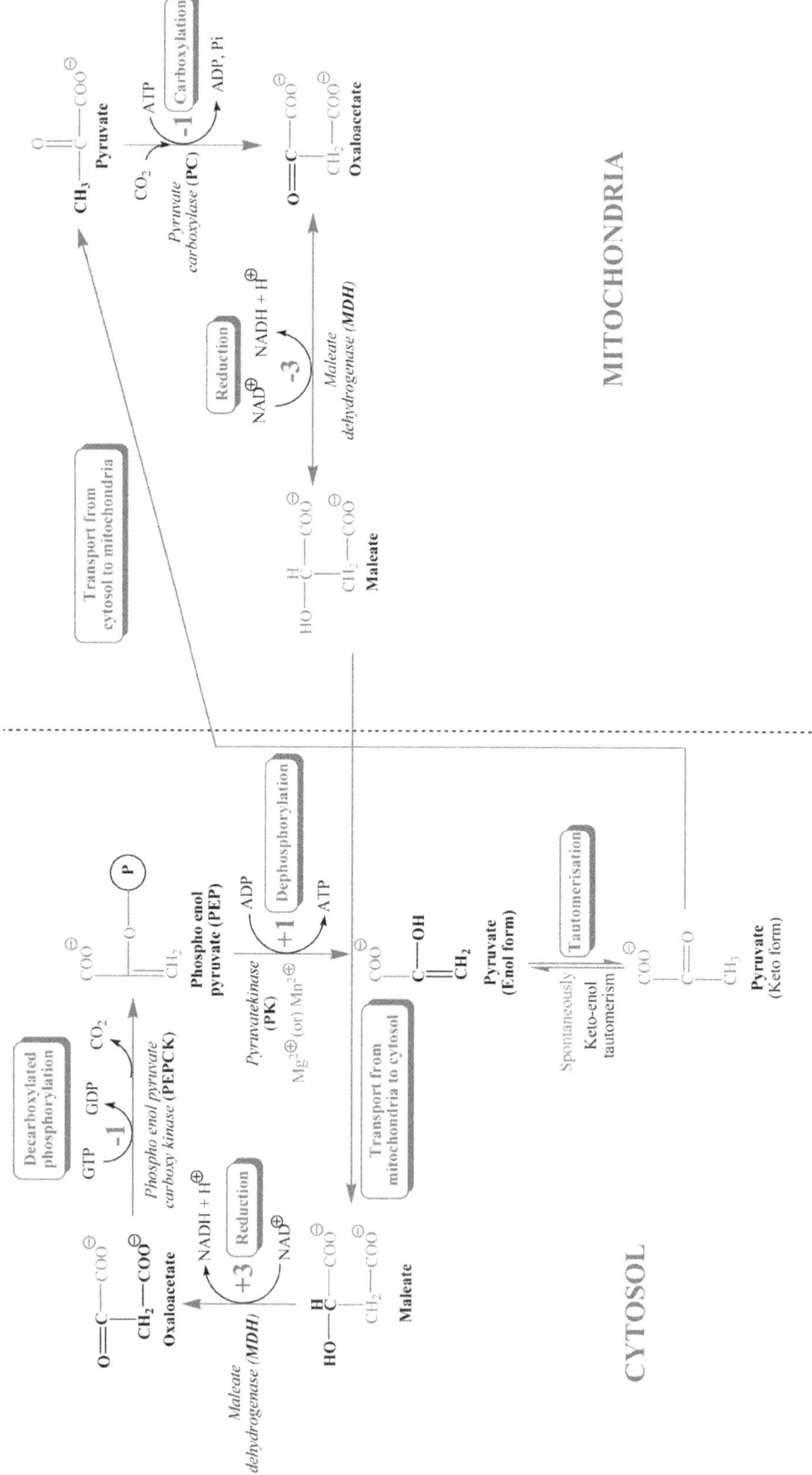
MITOCHONDRIA
Pyruvate
CO_2
ATP
-1
Carboxylation
ADP, Pi
Pyruvate carboxylase (PC)
Oxaloacetate
Reduction
NAD⊕
NADH + H⊕
-3
Maleate dehydrogenase (MDH)
Maleate
Transport from cytosol to mitochondria
CYTOSOL
Decarboxylated phosphorylation
GTP
GDP
CO_2
-1
Phospho enol pyruvate carboxy kinase (PEPCK)
Phospho enol pyruvate (PEP)
ADP
+1
Dephosphorylation
ATP
Pyruvatekinase (PK)
Mg2⊕ (or) Mn2⊕
Transport from mitochondria to cytosol
Pyruvate (Enol form)
Tautomerisation
Spontaneously
Keto-enol tautomerism
Pyruvate (Keto form)
Oxaloacetate
NADH + H⊕
+3
Reduction
NAD⊕
Maleate dehydrogenase (MDH)
Maleate

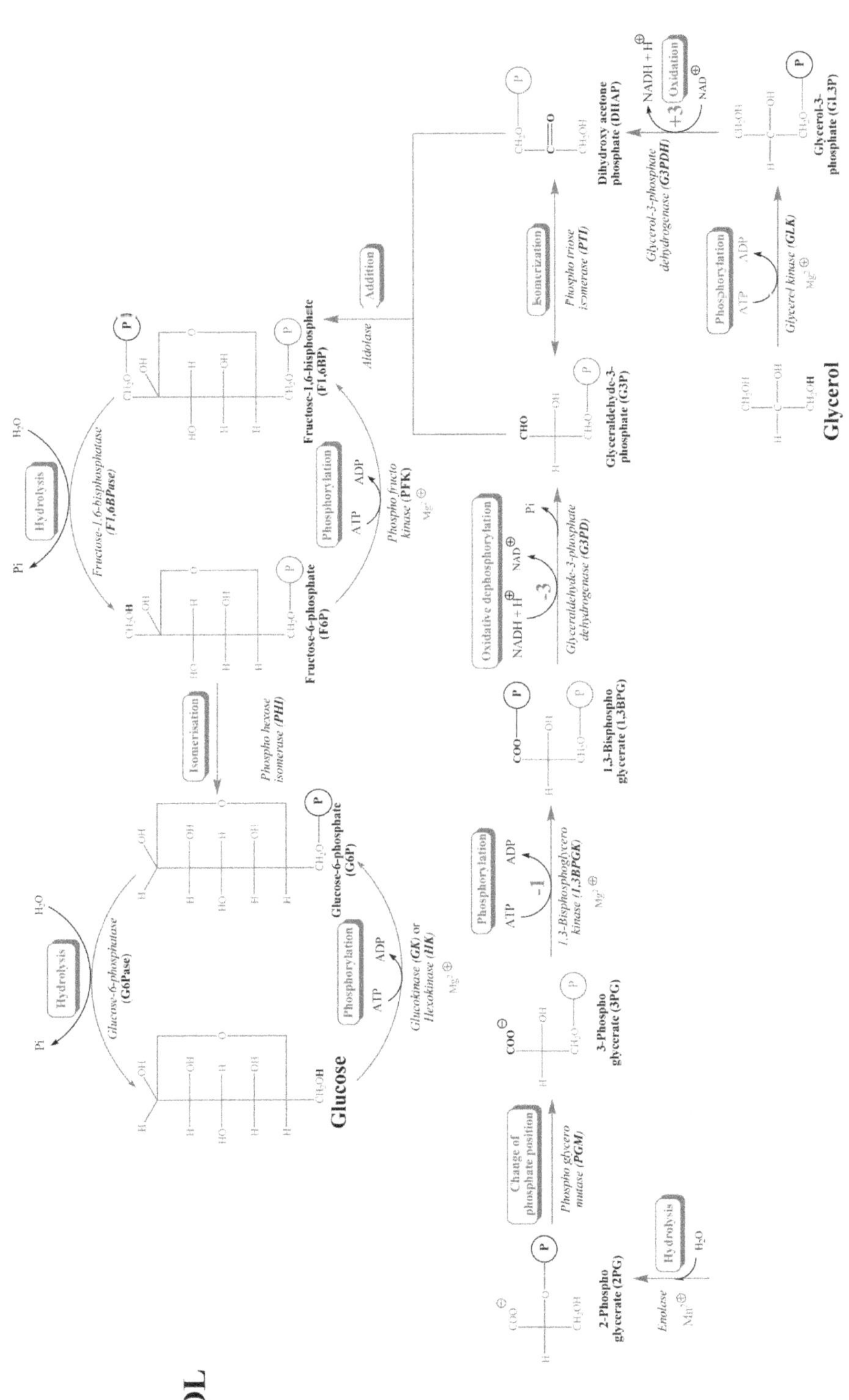
CYTOSOL
Glucose
Hydrolysis
Pi
H_2O
Glucose-6-phosphatase (G6Pase)
Phosphorylation
ATP
ADP
Glucokinase (GK) or Hexokinase (HK)
Glucose-6-phosphate (G6P)
Isomerisation
Phospho hexose isomerase (PHI)
Fructose-6-phosphate (F6P)
Fructose-1,6-bisphosphatase (F1,6BPase)
Phospho fructo kinase (PFK)
Fructose-1,6-bisphosphate (F1,6BP)
Aldolase
Addition
Glyceraldehyde-3-phosphate (G3P)
Isomerization
Phospho triose isomerase (PTI)
Dihydroxy acetone phosphate (DHAP)
Glycerol-3-phosphate dehydrogenase (G3PDH)
Oxidation
+3
NADH + H⊕
NAD⊕
Glycerol kinase (GLK)
Glycerol-3-phosphate (GL3P)
Glycerol
Oxidative dephosphorylation
Glyceraldehyde-3-phosphate dehydrogenase (G3PD)
-3
1,3-Bisphospho glycerate (1,3BPG)
1,3-Bisphosphoglycero kinase (1,3BPGK)
-1
3-Phospho glycerate (3PG)
Change of phosphate position
Phospho glycero mutase (PGM)
2-Phospho glycerate (2PG)
Enolase

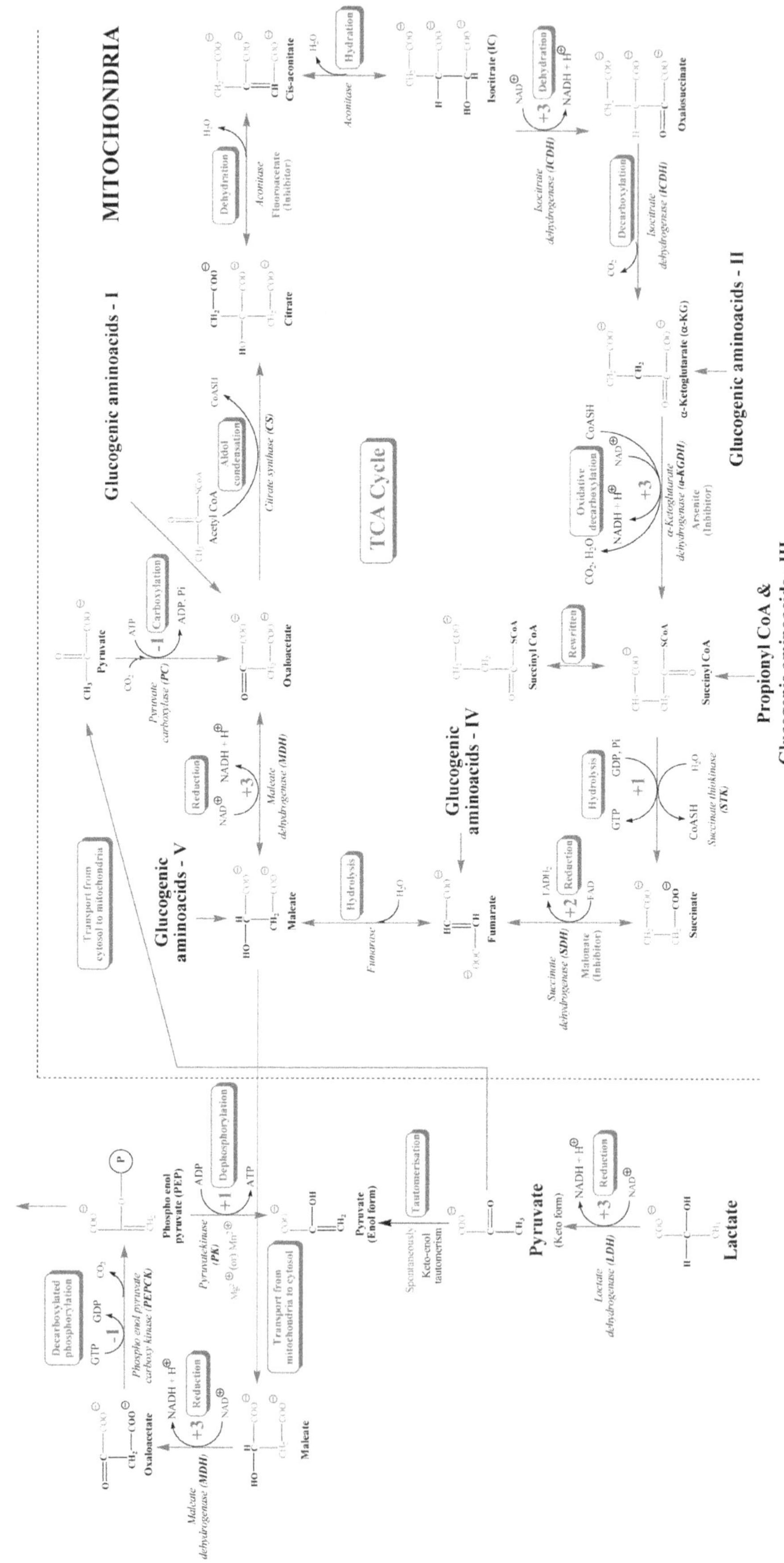
MITOCHONDRIA
TCA Cycle
Glucogenic aminoacids - I
Glucogenic aminoacids - II
Propionyl CoA &
Glucogenic aminoacids - III
Glucogenic aminoacids - IV
Glucogenic aminoacids - V
Pyruvate
Pyruvate carboxylase (PC)
Carboxylation
ATP
ADP, Pi
Oxaloacetate
Acetyl CoA
Aldol condensation
CoASH
Citrate synthase (CS)
Citrate
Dehydration
Aconitase
Flouroacetate (Inhibitor)
Cis-aconitate
Hydration
Isocitrate (IC)
Isocitrate dehydrogenase (ICDH)
NADH + H⊕
Oxalosuccinate
Decarboxylation
α-Ketoglutarate (α-KG)
Oxidative decarboxylation
α-Ketoglutarate dehydrogenase (α-KGDH)
Arsenite (Inhibitor)
Succinyl CoA
Rewritten
Hydrolysis
GTP
GDP, Pi
Succinate thiokinase (STK)
Succinate
Succinate dehydrogenase (SDH)
Malonate (Inhibitor)
Reduction
FADH₂
FAD
Fumarate
Fumarase
Maleate
Maleate dehydrogenase (MDH)
NAD⊕
Transport from cytosol to mitochondria
Transport from mitochondria to cytosol
Phospho enol pyruvate carboxy kinase (PEPCK)
Decarboxylated phosphorylation
Phospho enol pyruvate (PEP)
Pyruvatekinase (PK)
Dephosphorylation
Pyruvate (Enol form)
Tautomerisation
Spontaneously
Keto-enol tautomerism
Pyruvate (Keto form)
Lactate dehydrogenase (LDH)
Lactate

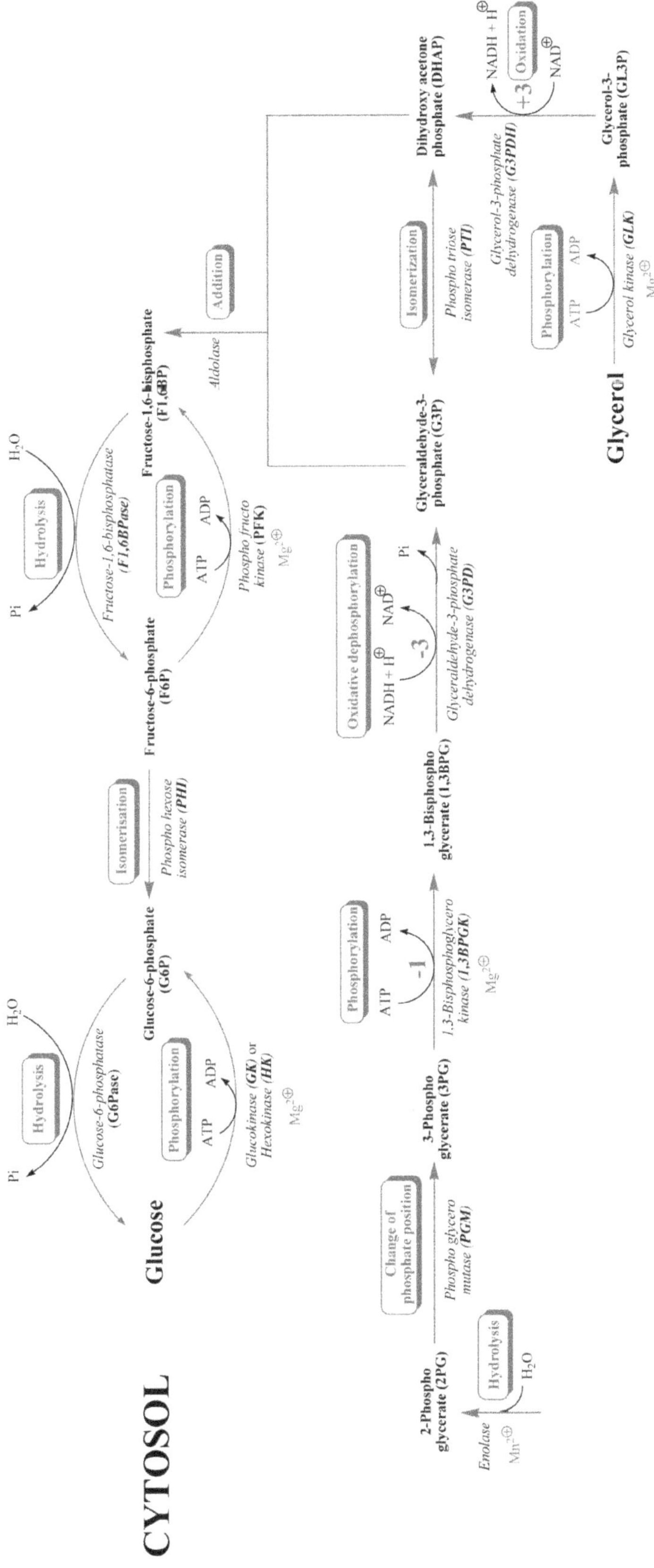
CYTOSOL
Glucose
Hydrolysis
Pi
H_2O
Glucose-6-phosphatase (G6Pase)
Phosphorylation
ATP
ADP
Glucokinase (GK) or Hexokinase (HK)
Mg^{2+}
Glucose-6-phosphate (G6P)
Isomerisation
Phospho hexose isomerase (PHI)
Fructose-6-phosphate (F6P)
Hydrolysis
Pi
H_2O
Fructose-1,6-bisphosphatase (F1,6BPase)
Phosphorylation
ATP
ADP
Phospho fructo kinase (PFK)
Mg^{2+}
Fructose-1,6-bisphosphate (F1,6BP)
Addition
Aldolase
Glyceraldehyde-3-phosphate (G3P)
Isomerization
Phospho triose isomerase (PTI)
Dihydroxy acetone phosphate (DHAP)
Oxidation
+3
NADH + H^+
NAD^+
Glycerol-3-phosphate dehydrogenase (G3PDH)
Glycerol-3-phosphate (GL3P)
Phosphorylation
ATP
ADP
Glycerol kinase (GLK)
Mg^{2+}
Glycerol
Oxidative dephosphorylation
-3
NADH + H^+
NAD^+
Pi
Glyceraldehyde-3-phosphate dehydrogenase (G3PD)
1,3-Bisphospho glycerate (1,3BPG)
Phosphorylation
-1
ATP
ADP
1,3-Bisphosphoglycero kinase (1,3BPGK)
Mg^{2+}
3-Phospho glycerate (3PG)
Change of phosphate position
Phospho glycero mutase (PGM)
2-Phospho glycerate (2PG)
Hydrolysis
H_2O
Enolase
Mn^{2+}

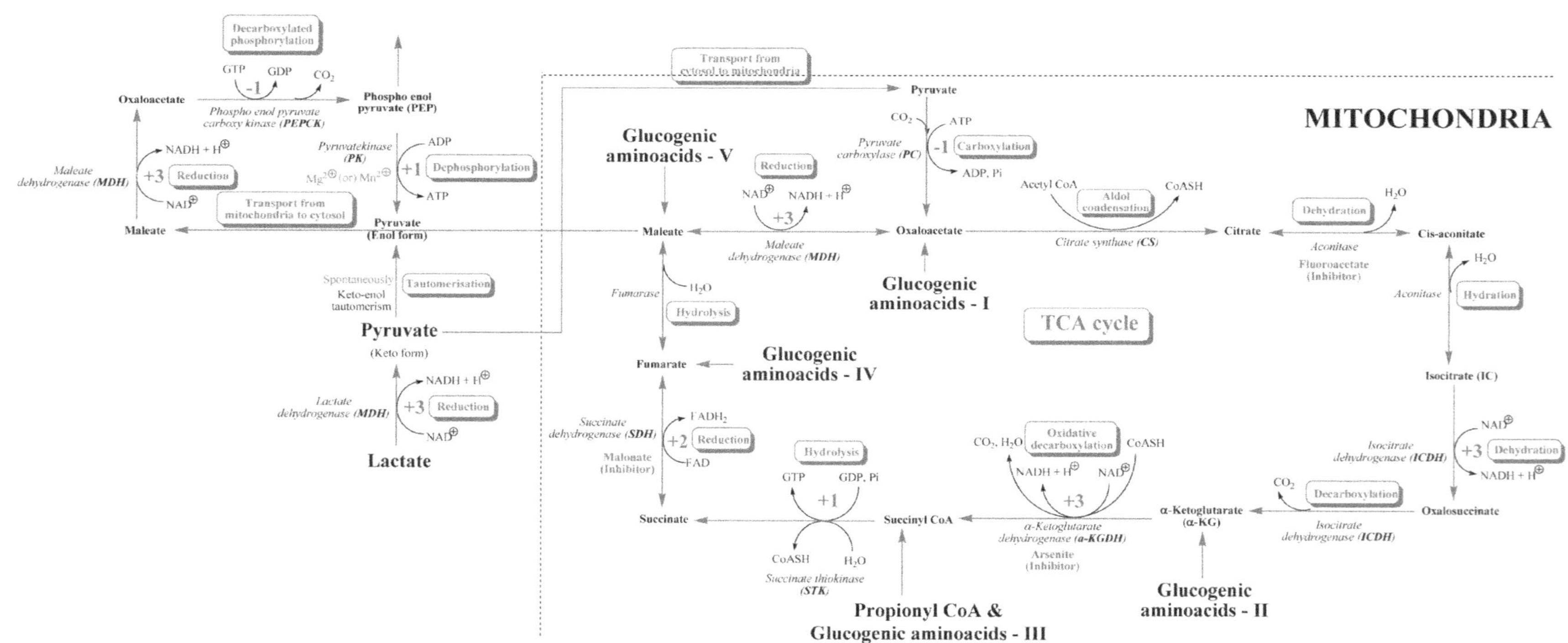
MITOCHONDRIA
TCA cycle
Oxaloacetate
Decarboxylated phosphorylation
GTP
GDP
CO_2
-1
Phospho enol pyruvate carboxy kinase (PEPCK)
Phospho enol pyruvate (PEP)
Maleate dehydrogenase (MDH)
+3
Reduction
NADH + H⊕
NAD⊕
Maleate
Transport from mitochondria to cytosol
Pyruvatekinase (PK)
Mg^{2+} (or) Mn^{2+}
+1
Dephosphorylation
ADP
ATP
Pyruvate (Enol form)
Spontaneously
Keto-enol tautomerism
Tautomerisation
Pyruvate
(Keto form)
Lactate dehydrogenase (MDH)
+3
Reduction
NADH + H⊕
NAD⊕
Lactate
Transport from cytosol to mitochondria
Pyruvate
CO_2
ATP
Pyruvate carboxylase (PC)
-1
Carboxylation
ADP, Pi
Glucogenic aminoacids - V
Reduction
NAD⊕
NADH + H⊕
+3
Maleate
Maleate dehydrogenase (MDH)
Oxaloacetate
Glucogenic aminoacids - I
Acetyl CoA
Aldol condensation
CoASH
Citrate synthase (CS)
Citrate
Dehydration
H_2O
Aconitase
Fluoroacetate (Inhibitor)
Cis-aconitate
H_2O
Aconitase
Hydration
Isocitrate (IC)
Fumarase
H_2O
Hydrolysis
Fumarate
Glucogenic aminoacids - IV
Succinate dehydrogenase (SDH)
Malonate (Inhibitor)
+2
Reduction
$FADH_2$
FAD
Succinate
Hydrolysis
GTP
GDP, Pi
+1
CoASH
H_2O
Succinate thiokinase (STK)
Succinyl CoA
Propionyl CoA & Glucogenic aminoacids - III
CO_2, H_2O
Oxidative decarboxylation
CoASH
NADH + H⊕
NAD⊕
+3
α-Ketoglutarate dehydrogenase (α-KGDH)
Arsenite (Inhibitor)
α-Ketoglutarate (α-KG)
Glucogenic aminoacids - II
CO_2
Decarboxylation
Isocitrate dehydrogenase (ICDH)
Oxalosuccinate
Isocitrate dehydrogenase (ICDH)
+3
Dehydration
NAD⊕
NADH + H⊕

List of glucogenic amino acids:

The followings are the list of various glucogenic amino acids entered into citric acid cycle at various stages and produces glucose through gluconeogenesis.

1. Glucogenic amino acids – I: Alanine, glycine, serine, cysteine, threonine and tryptophan
2. Glucogenic amino acids – II: Asparagine and aspartate
3. Glucogenic amino acids – III: Glutamate, glutamine, arginine, histidine and proline
4. Glucogenic amino acids – IV: Isoleucine, methionine and valine
5. Glucogenic amino acids – V: Phenyl alanine and tyrosine

Significance:

1. Continuous supply of glucose is very essential for the biological systems as it occupies a major position in metabolism.
2. For continuous supply of energy, organs like brain, CNS, erythrocytes, testes and kidney medulla is dependent on glucose. Per day 160 g of glucose is needed for the whole body. Out of this around 120 g is utilized by brain only.
3. Under aerobic condition glucose only supplies energy to the skeletal muscle.
4. Other carbohydrates such as lactose, amino sugars, etc. are bio-synthesized from glucose only.
5. Glucose is also utilized for the synthesis of fat by converting into glycerol.
6. In fasting condition more than a day, gluconeogenesis is essential for the survival of animals in order to meet the basal requirements of the biological systems for glucose and to maintain intermediate of TCA cycle.
7. Gluconeogenesis effectively clears some metabolites like lactate, glycerol, propionate, etc. produced in tissues which will accumulate in blood.

Regulation:

Gluconeogenesis is regulated by the hormone glucagon (hormone secreted by α-cells of islets of pancreas). Glucagon stimulates gluconeogenesis by inactivating *pyruvate kinase (PK)*, inhibiting *phospho fructo kinase (PFK)* and activating *fructose-1,6-bisphosphatase (F1,6BPase)*. In addition, glucogenic amino acids and acetyl CoA stimulate gluconeogenesis as it allosterically activates *pyruvate carboxylase (PC)*. *Glucose-6-phosphatase (G6Pase)*, *fructose-1,6-bisphosphatase (F1,6BPase)*, and *phospho enol pyruvate carboxy kinase (PEPCK)* are the **rate limiting enzymes of gluconeogenesis**. Hence it also regulates gluconeogenesis.

HEXOSE MONO PHOSPHATE (HMP) SHUNT

Other Names: Pentose phosphate pathway or Phospho gluconate pathway

Definition: For oxidation of glucose, HMP shunt is an alternative oxidative pathway for glycolysis and citric acid cycle. This pathway is concerned with the biosynthesis of pentose sugars and reducing equivalent NADPH; hence it is more anabolic in nature. **HMP pathway is defined as direct complete oxidation of glucose into carbon dioxide with the production of NADPH + H⁺.** Out of 6 moles of glucose-6-phosphate (G6P) entered in HMP shunt, one mole is completely oxidized into carbon dioxide and the rest of five moles are regenerated.

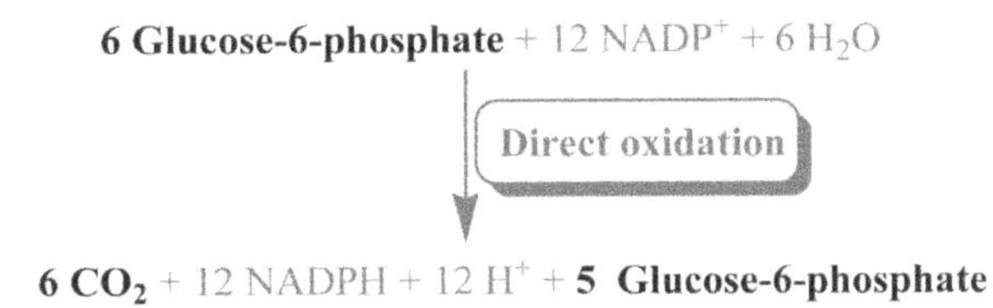

Pathway: HMP shunt takes place in tissues like liver, adipose tissue, testes, erythrocyte, adrenal gland and lactating mammary gland which are involved in the synthesis of steroids and fatty acids. The necessary enzymes are present in cytosol fraction of the cell. HMP shunt pathway is divided into two different phases as (a) oxidative phase and (b) non-oxidative phase.

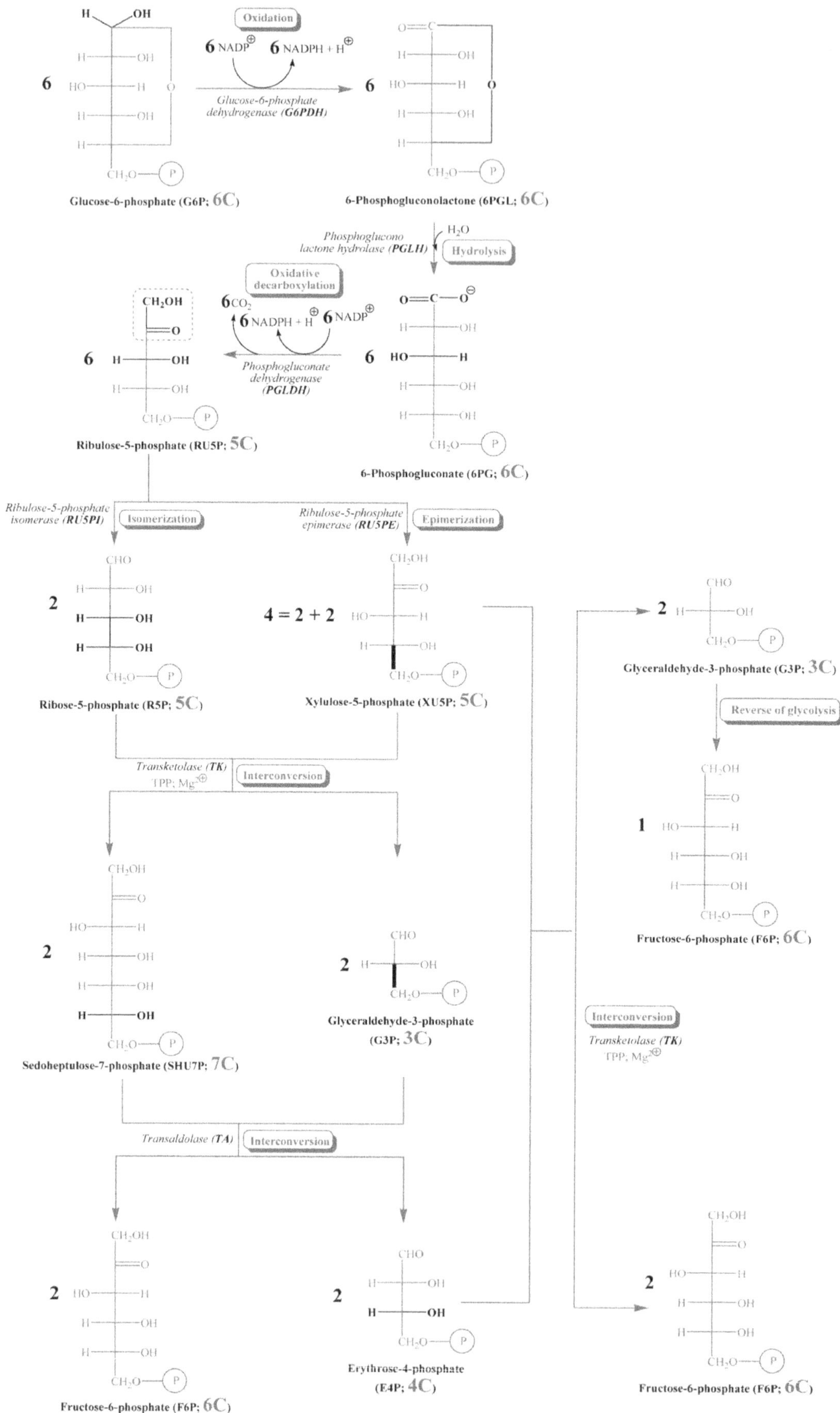
Oxidation
6 NADP⊕
6 NADPH + H⊕
Glucose-6-phosphate dehydrogenase (G6PDH)
Glucose-6-phosphate (G6P; 6C)
6-Phosphogluconolactone (6PGL; 6C)
Phosphoglucono lactone hydrolase (PGLH)
H2O
Hydrolysis
Oxidative decarboxylation
6CO2
6 NADPH + H⊕
6 NADP⊕
Phosphogluconate dehydrogenase (PGLDH)
Ribulose-5-phosphate (RU5P; 5C)
6-Phosphogluconate (6PG; 6C)
Ribulose-5-phosphate isomerase (RU5PI)
Isomerization
Ribulose-5-phosphate epimerase (RU5PE)
Epimerization
4 = 2 + 2
Ribose-5-phosphate (R5P; 5C)
Xylulose-5-phosphate (XU5P; 5C)
Glyceraldehyde-3-phosphate (G3P; 3C)
Reverse of glycolysis
Fructose-6-phosphate (F6P; 6C)
Transketolase (TK)
TPP; Mg2⊕
Interconversion
Sedoheptulose-7-phosphate (SHU7P; 7C)
Glyceraldehyde-3-phosphate (G3P; 3C)
Interconversion
Transketolase (TK)
TPP; Mg2⊕
Transaldolase (TA)
Interconversion
Fructose-6-phosphate (F6P; 6C)
Erythrose-4-phosphate (E4P; 4C)
Fructose-6-phosphate (F6P; 6C)

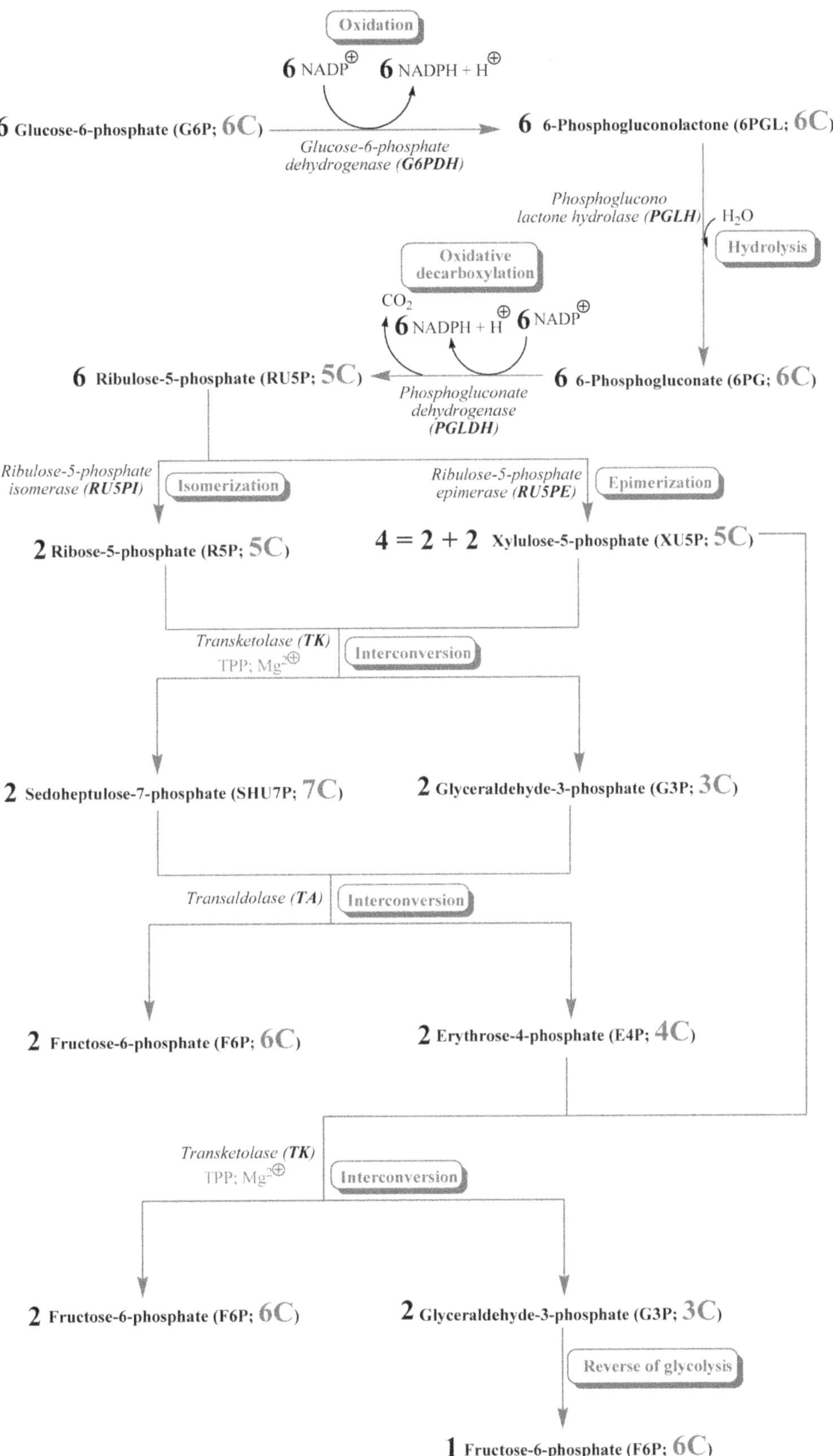

Oxidation
6 NADP⊕
6 NADPH + H⊕
6 Glucose-6-phosphate (G6P; 6C)
Glucose-6-phosphate dehydrogenase (G6PDH)
6 6-Phosphogluconolactone (6PGL; 6C)
Phosphoglucono lactone hydrolase (PGLH)
H_2O
Hydrolysis
Oxidative decarboxylation
CO_2
6 NADPH + H⊕
6 NADP⊕
6 Ribulose-5-phosphate (RU5P; 5C)
6 6-Phosphogluconate (6PG; 6C)
Phosphogluconate dehydrogenase (PGLDH)
Ribulose-5-phosphate isomerase (RU5PI)
Isomerization
Ribulose-5-phosphate epimerase (RU5PE)
Epimerization
2 Ribose-5-phosphate (R5P; 5C)
4 = 2 + 2 Xylulose-5-phosphate (XU5P; 5C)
Transketolase (TK)
TPP; Mg2⊕
Interconversion
2 Sedoheptulose-7-phosphate (SHU7P; 7C)
2 Glyceraldehyde-3-phosphate (G3P; 3C)
Transaldolase (TA)
Interconversion
2 Fructose-6-phosphate (F6P; 6C)
2 Erythrose-4-phosphate (E4P; 4C)
Transketolase (TK)
TPP; Mg2⊕
Interconversion
2 Fructose-6-phosphate (F6P; 6C)
2 Glyceraldehyde-3-phosphate (G3P; 3C)
Reverse of glycolysis
1 Fructose-6-phosphate (F6P; 6C)

(a) **Oxidative phase:** This phase starts from glucose-6-phosphate (G6P) and ends in the formation of ribose-5-phosphate (R5P). During this phase, compounds undergo oxidation in presence of reducing equivalent $NADP^+$.

1. Initially, glucose-6-phosphate (G6P) is oxidized at C-1 and produced 6-phosphogluconolactone (6PGL) by *glucose-6-phosphate dehydrogenase (G6PDH)* (In NAD^+ / $NADP^+$ / FAD involved reactions, the enzymes acted are "*dehydrogenase*" and the substrate is "glucose-6-phosphate"). **During this reaction one molecule of $NADP^+$ is reduced to NAPH + H^+.**
2. The formed 6-phosphogluconolactone (6PGL) undergoes hydrolysis by reacting with water in presence of *phosphoglucono lactone hydrolase (PGLH)* (Substrate is "6-phosphogluconolactone" and the type of reaction is "hydrolysis") results in formation of 6-phosphogluconate (6PG).
3. Oxidative decarboxylation of 6-phosphogluconate (6PG) produces pentose sugar ribulose-5-phosphate (RU5P). **One mole of carbon dioxide is eliminated** in the presence of *phosphogluconate dehydrogenase (PGLDH)* (In NAD^+ / $NADP^+$ / FAD involved reactions, the enzymes acted are "*dehydrogenase*" and the substrate is "6-phosphogluconate"). **During this reaction one molecule of $NADP^+$ is reduced to NAPH + H^+.**
4. In the next step, ribulose-5-phosphate (RU5P) is isomerized into ribose-5-phosphate (R5P) by "*ribulose-5-phosphate isomerase (RU5PI)*" (Substrate is "ribulose-5-phosphate" and the type of reaction is "isomerization"). In another way, ribulose-5-phosphate (RU5P) is epimerized into xylulose-5-phosphate (XU5P) by "*ribulose-5-phosphate epimerase (RU5PE)*" (Substrate is "ribulose-5-phosphate" and the type of reaction involved is "epimerization"). In HMP shunt, ribulose-5-phosphate (RU5P) undergoes isomerization and epimerization reaction in the ratio of 1:2.

(b) **Non-oxidative phase:** This phase starts from ribose-5-phosphate (R5P) and ends in the formation of fructose-6-phosphate (F6P). During this phase compounds do not undergo oxidation and only inter conversion of 3, 4, 5 and 7 carbon sugar molecules takes place.

1. 5 Carbon ribose-5-phosphate (R5P) reacts with 5 carbon xylulose-5-phosphate (XU5P) in the presence of *transketolase (TK)* (Transfer takes place from aldose to ketose sugar) and produces 7 carbon sedoheptulose-7-phosphate (SHU7P) and 3 carbon glyceraldehyde-3-phosphate (G3P). *Transketolase* (TK) needs thiamine pyrophosphate (TPP) and magnesium ion as co-enzyme for activity.
2. Later, 7 carbon sedoheptulose-7-phosphate (SHU7P) reacts with 3 carbon glyceraldehyde-3-phosphate (G3P) in the presence of *transaldolase (TA)* (Transfer takes place from ketose to aldose sugar) and produces 6 carbon fructose-6-phosphate (F6P) and 4 carbon erythrose-4-phosphate (E4P). Unlike *transketolase (TK)* enzymes, *transaldolase (TA)* do not need any co-enzyme for its activity.
3. The formed 4 carbon erythrose-4-phosphate (E4P) reacts with another mole of 5 carbon xylulose-5-phosphate (XU5P; earlier synthesized in oxidative phase) and produces 6 carbon fructose-6-phosphate (F6P) and 3 carbon glyceraldehyde-3-phosphate (G3P) in presence of *transketolase (TK)* (Transfer takes place from aldose to ketose sugar).
4. Glyceraldehyde-3-phosphate (G3P) produces fructose-6-phosphate (F6P) by gluconeogenesis pathway (2 mole of glyceraldehyde-3-phosphate (G3P) produce one mole of fructose-6-phosphate (F6P)).
5. Fructose-6-phosphate (F6P) and glyceraldehyde-3-phosphate (G3P) can be further catabolized through glycolysis and TCA cycle. Alternatively, glucose may also be synthesized from these two compounds.

Significance:

1. As such in HMP shunt pathway ATP is neither synthesized nor utilized directly which is uniqueness of this pathway.
2. Several inter convertible substances are produced in HMP shunt and these compounds may proceed in different directions in metabolic reactions. This is another uniqueness of HMP shunt pathway.
3. In this pathway 3, 4, 5 and 7 carbon sugar molecules undergo inter conversion.

4. Out of 6 moles of glucose-6-phosphate (G6P) entered in HMP shunt, one mole is completely oxidized into carbon dioxide and the rest of five moles are regenerated.
5. Two important compounds are biosynthesized in HMP shunt pathway namely pentose sugar and NADPH.
6. **Pentose sugar:** Three pentose sugars such as ribulose-5-phosphate (RU5P), ribose-5-phosphate (R5P) and xylulose-5-phosphate (XU5P) are biosynthesized in pentose phosphate pathway. Among this ribose-5-phosphate (R5P) is more important because this pentose or its derivatives are used for the synthesis of nucleic acid (RNA and DNA) and many nucleotides like ATP, NAD^+, FAD and co-enzyme A. For the synthesis of pentoses through HMP shunt, complete pathway may not be required. Hence, pentoses are synthesized in skeletal muscle even though it contains only first few enzymes of pathway.
7. **NADPH:** Reductive biosynthesis of steroids and fatty acids are dependent on NADPH. *Glutamate dehydrogenase* (GDH) is an enzyme useful for the synthesis of certain amino acid also needs NADPH for its activity. In anti-oxidant reactions, NADPH is necessary for the conversion of hydrogen peroxide (damages DNA, unsaturated lipids and proteins) into water molecule. Cytochrome P_{450} (It is a microsomal enzyme involved in oxidation reactions for detoxification of foreign compounds) are dependent on NADPH. It is also necessary for phagocytosis (engulfment of foreign particles including micro-organism). Reduced form of glutathione (necessary for the maintenance of integrity of RBC) in RBC was maintained by NADPH only. It also prevents the accumulation of methemoglobin by maintaining ferrous ion of hemoglobin in reduced form.

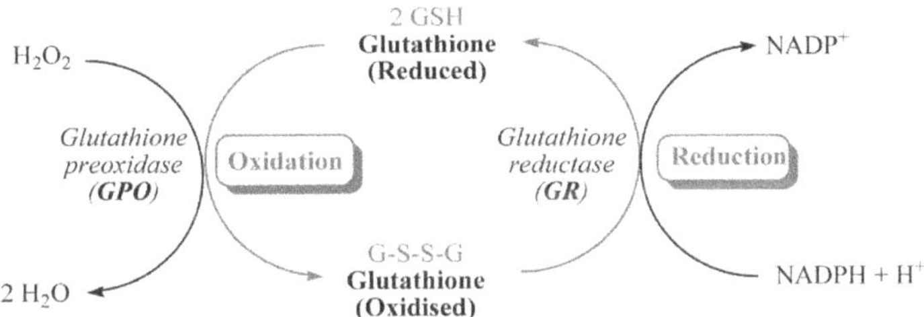

Metabolic disorder:

1. ***Glucose-6-phosphate dehydrogenase* (G6PD) deficiency or Hemolysis:** Deficiency of *G6PD* results in decreased synthesis of NADPH in RBC. Hence, peroxides and methemoglobins are accumulated in erythrocytes results in hemolysis. Severe conditions may lead to hemolytic anemia. In these patients hemolytic jaundice is produced by drugs like primaquine, sulfamethoxazole and acetanilide. *Glucose-6-phosphate dehydrogenase* (*G6PD*) deficiency is associated with resistance to *plasmodium falciparum* caused malaria because these micro-organisms are dependent on HMP shunt for reduced form of glutathione which is needed for their optimum growth in RBC.
2. **Wernicke-Korsakoff syndrome:** It is due to one tenth of reduced affinity of thiamine pyrophosphate (TPP) with *transketolase* (*TK*). Mental disorder, partial paralysis and loss of memory are the symptoms of this syndrome. Symptoms are manifested in alcoholics whose diet is vitamin deficient. Erythrocyte *transketolase* (*TK*) activity is increased in pernicious anemia.

Regulation: Glucose-6-phosphate dehydrogenase (*G6PD*) which catalyzes irreversible step is a **rate limiting enzymes** of HMP shunt pathway. Consequently, it regulates the HMP pathway. Moreover, NADPH competitively inhibits *glucose-6-phosphate dehydrogenase* (*G6PD*). Hence, the flux of cycle is determined by the ratio of NADPH / $NADP^+$.

GLYCOGEN METABOLISM

Glycogen: Glycogen is the storage form of glucose in animals like starch in plants. Glycogen is mainly stored in liver (6-8 %) and muscles (1-2 %); but the quantity of glycogen stored in muscle (250 g) is approximately 3 times more than liver glycogen (75 g) due to more muscle mass. Liver glycogen maintains or regulates blood glucose level particularly between meals whereas muscle glycogen is utilized for ATP supply during muscle contraction.

Glycogen is composed of α-D-glucose (Approximately 1,00,000 residues/molecules). Glucose molecules are attached to another glucose molecules by 1,4-α-glycosidic linkage. After every 8-10 glucose molecules branching takes place. In the branching point the glucose molecules are linked by 1,6-α-glycosidic linkage. Glycogen is stored as granules in cytosol where most of the enzymes of glycogen synthesis and breakdown are present. Glycogen metabolism includes two pathways namely,

1. Glycogenesis (Anabolic pathway - Synthesis of glycogen)
2. Glycogenolysis (Catabolic pathway - Breakdown of glycogen).

GLYCOGENESIS

Definition: Glyco indicates "glycogen" and in Greek genesis means "synthesis / production". **It is defined as synthesis of glycogen from glucose with utilization of ATP and UTP**. It takes place in cytosol fraction of the cell.

$$\textbf{n Glucose} + \text{UTP} + \text{ATP} \xrightarrow{\text{Synthesis}} \textbf{Glycogen} + \text{UDP} + \text{ADP} + 2\text{Pi}$$

Pathway:

1. The first step in glycogenesis is a simple phosphorylation reaction. In this step glucose is phosphorylated at 6th position in presence of enzyme called "*hexokinase* (*HK*) or *glucokinase* (*GK*)" (In ATP / GTP involved reactions, the enzymes acted are "*kinase*" and the substrate is "glucose' which is a "hexose sugar") and produces glucose-6-phosphate (G6P). *Kinase* enzyme needs magnesium ion as co-factor for its activity. In this step one ATP is converted into ADP **(1 ATP is utilized)**.
2. Further, the phosphate group present in 6th position of glucose-6-phosphate (G6P) is shifted to 1st position and produces glucose-1-phosphate (G1P). The enzyme responsible is *phospho gluco mutase* (*PGM*) (In change of position of phosphate group involved reactions, the enzymes acted are "*mutase*" and the substrate is "glucose-1-phosphate). **These two steps are similar to glycolysis first two steps**.
3. In the next step, glucose-1-phosphate (G1P) reacts with UTP and produces glucose carrier molecule uridine diphosphate glucose (UDPG) in presence of *UDP-glucose pyrophosphorylase* (*UDPGPP*) (The product is "UDP-glucose (UDPG)" and "pyrophosphate" is removed). The pyrophosphate is immediately broken into two inorganic phosphate by *pyrophosphatase* (*PPase*) (Substrate is "pyrophosphate" and type of reaction is "hydrolysis") through hydrolysis reaction. Otherwise the backward reaction takes place because it is reversible reaction.
4. A small fragment of pre-existing glycogen must act as a "primer" to initiate glycogen synthesis. Glycogen primer is necessary for initiation of glycogen synthesis. In case, if it is not available it is synthesized from UDP-glucose (UDPG) by reacting with tyrosine moiety of glycogenin with the removal of UDP in presence of *glycogen initiator synthase* (*GIS*) (Product formed is "glycogen" and the type of reaction is "synthesis initiation"). UDP can be converted to UTP by *nucleoside diphosphate kinase* (*NDPK*) (In ATP / GTP involved reactions, the enzymes acted are "*kinase*" and the substrate is "UDP" which is "nucleoside diphosphate") **(1 ATP is utilized)**.
5. In the next step, glycogen primer was reacted with more UDP-glucose (UDPG) in presence of *glycogen synthase* (*GS*) (Product is "glycogen" and the type of reaction is "synthesis") with a loss of UDP. The glucose molecules are linked to each other by 1,4-α-glycosidic linkage. The reaction will continue up to 16 glucose molecules in chain. Later, *glycogen synthase* is not able to increase the chain length.
6. After every 8 to 10 glucose molecules branching takes place by *branching enzyme* (*BE*) (Type of reaction is "branch production"). *Branching enzymes* (*BE*) otherwise known as "*glucosyl-α-4,6-transferase* (*G4,6T*) or *amylo-α-1,4 to α-1,6-transglucosidase* (*A1,4T1,6TG*) (Glucose is transferred from "α-1,4 linkage to α-1,6 linkage") transfer a small fragment of 5-8 glucose residues from non-reducing end of

glycogen chain to another glucose residue where it is linked by 1,6-α-glycosidic linkage. Only in the branching point the type of linkage is α-1,6-glycosidic linkage; whereas in rest of case it is α-1,4-glycosidic linkage.

7. Later, the chain length is increased by "*glycogen synthase (GS)*" and more branching are formed by *branching enzymes* (*BE*) which results in formation of homopolysaccharide "glycogen".
8. Totally 2 ATP are consumed for the attachment of single glucose residue. Out of these two, one ATP is needed for phosphorylation of glucose and another one is needed for conversion of UDP to UTP. The overall reactions of glycogenesis are summarized as follows

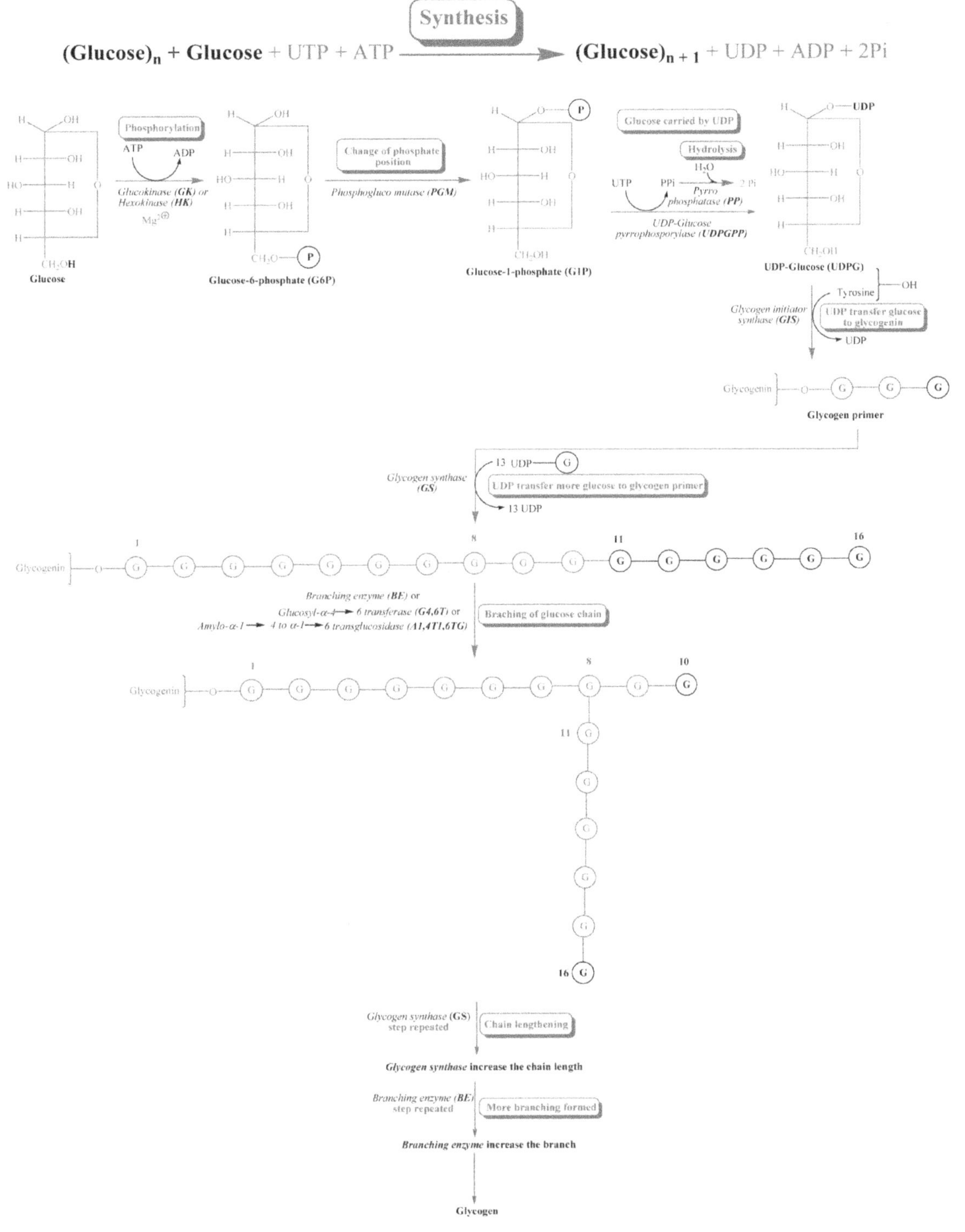

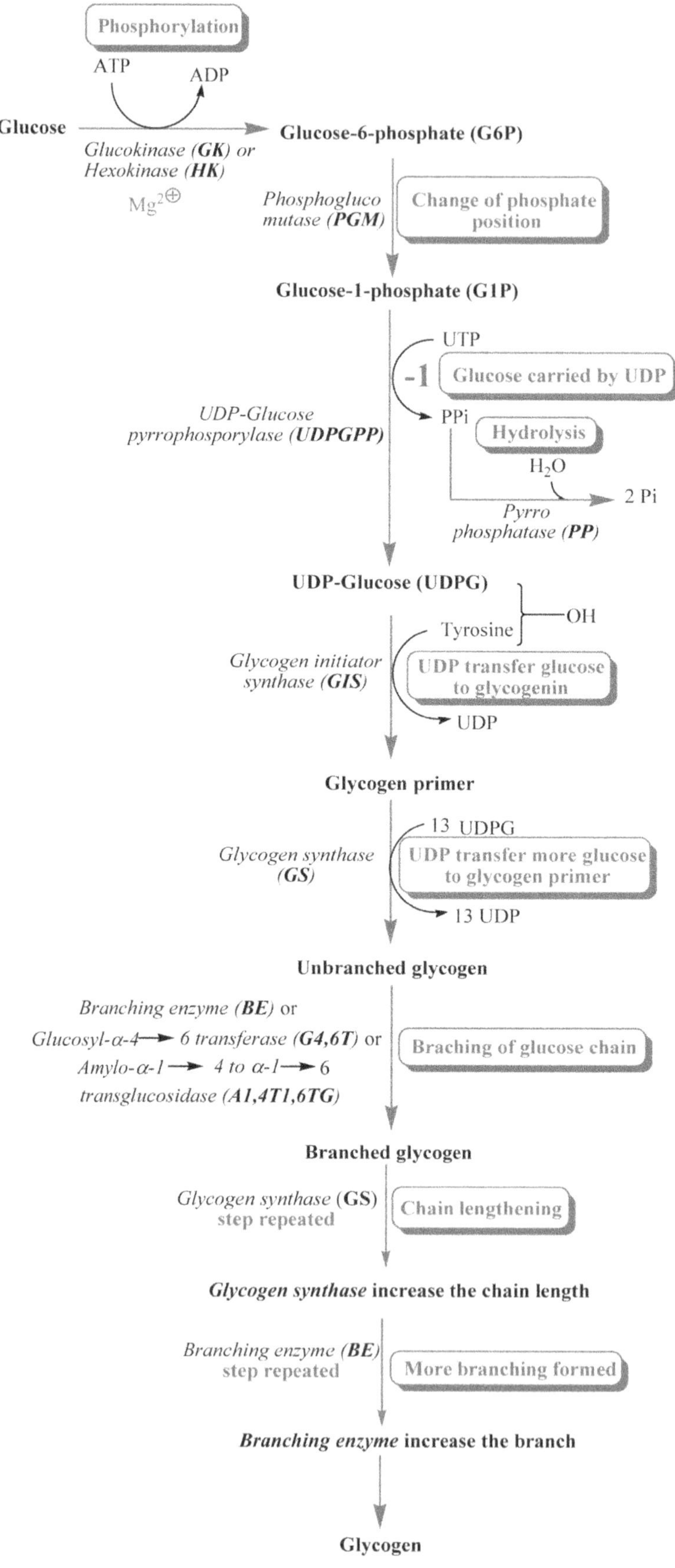

Phosphorylation
ATP
ADP
Glucose
Glucose-6-phosphate (G6P)
Glucokinase (GK) or Hexokinase (HK)
$Mg^{2\oplus}$
Phosphogluco mutase (PGM)
Change of phosphate position
Glucose-1-phosphate (G1P)
UTP
-1
Glucose carried by UDP
PPi
UDP-Glucose pyrrophosporylase (UDPGPP)
Hydrolysis
H_2O
2 Pi
Pyrro phosphatase (PP)
UDP-Glucose (UDPG)
OH
Tyrosine
Glycogen initiator synthase (GIS)
UDP transfer glucose to glycogenin
UDP
Glycogen primer
13 UDPG
Glycogen synthase (GS)
UDP transfer more glucose to glycogen primer
13 UDP
Unbranched glycogen
Branching enzyme (BE) or
Glucosyl-α-4→6 transferase (G4,6T) or
Amylo-α-1→ 4 to α-1→6
transglucosidase (A1,4T1,6TG)
Braching of glucose chain
Branched glycogen
Glycogen synthase (GS) step repeated
Chain lengthening
Glycogen synthase increase the chain length
Branching enzyme (BE) step repeated
More branching formed
Branching enzyme increase the branch
Glycogen

GLYCOGENOLYSIS

Definition: Glycogeno indicates "glycogen" and in Greek lysis means "breakdown / dissolution". **It is defined as breakdown of stored glycogen in liver and muscle into glucose.**

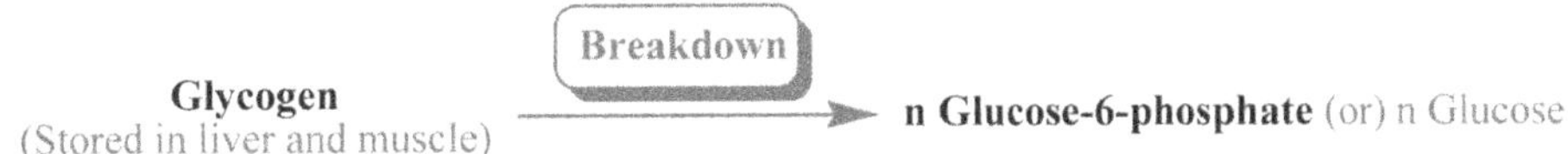

Pathway:

1. In the first step of glycogenolysis, glycogen undergoes phosphorylation reaction by reacting with inorganic phosphate in presence of *glycogen phosphorylase* (*GP*) (Substrate is "glycogen" and the type of reaction is "phosphorolysis") and liberates glucose-1-phosphate (G1P). This process of phosphorolysis continues until four glucose residues remains on either side of branching point. The molecule which contains four glucose residues on either side of branching point is called as "limit dextrin" which cannot be further degraded by *glycogen phosphorylase* (*GP*).
2. In the next step, *glucosyl-4,4-transferase* (*G4,4T*) (Glucose is transferred from α-1,4 linkage to α-1,4 linkage) removes 3 to 4 residues of glucose and transfer them to other chain. The linkage in both the breaking point and attaching point is α-1,4 linkage. ***Glucosyl-4,4-transferase* (*G4,4T*) is the first *debranching enzyme* (*DB*) of glycogenolysis.**
3. **The second *debranching enzyme* (*DB*) i.e., "*amylo-α-1,6-glucosidase*" (*A1,6G*)** (Break of α-1.6 glycosidic linkage) debranches the branching point glucose and removes as free glucose not as glucose phosphate. It only breaks the α-1,6 linkage and not transfers unlike *glucosyl-4,4-transferase* (*G4,4T*).
4. The resulted intermediate is again attacked by *glycogen phosphorylase* (*GP*) and produces glucose-1-phosphate (G1P).
5. Further, phosphate group present in 1st position of glucose-1-phosphate (G1P) is shifted to 6th position and produces glucose-6-phosphate (G6P). The enzyme responsible is *phospho gluco mutase* (*PGM*) (In change of position of phosphate group involved reactions, the enzymes acted are "*mutase*" and the substrate is "glucose-1-phosphate (G1P)").
6. Glucose-6-phosphate (G6P) can either undergo glycolysis or converted to glucose. *Glucose-6-phosphatase* (*G6Pase*) is present in liver, kidney and intestine thereby leads to glucose. Liver is the major glycogen storage organ to provide glucose into circulation to be utilized by various other tissues. In case of muscle and brain *glucose-6-phosphatase* (*G6Pase*) is absent thereby leads to glycolysis. Even though some free glucose is produced in these organs by *amylo-α-1,6-glucosidase* (*A1,6Gase*) enzyme.
7. The ratio of glucose-1-phosphate (G1P) and free glucose produced in glycogenolysis by combined effects of *glycogen phosphorylase* (*GP*) and *debranching enzyme* (*DB*) is 8:1. *Debranching enzyme* (*DB*) cleaves the glycogen branches by two enzyme activities present on a single polypeptide; hence it is a bifunctional enzyme.
8. *Lysosomal acid maltase* (*LAM*) or *acid maltase* (*AM*) or *α-1,4-glucosidase* (α1,4G) (Breaking of α-1.6 glycosidic linkage) is a lysosomal enzyme which continuously degrades a small quantity of glycogen. Significance of this pathway is not clear. However, deficiency of this enzyme cause glycogen accumulation and leads to serious glycogen storage disease type – II or Pompe's disease.

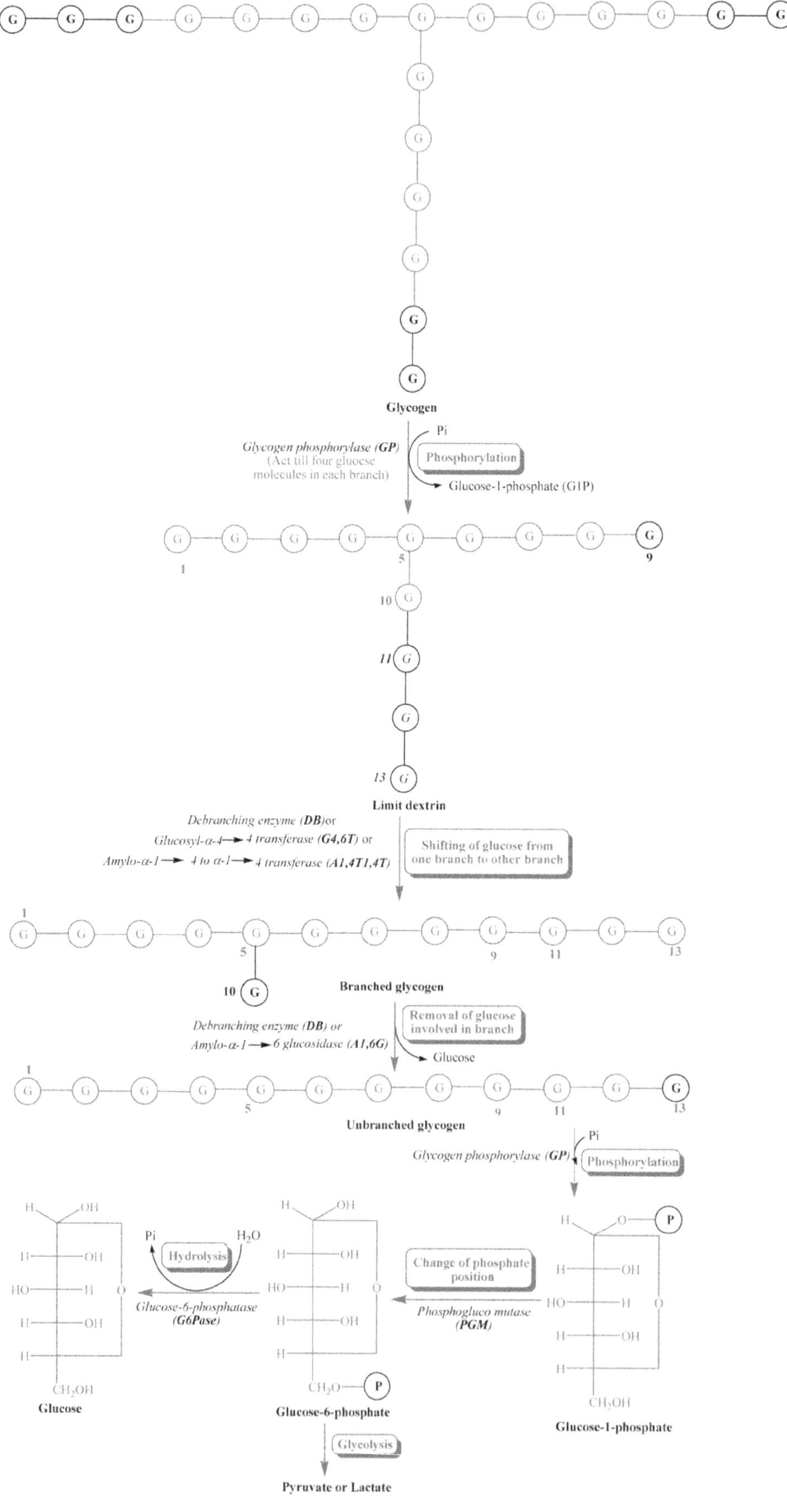
Glycogen
Pi
Glycogen phosphorylase (GP)
(Act till four glucose molecules in each branch)
Phosphorylation
Glucose-1-phosphate (G1P)
Limit dextrin
Debranching enzyme (DB) or
Glucosyl-α-4→4 transferase (G4,6T) or
Amylo-α-1→4 to α-1→4 transferase (A1,4T1,4T)
Shifting of glucose from one branch to other branch
Branched glycogen
Debranching enzyme (DB) or
Amylo-α-1→6 glucosidase (A1,6G)
Removal of glucose involved in branch
Glucose
Unbranched glycogen
Pi
Glycogen phosphorylase (GP)
Phosphorylation
Change of phosphate position
Phosphogluco mutase (PGM)
Pi
H2O
Hydrolysis
Glucose-6-phosphatase (G6Pase)
Glucose
Glucose-6-phosphate
Glucose-1-phosphate
Glycolysis
Pyruvate or Lactate

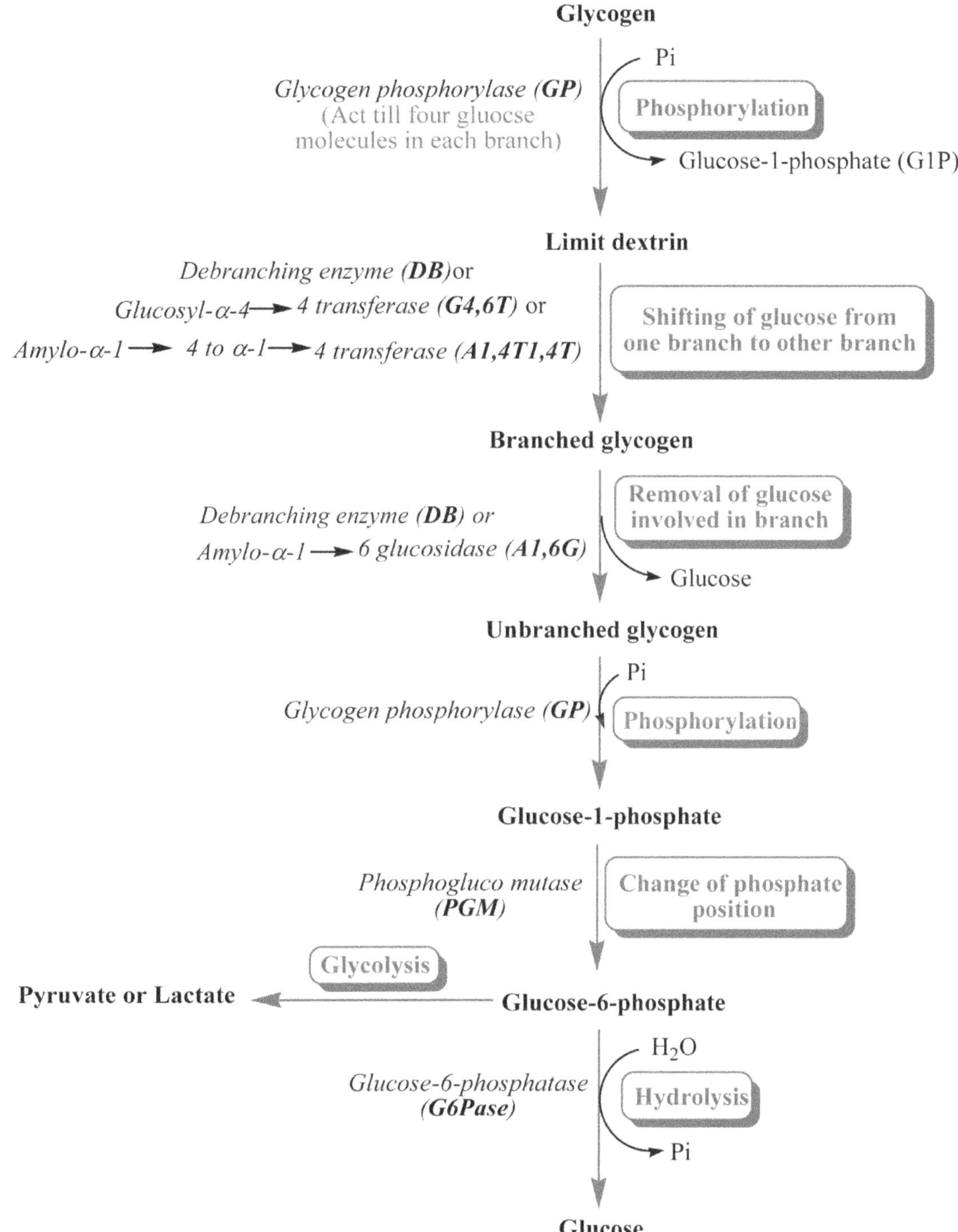

GLYCOGEN STORAGE DISEASES

The diseases which are related to glycogenesis and glycogenolysis are commonly known as glycogen storage diseases. The various glycogen storage diseases are summarized in Table 3.7 along with its responsible enzyme.

Table 3.7 Glycogen storage diseases & their characteristic features.

S. No.	Type of glycogen storage diseases	Disease name	Enzyme responsible	Characteristic features
1	Type – I	Von-Gierke's disease or Type – I glycogenosis	*Glucose-6-phosphatase* (*G6Pase*)	Glycogen accumulates in liver and kidney leads to fasting hypoglycemia, lactic acidemia, hyperlipidemia and hyperuricemia.
2	Type – II	Pompe's disease	*Lysosomal α-1,4-glucosidase* (*α1,4G*) or *acid maltase* (*AM*)	Increased glycogenesis leads to accumulation of glycogen in all tissues particularly heart
3	Type – III	Cori's disease or Forbe's disease or Limit dextrinosis	*Debranching enzyme* (*DE*) or *Amylo-α-1,6-glucosidase* (*A1,6G*)	Decreased debranching of limit dextrin leads to accumulation of branched chain glycogen (Similar to Type – I but mild).
4	Type – IV	Anderson's disease or Amylopectinosis	*Glucosyl-α-4,6-transferase* (*G4,6T*) or *Amylo-α-1,4 to α-1,6-transglucosidase* (*α1,4T1,6TG*)	Increased concentration of un branched glycogen and accumulates in liver.
5	Type – V	Mc Ardle's disease or Type – V glycogenosis	*Glycogen phosphorylase* (*GP*) (In muscle)	Decreased muscle contraction leads to muscle cramps. Storage of glycogen in muscle increases.
6	Type – VI	Her's disease	*Glycogen phosphorylase* (*GP*) (In liver)	Blood glucose level decreased leads to liver enlargement. Mild hypoglycemia and ketosis also seen.
7	Type – VII	Taruis disease	*Phospho fructo kinase* (*PFK*)	Increased glucose-6-phosphate (G6P) and muscle cramps due to exercise.
8	Type – VIII, Type –IX, Type – X, Type – XI	---------	Enzymes involved in activating and deactivating liver phosphorylase	Rare.

Von-Gierke's disease:

It is due to lack of *glucose-6-phosphatase* (***G6Pase***) enzyme hence glucose-6-phosphate (G6P) is not converted into glucose. It leads to the following clinical conditions.

1. **Fasting hypoglycemia:** During fasting period, biological system depends on non-carbohydrate sources for its glucose demand. Due to lack of *glucose-6-phosphatase* (*G6Pase*), non-carbohydrate sources are not converted into glucose and thereby not enough glucose is released from liver into blood. Hence blood glucose level is decreased.
2. **Lactic acidemia:** Due to lack of *glucose-6-phosphatase* (*G6Pase*), glucose is not synthesized from lactate. Hence, concentration of lactate in blood is increased and pH is lowered.
3. **Hyperlipidemia:** Due to blockage of gluconeogenesis, more fats are mobilized to meet the energy requirements which results in increased plasma free fatty acids and ketone bodies.
4. **Hyperuricemia:** In other way, accumulated glucose-6-phosphate (G6P) is diverted to HMP pathway leads to production of ribose-5-phosphate (R5P) which increases the cellular level of phospho ribosyl pyrophosphate (PRPP) and increases the purine metabolism to uric acid. Elevated level of uric acid is associated with deposition of uric acid crystals in soft tissues that leads to a disease called gouty arthritis.

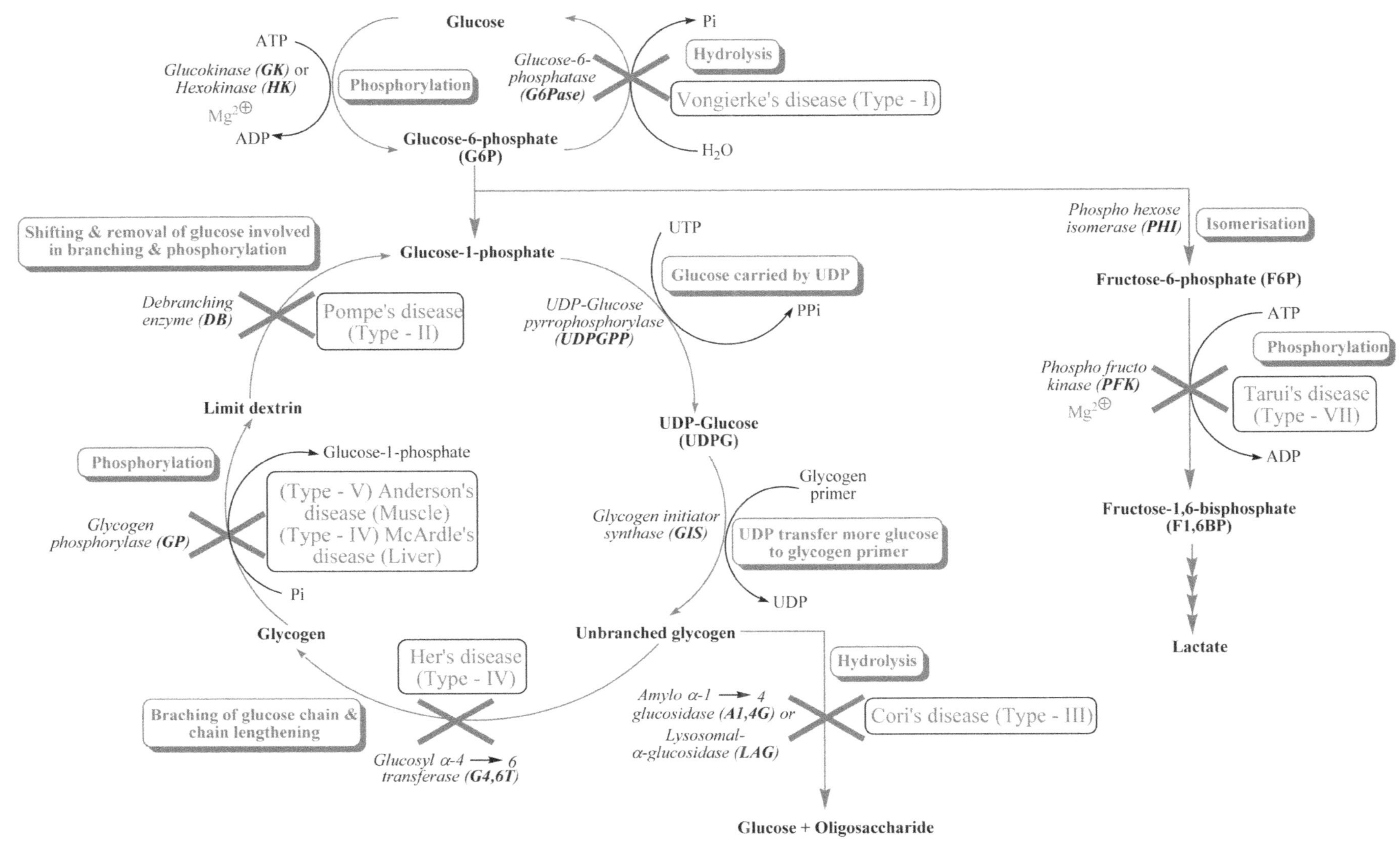
Glucose
ATP
Glucokinase (GK) or
Hexokinase (HK)
Mg2⊕
ADP
Phosphorylation
Glucose-6-phosphate
(G6P)
Glucose-6-
phosphatase
(G6Pase)
Pi
Hydrolysis
Vongierke's disease (Type - I)
H2O
Phospho hexose
isomerase (PHI)
Isomerisation
Fructose-6-phosphate (F6P)
ATP
Phosphorylation
Phospho fructo
kinase (PFK)
Mg2⊕
Tarui's disease
(Type - VII)
ADP
Fructose-1,6-bisphosphate
(F1,6BP)
Lactate
Shifting & removal of glucose involved
in branching & phosphorylation
Glucose-1-phosphate
Debranching
enzyme (DB)
Pompe's disease
(Type - II)
UTP
Glucose carried by UDP
PPi
UDP-Glucose
pyrrophosphorylase
(UDPGPP)
UDP-Glucose
(UDPG)
Limit dextrin
Phosphorylation
Glucose-1-phosphate
(Type - V) Anderson's
disease (Muscle)
(Type - IV) McArdle's
disease (Liver)
Glycogen
phosphorylase (GP)
Pi
Glycogen
primer
Glycogen initiator
synthase (GIS)
UDP transfer more glucose
to glycogen primer
UDP
Glycogen
Unbranched glycogen
Hydrolysis
Her's disease
(Type - IV)
Braching of glucose chain &
chain lengthening
Glucosyl α-4 → 6
transferase (G4,6T)
Amylo α-1 → 4
glucosidase (A1,4G) or
Lysosomal-
α-glucosidase (LAG)
Cori's disease (Type - III)
Glucose + Oligosaccharide

DIABETES MELLITUS

Diabetes mellitus also called as diabetes, is a carbohydrate metabolic disorder in which blood glucose levels are elevated due to decreased circulating insulin level. The following are the symptoms of diabetes mellitus such as a) Polyuria (frequent urination), b) Polydipsia (excessive thirst), c) Polyphagia (excessive hunger), d) Excess sweating, e) Hyperlipidemia, f) Dry mouth and itching skin, g) Blurred vision, h) Yeast infections, i) Slow healing sores or cuts, j) Pain or numbness in feet or legs and k) Weight loss.

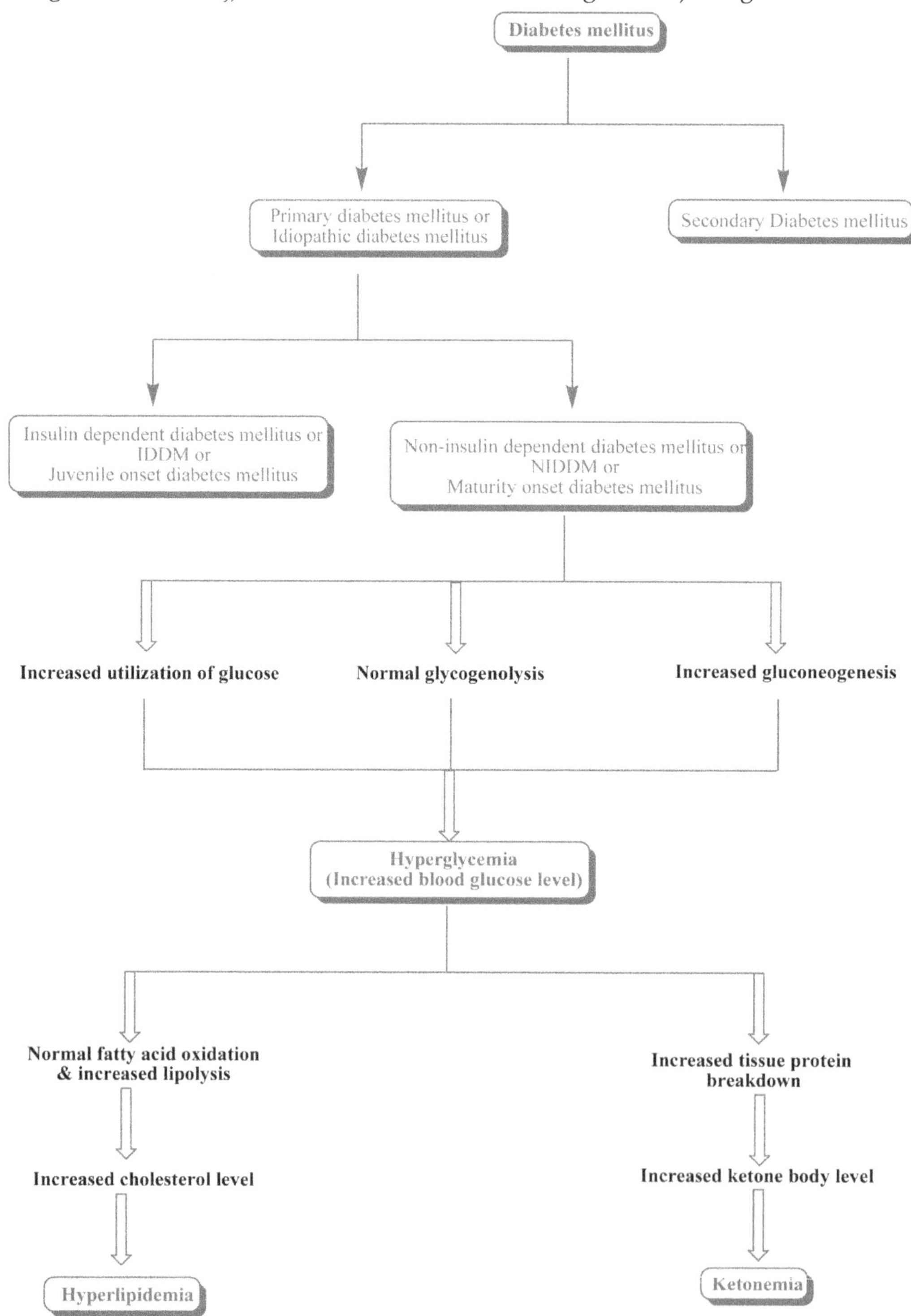

Classification

Diabetes mellitus are broadly classified into two major types namely 1) Primary diabetes mellitus, 2) Secondary diabetes mellitus. Clinically primary diabetes mellitus also known as idiopathic diabetes mellitus is more important than secondary diabetes mellitus. It is due to defect in insulin secretion. It is further classified into 1) Type – I diabetes mellitus and 2) Type–II diabetes mellitus.

Type – I diabetes mellitus: Also known as insulin dependent diabetes mellitus or IDDM or Juvenile onset diabetes mellitus. This diabetes mellitus is dependent on insulin. It is more common in younger people between 10-15 years. In this type of diabetes, there is a complete destruction of β-cells of islets of langerhans. Hence, circulating insulin level is low to very low. This leads to increased blood glucose level. Treatment for IDDM is administration of insulin.

Type – II diabetes mellitus: Also known as non-insulin dependent diabetes mellitus or NIDDM or maturity onset diabetes mellitus. This diabetes mellitus is not dependent on insulin. This type of diabetes mellitus is most common. It is common in elder people (more than 40 years). In this type of diabetes, there is no complete destruction of β-cells of islets of langerhans. Hence circulating insulin level is low. This leads to increased blood glucose level. Treatment for NIDDM is administration of oral hypoglycemic agents.

REGULATION OF CARBOHYDRATE METABOLISM or REGULATION OF BLOOD GLUCOSE LEVEL

The rate limiting enzyme of glycogenesis is *glycogen synthase* (*GS*) and the rate limiting enzyme of glycogenolysis is *glycogen phosphorylase* (*GP*). Hence *glycogen synthase* (*GS*) and *glycogen phosphorylase* (*GP*) regulate the carbohydrate metabolism. These enzymes are regulated by the three different mechanisms.

1. Allosteric regulation.
2. Hormonal regulation (Insulin stimulates glycogenesis and inhibits glycogenolysis whereas glucagon and nor-epinephrine inhibit glycogenesis and stimulates glycogenolysis)
3. Effect of calcium (Calcium stimulates glycogenolysis)

1. **Allosteric Regulation**

   The process of regulating carbohydrate metabolism by the availability of substrate and energy level is known as allosteric regulation. When glucose and energy levels are available in high amount, *glycogen synthase* (*GS*) (glycogenesis) is activated and *glycogen phosphorylase* (*GP*) (glycogenolysis) is inhibited. On the other hand, when glucose and energy levels are available in low amount *glycogen synthase* (*GS*) (glycogenesis) is inhibited and *glycogen phosphorylase* (*GP*) (glycogenolysis) is activated. Allosteric regulation of blood glucose level is depicted in Figure 3.3.

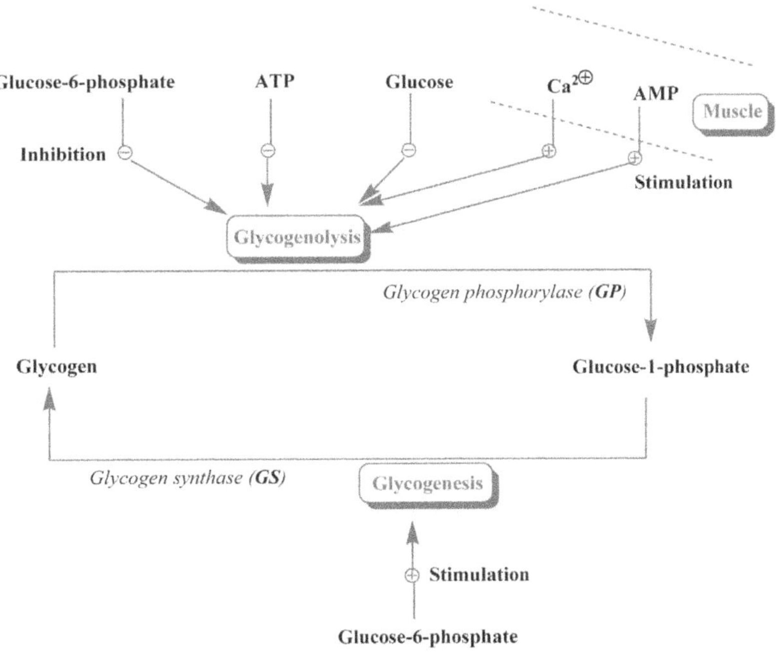

Figure 3.3 Allosteric regulation of blood glucose level.

2. **Hormonal Regulation**

Enzyme proteins are covalently modified by hormones by either phosphorylation or dephosphorylation which results in glycogenesis or glycogenolysis. In general, phosphorylation leads to degradation of glycogen and dephosphorylation leads to synthesis of glycogen. Overall effects of hormones in carbohydrate metabolism are summarized into two major categories.

1. **Insulin:** Increased level of insulin stimulates glycogenesis and inhibits glycogenolysis because insulin inhibits the conversion of active form of *adenylate cyclase* from inactive form of *adenylate cyclase* in plasma membrane.
2. **Glucagon and epinephrine:** Increased level of glucagon, nor-epinephrine and epinephrine inhibits glycogenesis and stimulates glycogenolysis because in plasma membrane it promotes the conversion of active form of *adenylate cyclase* from its inactive form. Effect of glucagon and epinephrine on glycogenesis and glycogenolysis is presented in Figure 3.4 and Figure 3.5, respectively. In addition, effect of insulin on glycogenesis and glycogenolysis is presented in Figure 3.6.

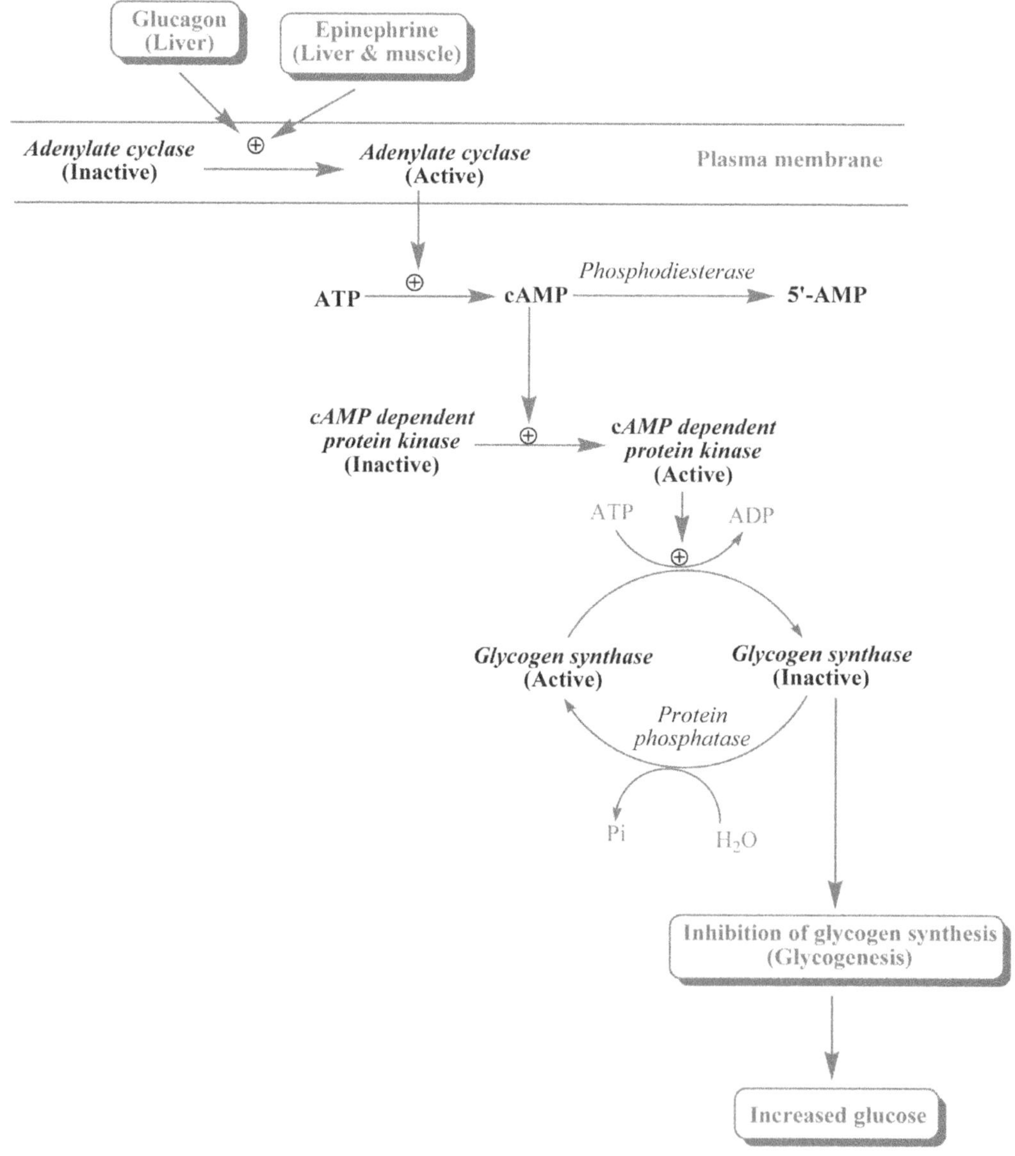

Figure 3.4 Effect of glucagon and epinephrine on glycogenesis.

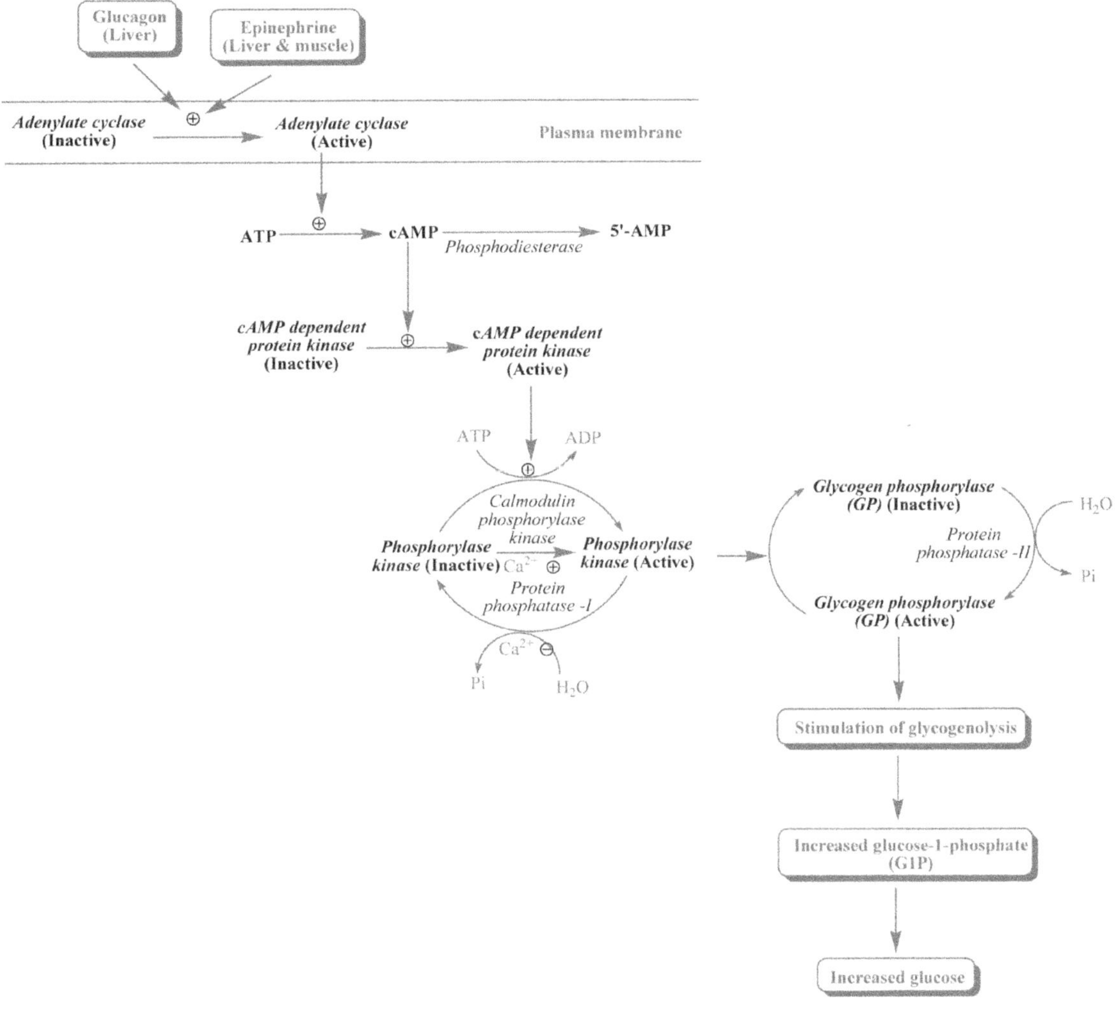

Figure 3.5 Effect of glucagon and epinephrine on glycogenolysis.

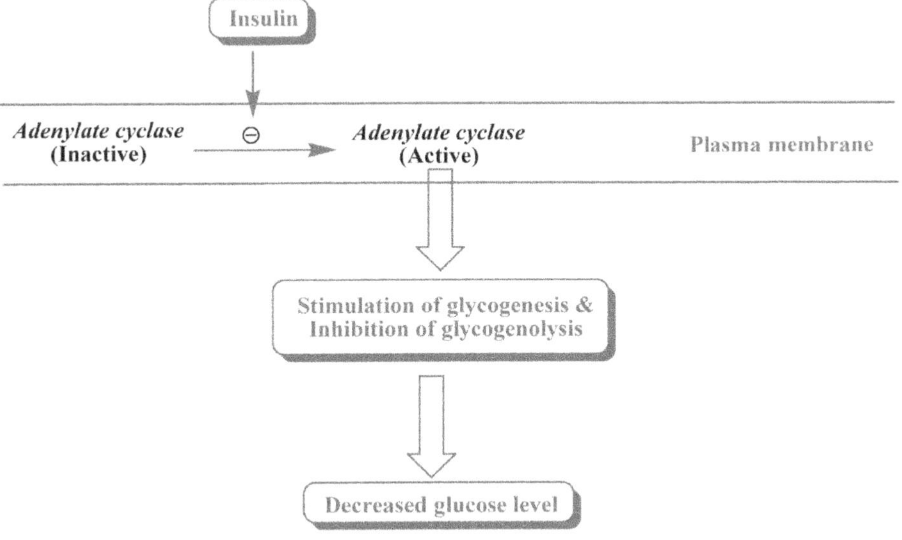

Figure 3.6 Effect of insulin on glycogenesis and glycogenolysis.

3. **Effect of Calcium**

   Generally, release of calcium from sarcoplasmic reticulum leads to reaction with a protein called calmodulin and produces calcium-calmodulin complex. This formed complex activates *glycogen phosphorylase* (*GP*) which leads to stimulation of glycogenolysis ultimately glucose level increased.

GLUCOSE TOLERANCE TEST (GTT)

Glucose tolerance is defined as the ability of the body to metabolize an additional load of glucose. This test is useful to assess the status of carbohydrate tolerance of a person. A decreased glucose tolerance is seen in diabetes mellitus, hyperpituitarism, hyperthyroidism and hyper function of adrenal cortex. It is also known as oral glucose tolerance test (OGTT). A glucose tolerance test measures how well your body's cells are able to absorb glucose (sugar) after you consume a specific amount of sugar. OGTT is a medical blood test used to find out how fast is glucose cleared from blood when given orally. It is used to detect or diagnose diabetes, impaired β-cell function, insulin resistance, rare carbohydrate metabolic disorder, acromegaly and reactive hypoglycemia.

Preparation of subject: Preparing for the glucose tolerance test involves the following steps.

1. Continue to eat a normal carbohydrates rich diet for at least 3 days prior to test.
2. Some medications, such as corticosteroids, beta-blockers, diuretics and antidepressants can interfere with the results. Hence at least 2 days before these drugs which effect carbohydrate metabolisms must be avoided.
3. At least one day before the test, severe exercise must be avoided.
4. Fasting for at least eight hours before the scheduled test. Except water, other beverages, including coffee and caffeinated tea should be avoided, as these can interfere with the results.
5. Avoid using bathroom just before the procedure because urine sample may required for the test.

Procedure:

The suitable time for OGTT is preferably morning i.e., 9-11 am. The test should be done in a comfortable seating position. Fasting blood glucose level and urine are collected for testing the presence of glucose qualitatively.

(a) **OGTT for diabetes:** Dissolve 75 gm of glucose in 300 ml of water and give to drink within 5 min period of time. Every half an hour after taking glucose, collect blood samples and urine samples until 2 hours. Estimate plasma blood glucose levels and test urine qualitatively for glucose. From the following table diabetes and impaired glucose tolerance can easily be identified from measured plasma glucose level. Urine must not contain glucose. Diagnostic criteria for OGTT is given in Table 3.8.

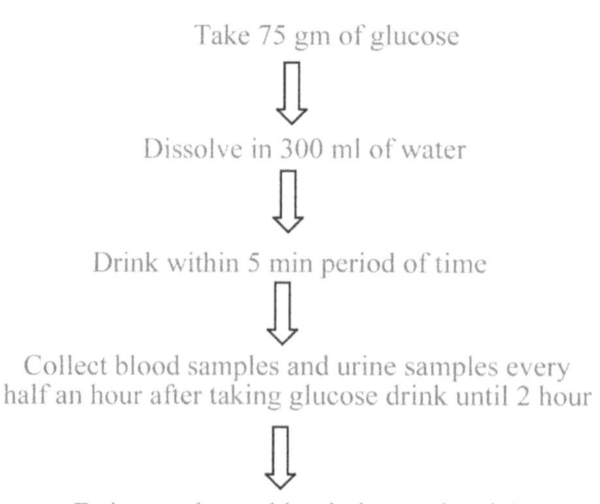

Table 3.8 Diagnostic criteria for OGTT.

Time of blood withdrawal	Plasma glucose level			
	Normal	Impaired glucose tolerance (pre-diabetes)	Diabetes	Gestational diabetes
Fasting	< 6.1 mmol/l or 110 mg/dl)	6.1-7.0 mmol/l or 110-126 mg/dl	> 7.0 mmol/l or 126 mg/dl	> 95 mg/dl
After 1 hour	-----------	-----------	------------	> 180 mg/dl
After 2 hours	< 7.8 mmol/l or 140 mg/dl)	7.8-11.1 mmol/l or 140-200 mg/dl	> 11.1 mmol/l or 200 mg/dl	> 153 mg/dl

(b) **OGTT for gestational diabetes:** Two OGTT tests are used for gestational diabetes. The first test is same as OGTT for diabetes as explained above and blood is withdrawn at both 1 h and 2 h mark. The second test involves two steps. In first step, 1 h screening and 3 h glucose tolerance test if the 1 h screening levels are elevated. Dissolve 50 gm of glucose in 300 ml of water and give to drink within 5 min period of time. Every one hour after glucose drink, collect blood samples until 2 h. Estimate plasma blood glucose levels. If one-hour results are equal to or greater than 135 or 140 mg/dl, then conduct second step of the test.

In the second step, dissolve 100 gm of glucose in 300 ml of water and give to drink within 5 min period of time. Every one hour after taking glucose, collect blood samples until 3 h. Estimate plasma blood glucose levels. If two of the four blood glucose levels are higher than those listed below, then it will diagnosed as gestational diabetes. Diagnostic criteria for OGTT for gestational diabetes are given in Table 3.9.

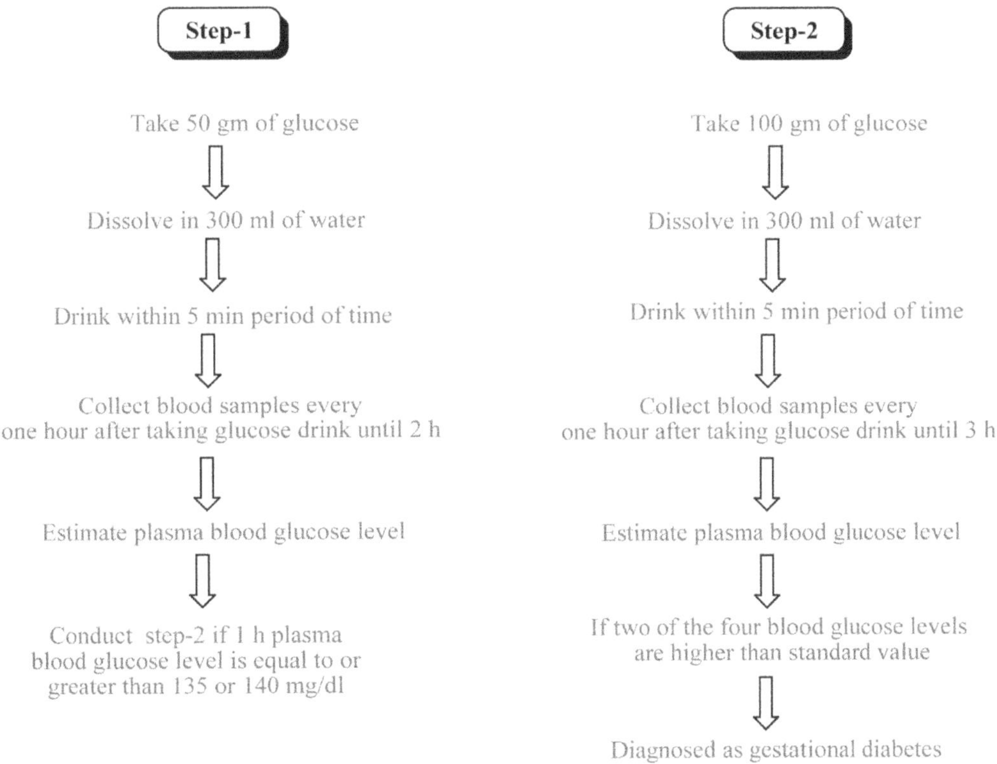

Table 3.9 Diagnostic criteria for OGTT for gestational diabetes

S. No	Time of blood withdrawal	Plasma glucose level
1	Fasting	> 95 mg/dl
2	After 1 h	> 180 mg/dl
3	After 2 h	> 155 mg/dl
4	After 3 h	> 140 mg/dl

GALACTOSE TOLERANCE TEST

Galactose tolerance test is one of the liver function tests which is based on the ability of the liver to convert galactose to glucose, measured by the rate of excretion of galactose following ingestion or intravenous injection of a known amount. It is used to assess the functioning of the liver. The normal half life of galactose is 10-15 min. Galactose tolerance test can be done in two ways 1) Oral method; 2) Intravenous (IV) method. Out of these, IV method is preferred because it is accurate and takes less time (2 h) whereas oral method takes 5 h time.

Procedure: Administer 300 mg/kg of galactose intravenously. Measure blood galactose levels for every 10 min till 2 h. In normal conditions, within 45 min all galactose is cleaned whereas, if liver is not functioning properly the blood galactose levels is elevated. Elevated blood galactose level indicates impaired liver function (hepatocellular damage) such as infective hepatitis and liver cirrhosis.

Administer 300 mg/kg of galactose intravenously

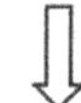

Measure blood galactose levels for every 10 min till 2 hour

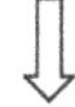

In normal conditions, within 45 min all galactose is cleaned

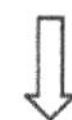

The blood galactose levels is elevated
if liver is not functioning properly

PROBABLE QUESTIONS

PART – A: Multiple Choice Questions

1. Which of the following is the general formula for polysaccharides?
   (a) $(C_6H_{10}O_5)n$ (b) $(C_6H_{12}O_5)n$
   (c) $(C_6H_{10}O_6)n$ (d) $(C_6H_{12}O_6)n$
2. Out of the following polysaccharide which one is homopolysaccharide?
   (a) Inulin (b) Heparin
   (c) Hyaluronic acid (d) Keratan sulfate
3. Which of the following one is aldose sugar?
   (a) Glycerose (b) Ribulose
   (c) Erythrulose (d) Dihydoxyacetone
4. Which of the following one is a triose sugar?
   (a) Glycerose (b) Ribose
   (c) Erythrose (d) Fructose
5. Which of the following one is a pentose sugar?
   (a) Dihydroxyacetone (b) Ribulose
   (c) Erythrose (d) Glucose
6. How many isomers are possible for glucose?
   (a) 2 (b) 4
   (c) 8 (d) 16

7. ________________ are compounds having the same structural formula but differing in spatial configuration.
   (a) Stereoisomers (b) Anomers
   (c) Optical isomers (d) Epimers
8. In semen which sugar is present abundant?
   (a) Glucose (b) Lactose
   (c) Galactose (d) Fructose
9. In solution, glucose is present predominantly in which form.
   (a) Acyclic form (b) Glucopyranose
   (c) Glucofuranose (d) Hydrated acyclic form
10. Which of the following sugars are not an oligosaccharide?
    (P) Raffinose (Q) Stachyose
    (R) Glucoheptose (S) Sedoheptulose.
    Choose the correct option.
    (a) P and Q (b) R and S
    (c) P and S (d) Q and S
11. Which of the following sugar does not form osazone?
    (a) Maltose (b) Sucrose
    (c) Lactose (d) Glucose
12. Which is a sweetener used in sugarless gums and candies?
    (a) Sorbitol (b) Ribitol
    (c) Myoinositol (d) Xylitol
13. Out of the following pathways which one is not an oxidative pathway?
    (a) Glycolysis (b) HMP shunt pathway
    (c) Glycogenesis (d) Uronic acid pathway
14. In which of the following category the degradative process will come.
    (P) Anabolism (Q) Catabolism
    (R) Metabolism (S) Excretion.
    Choose the correct option.
    (a) P and Q is correct (b) R and S is correct
    (c) P is correct (d) Q is correct
15. Which one of the following statement is false for glycolysis?
    (a) It is an oxidative pathway (b) ATPs are generated
    (c) Operative only in presence of oxygen (d) It is very essential for brain
16. In which of the following organs insulin dependent glucose transport is occurring?
    (P) Skeletal muscle (Q) Adipose tissue
    (R) Erythrocyte (S) Brain.
    Choose the correct one.
    (a) P and Q (b) P and S
    (c) Q and R (d) R and S
17. Which of the following substance inhibits phosphotriose isomerase enzyme?
    (a) Iodoacetate (b) Arsenite
    (c) Fluoride (d) Bromohydroxy acetone phosphate

18. For optimum activity of *pyruvate dehydrogenase* & *α-ketoglutarate dehydrogenase* which one is correct?
    (P) THF (Q) NAD^+
    (R) Lipoamide (S) TPP
    Choose the correct option.
    (a) P is not required and Q, R & S are required
    (b) Q is not required and P, R & S are required
    (c) R is not required and P, Q & S are required
    (d) S is not required and P, Q & R are required
19. How many ATPs are generated in TCA cycle?
    (a) 24 (b) 30
    (c) 12 (d) 8
20. Citric acid cycle is regulated by which enzyme?
    (P) *Citrate synthase* (Q) *Aconitase*
    (R) *α-Ketoglutarate dehydrogenase* (S) *Isocitrate dehydrogenase.*
    Choose the correct option.
    (a) P, Q & R (b) Q, R & S
    (c) P, R & S (d) P, Q & S
21. Which intermediate of TCA cycle is involved in lipid metabolism?
    (a) Oxaloacetate (b) Citrate
    (c) α-Ketoglutarate (d) Succinate
22. Which of the following takes place in glyoxylate cycle?
    (a) Glucose to pyruvate (b) Glucose to glycogen
    (c) Fat to glucose (d) Glucose to fat
23. One of the following enzyme(s) in glycolysis catalyzes an irreversible reaction.
    (P) *Hexokinase* (Q) *Phosphofructokinase*
    (R) *Pyruvate kinase* (S) *Aldolase.*
    Choose the correct option.
    (a) P, Q & R (b) Q, R & S
    (c) P, R & S (d) P, Q & S
24. Muscle can't be utilize pyruvate / lactate for the synthesis of glucose. What is the reason behind this?
    (P) *Glucose-6-phosphatase* (Q) *Frutose-1,6-bisphosphatase*
    (R) *Glucose-1,6-bisphosphatase* (S) *Fructose-6-phosphatase.*
    Choose the correct option.
    (a) Absence of Q & R (b) Absence of R & S
    (c) Absence of P & S (d) Absence of P & Q
25. Synthesis of 2,3-bisphosphoglycerate occurs in which of the following tissue?
    (a) Liver (b) Kidney
    (c) Erythrocyte (d) Brain
26. How many ATPs are generated when one glucose molecule is completely oxidized in anaerobic condition?
    (a) 38 (b) 24
    (c) 2 (d) 8

27. Why TCA cycle is the central pathway of metabolism of the cell?
    (a) It occurs in the center of the cell
    (b) Its intermediates are commonly used by other metabolic reactions
    (c) All other metabolic pathways depend upon it
    (d) None of the above
28. In what form does the product of glycolysis enter the TCA cycle?
    (a) Acetyl CoA (b) Pyruvate
    (c) NADH (d) Glucose
29. Why does the glycolytic pathway continue in the direction of glucose catabolism?
    (a) There are essentially three irreversible reactions that act as the driving force for the pathway
    (b) High levels of ATP keep the pathway going in a forward direction
    (c) The enzymes of glycolysis only function in one direction
    (d) Glycolysis occurs in either direction
30. What is the role of *kinase* enzyme?
    (P) Removes phosphate groups of substrates
    (Q) Uses ATP to add a phosphate group to the substrate
    (R) Uses NADH to change the oxidation state of the substrate
    (S) Removes water from a double bond.

    Choose the correct option.
    (a) P & Q (b) R & S
    (c) P & R (d) Q & S
31. Which of the following is not a good source for carbohydrate synthesis?
    (P) Pyruvate (Q) Glycerol
    (R) Odd chain fatty acid (S) Even chain fatty acid.

    Choose the correct option.
    (a) Only R (b) Only S
    (c) Both R & S (d) Both P & Q
32. How many ATPs are needed for the addition of each glucose residue in glycogenesis?
    (a) 1 (b) 2
    (c) 3 (d) 4
33. How many ATPs are generated & utilized in conversion of phosphoenol pyruvate to pyruvate & vice versa, respectively?
    (P) One generated (Q) Two generated
    (R) One utilized (S) Two utilized.

    Choose the correct option.
    (a) P & S (b) Q & R
    (c) P & R (d) Q & S
34. Which of the following enzyme regulates glycogenesis?
    (a) *Glycogen synthase* (b) *Glycogen phosphorylase*
    (c) *Hexokinase* (d) *Phosphogluco mutase*

35. Deficiency of *glucose-6-phosphatase* causes which disease?
    (a) Pompe's disease (b) Cori's disease
    (c) Anderson's disease (d) Von-Gierke's disease
36. Which of the following one is correct?
    (P) Glucagon stimulates gluconeogenesis
    (Q) Glucogenic amino acids stimulates gluconeogenesis
    (R) Glucose stimulates gluconeogenesis
    (S) Acetyl CoA stimulates gluconeogenesis.
    Choose the correct option.
    (a) P, Q & R is correct; S is wrong (b) Q, R & S is correct; P is wrong
    (c) P, Q & S is correct; R is wrong (d) P, R & S is correct; Q is wrong
37. Her's disease is due to deficiency of which of the following enzyme?
    (a) *Glycogen phosphorylase* (b) *Phosphofructo kinase*
    (c) *Lysosomal-α-glucosidase* (d) *Glucosyl-(4,6)-transferase*
38. Which of the following linkages are present in glycogen?
    (P) α-1,4-Glycosidic linkage (Q) β-1,4-Glycosidic linkage
    (R) α-1,6-Glycosidic linkage (S) β-1,6-Glycosidic linkage.
    Choose the correct option.
    (a) Both P & Q (b) Both P & R
    (c) Both P & S (d) Both Q & S
39. In which of the following metabolic pathways ATPs are not directly utilized or produced?
    (a) Glycolysis (b) Uronic acid pathway
    (c) HMP shunt (d) Glycogenolysis
40. Which is the connecting link between HMP shunt & lipid synthesis?
    (a) Ribose (b) NADPH
    (c) Sedoheptulose-7-phosphate (d) NADH
41. Wernicke-Korsakoff syndrome is due to the alteration of which of the following?
    (a) *Transketolase* (b) *Transaldolase*
    (c) *Glucose-6-phosphate dehydrogenase* (d) *Gluconolactone hydrolase*
42. Which of the following enzyme is a lysosomal enzyme?
    (P) *Amylo-α-1,6-glucosidase* (Q) *Amylo-α-1,4-glucosidase*
    (R) *Glucosyl-(α-4-6)-transferase* (S) *Glucosyl-(α-4-4)-transferase.*
    Choose the correct option.
    (a) Only P (b) Both P & Q
    (c) Both R & S (d) Only Q
43. In which of the following metabolic pathways free sugar / sugar acids are involved?
    (a) Glycolysis (b) Uronic acid pathway
    (c) HMP shunt (d) Glycogenolysis
44. Deficiency of which of the following causes essential pentoseuria?
    (a) *Glucuronidase* (b) *L-Gulonolactone oxidase*
    (c) *Xylitol dehydrogenase* (d) *Phosphogluco mutase*

45. Which of the following non-vitamin co-enzyme is a carrier of monosaccharide in glycogen synthesis?
   (P) UDP (Q) CDP
   (R) ATP (S) SAM.
   Choose the correct option.
   (a) Only P (b) Only Q
   (c) Both R & S (d) Both P & Q

46. Which of the following enzyme is absent in primates which is responsible for the synthesis of ascorbic acid?
   (a) *Glucuronidase* (b) *L-Gulonolactone oxidase*
   (c) *Xylitol dehydrogenase* (d) *Phosphogluco mutase*

47. Which is a good precursor for glucosamine?
   (a) Galactose-1-phosphate (b) Galactose-6-phosphate
   (c) Fructose-1-phosphate (d) Fructose-6-phosphate

48. Which of the following are characteristic features of Von Gierke's disease?
   (P) Fasting hypoglycemia (Q) Hypolipidemia
   (R) Lactic acidemia (S) Gouty arthritis.
   Choose the correct option.
   (a) P, Q & R (b) Q, R & S
   (c) P, R & S (d) P, Q & S

49. Dietary xylulose can participate in other metabolisms by entering through which of the following pathway?
   (a) HMP shunt pathway (b) Sorbitol pathway
   (c) Uronic acid pathway (d) Glycolysis

50. Essential fructosuria is due to deficiency of which of the following enzyme?
   (a) *Aldose reductase* (b) *Sorbitol dehydrogenase*
   (c) *Aldolase B* (d) *Fructokinase*

Key for Multiple Choice Questions

1. (a)	2. (a)	3. (a)	4. (a)	5. (b)
6. (d)	7. (a)	8. (d)	9. (b)	10. (b)
11. (b)	12. (d)	13. (c)	14. (d)	15. (c)
16. (a)	17. (d)	18. (a)	19. (c)	20. (c)
21. (b)	22. (c)	23. (a)	24. (d)	25. (c)
26. (c)	27. (b)	28. (a)	29. (a)	30. (a)
31. (b)	32. (b)	33. (a)	34. (a)	35. (d)
36. (c)	37. (a)	38. (b)	39. (c)	40. (b)
41. (a)	42. (d)	43. (b)	44. (c)	45. (a)
46. (b)	47. (d)	48. (c)	49. (c)	50. (d)

PART – B: Short Answers

1. Write briefly about the metabolic derangements in diabetes mellitus.
2. Write a note on glycogen storage diseases.
3. Write the significance of glucose tolerance test.
4. Write a note on glucose tolerance test and its clinical significance.
5. Write the reactions of Kreb's cycle.
6. What are the glycogen storage diseases?
7. Explain the terms: a) Hypoglycemia; b) Gluconeogenesis.
8. Write short notes on diabetes mellitus.
9. Write short notes on glycogen storage diseases.
10. Write a short note on hormonal regulation of blood glucose levels & diabetes mellitus.
11. Write about glycolysis pathway, energetic & significance.
12. Write the sequence of glycolysis reactions.
13. Explain pentose phosphate pathway.
14. Describe the process of gluconeogenesis in carbohydrate metabolism.
15. Define gluconeogenesis & glycogenolysis.
16. Give the significance of pentose phosphate pathway.
17. Explain the salient features of gluconeogenesis & its regulation.
18. Define and classify carbohydrates with suitable examples.
19. Write a note on structural aspects of carbohydrates.
20. Write a note on chemical reactions of monosaccharide.
21. Write a note on biological significance of carbohydrates.
22. Write short notes on a) Epimer, b) Anomer.
23. Explain optical activity and D- & L-isomer of monosaccharides.
24. Write a note on reducing properties of monosaccharides.
25. What is the basic principle involved in osazone test?

PART – C: Long Answers

1. Explain HMP pathway and its significance.
2. Write the procedure and interpretation of OGTT. Explain the role of hormones in carbohydrate metabolism.
3. Explain the steps involved in gluconeogenesis and explain its significance.
4. Explain Kreb's cycle with its regulation.
5. Explain the steps involved in glycolytic pathway and mention the energetic under aerobic and anaerobic conditions.
6. How does insulin and epinephrine regulate glycogen metabolism?
7. Outline the steps involved in glycolysis. The role of HMP shunts in the carbohydrate metabolism.
8. Write in detail about the difference between the gluconeogenesis and glycogenesis.
9. Explain how does hormones regulate glycogenesis.
10. Outline the hormonal regulations of carbohydrate metabolism.
11. Write short notes on glucose tolerance test. Describe Kreb's citric acid cycle with a neat diagram.
12. Write about citric acid cycle pathway, energetic & significance.
13. Explain pentose phosphate pathway & its significance.
14. Explain any two of the following: a) Glycogenolysis, b) HMP shunt, c) Glycogenesis.

15. Explain the following: a) TCA cycle, b) Glycolysis
16. Explain the citric acid cycle.
17. Write a brief account of glycolysis.
18. Write a detailed note on gluconeogenesis.
19. Describe about TCA cycle and add a note on effect of inhibitors and regulation of TCA cycle.
20. Describe the TCA cycle, its regulation & energy yield in it.
21. Sketch the pentose phosphate pathway & explain its physiological significance.
22. Define carbohydrates and explain its various structural aspects with special emphasize on anomer and mutarotation.
23. List out various chemical reactions of monosaccharide and explain any four reactions in detail.
24. Explain the following tests: a) OGTT, b) Galactose tolerance test,
25. How does blood glucose levels are regulated? Explain the different methods of regulation in detail.

4

Lipids & Its Metabolism

In Greek, lipos means "fat". **Lipids are defined as organic compounds which are relatively insoluble in water and soluble in organic solvents like alcohol, ether, etc, potentially related to fatty acids and utilized by the living cells**. Chemically, lipids are esters of fatty acids.

The polar groups present in lipids are much smaller than their non-polar portion, hence, they are insoluble in water. Although they have several uses in medicine and industries, the function of oils and fats is mainly the storage of energy. Lipids are the chief concentrated storage form of energy and they play a role in cellular structure and various other biochemical functions. It is a heterogeneous group of compounds and are mostly small molecules. Lipids differ from the rest of body compounds because of their hydrophobic and non-polar nature. Lipids are not polymers like polysaccharides, proteins and nucleic acid.

Throughout the plant and animal kingdom, lipids are distributed widely. In plants, they occur in the seeds, nuts and fruits. In animals, lipids are stored in adipose tissues, nervous-tissues, and bone marrow. Neutral lipids are uncharged lipids. **Example:** Monoacylglycerol, diacylglycerol, triacylglycerol, cholesterol and cholesteryl esters.

Classification of Lipids

Based on the composition, lipids are broadly classified into four major types as follows.

They are,

1. Simple lipids
2. Compound lipids (or) Complex lipids
3. Derived lipids
4. Miscellaneous lipids

1. **Simple lipids:**

   These lipids, upon hydrolysis, yield one or more fatty acids and an alcohol. Generally, simple lipids are esters of fatty acids. The simple lipids are further classified based on nature of the alcohol present into two major types as,

   (a) Fats & oils

   (b) Waxes

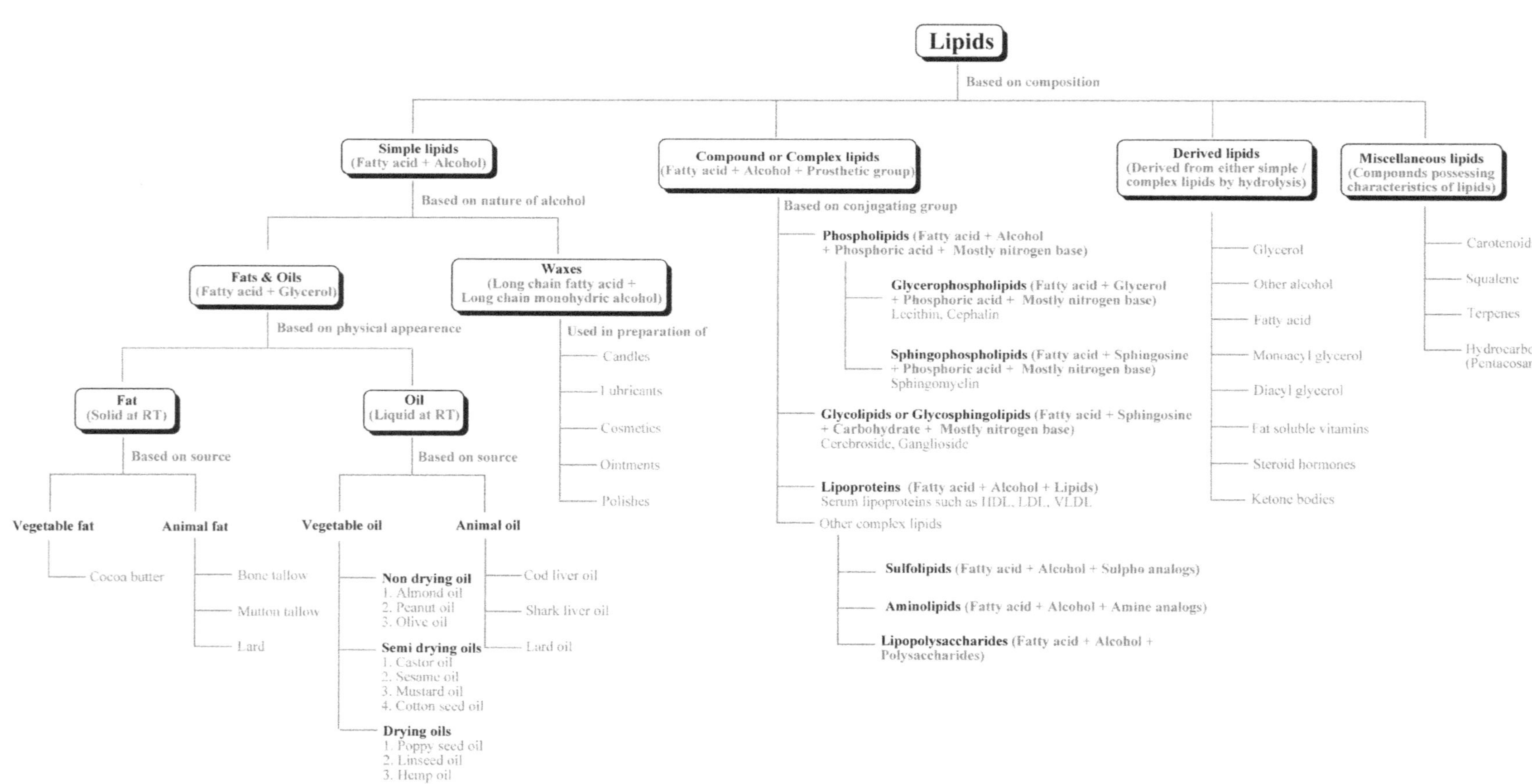
Lipids
Based on composition
Simple lipids
(Fatty acid + Alcohol)
Based on nature of alcohol
Fats & Oils
(Fatty acid + Glycerol)
Based on physical appearence
Fat
(Solid at RT)
Based on source
Vegetable fat
Cocoa butter
Animal fat
Bone tallow
Mutton tallow
Lard
Oil
(Liquid at RT)
Based on source
Vegetable oil
Non drying oil
1. Almond oil
2. Peanut oil
3. Olive oil
Semi drying oils
1. Castor oil
2. Sesame oil
3. Mustard oil
4. Cotton seed oil
Drying oils
1. Poppy seed oil
2. Linseed oil
3. Hemp oil
Animal oil
Cod liver oil
Shark liver oil
Lard oil
Waxes
(Long chain fatty acid +
Long chain monohydric alcohol)
Used in preparation of
Candles
Lubricants
Cosmetics
Ointments
Polishes
Compound or Complex lipids
(Fatty acid + Alcohol + Prosthetic group)
Based on conjugating group
Phospholipids (Fatty acid + Alcohol
+ Phosphoric acid + Mostly nitrogen base)
Glycerophospholipids (Fatty acid + Glycerol
+ Phosphoric acid + Mostly nitrogen base)
Lecithin, Cephalin
Sphingophospholipids (Fatty acid + Sphingosine
+ Phosphoric acid + Mostly nitrogen base)
Sphingomyelin
Glycolipids or Glycosphingolipids (Fatty acid + Sphingosine
+ Carbohydrate + Mostly nitrogen base)
Cerebroside, Ganglioside
Lipoproteins (Fatty acid + Alcohol + Lipids)
Serum lipoproteins such as HDL, LDL, VLDL
Other complex lipids
Sulfolipids (Fatty acid + Alcohol + Sulpho analogs)
Aminolipids (Fatty acid + Alcohol + Amine analogs)
Lipopolysaccharides (Fatty acid + Alcohol +
Polysaccharides)
Derived lipids
(Derived from either simple /
complex lipids by hydrolysis)
Glycerol
Other alcohol
Fatty acid
Monoacyl glycerol
Diacyl glycerol
Fat soluble vitamins
Steroid hormones
Ketone bodies
Miscellaneous lipids
(Compounds possessing
characteristics of lipids)
Carotenoids
Squalene
Terpenes
Hydrocarbons
(Pentacosane)

(a) **Fats and oils or triacylglycerols:** These are esters of fatty acids with glycerol. Fats and oils are glyceryl esters of higher fatty acids like palmitic, stearic, oleic, linoleic, and linolenic acids. In fats and oils (triglyceride), one molecule of glycerol is linked with three molecules of higher fatty acids by ester linkage.

$$\underset{\textbf{Glycerol}}{\begin{array}{l} CH_2-OH \\ HO-CH \\ CH_2-OH \end{array}} + \underset{\textbf{Fatty acids}}{\begin{array}{l} HO-C(=O)-R_1 \\ HO-C(=O)-R_2 \\ HO-C(=O)-R_3 \end{array}} \xrightarrow[-\,3\,H_2O]{\text{Esterification}} \underset{\textbf{Triglycerides or Triacylglycerol}}{\begin{array}{l} CH_2-O-C(=O)-R_1 \\ R_2-C(=O)-O-CH \\ CH_2-O-C(=O)-R_3 \end{array}}$$

Triglycerides are of two types based on the nature of fatty acids. If all the three fatty acids attached to glycerol are identical or same, then the triglycerides are known as simple triglycerides. Incase if three fatty acids attached to glycerol are not identical or different, then the triglycerides are known as mixed triglycerides. Natural fats are mainly composed of mixed triglycerides. As these glycerides have no free acidic or basic groups, they are often termed as neutral fats.

The composition of fats and oils are the same but they differ in their physical appearance at room temperature (RT). They are distinguished on the basis of their melting ranges. The oils are liquids at ordinary temperature while the fats are solids or semisolids (This distinction is not quite sharp and depends upon the climate and seasonal variation. **Example:** Coconut oil, sesame oil, and ghee are liquids in summer and solids in winter in our country). Fats are solid at room temperature and contain mostly saturated fatty acids like stearic and palmitic acids. Hence, melts at higher temperature. (**Example:** Vegetable fats like cocoa butter and animal fats like bone tallow, mutton tallow and lard).

Oils are liquid at room temperature and contain mostly unsaturated fatty acids like oleic acid. Hence, melts at lower temperature. (**Example:** Non-drying oils like almond oil, peanut oil, and olive oil, semi drying oils like castor oil, sesame oil, mustard oil and cotton seed oil, and drying oils like poppy seed oil, linseed oil and hemp oil).

(b) **Waxes:** These are esters of long chain fatty acids and long chain monohydric alcohols or sterols. The alcohols present in the waxes are other than glycerol. This alcohol may be aliphatic or alicyclic in nature. In general, the waxes are used in many industries for the production of candles, lubricants, cosmetics, ointments, polishes, etc.

2. **Complex lipids (or) compound lipids:**

These lipids contain additional or prosthetic groups such as phosphoric acid, proteins, carbohydrates, sulphate, nitrogen base, etc. along with fatty acids and alcohol. Based on the nature of additional groups present, the complex lipids are further subdivided into many types as follows.

(a) **Phospholipids:** In this complex lipid, the prosthetic group present is phosphoric acid. Most of the phospholipids also contain nitrogen bases. Based on the alcohol present in the phospholipids, it was further subdivided into two categories as,

1. **Glycerophospholipids:** It is composed of fatty acids, glycerol, phosphoric acid, and nitrogen bases. **Example:** Lecithin and cephalin.
2. **Sphingophospholipids:** It is composed of fatty acids, sphingosine (alcohol), phosphoric acid and nitrogen bases. **Example:** Sphingomyelin.

(b) **Glycolipids:** It is otherwise known as glycosphingolipids because of the presence of alcohol sphingosine. It is composed of fatty acids, sphingosine (alcohol), carbohydrate and nitrogen bases. **Example:** Cerebroside and ganglioside.

(c) **Lipoproteins:** It is composed of fatty acids, alcohol and lipids. **Example:** Serum lipoproteins such as HDL, LDL and VLDL.

(d) **Other complex lipids:** Among various other complex lipids, sulpholipids, aminolipids, and lipopolysaccharides are important.

3. **Derived lipids:** These compounds possess characteristics of lipids and are obtained either from simple or complex lipids by hydrolysis. **Example:** Glycerol, fatty acid, other alcohol, monoacylglycerol, diacylglycerol, fat soluble vitamin, steroid hormones and ketone bodies.
4. **Miscellaneous lipids:** Large numbers of compounds possess the characteristics of lipids and these compounds come under miscellaneous lipids. **Example:** Carotenoids, squalene, hydrocarbons like pentacosane, terpenes, etc.

Biological Significance of Lipids

The various biological significance of lipid are as follows:

1. Lipids are the concentrated fuel reserve of the body which is the most important role of lipids.
2. Lipid also acts as an insulating material and protects the internal organs.
3. In addition, lipids also give shape and smooth appearance to the body.
4. Dietary fat is important for the sufficient absorption of the essential fatty acid and fat-soluble vitamins from the food.
5. Lipids, particularly phospholipids and cholesterol are the major constituents of biological membrane structure and regulates the membrane permeability.
6. Lipids serve as a source of fat-soluble vitamins such as vitamin A, D, E, and K.
7. Some biologically active materials which serve as important building blocks of compounds like acetic acid are derived from lipids.
8. Lipids, especially steroid hormones and prostaglandins are important cellular metabolic regulators.
9. The cellular respiration and the conformation of ETC is maintained by the phospholipids particularly lecithin, cephalin and cardiolipin.
10. From the intestine, fats are absorbed by the participation of phospholipids.
11. Lipoproteins are involved in the transport of lipids and the phospholipids are necessary for the synthesis of different lipoproteins.
12. Phospholipids are regarded as lipotropic factors because in the liver it prevents the accumulation of fat.
13. Unsaturated fatty acids and arachidonic acids are released from phospholipids only. Eicosanoids such as prostaglandins, thromboxane, prostacyclins, etc. are biosynthesized from archidonic acid and unsaturated fatty acids only.

Fatty Acids

The simplest forms of lipids are fatty acids. In natural fats and oils, fatty acids occur mainly as esters but do occur in the unesterified form as free fatty acids. Fatty acids are carboxylic acids with hydrocarbon side chains. Fatty acids of natural fats are usually straight chain derivatives, containing even numbers of carbon atoms, as they are synthesized from two carbon units. The chain may be saturated or unsaturated. Compared to plant origin fatty acids (contain epoxy, keto and hydroxyl group and cyclopentane ring in structure), animal origin fatty acids possess a simple structure.

Classification of Fatty Acids

Fatty acids are classified in many different ways as follows,

1. Classification based on total number of carbon atoms
2. Classification based on length of hydrocarbon chain
3. Classification based on nature of hydrocarbon chain

1. **Classification based on total number of carbon atoms**

   Fatty acids are broadly classified into two major types based on the total number of carbon atoms present is even number or odd number.

   (a) **Even number of carbon atom chain fatty acids:** The total number of carbons present in this fatty acid is an even number (2, 4, 6 and similar series). In general, even carbons (14 to 20 carbons) are present in most of the fatty acids that occur in natural lipids. The reason behind this concept is the occurrence of fatty acid biosynthesis with sequential addition of two carbon units. **Example:** Palmitic acid (contains 16 carbons in total), stearic acid (contains 18 carbons in total), etc.

   (b) **Odd number of carbon atom chain fatty acids:** The total number of carbons present in this fatty acid is an odd number (1, 3, 5 and similar series). Odd numbered fatty acids are present in milk and are also found in microbial cell walls. **Example:** Propionic acid (contains 3 carbons in total), valeric acid (contains 5 carbons in total), etc.

2. **Classification based on length of hydrocarbon chain**

   Based on the length of the hydrocarbon chain present in fatty acid, it was broadly classified into three major types. They are,

   (a) **Short chain fatty acids:** This fatty acid consists of 2 to 7 carbon atoms.

   (b) **Medium chain fatty acids:** This fatty acid consists of 8 to 15 carbon atoms.

   (c) **Long chain fatty acids:** This fatty acid consists of 16 and above (usually up to 24) carbon atoms.

3. **Classification based on nature of hydrocarbon chain**

   Fatty acids are subdivided into two major groups based on the nature of hydrocarbon chains, particularly saturation conditions. They are,

   (a) **Saturated fatty acids:** Unsaturation (double or triple bonds) is absent in these fatty acids. CH_3-$(CH_2)_n$-COOH is the general structural formula of saturated fatty acids. They are named by adding the suffix "-anoic" after the hydrocarbon with the same number of carbon atoms. **Example:** Propanoic acid, pentanoic acid or valeric acid, n-hexadecanoic acid or palmitic acid, n-octadecanoic acid or stearic acid, etc.

   (b) **Unsaturated fatty acids:** Unsaturation (double or triple bonds) is present in these fatty acids. In systematic name, the suffix "-enoic" is added after the hydrocarbon with the same number of carbon atoms. Depending on the number of unsaturated bonds present or the degree of unsaturation, it is further classified into two different types as follows,

      1. **Monounsaturated (Monoethenoid, monoenoic) fatty acids:** Contains one double bond. **Example:** Palmitoleic acid and oleic acid.

      2. **Polyunsaturated (polyethenoid, polyenoic) fatty acids:** It is commonly known as PUFA and contains two or more double bonds. These fatty acids are not synthesized by the body due to the lack of double bond introducing enzymes beyond 9 to 10 carbons. It is necessary to take through dietary sources. Hence, PUFA is also called as **essential fatty acid. Example:** Linoleic acid, linolenic acid and arachidonic acid.

Nomenclature of Fatty Acids

1. Systematic nomenclature of fatty acids is based on the name of hydrocarbons with the same number of carbon atoms. In systematic nomenclature, the final 'e' in the name of the hydrocarbon is replaced by the suffix 'oic acid'. **Example:** Propanoic acid (the corresponding hydrocarbon is 'propane'. In this, final 'e' is replaced by the suffix 'oic acid' i.e., "propane – e + oic acid = propanoic acid")
2. In general, saturated fatty acids end with a suffix 'anoic acid'. **Example:** Octanoic acid and decanoic acid. Similarly, unsaturated fatty acids with double bonds end with a suffix 'enoic acid'. **Example:** Octadecenoic acid (oleic acid) and hexadecenoic acid (palmitoleic acid).

3. The C-1 would be carboxyl carbon of a fatty acid and the C-2 would be α-carbon, the C-3, C-4, C-5 and C-6 would be β, γ, δ and ε carbon, respectively. The end methyl carbon is known as the ω carbon or n-carbon atom.

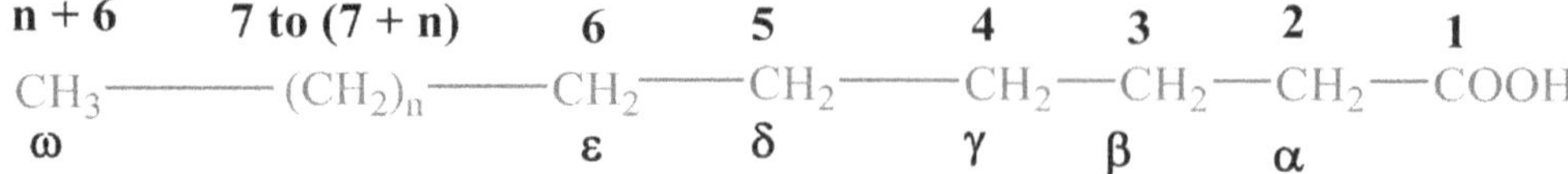

Table 4.1 List of biochemically important fatty acids.

S.No.	Common name	IUPAC name	Structure	Codes
I. Saturated fatty acids				
1	Acetic acid	n-Ethanoic acid	CH_3COOH	2: 0
2	Propionic acid	n-Propanoic acid	CH_3-CH_2-COOH	3: 0
3	Butyric acid	n-Butanoic acid	CH_3-$(CH_2)_2$-COOH	4: 0
4	Valeric acid	n-Pentanoic acid	CH_3-$(CH_2)_3$-COOH	5: 0
5	Caproic acid	n-Hexanoic acid	CH_3-$(CH_2)_4$-COOH	6: 0
6	Caprylic acid	n-Octanoic acid	CH_3-$(CH_2)_6$-COOH	8: 0
7	Capric acid	n-Decanoic acid	CH_3-$(CH_2)_8$-COOH	10: 0
8	Lauric acid	n-Dodecanoic acid	CH_3-$(CH_2)_{10}$-COOH	12: 0
9	Myristic acid	n-Tetradecanoic acid	CH_3-$(CH_2)_{12}$-COOH	14: 0
10	Palmitic acid	n-Hexadecanoic acid	CH_3-$(CH_2)_{14}$-COOH	16: 0
11	Stearic acid	n-Octadecanoic acid	CH_3-$(CH_2)_{16}$-COOH	18: 0
12	Arachidic acid	n-Eicosanoic acid	CH_3-$(CH_2)_{18}$-COOH	20: 0
13	Behenic acid	n-Docosanoic acid	CH_3-$(CH_2)_{20}$-COOH	22: 0
14	Lignoceric acid	n-Tetracosanoic acid	CH_3-$(CH_2)_{22}$-COOH	24: 0
II. Unsaturated fatty acids				
15	Palmitoleic acid	cis-9-Hexadecenoic acid	CH_3-$(CH_2)_5$-CH=CH-$(CH_2)_7$-COOH	16: 1: 9
16	Oleic acid	cis-9-Octadecenoic acid	CH_3-$(CH_2)_7$-CH=CH-$(CH_2)_7$-COOH	18: 1: 9
17	Linoleic acid	cis, cis-9,12-Octadecadienoic acid	CH_3-$(CH_2)_4$-CH=CH-CH_2-CH=CH-$(CH_2)_7$-COOH	18: 2: 9, 12
18	Linolenic acid	All cis-9,12,15-Octadecatrienoic acid	CH_3-CH_2-CH=CH-CH_2-CH=CH-CH_2-CH=CH-$(CH_2)_7$-COOH	18: 3: 9, 12, 15
19	Arachidonic acid	All cis-5,8,11,14-Eicosatetraenoic acid	CH_3-$(CH_2)_4$-CH=CH-CH_2-CH=CH-CH_2-CH=CH-CH_2-CH=CH-$(CH_2)_3$-COOH	20: 4: 5, 8, 11, 14

4. For indicating the number and position of the double bonds, various conventions are used. **Example:** In fatty acids, the presence of a double bond between carbon atoms 9 and 10 is indicated by Δ^9. The number of carbon atoms, the number of double bonds, and the positions of the double bonds are widely indicated by using this convention only.

18 13 12 11 10 9 1
CH_3—$(CH_2)_4$—CH=CH—CH_2—CH=CH—$(CH_2)_7$—COOH

Linoleic acid [C_{18},$\Delta^{9,12}$]

18 17 16 15 14 13 12 11 10 9 1
CH_3—CH_2—CH=CH—CH_2—CH=CH—CH_2—CH=CH—$(CH_2)_7$—COOH

Linolenic acid [C_{18}, $\Delta^{9,12,15}$]

20 15 14 13 12 11 10 9 8 7 6 5 1
CH_3—$(CH_2)_4$—CH=CH—CH_2—CH=CH—CH_2—CH=CH—CH_2—CH=CH—$(CH_2)_3$—COOH

Arachidonic acid [C_{20}, $\Delta^{5,8,11,14}$]

5. In biochemistry, fatty acids are represented in shorthand notation using numbers instead of writing the full structures. The general rule followed is that the total number of carbon atoms are written first, followed by the number of double bonds present, and finally the first carbon position of the double bonds starting from the carbonyl end. **Example:** Palmitic acid is written as 16: 0, oleic acid is written as 18: 1: 9 and arachidonic acid is written as 20: 4: 5, 8, 11, 14.
6. Various saturated and unsaturated fatty acids which are biologically important are listed in the Table 4.1.

Biological Significance of Fatty Acids

1. Fatty acids are the cellular fuel sources of the body.
2. Fatty acids are the composition of hormones and lipids.
3. Fatty acids play a role in the modification of proteins.
4. Essential fatty acids are the major lipids present in the biological membrane and are required for the membrane structure and function.
5. Essential fatty acids are useful for the transportation of cholesterol.
6. Essential fatty acids prevent fatty liver.
7. Essential fatty acids are useful for the synthesis of eicosanoids such as prostaglandin, prostacycline, thromboxane, leukotriene, etc.
8. Fatty acids are involved in a wide range of biological signaling pathways.
9. Fatty acids play a role in signal-transduction pathways.
10. Some skin-care products contain fatty acids, which can helps to maintain healthy skin appearance and function.
11. Commercially fatty acids are used not only in the production of numerous food products but also in soaps, detergents, and cosmetics.
12. Fatty acids, particularly omega-3 fatty acids, are also commonly sold as dietary supplements.

Fatty Acid Oxidation

Fatty acid undergoes oxidation and produces small metabolites such as acetyl CoA (mostly). Fatty acid oxidation is broadly classified into four major types based on the position where the oxidation takes place as follows,

1. α-Oxidation
2. β-Oxidation
3. γ-Oxidation
4. ω-Oxidation

Out of these different types, the most predominant one occurring in the body is β-oxidation. The other types of fatty acid oxidations such as α-oxidation, γ-oxidation and ω-oxidation are minor pathways.

β-Oxidation of Fatty Acids

Definition:

In the body, fatty acids are mainly oxidized by β-oxidation. **It is defined as the oxidation that takes place on the β-carbon atom of the fatty acids with the sequential removal of two carbon fragments as acetyl**

CoA. In the body, fatty acid oxidation takes place in most of the tissues but for energy requirements, some tissues such as the brain, erythrocytes and adrenal medulla cannot utilize fatty acids.

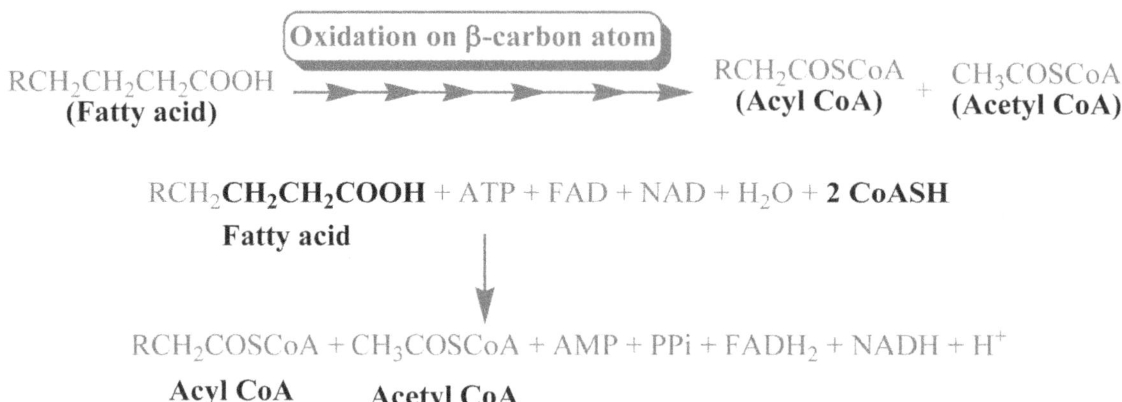

Stages involved:

There are three important steps involved in β-oxidation of fatty acids. They are,

1. Fatty acid activation in cytosol.
2. Transport of acyl CoA from cytosol to mitochondria.
3. Proper β-oxidation in mitochondrial matrix.

Stage 1 (Fatty acid activation in cytosol):

The active form of fatty acids is known as acyl CoA. In this stage, fatty acids are converted into acyl CoA in cytosol by the enzyme called "*acyl CoA synthetase* (*ACS*) or *thiokinase* (*TK*)". It involves two steps.

1. In the first step, fatty acid reacts with ATP in the presence of *acyl CoA synthetase* (*ACS*) or *thiokinase* (*TK*) that produces acyladenylate with the liberation of pyrophosphate (PPi). The total reaction is made irreversible by an immediate elimination of pyrophosphate into inorganic phosphate (Pi) through hydrolysis in the presence of *pyrophosphatase* (Substrate is "pyrophosphate" and the type of reaction is "hydrolysis").
2. In the next step, acyladenylate reacts with co-enzyme A to produce acyl CoA and AMP. This step is also catalyzed by the same enzyme involved in first step i.e., *acyl CoA synthetase* (*ACS*) (The product formed is "acyl CoA" and the type of reaction is "synthetic") or *thiokinase* (*TK*) (In ATP / GTP involved reactions, the enzymes acted are "*kinase*" and "sulphur" atom of co-enzyme A is also involved in reaction). *Kinase* enzyme needs magnesium ion as co-factors for its activity. In this step, one ATP is converted into AMP (2 ATP is utilized i.e., 1 ATP for ATP to ADP and other 1 ATP for ADP to AMP).

There are 3 different types of fatty acids based on length of the carbon chain. Hence, three different thiokinases are available to activate these fatty acids. They are,

(a) *Long chain thiokinase* (Activates fatty acid containing 9 to 20 carbon atoms)
(b) *Medium chain thiokinase* (Activates fatty acid containing 4 to 9 carbon atoms)
(c) *Short chain thiokinase* (Activates fatty acid containing less than 4 carbon atoms)

$$R-CH_2-CH_2-\overset{O}{\overset{||}{C}}-OH$$

Fatty acid
(Inactive form)

Acyl CoA synthetase or *Thiokinase*: ATP → PPi (- 2, Esterification or Transfer of AMP); PPi → 2 Pi (*Pyrophosphatase*, H_2O)

$$R-CH_2-CH_2-\overset{O}{\overset{||}{C}}-AMP$$

Acyladenylate

Acyl CoA synthetase or *Thiokinase*: CoASH → AMP (Substitution)

$$R-CH_2-CH_2-\overset{O}{\overset{||}{C}}-SCoA$$

Acyl CoA
(Active form of fatty acid)

Stage 2 (Transport of acyl CoA from cytosol to mitochondria):

Acyl CoA is impermeable to the inner mitochondrial membrane. Therefore, the transport of acyl CoA will not occur by a simple diffusion. Hence, a special transport system known as a **carnitine carrier system or carnitine shuttle** performs this one. Carnitine carrier system transfers acyl CoA from cytosol to mitochondria. This carrier system is a very good example for facilitated diffusion and the carnitine carrier system is presented in Figure 4.1. This stage involves four steps.

1. **Formation of acyl carnitine:** Carnitine is chemically β-hydroxy-γ-trimethyl aminobutyrate. In the first step, acyl group of acyl CoA is transferred to carnitine to produce acyl carnitine in the presence of *carnitine acyl transferase – I* or *CAT – I* (Substrate is "carnitine" and the group transferred is "acyl group"). *CAT– I,* is present in the outer surface of the inner mitochondrial membrane.
2. **Transport of acyl carnitine from cytosol to mitochondrial matrix:** Acyl carnitine is transported from cytosol to mitochondrial matrix by a specific carrier protein.
3. **Release of acyl CoA in mitochondrial matrix:** In this step, the acyl carnitine entered in the mitochondrial matrix liberates acyl CoA and carnitine by reacting with co-enzyme A in the presence of *carnitine acyl transferase – II* or *CAT – II* (Substrate is "carnitine" and the group transferred is "acyl group"). *CAT – II* is present in the inner mitochondrial membrane.
4. **Carnitine returns to cytosol:** Finally, released carnitine is transported from mitochondrial matrix to cytosol for reuse.

The cells have two separate pools of co-enzyme A i.e., cytosolic and mitochondrial. Hence, the co-enzyme A used for activation in the first stage is different from the one that combines with the acyl carnitine in the mitochondria to form acyl CoA. Malonyl CoA inhibits *carnitine acyl transferase – I* or *CAT – I*. Malonyl CoA is a key metabolite involved in the fatty acid synthesis that takes place in cytosol. In other words, while the fatty acid synthesis is in progress (reflected in high concentration of malonyl CoA), their oxidation does not occur because the carnitine shuttle is impaired.

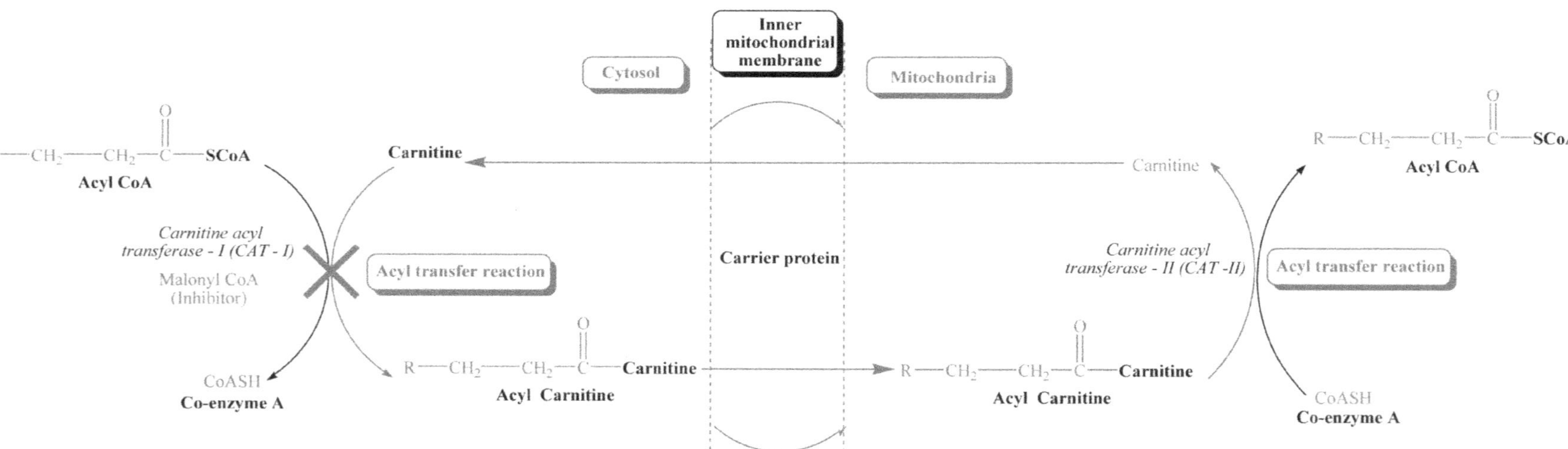

Figure 4.1 Carnitine shuttle or Carnitine carrier system.

Stage 3 (Proper β-oxidation in mitochondrial matrix):

Two carbon fragment "acetyl CoA" is liberated in each cycle of the proper β-oxidation. This stage involves four steps and the following are the sequence of four chemical reactions that take place in the mitochondrial matrix during proper β-oxidation. They are 1) Oxidation, 2) Hydration, 3) Oxidation, 4) Cleavage.

1. **Oxidation:** At first, acyl CoA undergoes oxidation with FAD by losing two hydrogen atoms in the presence of *acyl CoA dehydrogenase* (*ACAD*) (In NAD^+ / FAD involved reactions. the enzymes acted are "*dehydrogenase*" and the substrate is "acyl CoA"). One hydrogen is lost from α-carbon and the other hydrogen is lost from β-carbon. Hence, a double bond is formed between α- and β-carbon atoms and the product formed is known as α, β-unsaturated acyl CoA or Δ^2-trans enoyl CoA. ***Acyl CoA dehydrogenase* is the rate limiting enzyme of β-oxidation and it regulates the β-oxidation of fatty acid.** In this step, one FAD is converted into $FADH_2$ **(2 ATP is generated).**

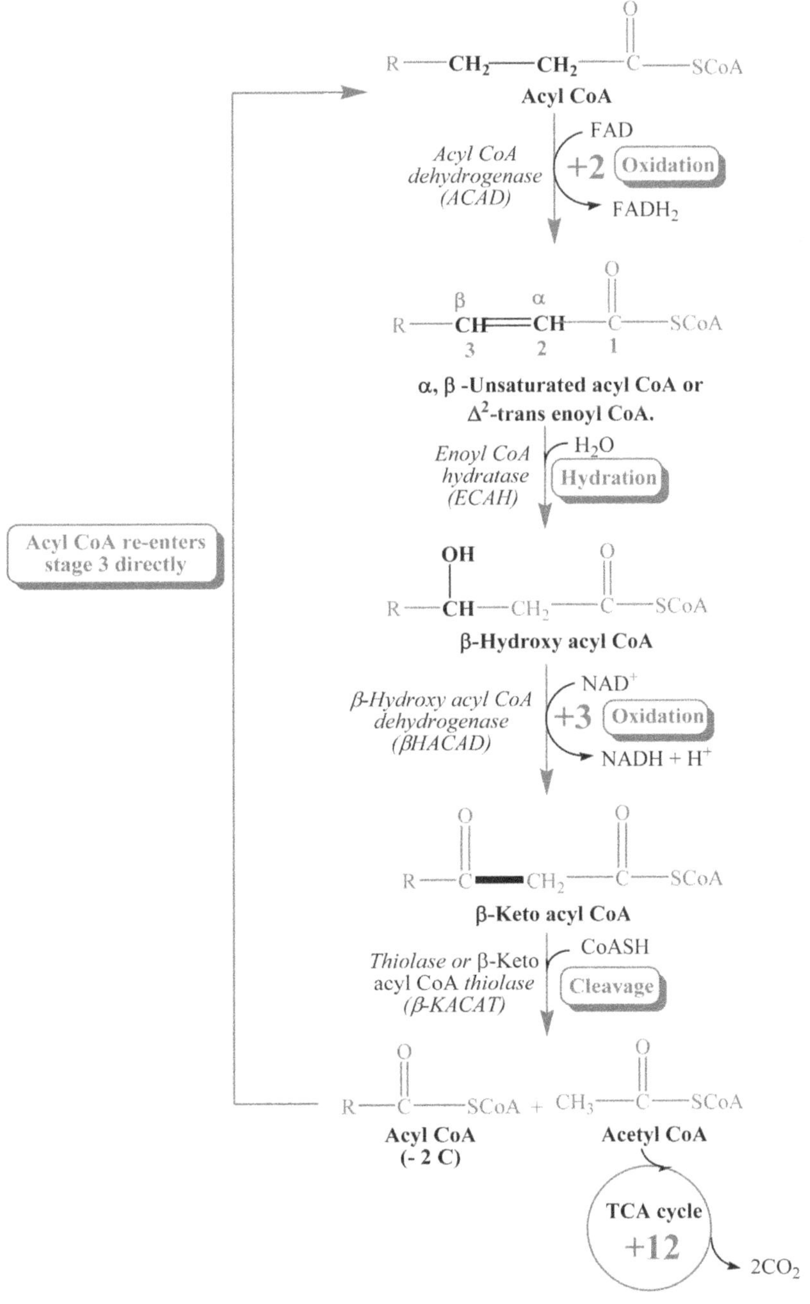

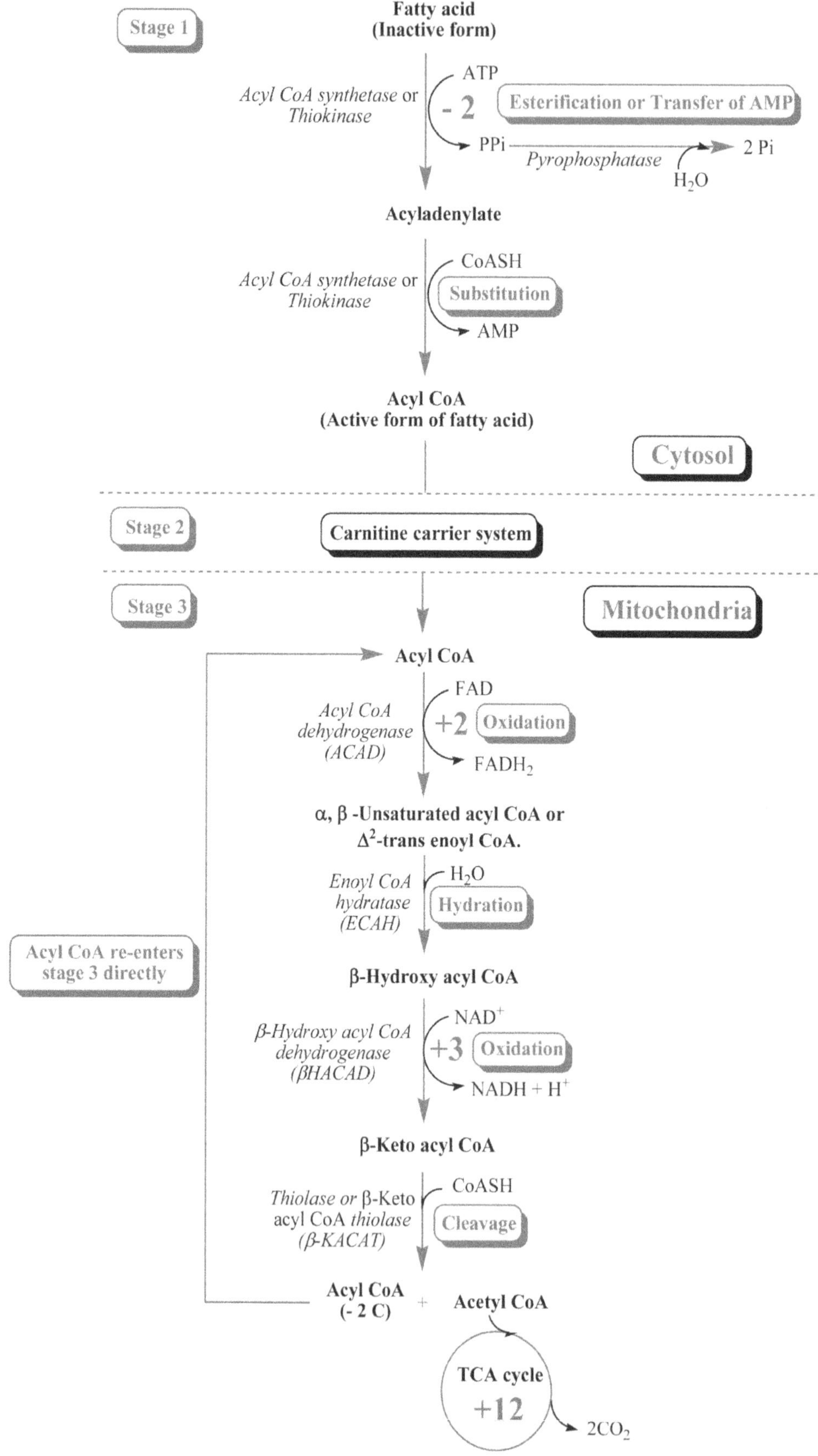
Stage 1
Fatty acid
(Inactive form)
ATP
Acyl CoA synthetase or Thiokinase
- 2
Esterification or Transfer of AMP
PPi
Pyrophosphatase
2 Pi
H_2O
Acyladenylate
CoASH
Acyl CoA synthetase or Thiokinase
Substitution
AMP
Acyl CoA
(Active form of fatty acid)
Cytosol
Stage 2
Carnitine carrier system
Stage 3
Mitochondria
Acyl CoA
FAD
Acyl CoA dehydrogenase (ACAD)
+2
Oxidation
$FADH_2$
α, β -Unsaturated acyl CoA or
Δ^2-trans enoyl CoA.
H_2O
Enoyl CoA hydratase (ECAH)
Hydration
Acyl CoA re-enters stage 3 directly
β-Hydroxy acyl CoA
NAD^+
β-Hydroxy acyl CoA dehydrogenase (βHACAD)
+3
Oxidation
$NADH + H^+$
β-Keto acyl CoA
CoASH
Thiolase or β-Keto acyl CoA thiolase (β-KACAT)
Cleavage
Acyl CoA
(- 2 C)
+
Acetyl CoA
TCA cycle
+12
$2CO_2$

2. **Hydration:** In this step, Δ^2-trans enoyl CoA is reacted with water molecules and produces β-hydroxy acyl CoA. Hydrogen is attached to α-carbon and the hydroxyl group is attached to β-carbon. This reaction is catalyzed by *enoyl CoA hydratase* (*ECAH*) (Substrate is "enoyl CoA" and the type of reaction is "hydration").
3. **Oxidation:** β-Hydroxy acyl CoA further oxidized by NAD^+ and produces β-keto acyl CoA in presence of *β-hydroxy acyl CoA dehydrogenase* (βHACAD) (In NAD^+ / FAD involved reactions, the enzymes acted are "*dehydrogenase*" and the substrate is "β-hydroxy acyl CoA"). In this oxidation, one hydrogen atom is lost from β-carbon and the other hydrogen is lost from the β-hydroxyl group. Hence, a double bond is formed between β-carbon and β-oxygen atoms. In other words, secondary alcohol is oxidized to keto group. In this step, one NAD^+ is converted into NADH + H^+ (3 ATP is generated).
4. **Cleavage:** This is the final reaction in which β-keto acyl CoA reacts with co-enzyme A in the presence of *thiolase* or *β-keto acyl CoA thiolase* (The type of reaction is "thiolytic cleavage" and the substrate is "β-keto acyl CoA") and produces acyl CoA with two carbon less than the original and liberates two carbon fragment acetyl CoA. The new acyl CoA re-enters proper β-oxidation step and it continues till the fatty acid is completely oxidized.

   The overall reaction involved in each cycle of proper β-oxidation can be written as follows.

Acyl CoA (with "n" carbon) + FAD + NAD^+ + H_2O + CoASH

↓ Proper β-oxidation (Per cycle)

Acyl CoA (with "n-2" carbon) + Acetyl CoA + $FADH_2$ + NADH + H^+

In the biological system, the most predominantly occurring β-oxidation is β-oxidation of saturated even carbon fatty acid. Hence, the above discussion is with respect to that one.

Oxidation of palmitic acid:

Palmitic is a sixteen-carbon containing fatty acid. It undergoes β-oxidation by the above method and produces energy.

$$CH_3—(CH_2)_{14}—\overset{\overset{\displaystyle O}{\|}}{C}—OH$$

Palmitic acid

In the first stage, palmitic acid is activated to its active form palmitoyl CoA with utilization of 2 ATP in cytosol by *thiokinase.* Later, palmitoyl CoA is transported from cytosol to mitochondrial matrix by facilitated diffusion through special carrier protein using a carnitine carrier system. The second stage is catalyzed by *carnitine acyl transferase* or *CAT*. In the final stage, the palmitoyl CoA undergoes proper β-oxidation in the mitochondrial matrix by a four-step process and liberates 2 carbon fragment acetyl CoA and acyl CoA with 2 carbon less than the original. This obtained acyl CoA (2 carbon less) further undergoes four-step proper β-oxidation again and produce corresponding acyl CoA (2 carbon less than substrate acyl CoA) and acetyl CoA. As palmitoyl CoA contains 16 carbons, the proper β-oxidation cycles are repeated for 7 times and produces 8 acetyl CoA totally. The produced acetyl CoA is oxidized to carbon dioxide by entering into TCA cycle and produce 12 ATP. The overall reaction involved in the oxidation of one mole of palmitic acid is summarized in the below equation.

$CH_3(CH_2)_{14}COOH$ + ATP + 7 FAD + 7 NAD + 7 H_2O + 8 CoASH
Palmitic acid

↓ β–Oxidation

8 $CH_3COSCoA$ + AMP + PPi + 7 $FADH_2$ + 7 NADH + 7 H^+
Palmitoyl CoA

Energetic of palmitic acid β-oxidation:

Energy generation is the ultimate aim in fatty acid metabolism. The energy obtained in complete β-oxidation of palmitic acid is summarized in Table 4.2 and Figure 4.2.

Table 4.2 Energetic of palmitic acid β-oxidation.

S. No	Mechanism or molecule involved	No. of ATP generated or utilized per cycle or mole	No. of cycles or moles involved	Total ATP generated or utilized
Proper β-oxidation cycle in mitochondrial matrix				
1	One FAD is reduced to $FADH_2$ (One $FADH_2$ is equals to 2 ATP)	+ 2	7	+ 14
2	One NAD^+ is reduced to NADH + H^+ (One NADH + H^+ is equals to 3 ATP)	+ 3	7	+ 21
TCA cycle				
3	One acetyl CoA is oxidized to carbondioxide	+ 12	8	+ 96
Total ATP generated by one mole of palmitic acid (+14 + 21 + 96)				**+ 131**
Activation of palmitic acid in cytosol				
4	One ATP is converted into AMP	- 2	1	- **2**
Net ATP generated by one mole of palmitic acid through complete **β-oxidation** (131 - 2)				**129**

The standard free energy of palmitic acid (one mole) = 2340 Cai

The energy yielded by β–oxidation of palmitic acid (one mole) = 129 ATP = 129 × 7.3 Cal = 941.7 Cal [1 ATP = 7.3 Cal]

The energey conversion efficiency of palmitic acid β-oxidation $= \frac{941.7}{2340} \times 100 = 40.24\ \%$

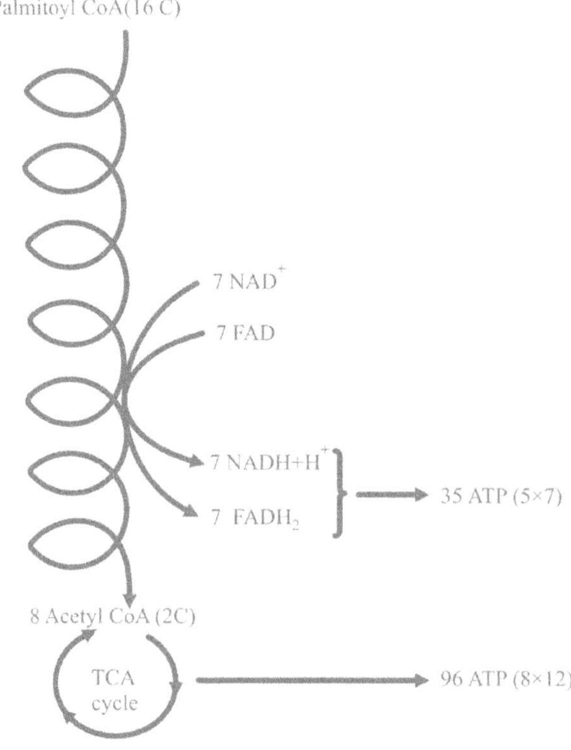

Figure 4.2 Energetic of palmitic acid β-oxidation - Overview.

Metabolic disorder:

1. **Sudden infant death syndrome (SIDS):** In general, an overnight unexpected death of healthy infants is known as SIDS and the real cause for this syndrome is not known. Now, it was identified that at least 10 % of SIDS is due to the deficiency of *medium chain acyl CoA dehydrogenase* (*MCACAD*). The frequency of this enzyme defect is 1 in 10,000 births and the prevalent is more than phenylketonuria. Soon after eating or feeding babies, glucose is the principle source of energy. The glucose utilization and its level are decreased after a few hours. Hence, simultaneously, the fatty acid oxidation must increase to meet the energy requirements. Hence, in infants blocking of β-oxidation due to the deficiency of *medium chain acyl CoA dehydrogenase* (*MCACAD*) leads to sudden death.
2. **Jamaican vomiting sickness:** This metabolic disorder is caused by eating unripe ackee fruit which contains an unusual toxic amino acid known as hypoglycin-A. *Acyl CoA dehydrogenase* (ACAD) is inhibited by this hypoglycin-A. Hence, fatty acid β-oxidation is blocked leads to several complications. Jamaican vomiting sickness is characterized by severe hypoglycemia, vomiting, and convulsion. In severe conditions, it produces coma and death, if untreated.

β-Oxidation of odd carbon chain fatty acids:

Odd carbon chain fatty acids are also metabolized in a similar way as described above like even carbon chain fatty acids. But in the final step, instead of two carbon fragment acetyl CoA, three carbon fragment propionyl CoA is produced. Later, propionyl CoA is converted to succinyl CoA by the following three step process.

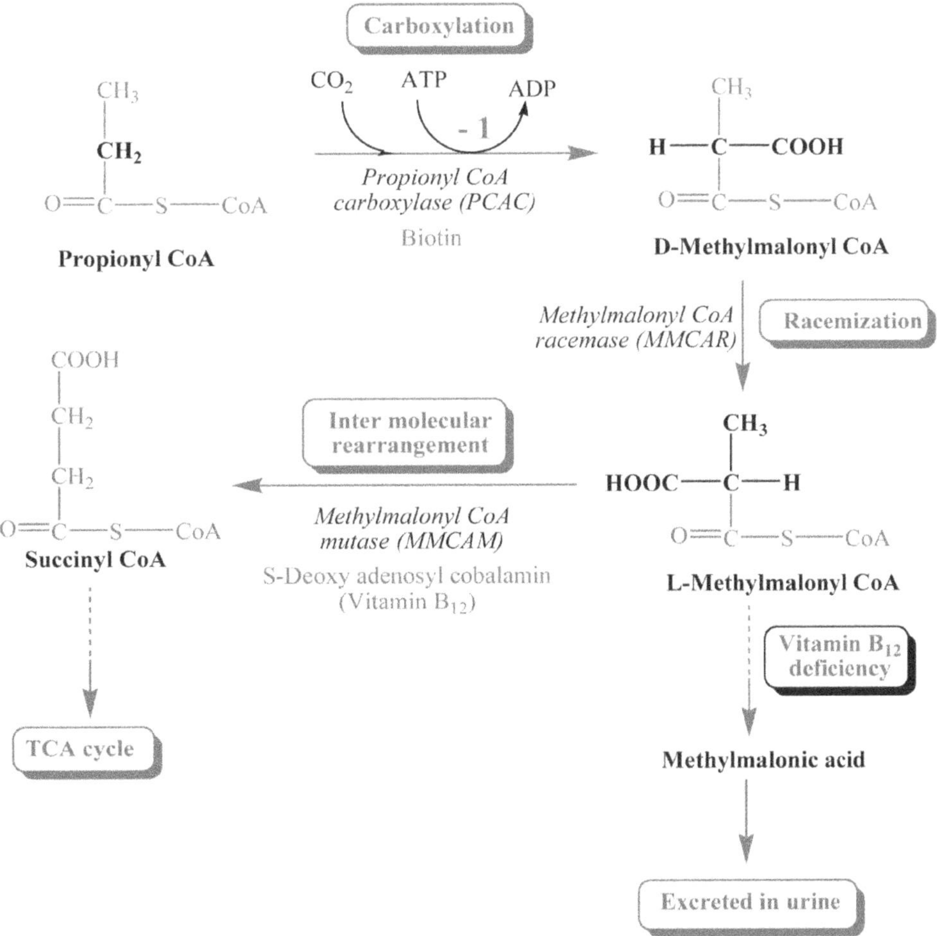

1. Initially, propionyl CoA undergoes carboxylation to produce D-methylmalonyl CoA in presence of *propionyl CoA carboxylase* (*PCAC*) (Substrate is "propionyl CoA" and the type of reaction is "carboxylation"). This enzyme needs biotin as co-enzyme for its activity. In this step, one ATP is converted into ADP **(1 ATP is utilized)**.

2. D-Methylmalonyl CoA is converted to L-methylmalonyl CoA by the enzyme *methylmalonyl CoA racemase* (*MMCAR*) (Substrate is "methylmalonyl CoA" and the type of reaction is "racemization"). This conversion is necessary to enter into the metabolic reactions of the body.
3. Finally, L-methylmalonyl CoA is converted into succinyl CoA in presence of *methylmalonyl CoA mutase* (*MMCAM*) (Substrate is "methylmalonyl CoA" and the type of reaction is "position changing"). This enzyme needs S-deoxy adenosyl cobalamin (vitamin B_{12}) as co-enzyme for its activity. This produces succinyl CoA as the component of the TCA cycle. Hence, it enters the TCA cycle.

Methylmalonic acidemia is the metabolic disorders of β-oxidation of odd carbon chain fatty acids due to deficiency of either vitamin B_{12} or *methylmalonyl CoA mutase* (*MMCAM*). In the body, methylmalonic acid is accumulated in both cases and excreted in urine. Increased methylmalonic acid generally causes severe metabolic acidosis, damages the CNS and retards the growth. In the early years of life, it is fatal.

β-Oxidation of unsaturated fatty acids:

Unsaturated fatty acids are not metabolized to the same extent like saturated fatty acids due to the presence of double bonds. Hence, less energy is provided by the oxidation of unsaturated fatty acids than that of the saturated fatty acids. The reactions are almost the same but the double bonds present create problems for the proceeding of β-oxidation. *Isomerase* and *epimerase* enzymes generally overcome this problem.

β-Oxidation of fatty acids in peroxisomes:

In most eukaryotic cells, the organelles peroxisomes are present. In peroxisomes, β-oxidation occurs in the modified form. The reducing equivalent $FADH_2$ produced by *acyl CoA dehydrogenase* (*ACAD*) in β-oxidation is not transferred to the electron transport chain (ETC). Instead, in peroxisomes, $FADH_2$ is directly handed over to the oxygen (O_2). Hence, hydrogen peroxide is formed which is cleaved by *catalase* and produces water and a nascent oxygen atom.

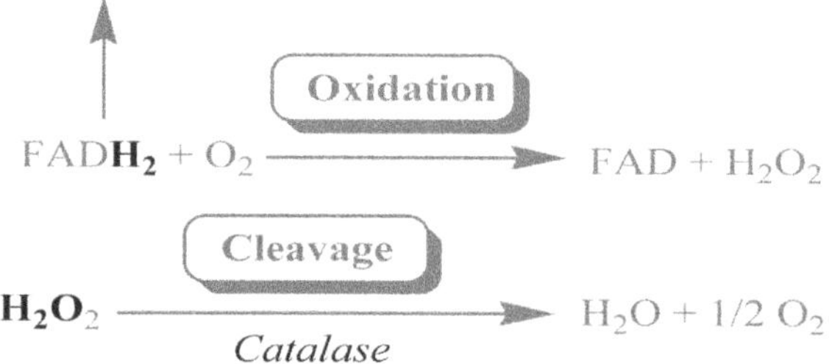

In peroxisomal β-oxidation of fatty acids, no ATP is synthesized because the reducing equivalents do not pass through ETC. However, heat is liberated. Now, it is believed that long chain fatty acid (more than 20 carbons) initially undergoes peroxisomal β-oxidation followed by mitochondrial oxidation. Hypolipidemic drugs like clofibrate and high fat diet induce peroxisomal β-oxidation.

Zellweger syndrome or Cerebrohepatorenal syndrome: In this syndrome, peroxisomes are absent in almost all tissues. Hence, long chain fatty acids (C_{26} to C_{38}) are not oxidized, resulting in the accumulation of long chain fatty acids in the tissues, especially in the brain, liver, and kidney. This is a rare metabolic disorder.

α-Oxidation of Fatty Acids

α-Oxidation of fatty acids is defined as the oxidation of fatty acids that takes place on an α-carbon atom with the removal of one carbon unit at a time as carbon dioxide. No energy is produced in α - oxidation and it does not involve the binding of fatty acid to co-enzyme A.

Refsum's disease: It is a severe and rare neurological disorder characterized by cerebral ataxia and peripheral neuropathy. In this condition, a large amount of an unusual fatty acid such as phytanic acid is accumulated in the body. Phytanic acid is mostly present in plant food and also in animal fats and milk lipid. It contains methyl groups at C-3. Hence, it cannot undergo β-oxidation. Initially, phytanic acid undergoes α-oxidation to lose its one carbon as carbon dioxide followed by β-oxidation. This disease is due to the deficiency of *phytanic acid α-oxidase* (PAαO) which is responsible for the conversion of phytanic acid into a compound that can be degraded by phytanic acid β-oxidation. Green leafy vegetables (chlorophyll) should not be consumed by its patients.

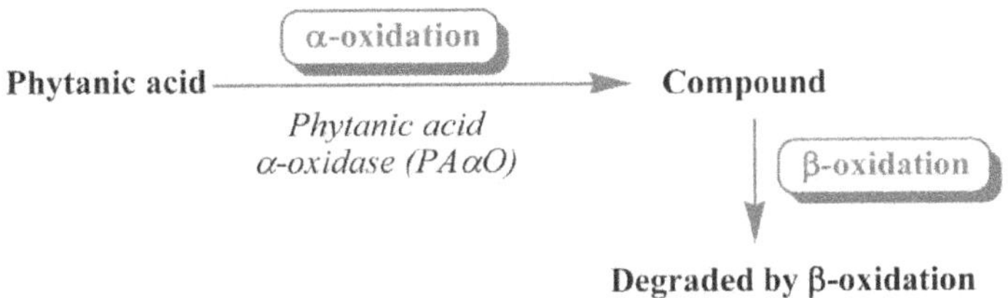

ω-Oxidation of Fatty Acids

This is another minor pathway for oxidation of fatty acids. The symbol "ω" indicates the last or terminal carbon atom. In a fatty acid, the terminal carbon is usually a methyl group. Hence, this methyl group is initially hydroxylated to produce primary alcohol followed by oxidation to produce carboxylic acid. *Cytochrome* P_{450}, NADPH + H^+ and oxygen molecule are needed for ω-oxidation of fatty acids.

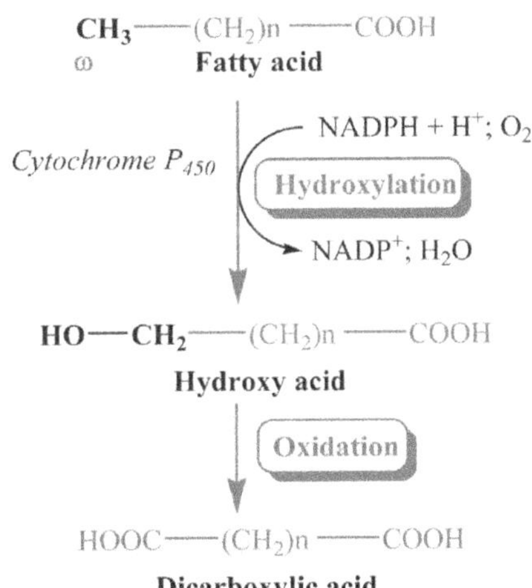

Metabolic water & fatty acid oxidation:

Water produced in fatty acid oxidation and other forms of aerobic respiration is known as metabolic water (**Example:** One mole of palmitic acid releases 16 water molecules in oxidation). In some animals, this metabolic water has great significance. A lipid stored in camel hump is a good source of water and energy supply. Hence, in deserts, camels can travel even for a longer period without food and water. A small animal, kangaroo rat is believed to live indefinitely without water. It consumes oil rich seeds only which produce metabolic water and is adequate to its water demands. However, the use of metabolic water is an adaptation and is accompanied by a reduced output of urine.

Ketone Bodies Metabolism

Ketone bodies are defined as a water-soluble chemical substance present in biological systems possessing carbonyl groups and yielding energy. Following are three important ketone bodies present in biological systems 1) Acetone, 2) Acetoacetate, 3) β-Hydroxybutyrate or 3-Hydroxybutyrate. Out of these three, acetone and acetoacetate are called as "true ketone bodies" because it contains carbonyl group; whereas β-hydroxybutyrate is not a true ketone body due to the lack of carbonyl keto group in structure. However, it is considered a ketone body due to its structural similarities or relationship with acetoacetate.

Except acetone, other two ketone bodies undergoe metabolism and produce energy. Acetone is not metabolized in the body. The summary of ketone body synthesis, utilization and excretion is presented in Figure 4.3.

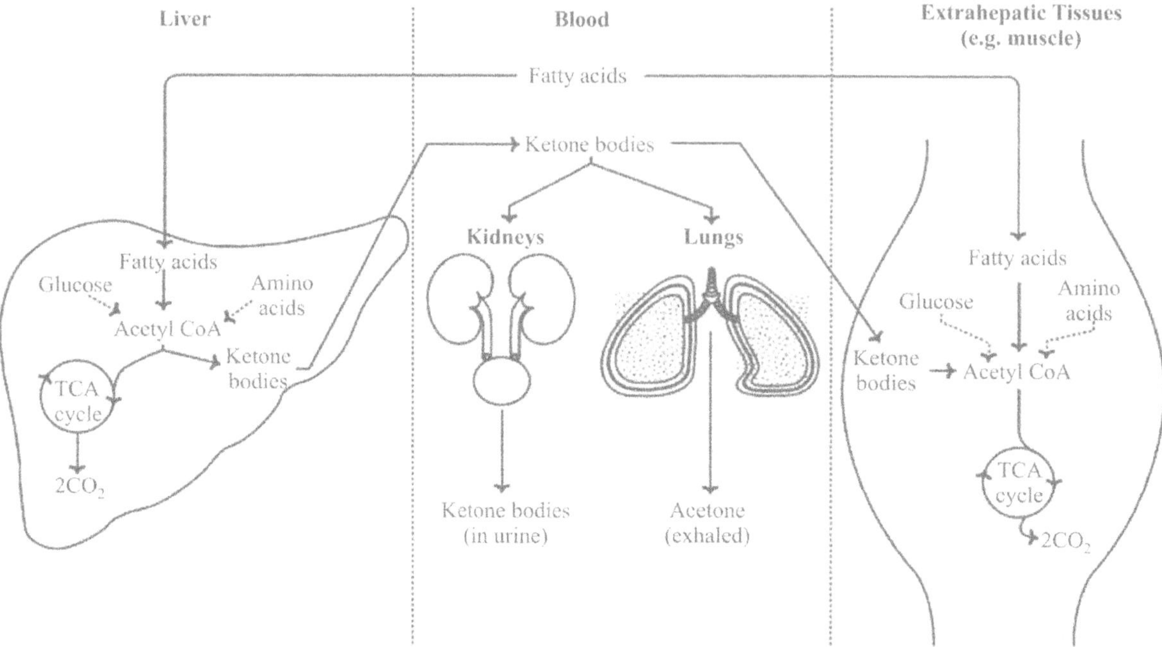

Figure 4.3 Summary of ketone body synthesis, utilization and excretion.

$CH_3-C(=O)-CH_3$

Acetone
(True ketone body;
Not metabolized)

$CH_3-C(=O)-CH_2-COOH$

Acetoacetate
(True ketone body;
Metabolized and yield energy)

$CH_3-\overset{\beta}{C}H(OH)-\overset{\alpha}{C}H_2-COOH$

β-Hydroxy butyrate
(Not true ketone body;
Metabolized and yield energy)

Ketone bodies metabolism is generally divided into 2 major pathways such as,

1. Ketogenesis
2. Ketolysis

Ketogenesis

It is defined as a series of chemical reactions occurring in the biological system to produce ketone bodies from acetyl CoA.

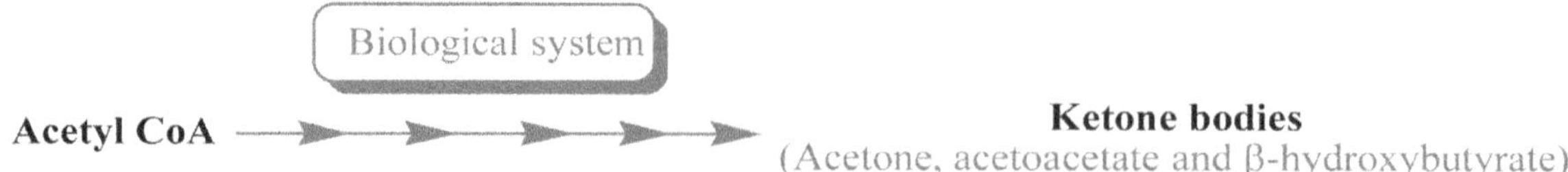

Mainly ketogenesis occurs in the liver and the enzymes involved in ketogenesis are present in the mitochondrial matrix. Acetyl CoA, needed for the synthesis of ketone bodies is generally obtained from the oxidation of fatty acids, pyruvate or some amino acids particularly ketogenic amino acids like leucine, lysine, phenylalanine, etc. (because they are degraded to acetoacetate and acetyl CoA). The following are the various reactions involved in ketogenesis.

1. Initially, two molecules of acetyl CoA are condensed together and produce acetoacetyl CoA with loss of co-enzyme A in presence of *β-ketoacyl CoA thiolase* (*βKACAT*) or *β-ketothiolase* (*βKT*) or simply *thiolase* (The type of reaction is "thiolytic cleavage" and the product is "acetoacetyl CoA" which is "β-keto acyl CoA"). This is the enzyme involved in the final step of proper β-oxidation of fatty acids. Hence, this reaction is considered as reverse reactions of *thiolase* catalyzed reaction in β-oxidation.

$CH_3-C(=O)-SCoA + CH_3-C(=O)-SCoA$

Acetyl CoA **Acetyl CoA**

β-Ketoacyl CoA thiolase (β-KACAT) or β-Keto thiolase (β-KT) or Thiolase

→ CoASH

Condensation

$CH_3-C(=O)-CH_2-C(=O)-SCoA$

Acetoacetyl CoA

H_2O

HMG CoA synthase

$CH_3-C(=O)-SCoA$

Acetyl CoA

Addition followed by hydrolysis

→ CoASH

$HO-C(=O)-CH_2-C(OH)(CH_3)-CH_2-C(=O)-SCoA$

β-Hydroxy-β-methylglutaryl CoA (HMG CoA)

HMG CoA lyase (HMGCAL)

→ $CH_3-C(=O)-SCoA$

Acetyl CoA

Breakdown

$HO-C(=O)-CH_2-C(=O)-CH_3$

Acetoacetate

β-Hydroxybutyrate dehydrogenase (β-HBD)

$NADH + H^+$

-3 Reduction

→ NAD^+

Spontaneous

→ CO_2

Decarboxylation

$HO-C(=O)-CH_2-C(OH)(H)-CH_3$

β–Hydroxybutyrate

$CH_3-C(=O)-CH_3$

Acetone

Rewritten

$CH_3-C(OH)(H)-CH_2-C(=O)-OH$

β–Hydroxybutyrate

2. Another molecule of acetyl CoA reacts with acetoacetyl CoA and one molecule of water in the presence of *HMG CoA synthase* (*HMGCAS*) (Product is "HMG CoA" and the type of reaction is "synthesis") and produce β-hydroxy-β-methylglutaryl CoA (HMG CoA) and co-enzyme A. The basic reaction involved in this step is addition followed by hydrolysis. This step is the rate limiting step of ketogenesis. Hence, ***HMG CoA synthase* (HMGCAS) regulates ketogenesis.**
3. In the succeeding step, HMG CoA undergoes breakdown reaction and produced one of the ketone body acetoacetate with liberation of one molecule of acetyl CoA. This reaction is catalyzed by *HMG CoA lyase* (*HMGCAL*) (Substrate is "HMG CoA" and the type of reaction is "lysis or breakdown").
4. From the ketone body acetoacetate, the remaining two ketone bodies are synthesized. Acetoacetate spontaneously undergoes decarboxylation with the removal of carbon dioxide from carboxylic group and produces the other ketone body "acetone".
5. In another way, acetoacetate is reduced using NADH + H^+ results in the formation of β-hydroxybutyrate and NAD^+ in presence of *β-hydroxybutyrate dehydrogenase* (*βHBD*) (In NAD^+ / $NADP^+$ involved reaction, the enzymes acted are "*dehydrogenase*" and the product is "β-hydroxybutyrate"). In this reaction, one mole of NADH + H^+ is converted to NAD^+ **(3 ATPs are utilized).**

From the liver, ketone bodies are easily transported to other tissues because they are water soluble. For peripheral tissues like skeletal muscle, cardiac muscle, renal cortex, etc., two ketone bodies namely acetoacetate and β-hydroxybutyrate serve as important sources of energy. Ketone bodies cannot be utilized by tissues that lack mitochondria such as erythrocytes. During starvation and diabetes mellitus, the supply of glucose to the tissues is short; hence in such situations ketone bodies production and utilization becomes more significant. For the brain and the other parts of CNS, ketone bodies are the major fuel source during prolonged starvation. Utilization of fatty acids by the brain for energy is very limited. 50 to 70 % of the brain's energy demands are rectified by ketone bodies only. During the period of food deprivation, this is an adaptation for the survival of the organism.

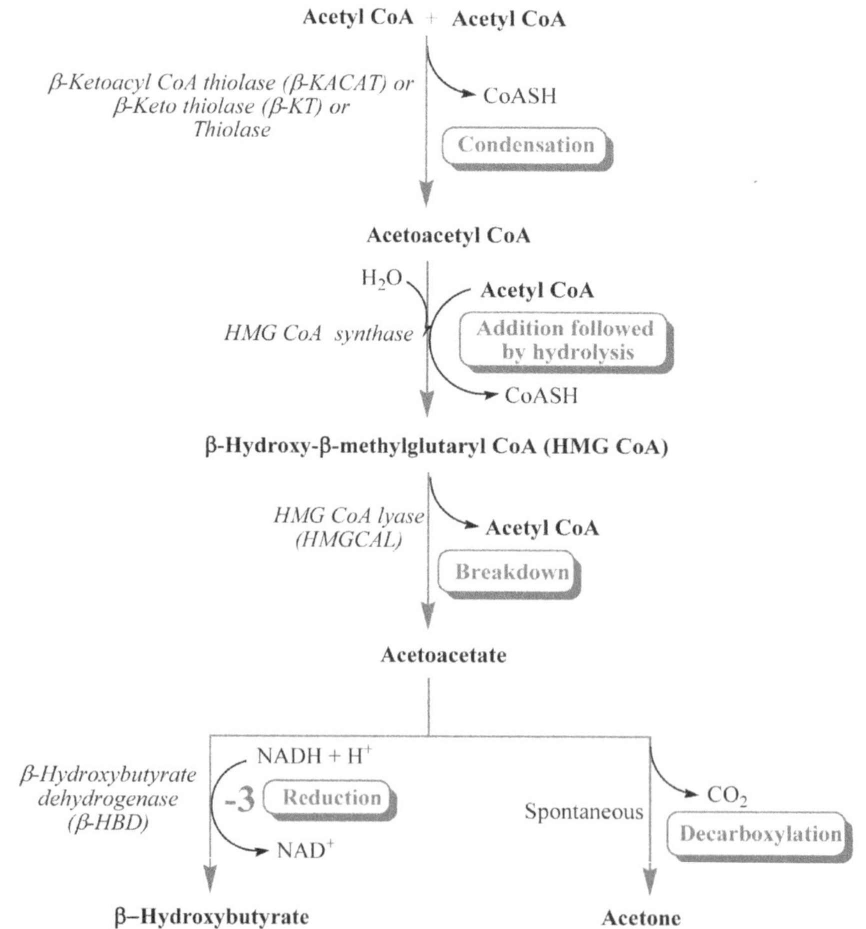

Regulation of ketogenesis:

Overproduction of ketonebodies take place when carbohydrates are not available to the tissues. This is due to excessive utilization of fatty acid to meet the energy requirements of the cells. Ketogenesis is stimulated by the hormone glucagon and inhibited by insulin. In diabetes mellitus, increased ratio of glucagon / insulin promotes ketogenesis due to disturbances in carbohydrate and lipid metabolism.

In general, ketogenic substances such as fatty acid and ketogenic amino acids like leucine, lysine, tyrosine, etc. promote ketogenesis. Conversely, anti-ketogenic substances such as glucose, glycerol and glucogenic amino acids like glycine, alanine, serine, glutamate, etc. inhibits ketogenesis.

Ketolysis

It is defined as a series of chemical reactions occurring in the biological system to break ketone bodies acetoacetate and β-hydroxybutyrate into acetyl CoA.

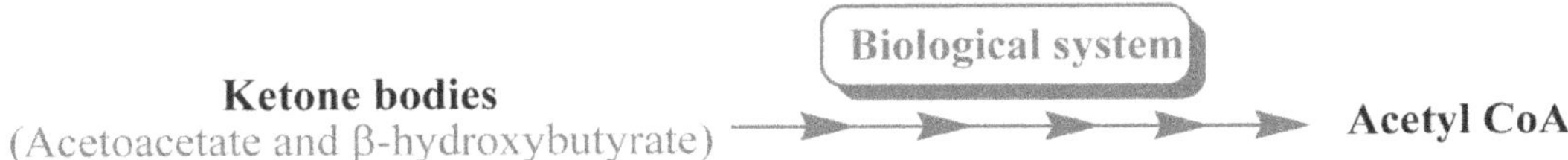

Ketolysis is the reverse of ketogenesis with a slight modification. The following are the various reactions taking place in conversion of ketone bodies like acetoacetate and β-hydroxybutyrate into acetyl CoA.

1. The first step is the reversal of the last step of ketogenesis. In this step, β-hydroxybutyrate is oxidized to acetoacetate using NAD^+ in presence of *β-hydroxybutyrate dehydrogenase* (*βHBD*) (In NAD^+ / $NADP^+$ involved reactions, the enzymes acted are "*dehydrogenase*" and the substrate is "β-hydroxybutyrate"). In this reaction, one mole of NAD^+ is converted to NADH + H^+ (**3 ATPs are generated**).
2. Later, acetoacetate is activated to its active form acetoacetyl CoA by succinyl CoA in the presence of mitochondrial enzyme *thiophorase* (TP) which is otherwise known *succinyl CoA acetoacetate CoA transferase* (*SCACT*) (Substrate is "acetoacetate and succinyl CoA" and the type of reaction is "transfer of co-enzyme A"). In this reaction, co-enzyme A is simply transferred from TCA cycle intermediate succinyl CoA to acetoacetate. After donating co-enzyme A, succinyl CoA is converted to succinate. Liver cannot utilize ketone bodies due to lack of *thiophorase* (*TP*).
3. Finally, acetoacetyl CoA reacts with co-enzyme A in presence of *β-ketoacyl CoA thiolase* (*βKACAT*) or *β-ketothiolase* (*βKT*) or simply *thiolase* (The type of reaction is "thiolytic cleavage" and the substrate is "β-keto acyl CoA") and produces 2 moles of acetyl CoA. This reaction is similar to *thiolase* catalyzed reaction in β-oxidation of fatty acid or reversal of the first step of ketogenesis.

Metabolic disorders of Ketone bodies metabolism

In healthy individuals, there is a constant synthesis of ketone bodies by the liver and their utilization by extrahepatic tissues. The normal level of ketone bodies in the blood is 1 mg/dl. Only very low quantities of ketone bodies are excreted in urine and cannot be detected by routine Rothera's test. When there is an imbalance between ketogenesis and ketolysis the following metabolic disorder may occur.

1. **Ketonemia:** It is defined as an increased level of ketone bodies in the blood due to their overproduction rather than the deficiency of their utilization (Rate of ketogenesis exceeds the rate of ketolysis).
2. **Ketonuria:** It is a clinical condition in which more quantities of ketone bodies are excreted in the urine. Generally, active fat metabolism is indicated by the appearance of ketone bodies in urine. Some body weight programs are designed to encourage a reduction in carbohydrate and total calorie intake until ketone bodies appear in the urine.
3. **Ketosis:** The combined effect of ketonemia and ketonuria is known as ketosis. The common feature of ketosis is the smell of acetone in breath. Usually, it is associated with starvation and uncontrolled diabetes mellitus.

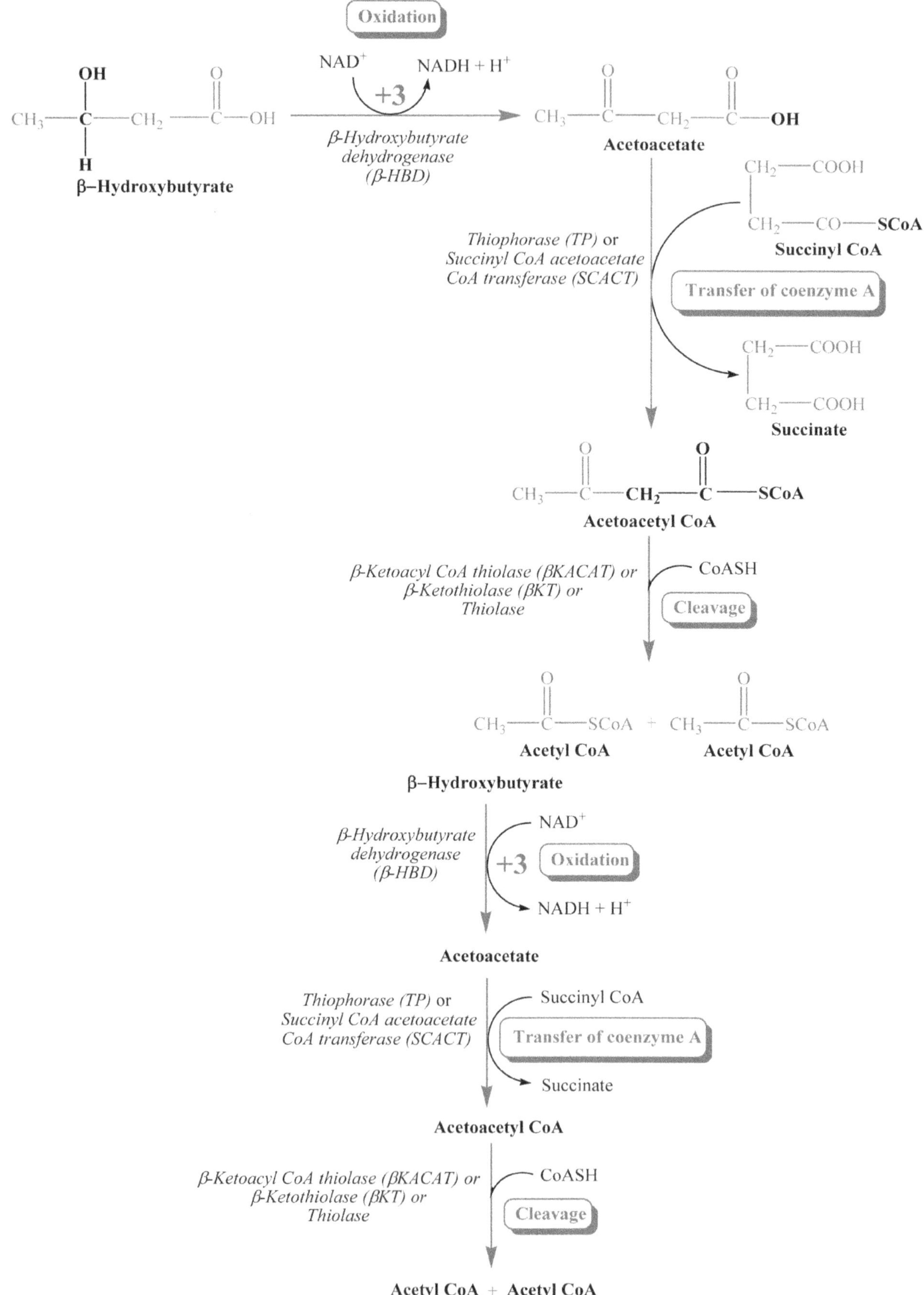
Oxidation
NAD+
NADH + H+
+3
OH
CH3—C—CH2—C—OH
H
β–Hydroxybutyrate
β-Hydroxybutyrate dehydrogenase (β-HBD)
CH3—C—CH2—C—OH
Acetoacetate
CH2—COOH
CH2—CO—SCoA
Succinyl CoA
Thiophorase (TP) or Succinyl CoA acetoacetate CoA transferase (SCACT)
Transfer of coenzyme A
CH2—COOH
CH2—COOH
Succinate
CH3—C—CH2—C—SCoA
Acetoacetyl CoA
β-Ketoacyl CoA thiolase (βKACAT) or β-Ketothiolase (βKT) or Thiolase
CoASH
Cleavage
CH3—C—SCoA + CH3—C—SCoA
Acetyl CoA
Acetyl CoA
β–Hydroxybutyrate
β-Hydroxybutyrate dehydrogenase (β-HBD)
NAD+
+3
Oxidation
NADH + H+
Acetoacetate
Thiophorase (TP) or Succinyl CoA acetoacetate CoA transferase (SCACT)
Succinyl CoA
Transfer of coenzyme A
Succinate
Acetoacetyl CoA
β-Ketoacyl CoA thiolase (βKACAT) or β-Ketothiolase (βKT) or Thiolase
CoASH
Cleavage
Acetyl CoA + Acetyl CoA

Fatty acid degradation is increased during starvation to meet the energy demands of the body. Hence, acetyl CoA is overproduced which cannot be fully handled by the TCA cycle. In addition, oxaloacetate deficiency (most of the oxaloacetate is diverted for the synthesis of glucose to meet essential requirements for tissues like the brain) also impairs the TCA cycle. Hence acetyl CoA is accumulated and it is diverted for the over synthesis of ketone bodies.

Diabetes mellitus is associated with insulin deficiency. In this condition, lipolysis is increased and carbohydrate metabolism is impaired which leads to the accumulation of acetyl CoA and increased ketogenesis. The ketone body concentration in blood and urine may reach 100 mg/dl and 500 mg/day, respectively in severe diabetes mellitus.

4. **Ketoacidosis:** Both acetoacetate and β-hydroxybutyrate are strong acids. Hence, increased concentration of ketone bodies decreases the pH and produce acidic condition known as ketoacidosis. Ketoacidosis combined with diabetes mellitus is commonly called **diabetic ketoacidosis** which is a dangerous disease. If untreated it may result in coma and death also. Ketosis due to starvation is not accompanied by ketoacidosis. Ketoacidosis is generally treated by using insulin which increases the glucose uptake by tissues and inhibits ketogenesis.

Denovo Synthesis of Fatty Acids

Fatty acids are synthesized and stored as triacylglycerols when excess dietary carbohydrates and amino acids are consumed. Cytosol fraction of the cell contains enzymes machinery for fatty acid synthesis and it is mainly takeing place in the liver, adipose tissue, kidney, and lactating mammary glands. For the synthesis of fatty acids, the three important components needed are, a) Acetyl CoA (provides carbon skeleton), b) ATP (provides energy), c) NADPH (provides reducing equivalent). Like β-oxidation of fatty acid, three stages are involved in the synthesis of fatty acid also. They are,

1. Synthesis of acetyl CoA and NADPH in cytosol.
2. Synthesis of malonyl CoA from acetyl CoA.
3. Reactions of *fatty acid synthase* (*FAS*) complex.

Stage 1 (Synthesis of acetyl CoA and NADPH in cytosol):

Synthesis of fatty acids needs acetyl CoA and NADPH as precursors. In mitochondria, oxidation of fatty acid and pyruvate, degradation of some amino acids carbon skeleton and catabolism of ketone bodies produces acetyl CoA. But mitochondrial membrane is impermeable to acetyl CoA. Hence, in mitochondria acetyl CoA reacts with oxaloacetate in presence of *citrate synthase* (CS) (Product is "citrate" and type of reaction is "synthesis") to produce citrate which is permeable to the mitochondrial membrane and transferred to the cytosol.

In cytosol, citrate undergoes breakdown to liberate acetyl CoA and oxaloacetate in presence of *citrate lyase* (*CL*) (Substrate is "citrate" and type of reaction is "lysis or breakdown"). The liberated oxaloacetate is converted into malate in presence of *malate dehydrogenase* (*MDH*) (In NAD^+ / $NADP^+$ involved reactions, the enzymes acted are "*dehydrogenase*" and the product is "malate"). Later, malate is converted to pyruvate in presence of *malic enzyme* (*ME*) or *malate dehydrogenase* (*MDH*) (In NAD^+ / $NADP^+$ involved reactions, the enzymes acted are "*dehydrogenase*" and the substrate is "malate") by oxidative decarboxylation. In this reaction, one mole of carbondioxide and NDPH + H^+ is synthesized which is utilized for the synthesis of fatty acid. The coupled transport of acetyl CoA with the production of carbon dioxide and NDPH + H^+ is highly advantageous to the cell for the biosynthesis of fatty acids.

Stage 2 (Synthesis of malonyl CoA from acetyl CoA):

This step is the rate-limiting step of the fatty acid synthesis. In this step, acetyl CoA undergoes carboxylation and produced malonyl CoA in presence of *acetyl CoA carboxylase* (*ACAC*) (Substrate is "acetyl

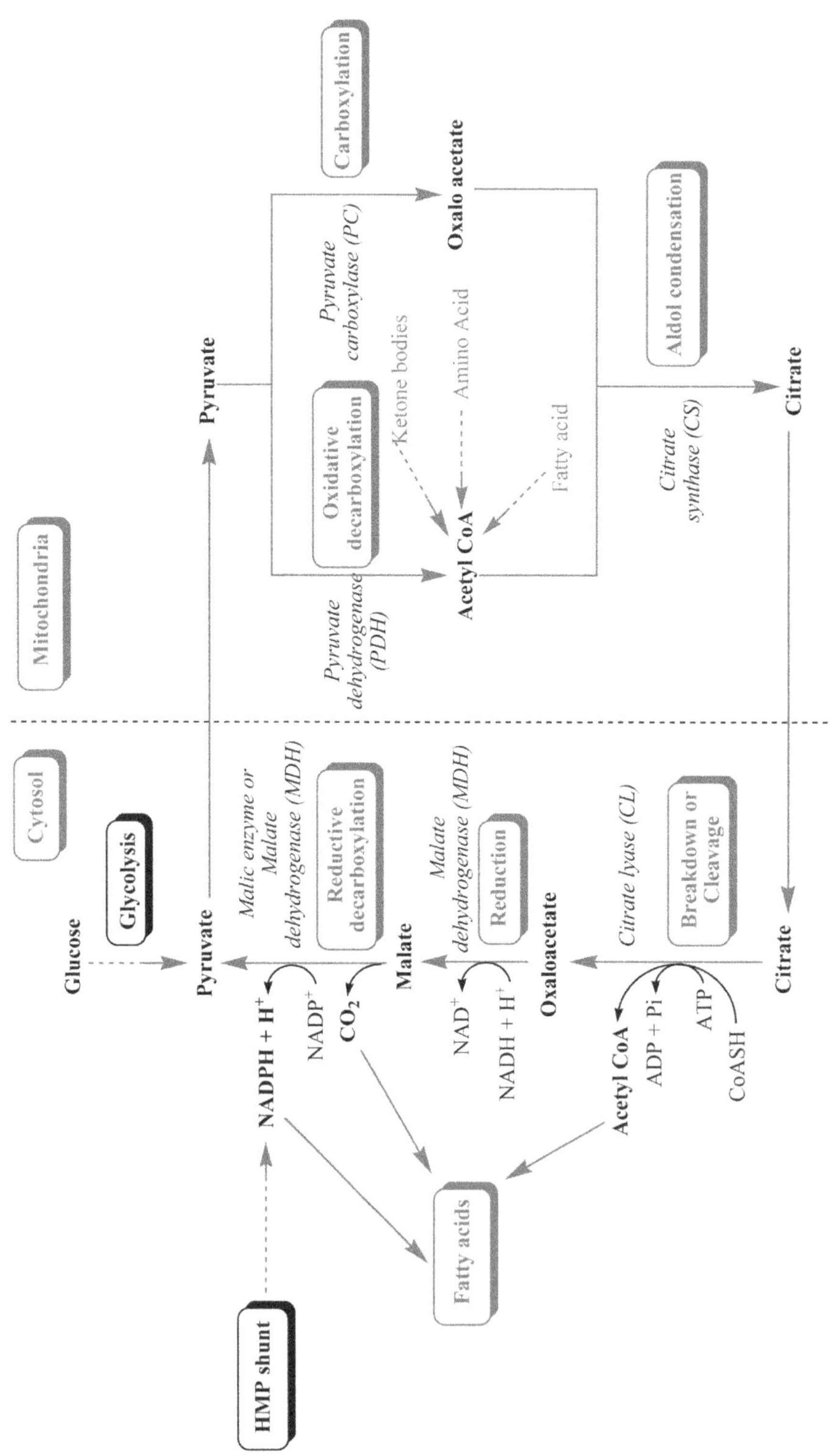
Mitochondria
Cytosol
Glycolysis
Glucose
Pyruvate
Pyruvate
Pyruvate dehydrogenase (PDH)
Oxidative decarboxylation
Pyruvate carboxylase (PC)
Carboxylation
Oxalo acetate
Ketone bodies
Amino Acid
Fatty acid
Acetyl CoA
Aldol condensation
Citrate synthase (CS)
Citrate
Citrate
Citrate lyase (CL)
Breakdown or Cleavage
ATP
CoASH
ADP + Pi
Acetyl CoA
Oxaloacetate
Malate dehydrogenase (MDH)
Reduction
NADH + H+
NAD+
Malate
Malic enzyme or Malate dehydrogenase (MDH)
Reductive decarboxylation
CO2
NADP+
NADPH + H+
Fatty acids
HMP shunt

CoA" and the type of reaction is "carboxylation"). *Acetyl CoA carboxylase* (*ACAC*) needs biotin as a co-enzyme. In a carboxylation reaction, biotin acts as a carrier molecule. Biotin-enzyme reacts with carbondioxide in the presence of ATP to form a carboxybiotin-enzyme complex. This high energy complex handed over the carbondioxide to acetyl CoA to produce succinyl CoA. In this step, one ATP is converted into ADP and inorganic phosphate to provide the energy needed for the reaction. The mechanism of action of *acetyl CoA carboxylase* (*ACAC*) is similar to *pyruvate carboxylase*(*PC*).

$$CH_3-\overset{\overset{O}{\|}}{C}-SCoA \xrightarrow{\text{Rewritten}} H-CH_2-\overset{\overset{O}{\|}}{C}-SCoA$$

Acetyl CoA → **Acetyl CoA**

Acetyl CoA carboxylase (ACAC), Biotin; CO_2, ATP → ADP + Pi (Carboxylation)

$$COOH-CH_2-\overset{\overset{O}{\|}}{C}-SCoA$$

Malonyl CoA

Stage 3 (Reactions of *fatty acid synthase* (*FAS*) complex):

Fatty acid synthase (*FAS*) complex is a multifunctional enzyme catalyzes the remaining reactions of fatty acid synthesis. *FAS* exists as a dimer with two identical units in eukaryotic cells including man. Seven different enzymes and a 4′-phosphopantetheine bound acyl carrier protein (ACP) is present in each monomer of the *FAS* complex. As a single unit this *FAS* complex catalyzes all seven reactions of stage 3 fatty acid synthesis; hence, dissociation of any one of *FAS* complex results in loss of enzyme activities. In eukaryotic cells (higher organism), an acyl carrier protein (ACP) is a part of the *FAS* complex; whereas in prokaryotic cells (lower organisms), ACP is not a part of the *FAS* complex and it is present separately. Seven reactions are catalyzed by seven different enzymes present in the *FAS* complex.

1. In the first step, ACP of *FAS* complex reacts with acetyl CoA and produces acetyl-S-ACP by transfer of acetyl group from acetyl CoA to ACP of the *FAS* complex. The reaction is catalyzed by *acetyl CoA-ACP transacylase* (Substrate is "acetyl CoA & ACP" of *FAS*, the type of reaction is "transfer" and the group transferred is "acetyl i.e., acyl"). Subsequently, the acetyl group is transferred to a cysteine residue of the enzyme from ACP to produce acetyl-S-enzyme. Hence, the ACP site becomes vacant.
2. Latter, malonyl CoA synthesized in stage 2 reacts with the above-formed acetyl-S-enzyme in presence of *malonyl CoA-ACP transacylase* (Substrate is "malonyl CoA & ACP" of *FAS*, the type of reaction is "transfer" and the group transferred is "malonyl") and produced acyl-S-ACP-malonyl-S-enzyme. In this step, the malonyl group is transferred from malonyl CoA to ACP of acetyl-S-enzyme.
3. In the next step, the acyl-S-ACP-malonyl-S-enzyme undergoes decarboxylation followed by addition to produce β-ketoacyl-S-ACP or simply β-ketoacyl-ACP. In this reaction initially, malonyl moiety attached to ACP loses the carboxyl group (added in stage 2 by *acetyl CoA carboxylase* (*ACAC*)) as carbondioxide and this carbondioxide is never incorporated into fatty acid carbon chain but the free energy lost by this decarboxylation is used for the addition takes place. Later, acetyl unit attached to cysteine is transferred to ACP and added to decarboxylated malonyl portion present in presence of *β-ketoacyl-ACP synthase* (The product formed is "β-ketoacyl-ACP" and the type of reaction is "synthesis").

Cys—SH
ACP—SH
***Fatty acid synthase (FAS)* complex**

CH_3—C(=O)—SCoA
Acetyl CoA
Acetyl CoA ACP transacylase
Transfer of acetyl group
CoASH

Cys—SH
ACP—S—C(=O)—CH_3
Acetyl-S-ACP

Transfer of acetyl group to cysteine

Cys—S—C(=O)—CH_3
ACP—SH
Acetyl-S-enzyme

COOH—CH_2—C(=O)—SCoA
Malonyl CoA
Malonyl CoA-ACP transacylase
Transfer of malonyl group
CoASH

Cys—S—C(=O)—CH_3
ACP—S—C(=O)—CH_2—COOH
Acyl-ACP-malonyl-S-enzyme

β-Ketoacyl-ACP synthase
Decarboxylation followed by transfer of acetyl group to ACP
CO_2

Cys—SH
ACP—S—C(=O)—CH_2—C(=O)—CH_3
α β
β-Ketoacyl-ACP

β-Ketoacyl-ACP reductase
NADPH + H^+
Reduction
$NADP^+$

Cys—SH
ACP—S—C(=O)—CH_2—CH(OH)—CH_3
α β
β-Hydroxyacyl-ACP

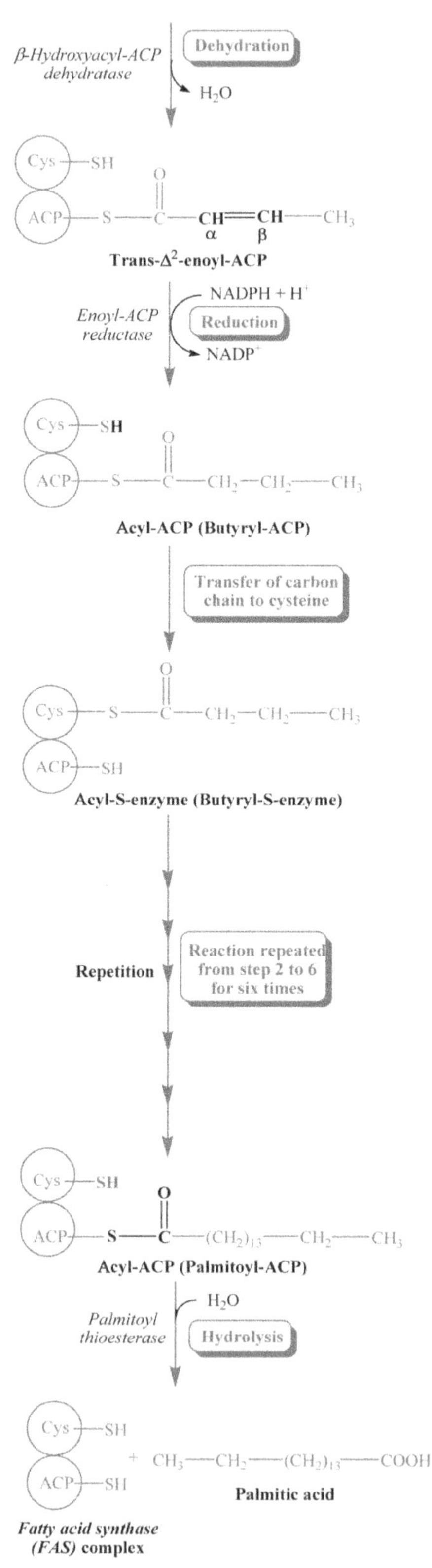

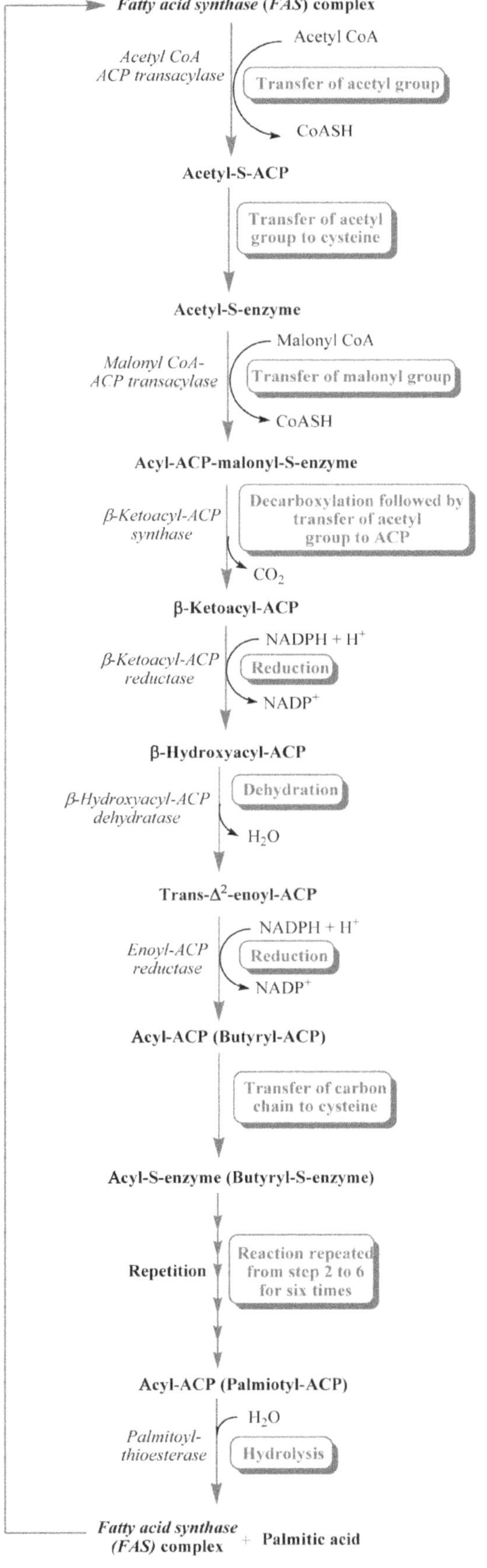

Fatty acid synthase (FAS) complex
Acetyl CoA ACP transacylase
Acetyl CoA
Transfer of acetyl group
CoASH
Acetyl-S-ACP
Transfer of acetyl group to cysteine
Acetyl-S-enzyme
Malonyl CoA-ACP transacylase
Malonyl CoA
Transfer of malonyl group
CoASH
Acyl-ACP-malonyl-S-enzyme
β-Ketoacyl-ACP synthase
Decarboxylation followed by transfer of acetyl group to ACP
CO_2
β-Ketoacyl-ACP
β-Ketoacyl-ACP reductase
NADPH + H^+
Reduction
$NADP^+$
β-Hydroxyacyl-ACP
β-Hydroxyacyl-ACP dehydratase
Dehydration
H_2O
Trans-Δ^2-enoyl-ACP
Enoyl-ACP reductase
NADPH + H^+
Reduction
$NADP^+$
Acyl-ACP (Butyryl-ACP)
Transfer of carbon chain to cysteine
Acyl-S-enzyme (Butyryl-S-enzyme)
Repetition
Reaction repeated from step 2 to 6 for six times
Acyl-ACP (Palmiotyl-ACP)
Palmitoyl-thioesterase
H_2O
Hydrolysis
Fatty acid synthase (FAS) complex
+ Palmitic acid

4. The keto group of β-ketoacyl-ACP is reduced to secondary alcohol to produce β-hydroxyacyl-ACP in presence of *β-ketoacyl-ACP reductase* (The substrate is "β-ketoacyl-ACP" and the type of reaction is "reduction"). NADPH supplies the reducing equivalents for this reaction.
5. The produced β-hydroxyacyl-ACP undergoes dehydration in presence of *β-hydroxyacyl-ACP dehydratase* (The substrate is "β-hydroxyacyl-ACP" and the type of reaction is "dehydration") and produced α,β-unsaturated acyl-ACP or Δ^2-trans enoyl acyl-ACP. Hydrogen is removed from α-carbon and the hydroxyl group is removed from β-carbon atom of β-hydroxy acyl-ACP to loss water molecule. Hence, a double bond is formed between α- and β-carbon.
6. In the sixth step, Δ^2-trans enoyl acyl-ACP undergoes NADPH dependent reduction to produce acyl-ACP (butyryl-ACP) and the reaction is catalyzed by *enoylacyl-ACP reductase* (The substrate is "Δ^2-trans enoylacyl-ACP" and the type of reaction is "reduction").

   Now, the carbon chain attached to ACP of acyl-ACP (butyryl-ACP) is transferred to cysteine residue and the reactions of step 2 to step 6 are repeated for six more times. Each time the length of the fatty acid chain is increased to two carbon units which are obtained from malonyl CoA. Hence, at the end of the seventh cycle palmitate (a 16 carbon fully saturated fatty acid) bound ACP is produced, and in this step fatty acid synthesis is completed.
7. Finally, palmitate is separated from the *FAS* complex by simple hydrolysis reaction and the *FAS* complex is used again for the synthesis of fatty acids. This final step is catalyzed by *palmitoyl thioesterase* (The product formed is "palmitate", the substrate is "thioester" i.e., palmitoyl-ACP and the type of reaction is "hydrolysis").

Two carbon of palmitate is obtained from acetyl CoA directly and the remaining 14 carbon is also obtained from acetyl CoA only but indirectly through malonyl CoA. Hence, the overall reactions of palmitate synthesis can be summarized as follows,

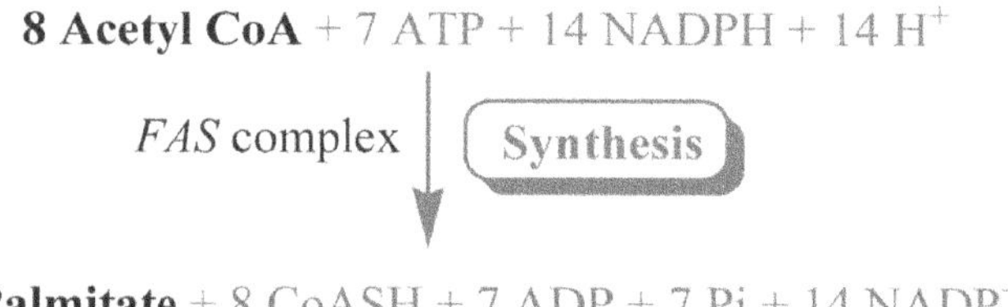

***Fatty acid synthase* (*FAS*) complex:**

FAS complex model is based on Wakil work and is tentative. *FAS* is a dimer containing two identical sub units i.e., monomer, each with 2,40,000 molecular weight. Each monomer is composed of seven different enzymes and an ACP with 4-phosphopantetheine sulfhydryl (-SH) group. Hence, each monomer possesses all enzyme activities of fatty acid synthesis. The two monomers are present in head to tail orientation i.e., lie in antiparallel orientation. The 4-phosphopantetheine sulfhydryl (-SH) group of one monomer is in close proximity to the cysteine sulfhydryl (-SH) group (of the *ketoacyl synthase* enzyme) of another monomer. Schematic representation of *fatty acid synthase* (*FAS*) complex is presentedin Figure 4.4.

Only the dimer of *FAS* is active because the functional unit consists of half of each sub unit interacting with the complementary half to the other. Hence, the *FAS* complex contains both functional division and subunit division. Simultaneously two fatty acids can be synthesized because; two functional subunits of *FAS* are independently operating. The followings are the various advantages of the *FAS* complex.

1. Great efficiency is offered by the *FAS* complex because no other cellular reactions are interfered with the fatty acid synthesis.
2. There are no permeability barriers for the several intermediates since the whole process is taking place in one complex.

3. Single gene codes the multi-enzyme polypeptide complex. Hence, there is good coordination in the synthesis of all seven enzymes of the *FAS* complex.

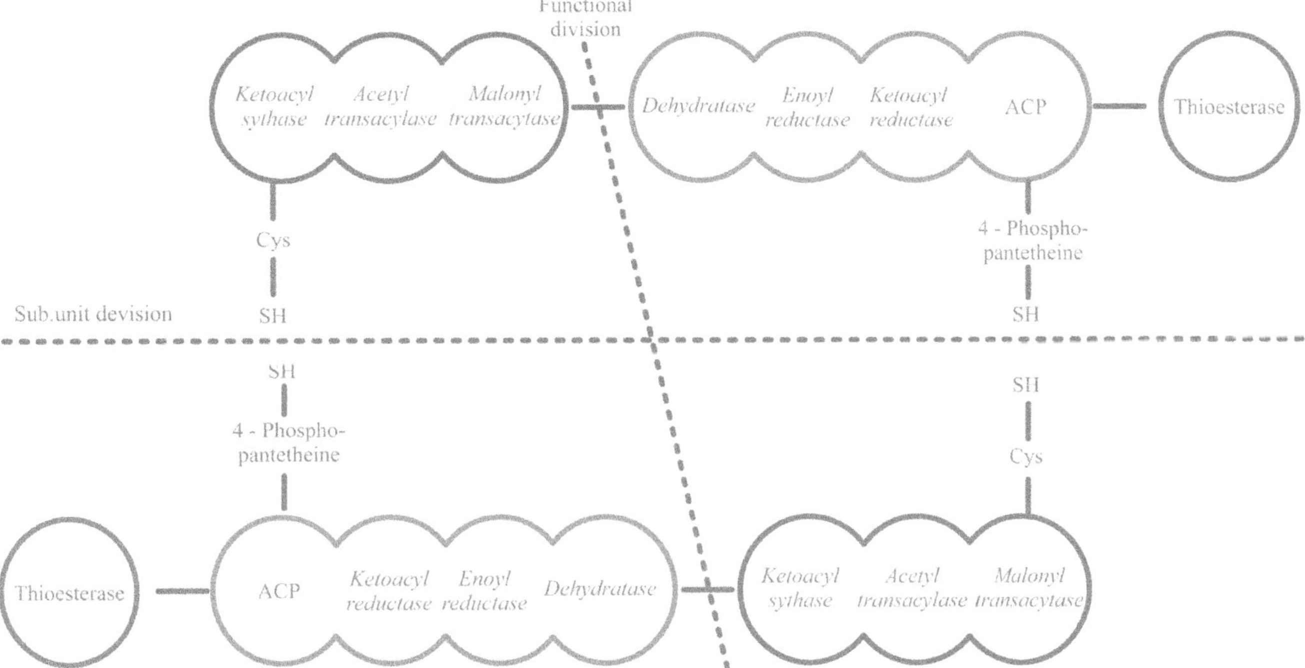

Figure 4.4 Schematic representation of *fatty acid synthase* (*FAS*) complex.

Regulation:

There are several substances such as enzymes, end products, metabolites, dietary manipulations and hormones regulate fatty acid synthesis. Regulation of fatty acid synthesis is presented in Figure 4.5.

1. ***Acetyl CoA carboxylase* (*ACAC*):** This is the rate limiting enzyme of fatty acid synthesis responsible for the production of malonyl CoA from acetyl CoA. It exists in two forms like inactive monomer (protomer) form and active polymer form. Citrate and malonyl CoA promote the polymeric form whereas palmityl CoA promotes monomeric form. Polymeric form increases the fatty acid synthesis and the monomeric forms inhibit fatty acid synthesis.
2. **Hormones:** *Acetyl CoA carboxylase* (*ACAC*) is regulated differently by hormones by a separate mechanism. The phosphorylated form of *acetyl CoA carboxylase* (*ACAC*) is inactive form and the dephosphorylated form is the active form. *Acetyl CoA carboxylase* is (*ACAC*) inactivated by glucagon, epinephrine and nor-epinephrine by cAMP dependent phosphorylation. On the other hand, insulin dephosphorylate the *acetyl CoA carboxylase* (*ACAC*) thereby promotes fatty acid synthesis. In addition, insulin also stimulates glucose uptake of tissues and conversion of pyruvate to acetyl CoA. This also favors fatty acid synthesis.
3. **Diet:** High carbohydrate rich diet or fat-free diet increases the production of *acetyl CoA carboxylase* (*ACAC*) and the *FAS* complex leads to increased fatty acid synthesis. Conversely, fat-rich diet or starvation decreases the production of the above two enzymes; hence it decreases the synthesis of fatty acids.
4. **NADPH availability:** NADPH is generally produced from HMP shunt and acetyl CoA (citrate) transport. HMP shunt provides 50 to 60 % NADPH required by fatty acid synthesis, hence it significantly regulates fatty acid synthesis.

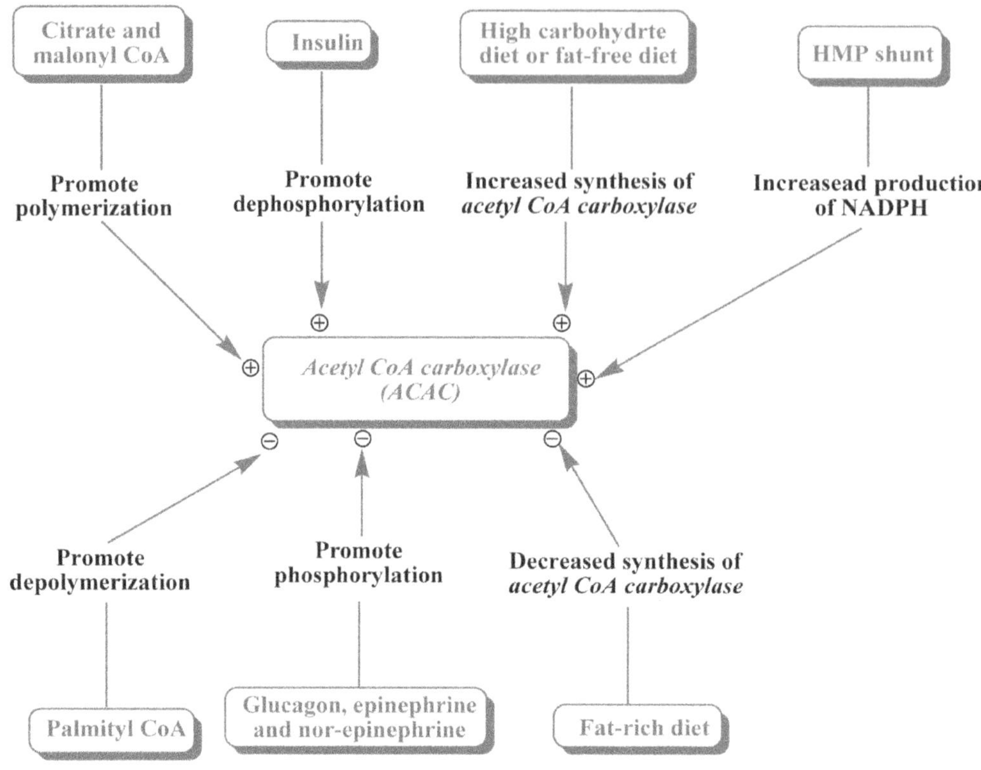

Figure 4.5 Regulation of fatty acid synthesis.

Synthesis of unsaturated fatty acid:

Unsaturated fatty acids are synthesized by a microsomal enzyme called *fatty acyl CoA desaturase*. This desaturation also needs flavin dependent *cytochrome b_5 reductase*, NADH, and molecular oxygen (O_2). Oleic acid and palmitoleic acid are monounsaturated fatty acids which are synthesized from saturated fatty acids stearic acid and palmitic acid, respectively.

In general, in mammals, polyunsaturated fatty acids (PUFA) like linoleic acid and linolenic acid are not synthesized due to lack of enzyme responsible to introduce double bond at C-10 and methyl terminal (ω-carbon) end. Hence, these PUFA is essential for human in the diet. However, arachidonic acid is synthesized form linoleic acid by desaturation and chain elongation. Arachidonic acid is the precursor for the synthesis of eicosanoids such as prostaglandin, thromboxane, etc.

Synthesis of long chain fatty acid:

Long chain fatty acids are generally synthesized from palmitate which is the end product of the *FAS* complex in cytosol. Further, either in mitochondria or microsomes (endoplasmic reticulum) chain elongation can take place by a separate mechanism. The predominant one is microsomal elongation with successive addition of malonyl CoA using NADPH. These reactions are similar to *FAS* catalyzed reactions. Fatty acid elongation can be done by a group of enzymes namely known as *elongase*. Almost reverse of β-oxidation of fatty acids, chain elongation is taking place in mitochondrial elongation. In this elongation, acetyl CoA is successively added with the involvement of reducing equivalent NADPH.

Comparison of fatty acid synthesis and β-oxidation of fatty acids:

Two distinct and independent pathways are involved in fatty acid synthesis and β-oxidation of fatty acids. The comparison of these two metabolic pathways is described in the Table 4.3.

Table 4.3 Synthesis and β-oxidation of fatty acids – A comparison.

S. No.	Parameter	Fatty acid synthesis	β-Oxidation of fatty acid
1	Subcellular site	Cytosol	Mitochondria
2	Major tissue	Liver and adipose tissue	Liver and muscle
3	Substrate or precursor	Acetyl CoA	Fatty acid (Acyl CoA)
4	Carbon units added or degraded	Malonyl CoA	Acetyl CoA
5	Transport system involved	Citrate from mitochondria to cytosol	Carnitine from cytosol to mitochondria
6	Co-enzyme required	NADPH (supplies reducing equivalent)	FAD and NAD^+ (undergoes reduction)
7	Intermediates bound to	Acyl carrier protein (ACP)	Co-enzyme A
8	End product	Palmitic acid	Acetyl CoA
9	Rate limiting enzyme	*Acetyl CoA carboxylase (ACAC)* (inhibited by long chain acyl CoA)	*Carnitine acyl transferase – I / CAT –I* (inhibited by malonyl CoA)
10	Dietary condition which promotes pathway	After carbohydrate rich diet	In starvation
11	Hormones which promotes pathway	High ratio of insulin / glucagon	Low ratio of insulin / glucagon
12	Type of enzyme	Multifunctional enzyme complex	Individual enzymes

Metabolism of Cholesterol

Cholesterol is commonly known as animal sterol because it is found exclusively in animals and is chemically steroidal alcohol. Cholesterol contains both hydrophilic and hydrophobic regions in the structure; hence it is amphipathic in nature. In adults, 2 g of cholesterol is present per kg of body weight i.e., the total cholesterol present in 70 kg adult is 140 g (2 × 70). The chemical structure of cholesterol with the numbering of carbon atom is given below.

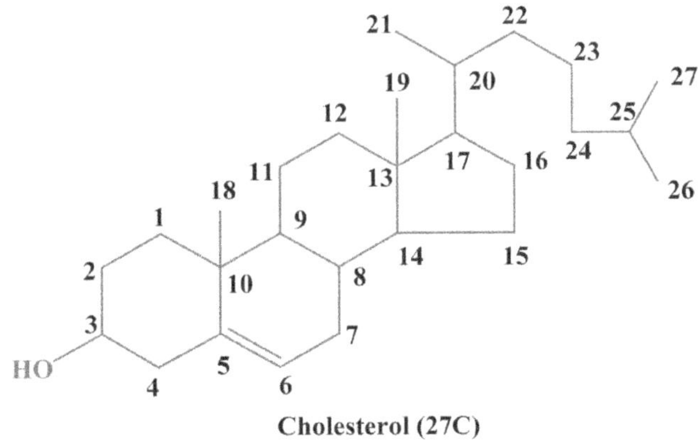

Cholesterol (27C)

Biosynthesis of Cholesterol

In cholesterol biosynthesis, almost all body tissues participate. Liver (50 %) and intestine (15 %) make the largest contribution followed by skin, adrenal cortex, reproductive tissue, etc. In adults, per day about 1 g of cholesterol is synthesized. Cytosol and microsomal fraction of the cell contains the enzymes necessary for the synthesis of cholesterol. The major components involved in the synthesis of cholesterol are,

1. Acetyl CoA (Source of carbon)
2. NADPH (Supplies reducing equivalent)
3. ATP (Source of energy)

For the synthesis of one mole of cholesterol, it requires 18 moles of acetyl CoA, 36 moles of ATP, and 16 moles of NADPH. In the entire molecule of cholesterol, the origins of carbon atoms are established by administering acetate with ^{14}C isotope label either methyl ($-CH_3$) group or carboxyl (-COOH) group. The source of the carbon atoms of cholesterol is presented in below structure.

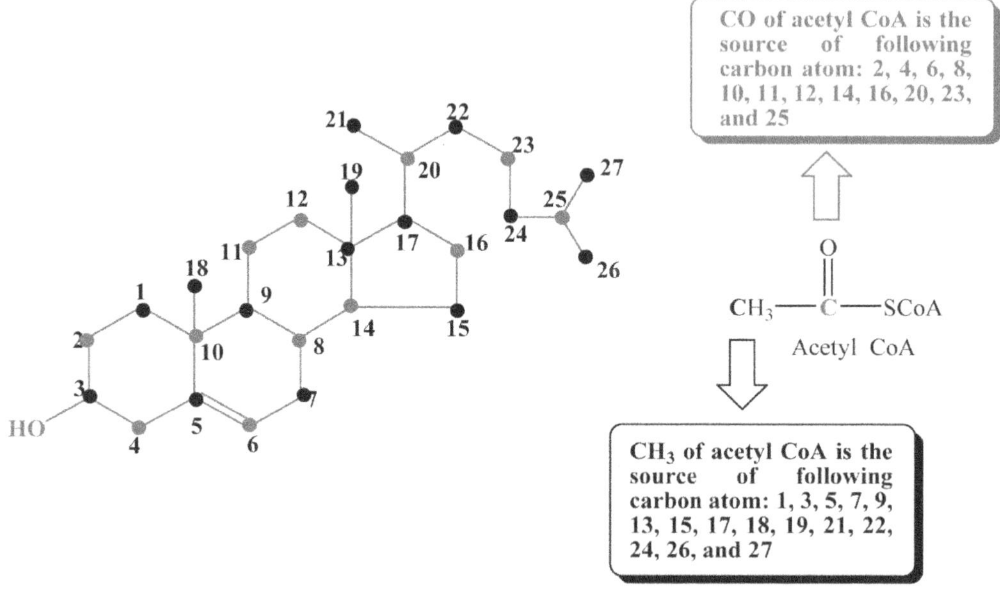

Five different stages are involved in the synthesis of cholesterol. They are,

1. Synthesis of HMG CoA
2. Production of mevalonate (6 carbons)
3. Formation of isoprenoid units (5 carbons)
4. Synthesis of squalene (30 carbons)
5. Conversion of squalene to cholesterol (27 carbons)

1. Synthesis of HMG CoA:

HMG CoA is biosynthesized from acetyl CoA and involves two steps.

1. Initially, two molecules of acetyl CoA are condensed together and produce acetoacetyl CoA with loss of co-enzyme A in the presence of *β-ketoacyl CoA thiolase* (*βKACAT*) or *β-ketothiolase* (*βKT*) or simply *thiolase* (The type of reaction is "thiolytic cleavage" and the product is "acetoacetyl CoA" which is "β-keto acyl CoA").
2. Another molecule of acetyl CoA is reacting with acetoacetyl CoA and one molecule of water in presence of *HMG CoA synthase* (*HMGCAS*) (Product is "HMG CoA" and the type of reaction is "synthesis") and produce β-hydroxy-β-methylglutaryl CoA (HMG CoA) and co-enzyme A. The basic reaction involved in this step is addition followed by hydrolysis.

In ketone body synthesis also, the same reactions are involved but the difference is, cholesterol synthesis takes place in cytosol; whereas, ketone bodies synthesis occurring in mitochondria. Two pools of HMG CoA exist in the cell. In addition, two isoenzymes of *HMG CoA synthase* (*HMGCAS*) are known. The cytosomal *HMG CoA synthase* (*HMGCAS*) is involved in the synthesis of cholesterol and the mitochondrial *HMG CoA synthase* (*HMGCAS*) is involved in the synthesis of ketone bodies.

2. Production of mevalonate (6 carbons):

HMG CoA is reduced to mevalonate and the reducing equivalent is provided by NADPH. In this step, initially, HMG CoA is hydrolyzed to β-hydroxy-β-methylglutarate (HMG) with the liberation of co-enzyme A. Later, the carboxylic acid group of HMG is reduced to aldehyde followed by primary alcohol i.e., mevalonate. Hence, 2 moles of NADPH are involved in this reaction (one mole for reduction of acid to aldehyde and another mole for reduction of aldehyde to primary alcohol). The enzyme involved in this reaction is *HMG CoA reductase* (*HMGCAR*) (Substrate is "HMG CoA" and the type of reaction is "reduction"). ***HMG CoA reductase* (*HMGCAR*) is present in the endoplasmic reticulum and is the rate limiting enzyme of cholesterol biosynthesis.**

3. **Formation of isoprenoid unit (5 carbons or multiples of 5 carbons):**

   Mevalonate undergoes phosphorylation to produce 3-phospho-5-pyrophospho mevalonate (PPPM) which involves three steps.

   1. In the first step, mevalonate is phosphorylated at 5th position by reacting with ATP to produce 5-phospho mevalonate (PM) in presence of enzyme *mevalonate kinase* (*MK*) (In ATP/ADP involved reactions, the enzymes acted are "*kinase*" and the substrate is "mevalonate"). *Kinase* enzyme needs magnesium cation (Mg^{2+}) as a co-factor. In this reaction one ATP is converted into ADP **(1 ATP is utilized)**.
   2. Latter, 5-phospho mevalonate (PM) is again phosphorylated at 5th position by reacting with ATP to produce 5-pyrophospho mevalonate (PPM) in presence of enzyme *phosphomevalonate kinase* (*PMK*) (In ATP/ADP involved reactions, the enzymes acted are "*kinase*" and the substrate is "5-phospho mevalonate (PM)"). *Kinase* enzyme needs magnesium cation (Mg^{2+}) as cofactor. In this reaction, one ATP is converted into ADP **(1 ATP is utilized).**
   3. Finally, 5-pyrophospho mevalonate (PPM) is phosphorylated at 3rd position by reacting with ATP to produce 3-phospho-5-pyrophospho mevalonate (PPPM) in the presence of enzyme *pyrophosphomevalonate kinase* (*PPMK*) (In ATP/ADP involved reactions, the enzymes acted are "*kinase*" and the substrate is "5-pyrophospho mevalonate (PPM)"). *Kinase* enzyme needs magnesium cation (Mg^{2+}) as cofactor. In this reaction, one ATP is converted into ADP **(1 ATP is utilized).**

   This 3-phospho-5-pyrophospho mevalonate (PPPM) undergoes decarboxylation followed by dephosphorylation and dehydration in the presence of *pyrophosphomevalonate decarboxylase (PPMD)* (Substrate is "3-phospho-5-pyrophospho mevalonate (PPPM)" which is "pyrophospho mevalonate (PPM)" derivative and the type of reaction is "decarboxylation") produced isoprenoid compound isopentenyl pyrophosphate (IPP). During this step, one mole of carbondioxide, inorganic phosphate, and a water molecule is removed. The formed isopentenyl pyrophosphate (IPP) undergoes isomerization and produces dimethylallyl pyrophosphate (DPP) in presence of *isopentenyl pyrophosphate isomerase* (IPPI) (Substrate is "isopentenyl pyrophosphate (IPP)" and the type of reaction is "isomerization"). IPP and DPP are 5-carbon isoprenoid units and are positional isomers (position of double bond differs).

4. **Synthesis of squalene (30 carbons):**

   In the next step, dimethylallyl pyrophosphate (DPP) and isopentenyl pyrophosphate (IPP) combined together by condensation and produce a 10-carbon geranyl pyrophosphate (GPP) in presence of *isoprenyl transferase* (*IPT*) (Substrate is "DPP & IPP" which are isoprene derivatives and the type of reaction is "transfer") with the liberation of one pyrophosphate (PPi). Later, geranyl pyrophosphate (GPP) condense with another molecule of isopentenyl pyrophosphate (IPP) and produced a 15-carbon farnesyl pyrophosphate (FPP) in presence of *isoprenyl transferase* (*IPT*) (Substrate is "GPP & IPP"which are isoprene derivatives and the type of reaction is "transfer") with the liberation of one pyrophosphate (PPi). Finally, farnesyl pyrophosphate (FPP) condensed with another molecule of farnesyl pyrophosphate (FPP) and produced 30-carbon squalene with the liberation of two pyrophosphates (PPi). This reaction is catalyzed by *squalene synthase* (*SS*) (Product is "squalene" and the type of reaction is "synthesis"). In this reaction, one mole of NADPH is oxidized to $NADP^+$ and the lost hydrogen is accepted by pyrophosphate (PPi).

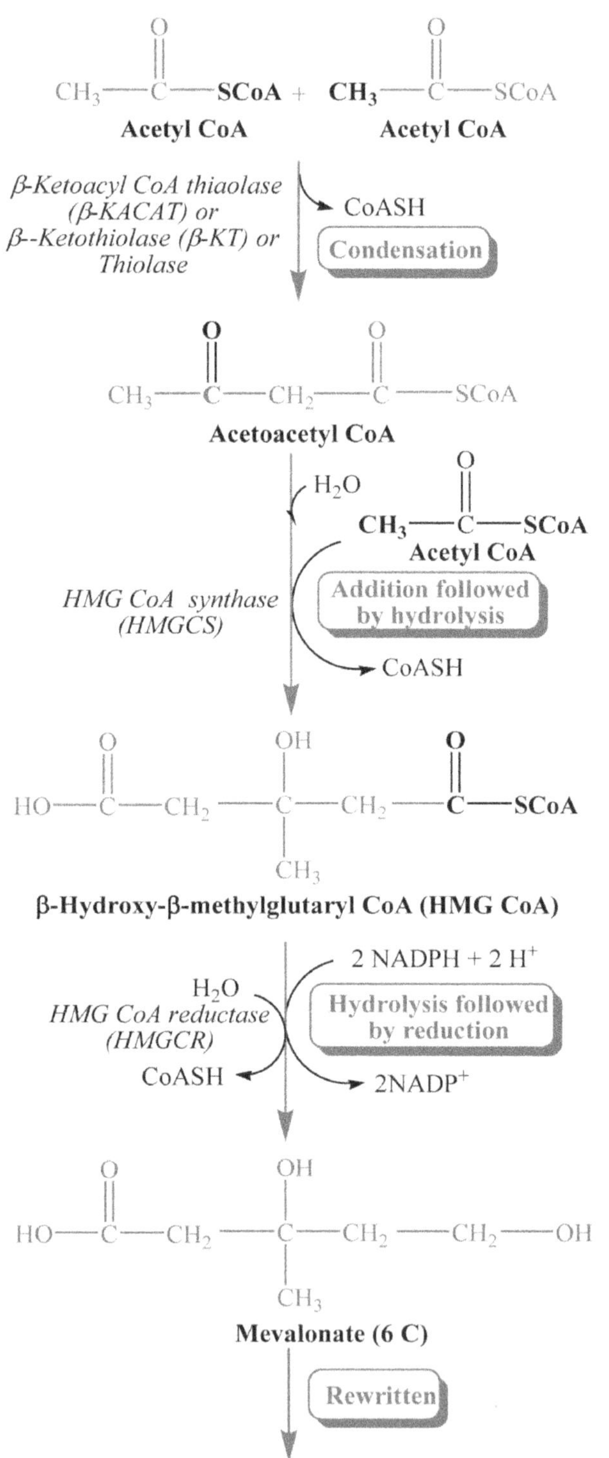

CH3—C(=O)—SCoA + CH3—C(=O)—SCoA
Acetyl CoA
Acetyl CoA
β-Ketoacyl CoA thiaolase (β-KACAT) or β--Ketothiolase (β-KT) or Thiolase
CoASH
Condensation
CH3—C(=O)—CH2—C(=O)—SCoA
Acetoacetyl CoA
H2O
CH3—C(=O)—SCoA
Acetyl CoA
HMG CoA synthase (HMGCS)
Addition followed by hydrolysis
CoASH
HO—C(=O)—CH2—C(OH)(CH3)—CH2—C(=O)—SCoA
β-Hydroxy-β-methylglutaryl CoA (HMG CoA)
2 NADPH + 2 H+
H2O
HMG CoA reductase (HMGCR)
Hydrolysis followed by reduction
CoASH
2NADP+
HO—C(=O)—CH2—C(OH)(CH3)—CH2—CH2—OH
Mevalonate (6 C)
Rewritten

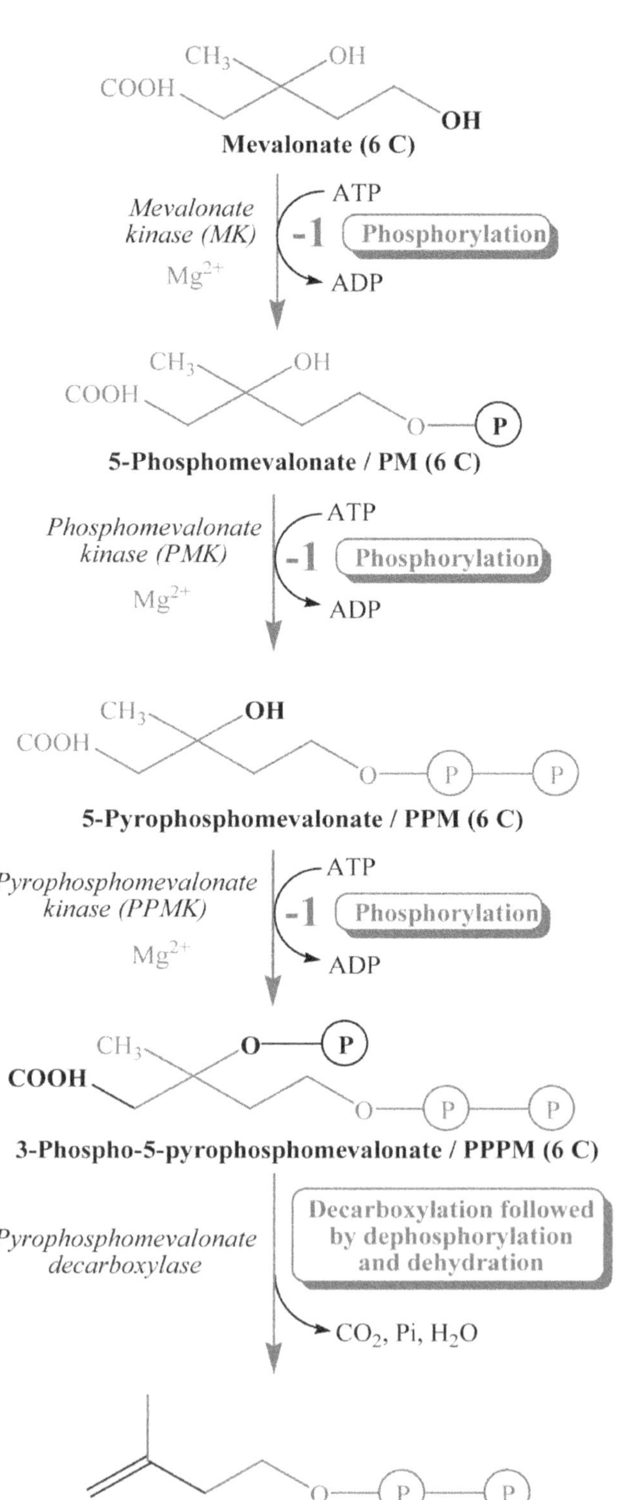

CH3
OH
COOH
OH
Mevalonate (6 C)
Mevalonate kinase (MK)
Mg2+
ATP
-1
Phosphorylation
ADP
5-Phosphomevalonate / PM (6 C)
Phosphomevalonate kinase (PMK)
Mg2+
ATP
-1
Phosphorylation
ADP
5-Pyrophosphomevalonate / PPM (6 C)
Pyrophosphomevalonate kinase (PPMK)
Mg2+
ATP
-1
Phosphorylation
ADP
3-Phospho-5-pyrophosphomevalonate / PPPM (6 C)
Pyrophosphomevalonate decarboxylase
Decarboxylation followed by dephosphorylation and dehydration
CO2, Pi, H2O
Isopentenyl pyrophosphate / IPP (5 C)

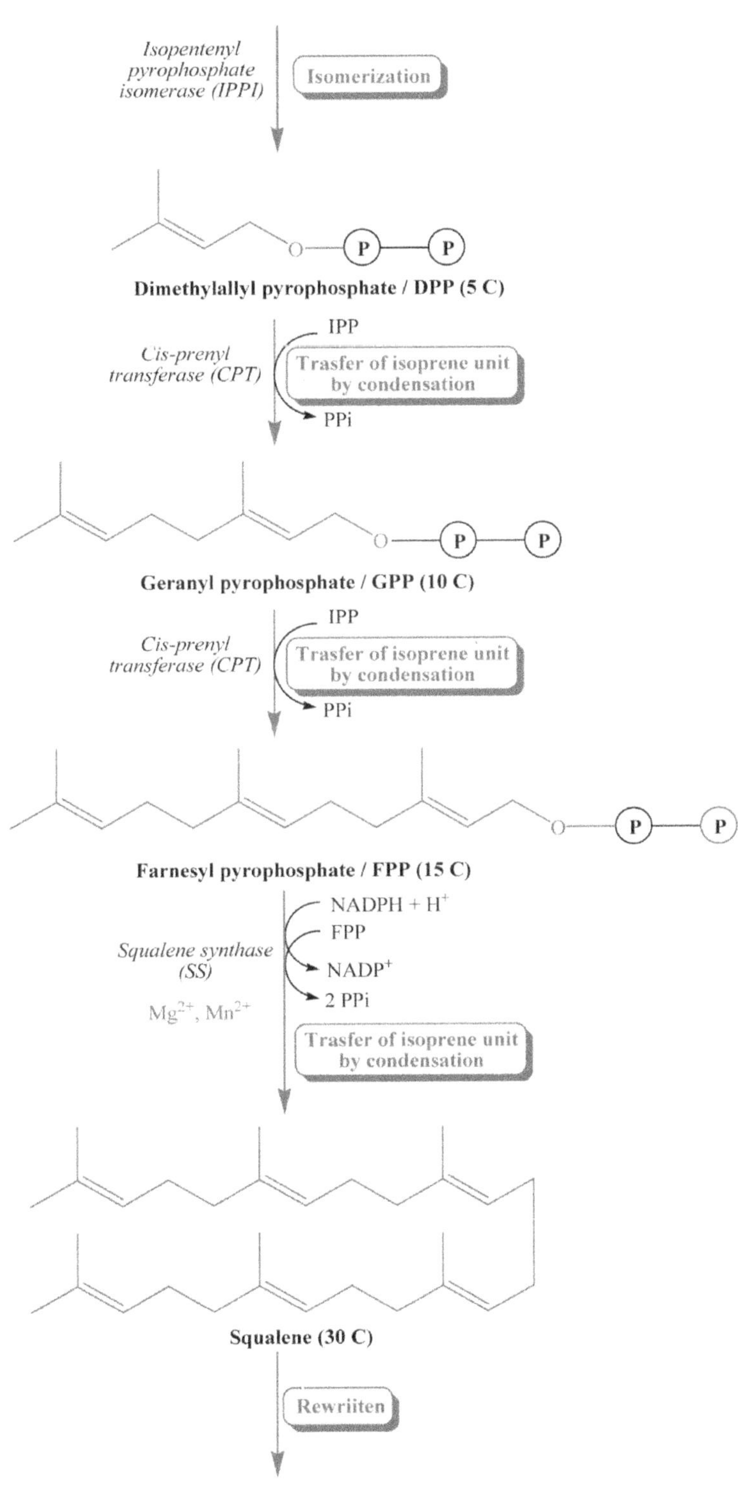

Squalene (30 C)

$NADPH + H^+$

O_2

Epoxidase

Hydroxylase

$NADP^+$

H_2O

Epoxidation
Hydroxylation
Cyclisation

HO

Lanosterol (30 C)

HCOOH

$2\ CO_2$

$NADPH + H^+, O_2$

$NADP^+$

A series of about 19 reactions

HO

Cholesterol (27 C)

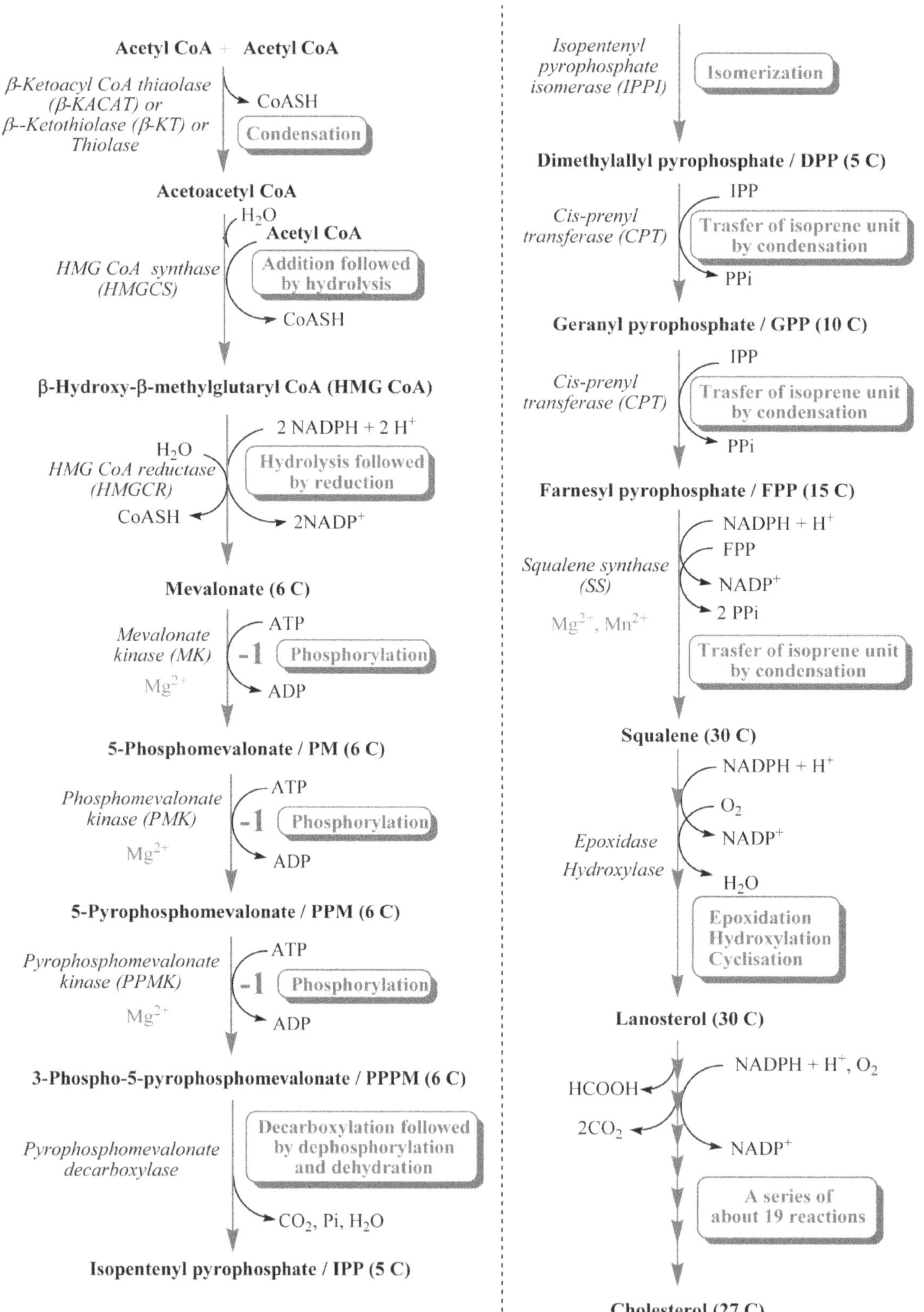
Acetyl CoA + Acetyl CoA
β-Ketoacyl CoA thiaolase (β-KACAT) or β-Ketothiolase (β-KT) or Thiolase
CoASH
Condensation
Acetoacetyl CoA
H_2O
Acetyl CoA
HMG CoA synthase (HMGCS)
Addition followed by hydrolysis
CoASH
β-Hydroxy-β-methylglutaryl CoA (HMG CoA)
2 NADPH + 2 H^+
H_2O
HMG CoA reductase (HMGCR)
Hydrolysis followed by reduction
CoASH
$2NADP^+$
Mevalonate (6 C)
Mevalonate kinase (MK)
Mg^{2+}
ATP
-1
Phosphorylation
ADP
5-Phosphomevalonate / PM (6 C)
Phosphomevalonate kinase (PMK)
Mg^{2+}
ATP
-1
Phosphorylation
ADP
5-Pyrophosphomevalonate / PPM (6 C)
Pyrophosphomevalonate kinase (PPMK)
Mg^{2+}
ATP
-1
Phosphorylation
ADP
3-Phospho-5-pyrophosphomevalonate / PPPM (6 C)
Pyrophosphomevalonate decarboxylase
Decarboxylation followed by dephosphorylation and dehydration
CO_2, Pi, H_2O
Isopentenyl pyrophosphate / IPP (5 C)
Isopentenyl pyrophosphate isomerase (IPPI)
Isomerization
Dimethylallyl pyrophosphate / DPP (5 C)
IPP
Cis-prenyl transferase (CPT)
Trasfer of isoprene unit by condensation
PPi
Geranyl pyrophosphate / GPP (10 C)
IPP
Cis-prenyl transferase (CPT)
Trasfer of isoprene unit by condensation
PPi
Farnesyl pyrophosphate / FPP (15 C)
NADPH + H^+
FPP
Squalene synthase (SS)
$NADP^+$
2 PPi
Mg^{2+}, Mn^{2+}
Trasfer of isoprene unit by condensation
Squalene (30 C)
NADPH + H^+
O_2
Epoxidase
Hydroxylase
$NADP^+$
H_2O
Epoxidation
Hydroxylation
Cyclisation
Lanosterol (30 C)
NADPH + H^+, O_2
HCOOH
$2CO_2$
$NADP^+$
A series of about 19 reactions
Cholesterol (27 C)

5. **Conversion of squalene to cholesterol (27 carbons):**

Squalene undergoes hydroxylation particularly epoxidation followed by cyclization to produce lanosterol in presence of *epoxidase* and *cyclase* (Type of reaction is "epoxidation" and "cyclization"). In this reaction, one mole of NADPH and molecular oxygen is involved. NADPH is oxidized to $NADP^+$ and the one of oxygen atom is removed as a water molecule and another one is incorporated in the steroid nucleus at the C-3 position of lanosterol.

Later, from lanosterol by multistep reaction (19 enzymatic reactions) cholesterol is biosynthesized and the following are some important structural changes that take place during this conversion.

1. The carbon atoms are reduced from 30 to 27.
2. Totally, three methyl groups are removed. At C-4, two methyl groups are removed and at C-14, one methyl group is removed.
3. Double bond present between C-8 and C-9 is shifted between C-5 and C-6.
4. The double bond present between C-24 and C-25 is reduced i.e., removed.

In the endoplasmic reticulum, these 19 enzymes which involved in the conversion of lanosterol to cholesterol is present. The various important intermediates formed during this conversion are 14-desmethyllanosterol, zymosterol, cholestadienol and desmosterol. In cholesterol biosynthesis, the penultimate (one before the last or second to last or last but one) product is 7-dehydrocholesterol which on reduction produces 27 carbons possessing cholesterol. 7-Dehydrocholesterol is the precursor used for the synthesis of vitamin-D_3 using sunlight.

Now it is believed that cholesterol biosynthesis is a part of other major metabolic pathways involved in synthesis of isoprenoid compounds. **Example:** Ubiquinone or co-enzyme Q in electron transport chain (ETC) and dolichol found in glycoprotein. Farnesyl pyrophosphate (FPP) is a precursor for the synthesis of both ubiquinone and dolichol.

Regulation:

In cholesterol biosynthesis, *HMG CoA reductase* is the rate-limiting enzyme and it is found in association with the endoplasmic reticulum. This enzyme is subjected to different metabolic controls such as 1) Feedback control, 2) Hormonal regulation, 3) Inhibition by drugs, and 4) Inhibition by other compounds, and food habits. The regulation of cholesterol biosynthesis by *HMG CoA reductase* (*HMGCAR*) is presented in the Figure 4.6.

1. **Feedback control:** By a feedback mechanism its own synthesis is controlled by the end product cholesterol. Synthesis of *HMG CoA reductase* (*HMGCAR*) is inhibited by an increased cellular concentration of cholesterol by decreasing the transcription of the gene responsible for the synthesis of *HMG CoA reductase* (*HMGCAR*). With regard to LDL cholesterol taken up by the cells, feedback regulation is investigated. Whenever the cellular cholesterol level is increased the same mechanism is believed to operate.
2. **Hormonal regulation:** Two interconvertible forms of *HMG CoA reductase* (*HMGCAR*) exist in body. Among these, a more active form is dephosphorylated form and less active form is phosphorylated form. Through cAMP, the hormone influences by a series of reaction which are comparable with the control of the enzyme *glycogen synthase* (*GS*). In general, insulin and thyroxine stimulate the production of the active form of *HMG CoA reductase* (*HMGCAR*) leads to increased synthesis of cholesterol; whereas, glucagon and glucocorticoids stimulate the production of the inactive form of *HMG CoA reductase* (*HMGCAR*) leads to decreased synthesis of cholesterol.
3. **Inhibition by drugs:** Clinically, competitive inhibitors of *HMG CoA reductase* (*HMGCAR*) are used in the treatment of hypercholesterolemia. **Example:** Statins particularly lovastatin (mevinolin) and compactin. Both drugs are fungal products and are reported to decrease about 50 to 60 % serum cholesterol levels when combined in use.
4. **Inhibition by other compounds and food habits:** Bile acid inhibits the activity of *HMG CoA reductase* (*HMGCAR*). Similarly, fasting also inhibits the activity of *HMG CoA reductase* (*HMGCAR*).

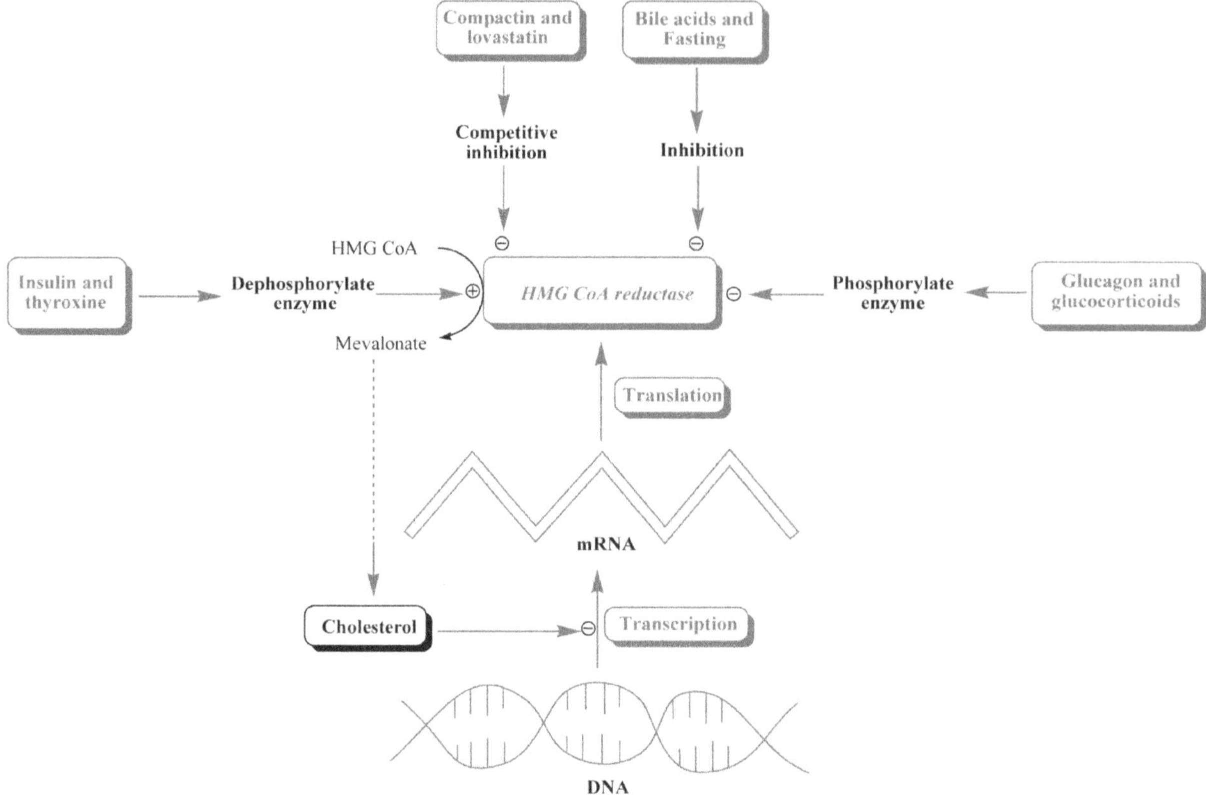

Figure 4.6 Regulation of cholesterol biosynthesis by *HMG CoA reductase.*

Biological Significance of Cholesterol

Cholesterol performs many important biological functions. Hence, it is essential for life. Following are some important biological significance of cholesterol.

1. Cholesterol is the structural component of cell membrane.
2. All other steroidal compounds in the body are biosynthesized from cholesterol only.
3. Steroidal hormones are biosynthesized from cholesterol.
4. Cholesterol acts as a precursor for the synthesis of vitamin-D.
5. In addition, from cholesterol bile acids also biosynthesized in the body.
6. In general, lipids are biosynthesized in the form of lipoprotein only. Cholesterol is the essential component in the lipoproteins.
7. To liver, fatty acids are transported for oxidation as cholesteryl esters.

Degradation of Cholesterol

In humans, the ring structure (steroidal nucleus) of cholesterol cannot be metabolized. Unlike other compounds, cholesterol is not metabolized into carbondioxide and water. Instead of that cholesterol (about 50 %) is

1. Converted to bile acids (excreted in feces)
2. Act as a precursor for the synthesis of steroid hormones
3. Serves as a precursor for the synthesis of vitamin-D, coprostanol, and cholestanol.

Cholesterol, coprostanol, and cholestanol are called fecal sterol because these are steroidal alcohol excreted in feces also. Major source of liver cholesterol and its utilization are summarized in Figure 4.7.

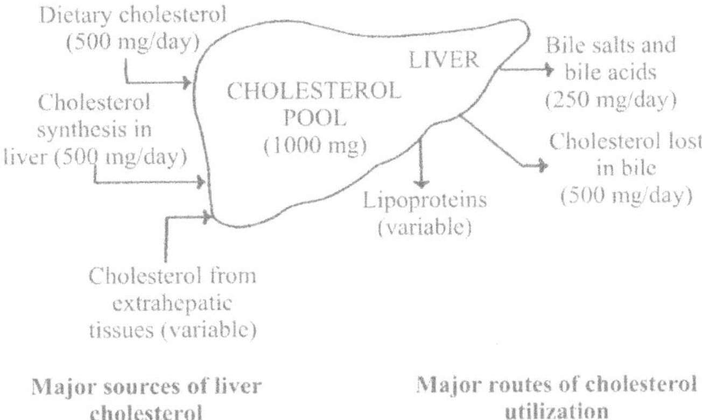

Figure 4.7 Summary of major sources of liver cholesterol and its utilization (values given in brackets are variable).

Synthesis of bile acids:

Bile acids are 24 carbon-containing steroidal compounds with two to three hydroxyl (-OH) group in the steroidal ring and a side chain ending in the carboxyl (-COOH) group. Like cholesterol, bile acids are also amphipathic in nature because it contains both hydrophilic and hydrophobic regions in the structure. In the intestine, bile acids are actively participate in the digestion and absorption of lipids as emulsifying

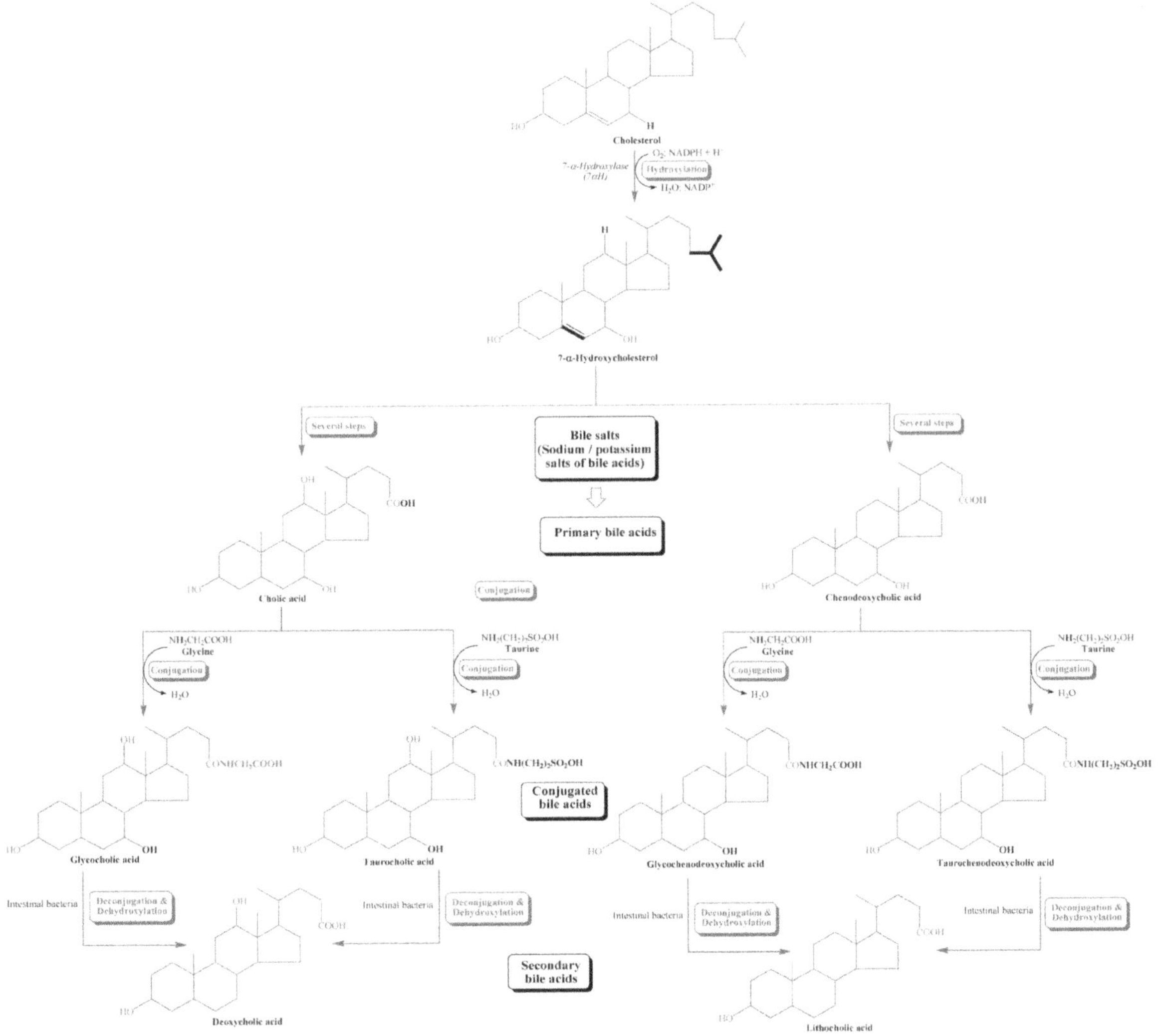

Cholesterol
7-α-Hydroxylase (7αH)
Hydroxylation
O_2, NADPH + H^+
H_2O, $NADP^+$
7-α-Hydroxycholesterol
Several steps
Bile salts (Sodium / potassium salts of bile acids)
Primary bile acids
Several steps
Cholic acid
Conjugation
Chenodeoxycholic acid
NH_2CH_2COOH Glycine
Conjugation
H_2O
$NH_2(CH_2)_2SO_2OH$ Taurine
Conjugation
H_2O
NH_2CH_2COOH Glycine
Conjugation
H_2O
$NH_2(CH_2)_2SO_2OH$ Taurine
Conjugation
H_2O
Glycocholic acid
Taurocholic acid
Conjugated bile acids
Glycochenodeoxycholic acid
Taurochenodeoxycholic acid
Intestinal bacteria
Deconjugation & Dehydroxylation
Intestinal bacteria
Deconjugation & Dehydroxylation
Secondary bile acids
Intestinal bacteria
Deconjugation & Dehydroxylation
Intestinal bacteria
Deconjugation & Dehydroxylation
Deoxycholic acid
Lithocholic acid

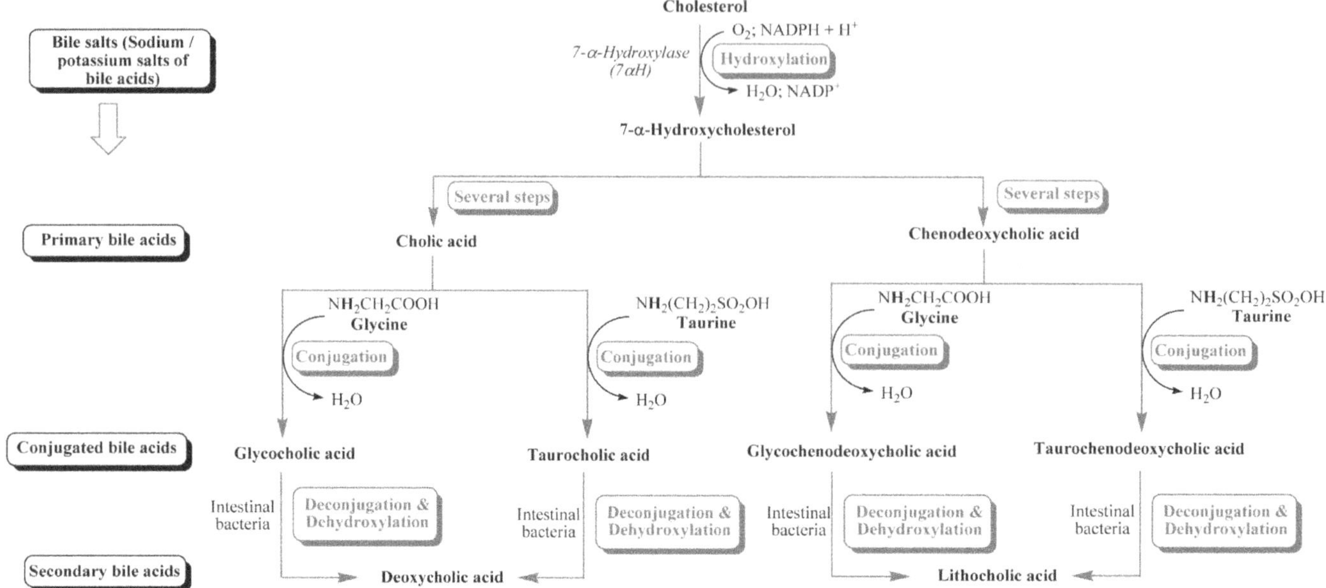

agents. Bile acids are biosynthesized in the liver by a series of a biochemical reaction. The following are some important steps involved in the biosynthesis of bile acids.

1. Initially, cholesterol undergoes hydroxylation at C-7 position to produce 7-α-hydroxy cholesterol in the presence of *7-α-hydroxylase* (*7αH*) (Type of reaction is "hydroxylation" and position of reaction is "7-α") with the involvement of NADPH and molecular oxygen. The NADPH is reduced to $NADP^+$ and one oxygen atom of molecular oxygen is removed as a water molecule and the other one is incorporated in C-7 position of cholesterol. **This step is a rate limiting step of bile acid production and the rate-limiting enzyme *7-α-hydroxylase* (*7αH*) is inhibited by bile acids.**
2. Later, through several biochemical reactions, primary bile acids such as cholic acid and chenodeoxycholic acid are synthesized from 7-α-hydroxy cholesterol. In bile, cholic acid is found in higher concentrations than chenodeoxycholic acid.
3. Conjugated bile acids such as glycocholic acid and taurocholic acid are synthesized when cholic acid is conjugated with amino acid glycine and taurine, respectively. Similarly, glycochenodeoxycholic acid and taurochenodeoxycholic acid are synthesized when chenodeoxycholic acid is conjugated with amino acid glycine and taurine, respectively. The conjugated bile acids are used as surfactants in the body. The sodium and potassium salts of conjugated bile acids are known as bile salts that are present in the bile.
4. In the intestine, secondary bile acids such as deoxycholic acid and lithocholic acid are produced by intestinal bacteria when a portion of conjugated bile acids undergoes deconjugation and dehydroxylation.

Enterohepatic circulation: In gall bladder, the conjugated bile acids produced in liver is accumulated. From there they are secreted into the small intestine where they serve as emulsifying agents for the digestion and absorption of fats and fat-soluble vitamins. Through portal vein, primary and secondary bile salts are reabsorbed and returned to the liver in large portions. Consequently, in a day several times, the bile salts are recycled and reused. This process is known as enterohepatic circulation. Each day about 15 to 30 g of bile salts are secreted into the intestine and reabsorbed. Though, in the feces, only a small portion (0.5 g/day) is lost. In the liver, an equal quantity (0.5 g/day) of bile salts is synthesized. The only route for the removal of cholesterol from the body is the fecal excretion of bile salts.

Cholelithiasis: Cholesterol is present in bile in a soluble form due to the presence of bile salts and phospholipids. Cholesterol crystals are deposited in the gall bladder due to the deficiency of bile salts (especially) and phospholipids results in cholelithiasis or cholesterol gall stone disease. Defective absorption of bile salts from the intestine, liver function impairment, and obstruction of the biliary tract is the major reason for cholelithiasis. In general, mild and moderate cholelithiasis are treated by administering chenodiol (chenodeoxycholic acid) which slowly but gradually dissolves the gall stones. In severe cholelithiasis, the only remedy is the surgical removal of gall bladder.

Synthesis of steroid hormones from cholesterol:

Cholesterol serves as a precursor for the synthesis of steroid hormones. The following are five classes of steroid hormones that are synthesized from cholesterol in the body.

1. Glucocorticoids (**Example:** Cortisol)
2. Mineralocorticoids (**Example:** Aldosterone)
3. Progestins (**Example:** Progesterone)
4. Androgens (**Example:** Testosterone)
5. Estrogens (**Example:** Estradiol)

At first, from 27 carbons containing cholesterol, 21 carbons containing pregnenolone are synthesized. Pregnenolone is the common precursor for the synthesis of all steroid hormones. From pregnenolone, 21 carbons containing progesterone (progestin) are produced. From this progesterone-only cortisol, aldosterone, and estradiol are biosynthesized. Out of these three, cortisol and aldosterone contain 21 carbons; whereas estradiol contains only 18 carbons. For the convenience, the synthesis of hormones from cholesterol is divided into two pathways as follows, 1) Synthesis of adrenocorticoids, 2) Synthesis of steroid sex hormones.

1. **Synthesis of adrenocorticosteroids:**

   Adrenocorticosteroids or adrenocorticoids are produced by the adrenal cortex in adrenal glands. Based on their biological actions, adrenocorticoids are broadly classified into three different classes as follows.

   1. **Glucocorticoids:** Theses are 21 carbon steroids produced by zona fasciculate. They are opposite in action to insulin and affects the metabolism of glucose, amino acid, and fat. Cortisol or hydrocortisone is the most important glucocorticoid in humans. In rats, predominantly corticosterone is present.
   2. **Mineralocorticoids:** Theses are 21 carbon steroids produced by zona glomerulosa. It regulates electrolyte and water balance. The most important mineralocorticoid is aldosterone.
   3. **Androgens and estrogens:** Small quantities of androgens (19 carbon steroids) and estrogens (18 carbon steroids) are produced from the innermost adrenal cortex zona reticularis. Mostly gonads produce these hormones and it affects sexual development and functions. In the adrenal cortex, dehydroepiandrosterone is synthesized which is a precursor for the synthesis of androgens.

   The various enzymes necessary for the synthesis of adrenocorticosteroids are present in mitochondria or endoplasmic reticulum and the reaction involved are explained below.

   1. Initially, cholesterol lost 6 carbon fragments and produced pregnenolone in the presence *cytochrome* P_{450} *side chain cleavage* enzyme. Adrenocorticotropic hormone (ACTH) promotes this reaction.
   2. Later, pregnenolone undergoes hydroxylation at C-17 position to produce 17-α-hydroxy pregnenolone in presence of *17-α-hydroxylase* (Type of reaction is "hydroxylation" and position of hydroxylation is "C-17α").
   3. This formed 17-α-hydroxy pregnenolone undergoes two different reactions. In one way, it losses the side chain attached at C-17 by *lyase* enzyme followed by oxidation of alcohol group present in C-17 to ketone group results in the formation of dehydroepiandrosterone. In other way, it undergoes dehydrogenation at C-3 (secondary alcohol converted to ketone) in presence of *dehydrogenase* followed by isomerization (Position of double bond shifted from C-5 to C-4) in presence of *isomerase* produced 17-α-hydroxy progesterone.
   4. In the next step, 17-α-hydroxy progesterone also reacts in two different ways. In one way it undergoes hydroxylation at C-21 position to produce 11-deoxycortisol in presence of C_{21} *hydroxylase* (Type of reaction is "hydroxylation" and position of hydroxylation is "C-21").

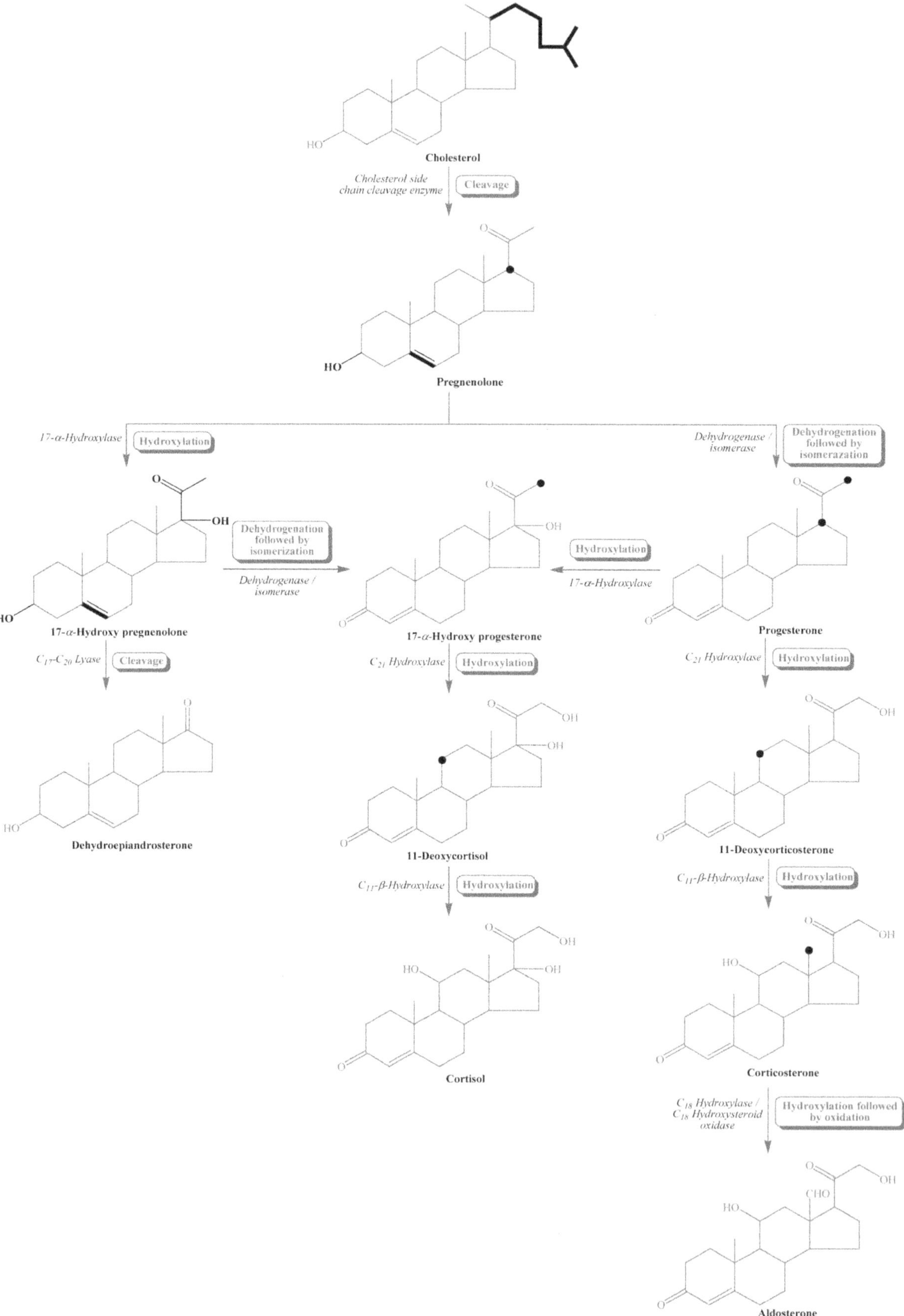
HO
Cholesterol
Cholesterol side chain cleavage enzyme
Cleavage
O
HO
Pregnenolone
17-α-Hydroxylase
Hydroxylation
Dehydrogenase / isomerase
Dehydrogenation followed by isomerazation
O
OH
HO
17-α-Hydroxy pregnenolone
Dehydrogenation followed by isomerization
Dehydrogenase / isomerase
O
OH
O
17-α-Hydroxy progesterone
Hydroxylation
17-α-Hydroxylase
O
O
Progesterone
C_{17}-C_{20} Lyase
Cleavage
C_{21} Hydroxylase
Hydroxylation
C_{21} Hydroxylase
Hydroxylation
O
HO
Dehydroepiandrosterone
O
OH
OH
O
11-Deoxycortisol
O
OH
O
11-Deoxycorticosterone
C_{11}-β-Hydroxylase
Hydroxylation
C_{11}-β-Hydroxylase
Hydroxylation
O
OH
HO
OH
O
Cortisol
O
OH
HO
O
Corticosterone
C_{18} Hydroxylase / C_{18} Hydroxysteroid oxidase
Hydroxylation followed by oxidation
O
OH
CHO
HO
O
Aldosterone

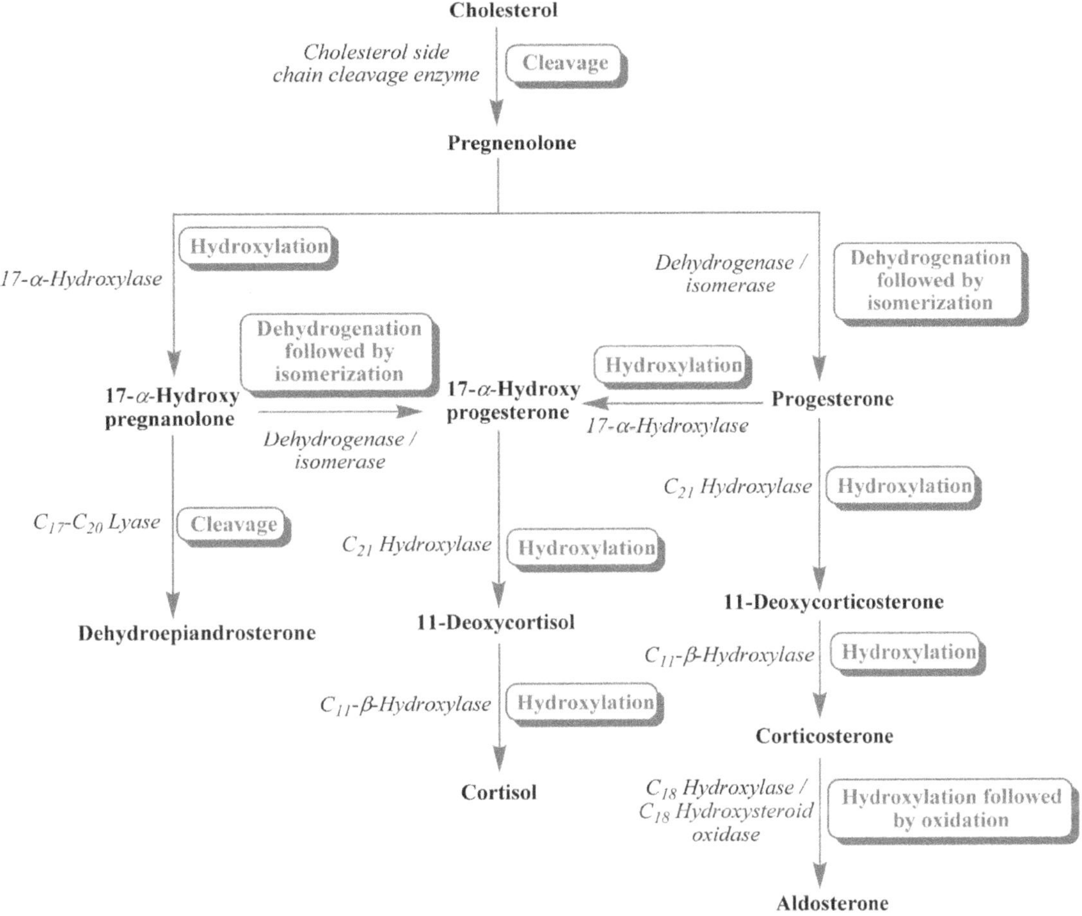

5. The formed 11-deoxycortisol undergoes hydroxylation at C-11β position to produce cortisol in presence of *C_{11}-β-hydroxylase* (Type of reaction is "hydroxylation" and position of hydroxylation is "C-11β").
6. The pregnenolone formed in the first step may undergo another reaction also. In this reaction pregnenolone undergoes dehydrogenation at C-3 (secondary alcohol converted to ketone) in presence of *dehydrogenase* followed by isomerization (Position of double bond shifted from C-5 to C-4) in presence of *isomerase* produced progesterone.
7. In the succeeding reactions, progesterone reacts in two different ways. In one way, it is hydroxylated at C-17 position by *17-α-hydroxylase* (Type of reaction is "hydroxylation" and position of hydroxylation is "C-17α") results in the formation of 17-α-hydroxy progesterone. In the second type of reaction, progesterone is hydroxylated at C-21 position by *C_{21} hydroxylase* (Type of reaction is "hydroxylation", and position of hydroxylation is "C-21") results in the formation of 11-deoxycorticosterone.
8. The formed 11-deoxycorticosterone further undergoes hydroxylation at C-11β position to produce corticosterone in presence of *C_{11}-β-hydroxylase* (Type of reaction is "hydroxylation" and position of hydroxylation is "C-11β").
9. Finally, aldosterone is synthesized from corticosterone by hydroxylation at C-18 position in presence of *C_{18} hydroxylase* (Type of reaction is "hydroxylation" and position of hydroxylation is "C-18") followed by oxidation of that C-18 primary alcohol to aldehyde in presence of *C_{18} hydroxysteroid oxidase* (Substrate is "C_{18} hydroxy steroid" and the type of reaction is "oxidation").

2. **Synthesis of steroid sex hormones:**

The steroid sex hormones are responsible for growth, development, maintenance, and regulation of the reproductive system. Three different sex hormones are present. They are,

1. **Androgens:** These are male sex hormones that are C-19 steroids and are produced mainly by Leydig cells of the testes. In both sexes, adrenal glands produce a minor quantity of androgens. In addition, small amounts are produced by ovaries also.
2. **Estrogens:** These are female sex hormones which are C-18 steroids and are synthesized by follicles and corpus luteum of the ovary. The ring A of the steroid nucleus is phenolic in nature and is devoid of the C-19 methyl group. These hormones are responsible for maintenance of the menstrual cycle and reproductive process in women.
3. **Progesterone:** These are C-21 steroids produced during the luteal phase of menstrual cycle and also during pregnancy. It is synthesized and secreted by corpus luteum and placenta. Luteinizing hormone controls the production of progesterone.

The various reactions involved in the synthesis of sex hormones are explained below.

1. 17-α-Hydroxy progesterone and dehydroepiandrosterone are produced in the same way as mentioned in the synthesis of adrenocorticoids.
2. Later, from both 17-α-hydroxy progesterone and dehydroepiandrosterone, androstenedione is produced. 17-α-Hydroxy progesterone losses the side chain attached at C-17 by C_{17} to C_{20} lyase enzyme followed by oxidation of alcohol group present in C-17 to ketone group results in formation of androstenedione. In addition, dehydroepiandrosterone undergoes dehydrogenation at C-3 (secondary alcohol converted to ketone) in presence of *dehydrogenase* followed by isomerization (Position of double bond shifted from C-5 to C-4) in presence of isomerase produced androstenedione.
3. Androstenedione undergoes two different reactions. In one reaction, it undergoes aromatization, and the ring A of steroid nucleus is aromatized to produce estrone by *aromatase* enzyme (The type of reaction is "aromatization"). In another reaction, androstenedione undergoes reduction at C-17 position in presence of *reductase* enzyme (The type of reaction is "reduction") and produced testosterone. During this reaction, the keto group present at C-17 is reduced to a secondary alcohol.
4. The estrone formed in the previous step undergoes hydroxylation at C-16α position to produce estriol in presence of 16-α-hydroxylase (The type of reaction is "hydroxylation" and position of hydroxylation is "C-16α").
5. Testosterone produced also undergoes two different reactions. At first, testosterone undergoes aromatization and the ring A of steroid nucleus is aromatized to produce 17-β-estradiol by *aromatase* enzyme (The type of reaction is "aromatization"). In another reaction, it undergoes reduction between C-4 and C-5 position in presence of *5-α-reductase* enzyme (The type of reaction is "reduction") and produced 5-α-dihydrotestosterone. During this reaction, double bond present between C-4 and C-5 is reduced.

3. **Synthesis of vitamin D:**

Vitamin D is synthesized in the body from cholesterol using ultraviolet (UV) rays present in sunlight. 7-Dehydrocholesterol is an intermediate compound present in cholesterol biosynthesis. The following are the sequence of reactions involved in the synthesis of active form of vitamin D.

1. When 7-dehydrocholesterol is exposed to UV rays present in sunlight converted to cholecalciferol or vitamin-D_3. The dietary source also contains vitamin-D as cholecalciferol only but it is inactive form. The active form of vitamin-D is biosynthesized from cholecalciferol.
2. In the next step, vitamin-D_3 undergoes hydroxylation at C-25 in the liver in presence of *calciol-25-hydroxylase* and produced 25-hydroxycholecalciferol or calcidiol.

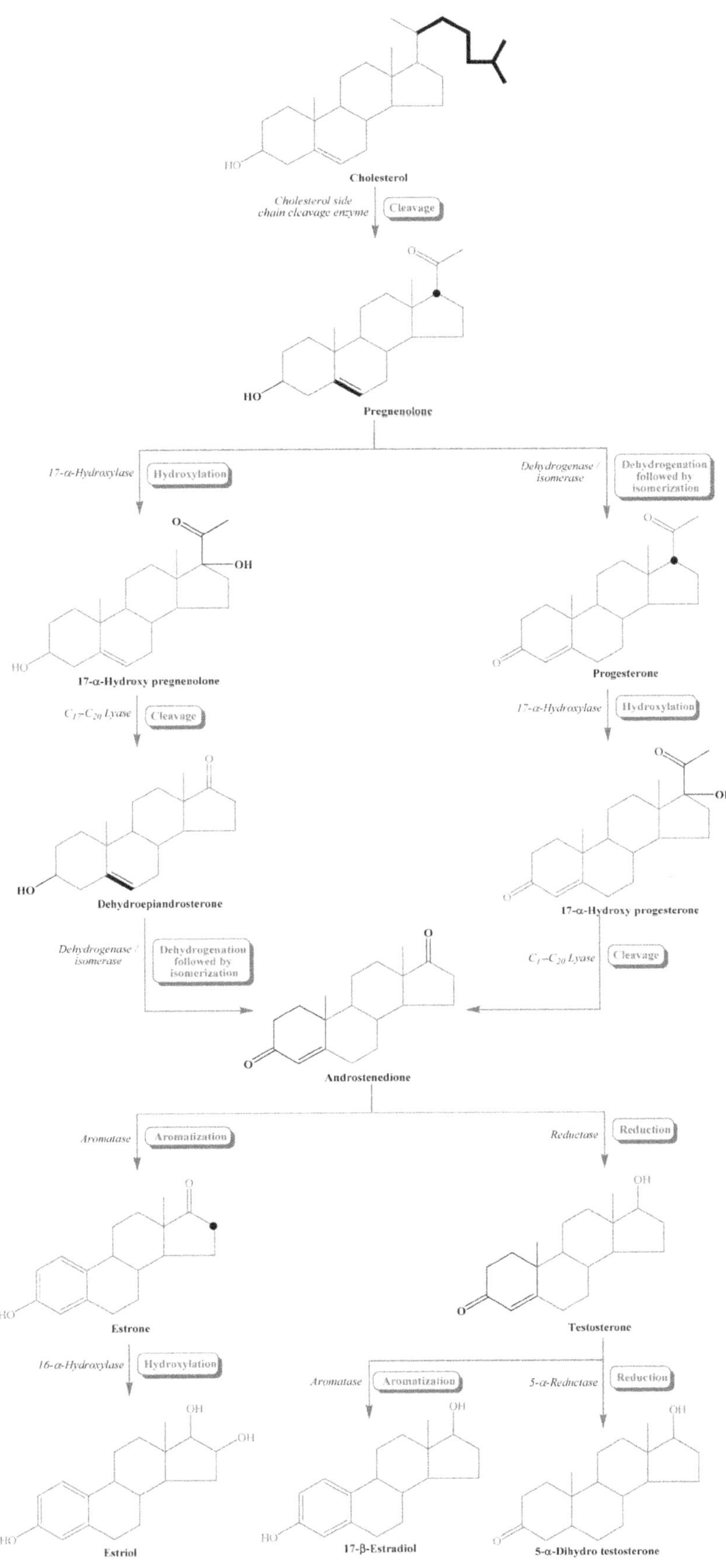

Cholesterol
Cholesterol side chain cleavage enzyme
Cleavage
Pregnenolone
17-α-Hydroxylase
Hydroxylation
Dehydrogenase / isomerase
Dehydrogenation followed by isomerization
17-α-Hydroxy pregnenolone
Progesterone
C17-C20 Lyase
Cleavage
17-α-Hydroxylase
Hydroxylation
Dehydroepiandrosterone
17-α-Hydroxy progesterone
Dehydrogenase / isomerase
Dehydrogenation followed by isomerization
C17-C20 Lyase
Cleavage
Androstenedione
Aromatase
Aromatization
Reductase
Reduction
Estrone
Testosterone
16-α-Hydroxylase
Hydroxylation
Aromatase
Aromatization
5-α-Reductase
Reduction
Estriol
17-β-Estradiol
5-α-Dihydro testosterone

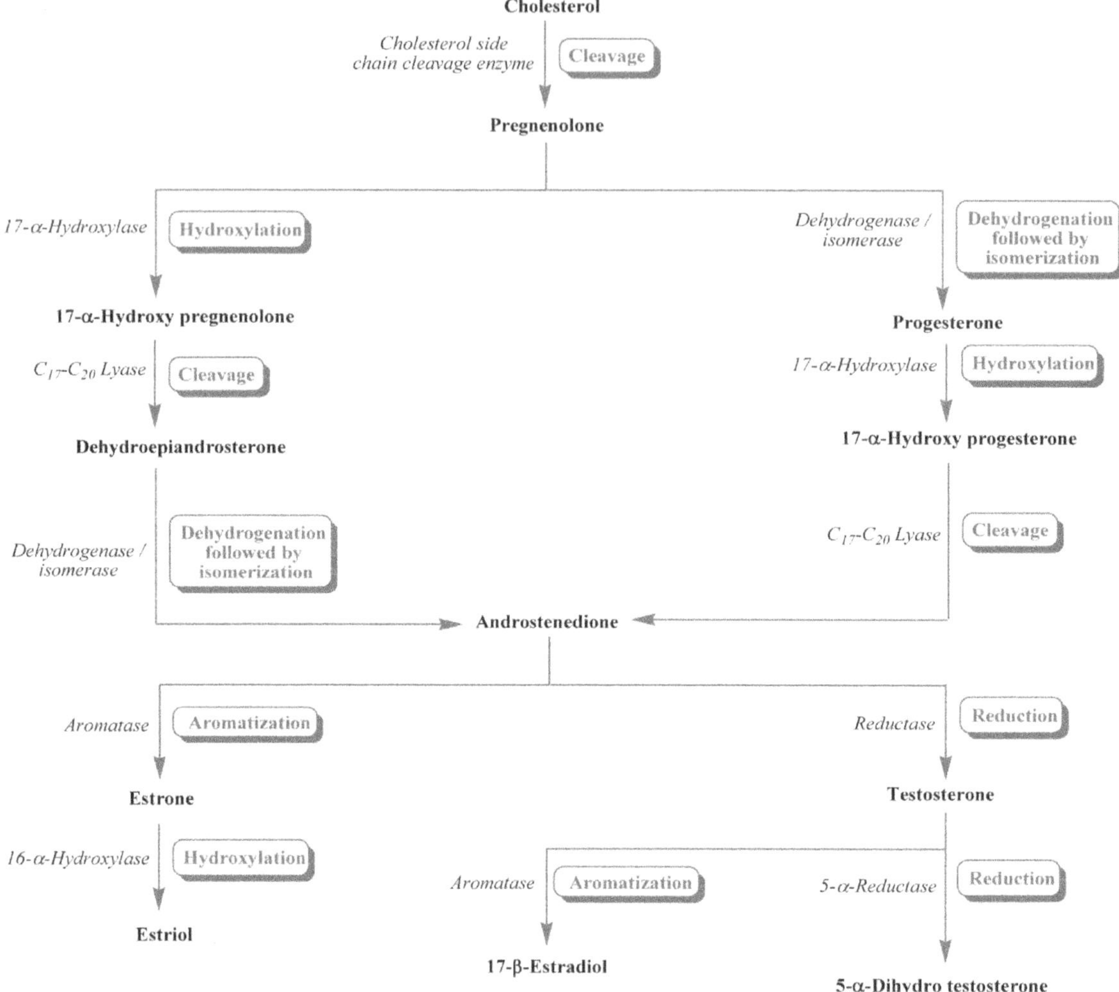

3. This formed calcidiol in kidney further undergoes hydroxylation at C-1 in presence of *calcidiol-1α-hydroxylase* produced the active form of vitamin-D i.e., 1,25-dihydroxycholecalciferol or calcitriol or 1,25-DHCC.

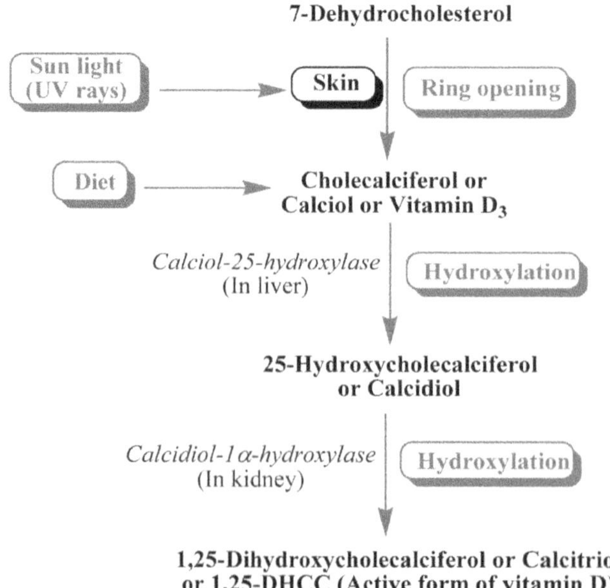

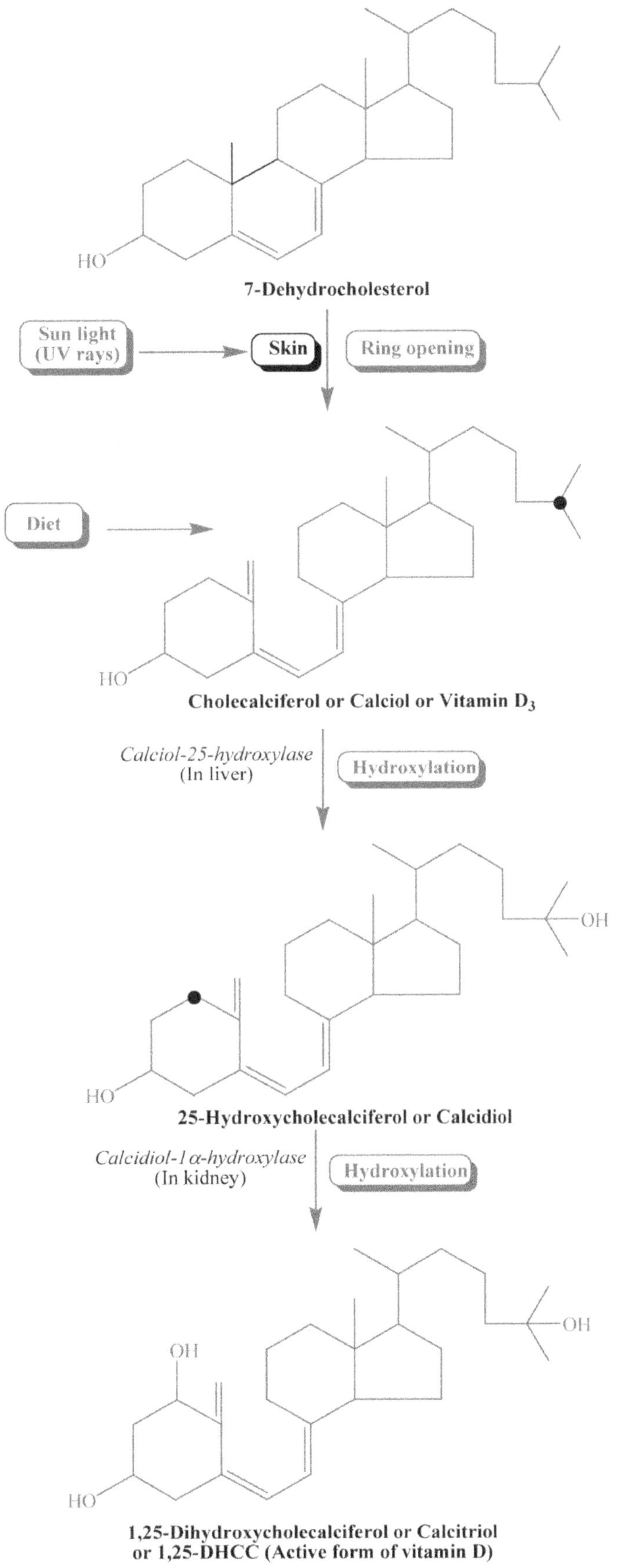

HO

7-Dehydrocholesterol

Sun light (UV rays) → Skin | Ring opening

Diet →

HO

Cholecalciferol or Calciol or Vitamin D_3

Calciol-25-hydroxylase (In liver) | Hydroxylation

OH

HO

25-Hydroxycholecalciferol or Calcidiol

Calcidiol-1α-hydroxylase (In kidney) | Hydroxylation

OH

OH

HO

1,25-Dihydroxycholecalciferol or Calcitriol or 1,25-DHCC (Active form of vitamin D)

Metabolic Disorders of Lipid Metabolism

The following are the major metabolic disorders of lipid metabolism. They are,

1. Hypercholesterolemia
2. Atherosclerosis
3. Fatty liver
4. Obesity

1. **Hypercholesterolemia:**

   Hypercholesterolemia is defined as an increased concentration of cholesterol in plasma (greater than 200 mg/dl). It is commonly observed in many disorders such as,

   (a) **Diabetes mellitus:** In diabetes mellitus, increased glucose increases the concentration of acetyl CoA leads to increased cholesterol synthesis.

   (b) **Hypothyroidism (Myxedema):** In hypothyroidism, cholesterol level is increased due to decreased HDL receptors on hepatocytes.

   (c) **Obstructive jaundice:** In obstructive jaundice, cholesterol level is increased due to obstruction in cholesterol excretion through bile.

   (d) **Nephrotic syndrome:** In nephrotic syndrome, cholesterol level is increased due to increased lipoprotein concentration in plasma. In nephrotic syndrome, plasma globulin concentration is increased.

   In general, hypercholesterolemia is associated with atherosclerosis and coronary heart disease (CHD). With respect to CHD, LDL cholesterol is positively correlated and HDL cholesterol is negatively correlated. Cholesterol is a natural metabolite performing a wide variety of functions like membrane structure, a precursor for steroid hormones, bile acid, vitamin D, etc. If cholesterol is present in high concentrations as LDL is considered bad because LDL is involved in atherosclerosis. Hence, LDL or low-density lipoprotein may regard as lethally dangerous lipoprotein or simply bad cholesterol. The most dangerous fraction of LDL is small dense low-density lipoprotein (sdLDL) because it is associated with CHD. On the other hand, HDL cholesterol is considered as good because it counteracts atherogenesis. Hence, HDL or high-density lipoprotein may regard as highly desirable lipoprotein or simply good cholesterol.

   In the development of CHD, individual lifestyle and habits influence due to its effect on serum cholesterol. Serum cholesterol level is increased by the parameters such as blood pressure, smoking, drinking of soft water against hard water, emotional stress, drinking of coffee, lack of exercise, obesity particularly abdomen, etc.

   The plasma cholesterol levels can be lowered by following the below guidelines.

   (a) **Consumption of polyunsaturated fatty acids (PUFA):** By *LCAT (Lecithin cholesterol acyltransferase)* mechanism PUFA is useful for the transport of cholesterol and its excretion from the body. PUFA is rich in cottonseed oil, soya bean oil, sunflower oil, corn oil, fish oil, etc. and it is poor in ghee and coconut oil.

   (b) **Dietary cholesterol:** The influence of dietary cholesterol on plasma cholesterol is minimal. Even though it is advised to avoid cholesterol-rich foods and the advisable dietary cholesterol level is < 300 mg/day, drugs like ezetimide inhibit the absorption of cholesterol in the intestine.

   (c) **Plant sterol:** Some plant sterol and their esters reduce plasma cholesterol by inhibiting cholesterol absorption in the intestine.

   (d) **Dietary fiber:** Similar to plant sterol, dietary fibers also reduce plasma cholesterol by inhibiting cholesterol absorption from the intestine.

   (e) **Avoiding a high carbohydrate diet:** It is better to avoid diets rich in carbohydrates to control hypercholesterolemia.

   (f) **Impact of life styles:** Adequate changes in lifestyle may decrease plasma cholesterol because increased serum cholesterol level is seen in people with blood pressure, smoking, drinking of soft water against hard water, emotional stress, drinking of coffee, lack of exercise, obesity particularly abdomen, etc.

(g) **Moderate alcohol consumption:** Besides low alcohol content, red wine is beneficial due to its antioxidant properties. The ill-effects of chronic alcoholism mask the beneficial effect of consuming moderate alcohol.

(h) **Use of drugs:** Statins decrease plasma cholesterol by inhibiting the synthesis of cholesterol through *HMG CoA reductase* (*HMGCAR*) inhibition. Drugs like cholestyramine and colestipol bind with bile acids and decrease their intestinal absorption. Hence, more cholesterol is converted to bile acids and excreted through feces. The activity of lipoprotein *lipase* is increased and plasma cholesterol and triacylglycerol level are decreased by clofibrate.

2. **Atherosclerosis:**

In Greek, "athere" means "mush" and atherosclerosis is a complex cardiac disorder defined as hardening or thickening of inner arterial walls due to accumulation of lipids (particularly cholesterol in a free and esterified form), collagen, fibrous tissues, proteoglycans, calcium deposits, etc. Atherosclerosis is a progressive disorder, hence, it may lead to narrowing of blocks and at one stage it completely blocks the arteries. Death of affected tissue due to the stoppage of blood flow is termed as infarction. If the infarction is taking place in coronary arteries (supplying blood to the heart) it is known as myocardial infarction and it is the most common one.

The risk of CHD and the development of atherosclerosis are directly correlated with plasma LDL and cholesterol. Conversely, HDL is inversely correlated with CHD. Diseases like diabetes mellitus, hyperlipoproteinemia, hypothyroidism, nephrotic syndrome, etc., are generally associated with atherosclerosis. The various probable causes of atherosclerosis are obesity, high consumption of saturated fat, excessive smoking, lack of physical exercise, hypertension, stress, etc.

In general, increased plasma HDL i.e., good cholesterol is correlated with a low incidence of cardiovascular disorders. Compared to men, women are less prone to heart disease because they have higher HDL. Estrogen present in women is responsible for higher HDL. The risk of CHD is reduced by increasing the concentration of HDL in the following ways like doing strenuous physical exercise, consuming moderate alcohol, consumption of PUFA, reducing body weight, etc.

LDL and lipoprotein-a (Lp-a) are identical in structure. Additional apoprotein-a (Apo-a) is present in lipoprotein-a (Lp-a) compared to LDL. Fibrinolysis is inhibited by lipoprotein-a (Lp-a). CHD risk is increased when the plasma lipoprotein-a (Lp-a) is elevated to more than 30 mg/dl. It is assumed that interfering with the plasminogen activation reduces the breakdown of blood clots when lipoprotein-a (Lp-a) is elevated. This leads to intravascular thrombosis and an increased risk of heart attacks. Compared to western people, Indians have higher levels of lipoprotein-a (Lp-a).

In general, the oxidation of LDL is decreased by antioxidants. Some evidences suggest that taking antioxidants such as vitamin-C, vitamin-E or β-carotene decreases the risk of atherosclerosis and CHD.

3. **Fatty liver:**

About 5 % of lipid (mostly phospholipid) is present in the liver normally. Unlike adipose tissue, the liver is not a storage organ for fat. But in some conditions lipids particularly triglycerides are excessively accumulated in the liver leading to the fatty liver [deposition of lipids in liver]. Generally, lipids are present in the form of droplets in Kupffer cells. But in fatty liver droplets of triacylglycerols are present throughout the entire cytoplasm of the hepatic cell. Hence, fatty liver may lead to impairment in metabolic functions of the liver. Fatty liver is usually associated with fibrotic changes and cirrhosis. The two major causes of fatty liver are 1) Increased synthesis of triacylglycerols, 2) Impairment in lipoprotein synthesis.

Increased synthesis of triacylglycerols: Mobilization of free fatty acids from adipose tissue and their influx into the liver is much higher than their utilization. Hence, triacylglycerides are overproduced and accumulated in the liver. Free fatty acid mobilizations are increased in clinical conditions such as diabetes mellitus, starvation, alcoholism, and a high-fat diet which often causes fatty liver. Fat synthesis and its deposition are promoted by inhibiting fatty acid oxidation by alcohol.

Impairment in lipoprotein synthesis: Phospholipids and apoprotein-B are required for the production of VLDL in the liver. The reasons for fatty liver caused by impaired lipoprotein synthesis are,

(a) A defect in phospholipid synthesis.

(b) A block in apoprotein formation.

(c) A failure in the formation or secretion of lipoprotein.

Usually, a defect in phospholipid synthesis is associated with dietary deficiency of lipotropic factors such as choline, betaine, inositol, etc. Production of phospholipid is decreased due to essential fatty acids deficiency. In addition, phospholipid synthesis is impaired by competition of excessive cholesterol consumption with essential fatty acids.

Fatty liver can also be caused by some chemicals such as puromycin, chloroform, lead, phosphorous, etc. These chemicals inhibit the synthesis of protein due to the blockade in the synthesis of apoprotein-B required for VLDL production. ATP is required for the synthesis and secretion of lipoprotein. Sometimes, in pyridoxine and pantothenic acid deficiency lipoprotein formation is impaired due to decreased availability of ATP. Ethionine reduces the availability of ATP, thereby, it takes part in the development of the fatty liver. Available adenosine (as adenosylethionine) is trapped when ethionine competes with methionine leads to decreased ATP levels. The deficiency of vitamin-E is associated with fatty liver. In such a condition, selenium acts as a protective agent. Hormones like adrenocorticotropic hormone (ACTH), insulin, thyroid hormones, adrenocorticoids promote the deposition of fat in the liver. Factors responsible for the development of fatty liver is summarized in Figure 4.8.

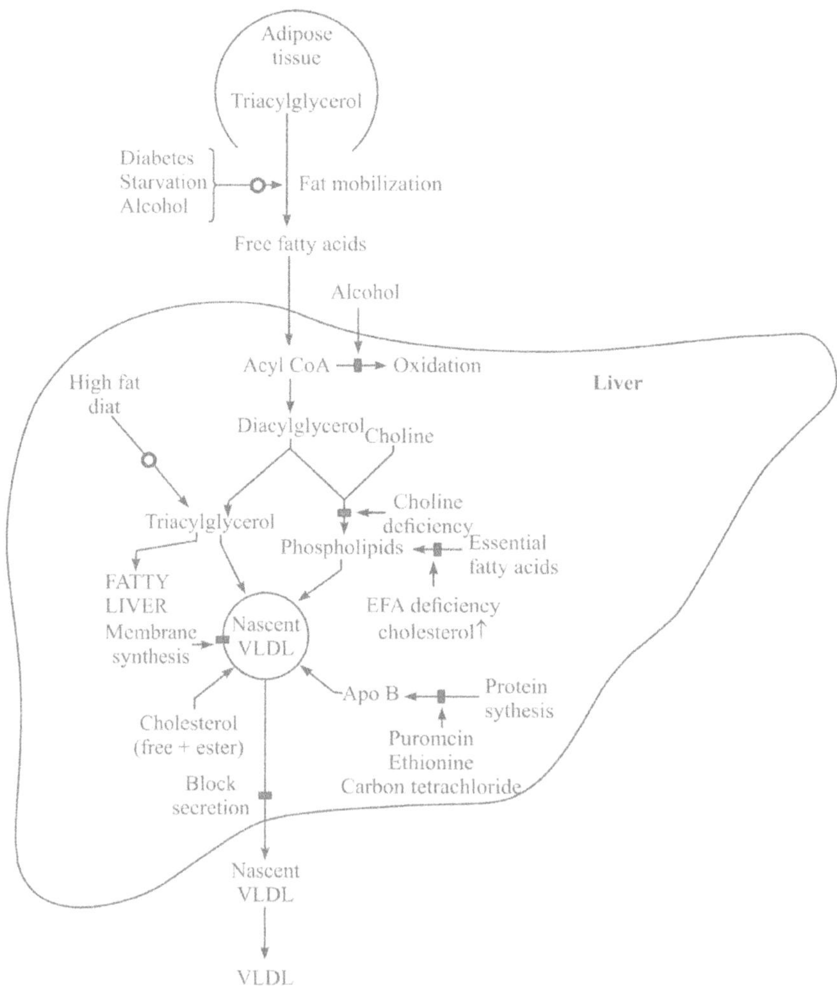

Figure 4.8 Factors responsible for the development of fatty liver.

4. **Obesity:**

Due to excessive fat deposition, an abnormal increase in body weight is known as obesity. When the weight of adipose tissue fat exceeds 20 % and 25 % of total body weight then the men and women are considered obese, respectively. Basically, obesity is a disorder of excess calorie intake or simply overeating. 1 g fat will deposit in the body and increases body weight for every 7 calories of excess intake. Obesity contributors are overeating coupled with a lack of physical exercise. Sometimes, a virus infection may be the reason for obesity. 15 % of people weighing more than 120 kg had antibodies to *adenovirus-36* in their blood. It implies that the virus infection by an unknown mechanism contributes to obesity. Surprisingly, serum cholesterol and other lipid parameters are normal in *adenovirus-36* infected peoples.

Body mass index (BMI): Body mass index (BMI) is generally used to represent clinical obesity. The following formula is used to estimate body mass index (BMI).

$$BMI\left(\frac{kg}{m^2}\right)=\frac{\text{Weight (in kg)}}{\text{Height (in m}^2\text{)}}$$

The healthy reference range for BMI is usually between 18.5 and 24.8 kg/m^2. Based on the body mass index (BMI), obesity is broadly classified into three different classes as follows.

(a) **Overweight or Grade – I obesity:** In this class, BMI is between 25 to 30 kg/m^2.

(b) **Clinical obesity or Grade – II obesity:** In this class, BMI is > 30 kg/m^2.

(c) **Morbid obesity or Grade – III obesity:** In this class, BMI is > 40 kg/m^2.

Generally, obesity is associated with many health issues like CHD, type – II diabetes mellitus, stroke, hypertension, arthritis, and gall bladder disease. The ratio between waist and hip sizes is more efficient than BMI for representing obesity. Hence, recently waist to hip ratio is used to represent the risk of heart disease. For men, the normal waist to hip ratio is < 0.9 and for women, it is < 0.85. If the waist to hip ratio is less then, the risk for health complications is less and leads to better health.

Obesity has genetic basis and there is a 75 % chance of being obese if a child born to two obese people. ob gene expressed in adipocytes (of white adipose tissue) producing a protein called leptin (16000 daltons molecular weight) is associated with obesity. Leptin is considered as a body weight regulatory hormone. It functions as a lipostat by binding with specific receptors in the brain. Leptin levels are high when the fat stores in adipose tissues are adequate. This leads to a restriction of feeding behavior and limits fat deposition. Also, lipolysis is stimulated and lipogenesis is inhibited by leptin. Any genetic defect in leptin or its receptor will lead to extreme overeating and obesity. In this case, the people can be treated by leptin to reverse obesity. Leptin levels fall during starvation which promotes feeding and fat production and its deposition.

Both the size and number of adipocytes (adipose tissues) are increased in obesity. Adipose tissues are two types namely white adipose tissue and brown adipose tissue. White adipose tissue is metabolically less active but stored fats is more; whereas, brown adipose tissue is metabolically very active but stored fats is less. The reason for high activity of brown adipose tissue is attributed to their high mitochondria and cytochrome proportion and low activity of *ATP synthase*. It is responsible for the diet induced thermogenesis and it is an active center for the oxidation of fat and glucose. The unique feature of brown adipose tissue mitochondria is that the oxidation and phosphorylation are not coupled. More heat and less ATP are produced in mitochondrial oxidation. In the inner membrane of these mitochondria, a specific protein known as thermogenin has been isolated. This thermogenin acts like an uncoupler and dissipiates the energy in the form of heat and blocks the formation of ATP. Mostly, brown adipose tissue is found in hibernating animals, and the animals exposed to cold, besides the newborn. In human adults it is located in the thoracic region though not a permanent tissue. In obese peoples this brown adipose tissue is almost absent. Fortunately, some people have active brown adipose tissue. They do not become obese due to eat and liberate it as heat.

Olestra and orlistat are the synthetic lipids used recently for the treatment of obesity. They are not digested, excreted unchangingly and taste like natural lipids.

Biosynthesis of Triglycerides or Triacylglycerols (TG)

Triacylglycerol is the most abundant lipid comprising about 85 to 90 % of body lipids. Mostly in liver and adipose tissue only triacylglycerols biosynthesis takes place and to a lesser extent it also takes place in other tissues also. Activation of fatty acid and glycerol is the primary request for the synthesis of triacylglycerol. The active form of fatty acid is acyl CoA and the active form of glycerol is glycerol-3-phosphate (GL3P).

Activation of fatty acid:

The active form of fatty acids is known as acyl CoA. In this stage, fatty acids are converted into acyl CoA in cytosol by the enzyme called "*acyl CoA synthetase* (*ACS*) or *thiokinase* (*TK*)". It involves two steps.

1. In the first step, fatty acid reacts with ATP in the presence of *acyl CoA synthetase* (*ACS*) or *thiokinase* (*TK*) *that* produces acyladenylate with the liberation of pyrophosphate (PPi). The total reaction is made irreversible by an immediate elimination of pyrophosphate into inorganic phosphate (Pi) through hydrolysis in the presence of *pyrophosphatase* (Substrate is "pyrophosphate" and the type of reaction is "hydrolysis").
2. In the next step, acyladenylate reacts with co-enzyme A to produce acyl CoA and AMP. This step is also catalyzed by the same enzyme involved in first step i.e., *acyl CoA synthetase* (*ACS*) (The product formed is "acyl CoA" and the type of reaction is "synthetic") or *thiokinase* (*TK*) (In ATP / GTP involved reactions, the enzymes acted are "*kinase*" and "sulphur" atom of co-enzyme A is also involved in reaction). *Kinase* enzyme needs magnesium ion as co-factors for its activity. In this step, one ATP is converted into AMP **(2 ATP is utilized)** because 1 ATP for conversion of ATP to ADP and other one is for ADP conversion into AMP.

$$R-CH_2-CH_2-\overset{O}{\overset{\|}{C}}-\mathbf{OH}$$

Fatty acid
(Inactive form)

Acyl CoA synthetase or *Thiokinase*

ATP → PPi (- 2) **Esterification or Transfer of AMP**

PPi → 2 Pi (*Pyrophosphatase*, H_2O)

$$R-CH_2-CH_2-\overset{O}{\overset{\|}{C}}-\mathbf{AMP}$$

Acyladenylate

Acyl CoA synthetase or *Thiokinase*

CoASH → AMP **Substitution**

$$R-CH_2-CH_2-\overset{O}{\overset{\|}{C}}-SCoA$$

Acyl CoA
(Active form of fatty acid)

Activation of glycerol:

Glycerol can be activated to its active form glycerol-3-phosphate in two different mechanisms.

1. **Mechanism-1:** In the liver, glycerol is reacted with ATP and produces glycerol-3-phosphate by phosphorylation reaction. The reaction is catalyzed by *glycerol kinase* (GLK) enzyme (In ATP / GTP involved reactions, the enzymes acted are "*kinase*" and the substrate is "glycerol"). *Kinase* enzyme needs magnesium ion as co-factors for its activity. In this reaction one ATP is converted into ADP **(1 ATP is utilized).**
2. **Mechanism-2:** In both liver and adipose tissue, the source of glycerol-3-phosphate (GL3P) is glucose. In glycolysis, dihydroxy acetone phosphate (DHAP) is produced from glucose. This formed dihydroxy acetone phosphate (DHAP) is reduced by reacting with NADH in presence of *glycerol-3-phosphate dehydrogenase* (*GL3PD*) (In NAD^+ / $NADP^+$ involved reactions, the enzymes acted are "*dehydrogenase*" and the product is "glycerol-3-phosphate (GL3P)") to produce glycerol-3-phosphate (GL3P) with liberation of NAD^+. In this reaction one NADH is reduced to NAD^+ (One NADH is equal to 3 ATP. Hence, **3 ATP is utilized).**

Addition of acyl groups for the formation of triacylglycerol:

The various reactions involved in the formation of triacylglycerol (TAG) are as follows.

1. Glycerol-3-phosphate (GL3P) is reacted with acyl CoA in presence of *glycerol-3-phosphate acyl transferase* (*GL3PAT*) (Substrate is "glycerol-3-phosphate (GL3P)" and the type of reaction is "acyl group transfer") and produced lysophosphatidic acid with liberation of co-enzyme A by acylation reaction.
2. In the similar manner, dihydroxy acetone phosphate (DHAP) is also reacted with acyl CoA and produced 1-acyl dihydroxyacetone phosphate (1ADHAP) in presence of *dihydroxy acetone phosphate acyl transferase* (*DHAPAT*) (Substrate is "dihydroxy acetone phosphate (DHAP)"and the type of reaction is "acyl group transfer").
3. Later, by reduction 1-acyl dihydroxyacetone phosphate (1ADHAP) is converted into lysophosphatidic acid (LPA) with involvement of NADPH. The reaction is catalyzed by *1-acyl dihydroxyacetone phosphate reductase* (*1ADHAPR*) (Substrate is "1-acyl dihydroxyacetone phosphate (1ADHAP)" and the type of reaction is "reduction"). In this reaction, one NADPH is reduced to $NADP^+$.
4. In the next step, lysophosphatidic acid (LPA) formed is further undergoes acylation by reacting with acyl CoA in presence of *lysophosphatidic acidacyl transferase* (*LPAAT*) (Substrate is "lysophosphatidic acid (LPA)" and the type of reaction is "acyl group transfer") and produced phosphatidic acid (PA) with liberation of co-enzyme A. Phosphatidic acid (PA) is chemically 1,2-diacylglycerol phosphate (1,2DAGLP).
5. Phosphatidic acid (PA) undergoes hydrolysis by reacting with one mole of water molecule and produces 1,2-diacylglycerol (1,2DAGL) with liberation of inorganic phosphate (Pi). The reaction is catalyzed by *phosphatase* enzyme (Substrate is "phosphatidic acid (PA) and the type of reaction is "hydrolysis"). The phosphatidic acid (PA) and the formed 1,2-diacylglycerol (1,2DAGL) are also utilized for the biosynthesis of phospholipids.
6. Finally, 1,2-diacylglycerol (1,2DAGL) is reacted with another molecule of acyl CoA in presence of *diacylglycerol acyl transferase* (*DAGLAT*) (Substrate is "diacylglycerol (DAGL)" and the type of reaction is "acyl group transfer") and produced triacylglycerol (TAG) with liberation of co-enzyme A by simple acylation reaction.

In general, the three fatty acids found in triacylglycerol are not of the same type. On C-1 saturated fatty acid is present, on C-2 unsaturated fatty acid is present and on C-3 either saturated or unsaturated fatty acid is present.

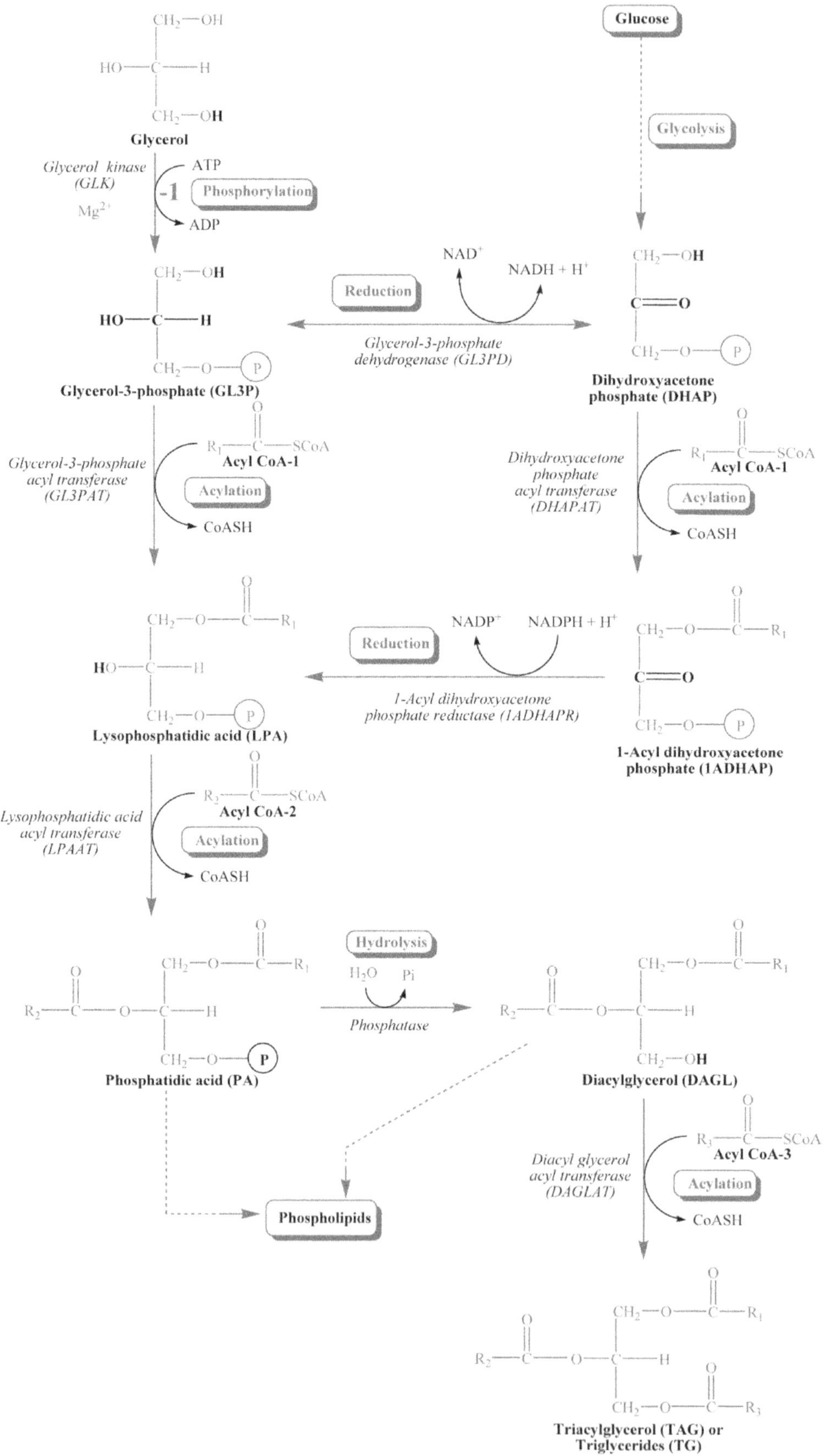

Glucose
Glycolysis
Glycerol
Glycerol kinase (GLK)
Mg^{2+}
ATP
ADP
Phosphorylation
NAD⁺
NADH + H⁺
Reduction
Glycerol-3-phosphate dehydrogenase (GL3PD)
Glycerol-3-phosphate (GL3P)
Dihydroxyacetone phosphate (DHAP)
Glycerol-3-phosphate acyl transferase (GL3PAT)
Acyl CoA-1
Acylation
CoASH
Dihydroxyacetone phosphate acyl transferase (DHAPAT)
NADP⁺
NADPH + H⁺
1-Acyl dihydroxyacetone phosphate reductase (1ADHAPR)
Lysophosphatidic acid (LPA)
1-Acyl dihydroxyacetone phosphate (1ADHAP)
Lysophosphatidic acid acyl transferase (LPAAT)
Acyl CoA-2
Hydrolysis
H_2O
Pi
Phosphatase
Phosphatidic acid (PA)
Diacylglycerol (DAGL)
Phospholipids
Diacyl glycerol acyl transferase (DAGLAT)
Acyl CoA-3
Triacylglycerol (TAG) or Triglycerides (TG)

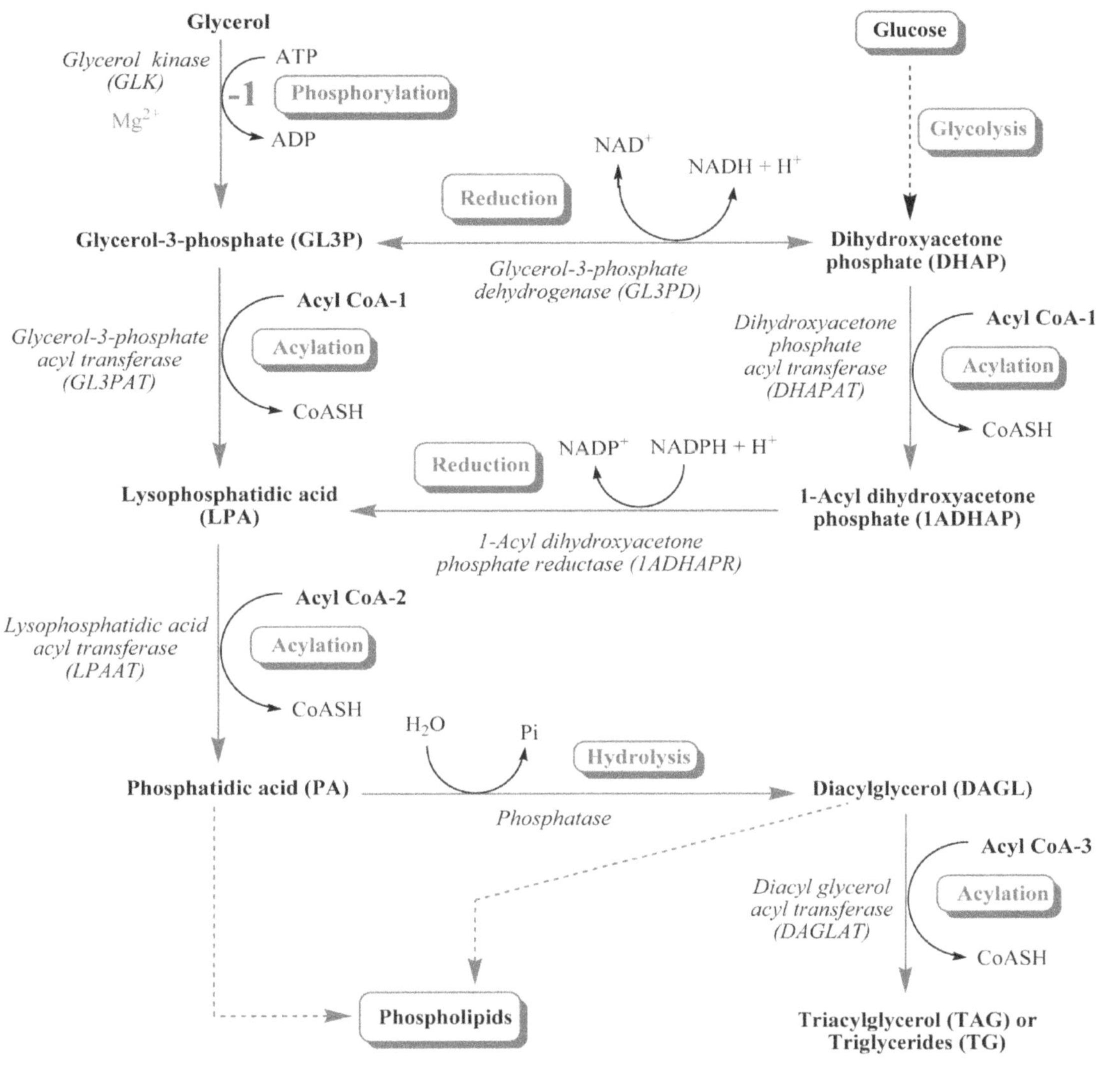

Biosynthesis of Phospholipids

Phospholipids are a special group of lipids and perform the following several important functions.

1. Membrane structure and function.
2. Play a role in blood clotting.
3. In synthesis of prostaglandin (PG), phospholipids supply arachidonic acid.

In smooth endoplasmic reticulum, phospholipids are biosynthesized from phosphatidic acid (PA), 1,2-diacylglycerol (1,2DAG) and intermediates in the synthesis of triacylglycerol (TAG).

The various important phospholipids are lecithin, cephalin, phosphatidylserine, phosphatidylinositol, phosphatidylglycerol, cardiolipin, plasmalogens and sphingomyelins. The various phospholipids are synthesized as follows.

1. **Synthesis of lecithin, cephalin:** Lecithin is chemically phosphatidylcholine and cephalin is chemically phosphatidylethanolamine. Initially, choline and ethanolamine are phosphorylated by reacting with ATP and produce phosphocholine and phosphoethanolamine, respectively with liberation of ADP. Later, phosphocholine and phosphoethanolamine are combined with CTP to produce CDP-choline and CDP-ethanolamine, respectively with removal of pyrophosphate (PPi). Finally, lecithin and cephalin is synthesized from CDP-choline and CDP-ethanolamine, respectively by condensing with

1,2-diacylglycerol (1,2DAG). Lecithin can be synthesized from cephalin by methylation reaction. Generally, from the pre-existing phospholipids only choline and ethanolamine are derived. Hence, the synthesis of phospholipids starting from choline and ethanolamine is regarded as a salvage pathway.

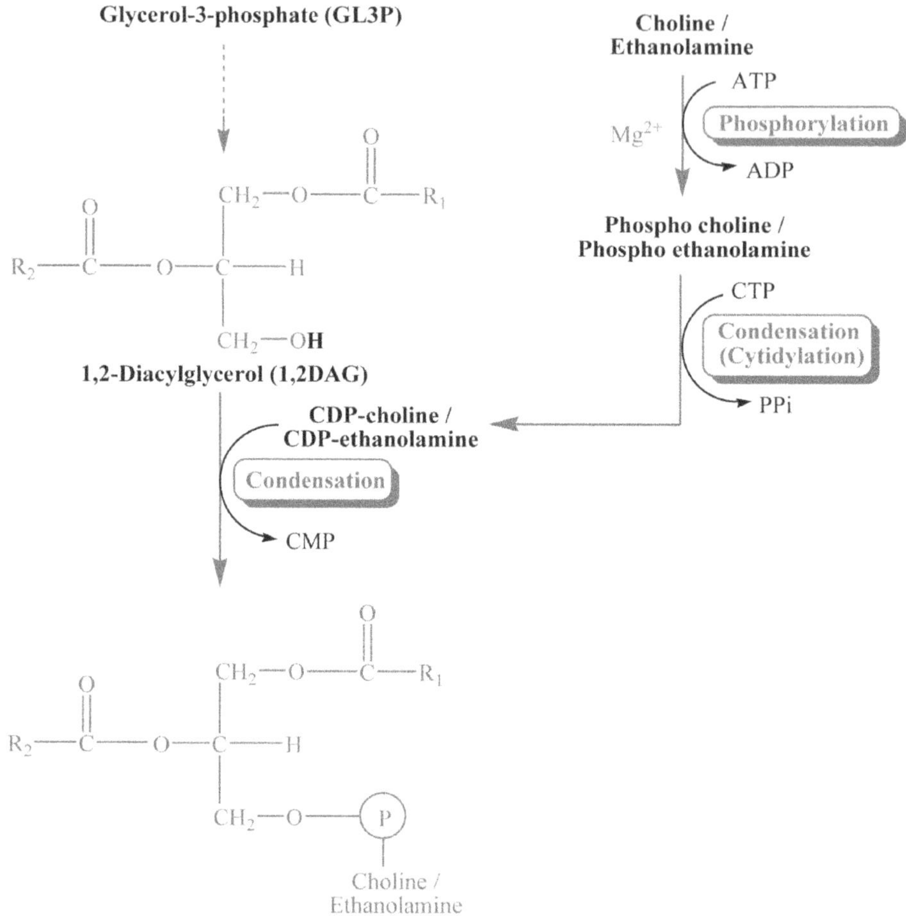

2. **Synthesis of phosphatidylserine:** When phosphatidylethanolamine (cephalin) is reacted with free serine, ethanolamine is replaced by serine resulting in formation of phosphatidylserine. On the other hand, from phosphatidylserine, phosphatidylethanolamine (cephalin) is produced by decarboxylation reaction.

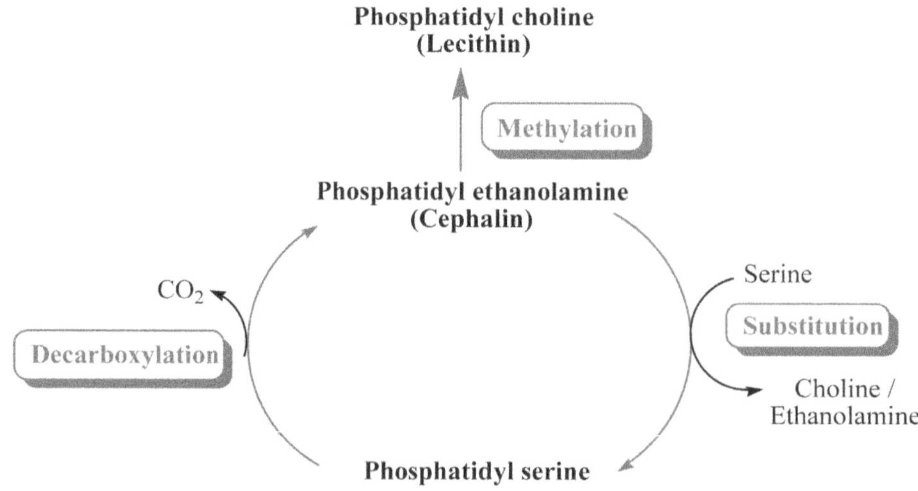

3. **Synthesis of phosphatidylinositol:** Initially, phosphatidic acid (PA) is condensed with CTP to produce CDP-diacylglycerol with pyrophosphate (PPi). Later, inositol condensed with above synthesized CDP-diacylglycerol results in formation of phosphatidylinositol with CMP. On C-2 of glycerol, arachidonic acid is present in phosphatidylinositol; hence, it serves as a substrate for the synthesis of prostaglandin (PG). In addition, phosphatidylinositol is also important for signal transmission across membranes.

Glycerol-3-phosphate (GL3P) or Dihydroxyacetone phosphate (DHAP) → **Phosphatidic acid (PA)**

CTP → Condensation (Cytidylation) → PPi

CDP-diacylglycerol (Cytidine)

Condensation: Inositol → CMP

Phosphatidyl inositol

4. **Synthesis of phosphatidylglycerol and cardiolipin:** The CDP-diacylglycerol formed above is reacted with glycerol-3-phosphate (GL3P) to produce phosphatidylglycerol-3-phosphate and CMP. Later, by hydrolysis phosphatidylglycerol-3-phosphate loses inorganic phosphate (Pi) and produces phosphatidylglycerol. Finally, cadiolipin is obtained when phosphatidylglycerol is reacted with another mole of phosphatidylglycerol with liberation of one glycerol. Chemically, cadiolipin is diphosphatidylglycerol and it is the only phospholipid possessing antigenic properties.

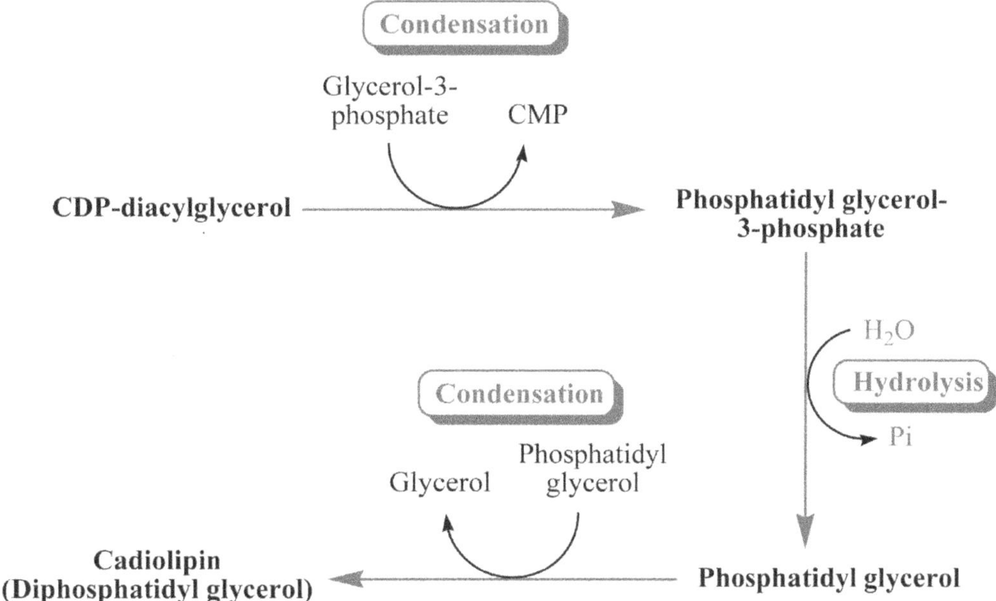

5. **Synthesis of plasmalogens:** Plasmalogens are the phospholipid contains ether linkage instead of ester linkage in C-1 of glycerol. 1-Alkenyl-2-acetylglycerol is the important plasmalogen causes blood platelet aggregation. Hence, it is referred to as platelet activating factor (PAF).

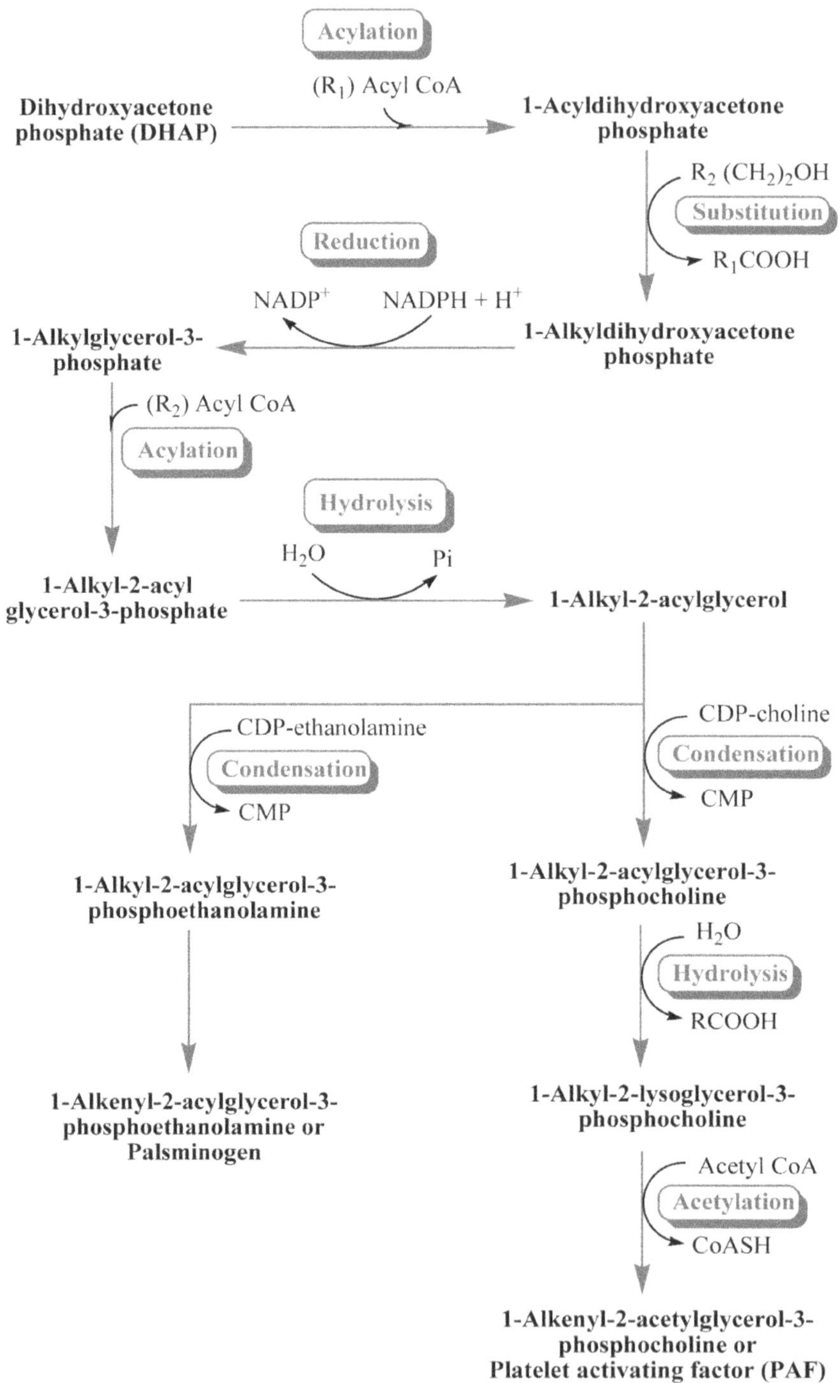

6. **Synthesis of sphingomyelins:** Sphingosine is a complex amino alcohol present in sphingomyelin instead of glycerol. Sphingosine is produced by a sequence of reactions from serine and palmityl CoA. Later, sphingosine undergoes acetylation by reacting with acetyl CoA and produced ceramide with co-enzyme A. Finally, sphingomyelin is obtained from ceramide by condensing with CDP-choline with liberation of CMP.

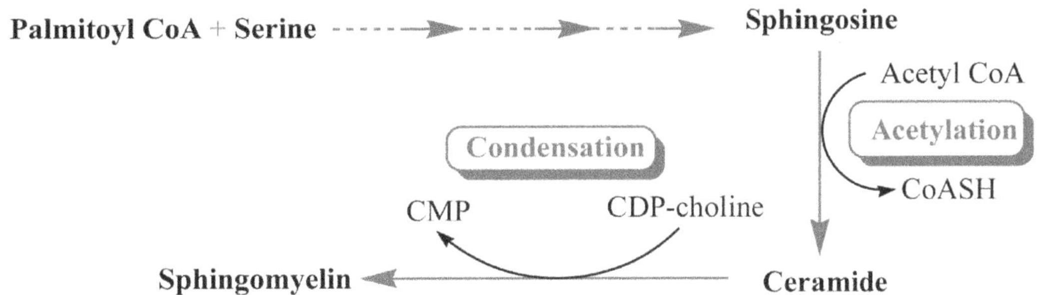

Hormonal Regulation in Lipid Metabolism

Triacylglycerol lipase or simply *TG-lipase* (Substrate is "triacylglycerol (TAG)" which is a "lipid" and type of reaction is "hydrolysis") is an enzyme responsible for lipolysis (hydrolysis) of triacylglycerol (TAG) to diacylglycerol (DAG), monoacylglycerol (MAG) and fatty acid. This enzyme is mostly controlled by hormones; hence it is named as *hormone sensitiveTG-lipase*. The phosphorylated form of *hormone sensitiveTG-lipase* is active form and the dephosphorylated form of *hormone sensitiveTG-lipase* is inactive form. The inactive form i.e., *hormone sensitiveTG-lipase-b* is phosphorylated and converted to its active form i.e., *hormone sensitiveTG-lipase-a* by cAMP dependent *protein kinase*. cAMP is obtained from ATP by an enzyme called *adenylate cyclase*(Substrate is "ATP" which is adenylate derivative and the type of reaction is "cyclization". Many enzymes such as epinephrine, nor-epinephrine, glucagon, glucocorticoids, thyroxine, growth hormones (GH), thyroid stimulating hormone (TSH) and adrenocorticotropic hormone (ACTH) stimulates the activity of *adenylate cyclase* leads to increased lipolysis. On the other hand, compounds like insulin, niacin and prostaglandin-E_1 (PG-E_1) inhibits the activity of *adenylate cyclase* leads to decreased cAMP levels and thereby inactivates *hormone sensitiveTG-lipase*. Insulin on the other side also increases cAMP levels by promoting the activity of *phosphodiesterase* which is responsible for degradation of cAMP to 5′-AMP. Caffeine increases cAMP levels by inhibiting *phosphodiesterase* activity leads to increased lipolysis.

Glycerol kinase (*GLK*) is not present in adipose tissue. Hence, glycerol produced by lipolysis is not phosphorylated in adipose tissue. Instead of that glycerol is transported to the liver where it is converted to its active form i.e., glycerol-3-phosphate (GL3P). This active form of glycerol is used for the synthesis of triacylglycerols and phospholipids. In addition, it also enters in glycolysis and is converted into dihydroxy acetone phosphate (DHAP).

In adipose tissue, the liberated fatty acids are entered in circulation and in bound form to albumin they are transported to various tissues. These entered fatty acids in various tissues are utilized for the energy. From the oxidation of fatty acids only about 95 % of total fat energy is obtained. Even though tissues such as the brain and erythrocytes cannot oxidize fatty acids for its energy demand.

During starvation, to provide energy to skeletal muscle and cardiac muscle triacylglycerols (TAG) stored in adipose tissue are hydrolyzed to produce free fatty acids for oxidation. Even though, a major quantity (about 65 %) of free fatty acids are re-esterified to triacylglycerol (TAG) and sent back to adipose tissue for deposition. This process of lipolysis of triacylglycerol (TAG) and re-esterification of free fatty acid to triacylglycerol (TAG) is known as triacylglycerol / free fatty acid cycle. Regulation of lipid metabolism by hormone is summarized in Figure 4.9.

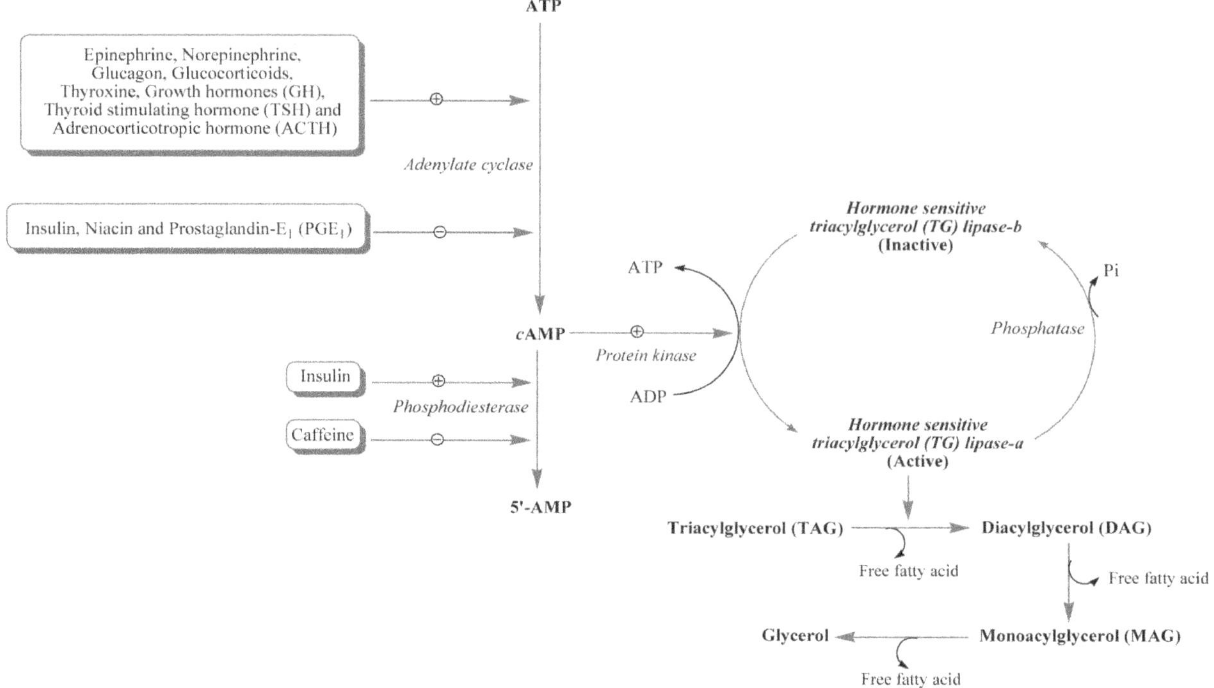

Figure 4.9 Regulation of lipid metabolism by hormone.

PROBABLE QUESTIONS

PART – A: Multiple Choice Questions

1. Esters of fatty acids with alcohols other than glycerol are commonly known by which of the following name? P) Fats Q) Oils R) Waxes S) Phospholipids. Choose the correct option.
   (a) P & Q (b) R & S
   (c) P only (d) R only
2. Which of the following fatty acids are hydroxy fatty acids? P) β-Hydroxy butyric acid Q) Cerebronic acid R) Recinoleic acid S) Linolenic acid. Choose the correct option.
   (a) Both P, Q & R (b) Both Q, R & S
   (c) Both R, S & P (d) Both S, P & Q
3. Which of the following are glycolipids? P) Lecithin Q) Cephalin R) Cerebrosides S) Gangliosides. Choose the correct option.
   (a) Both P & Q (b) Both R & S
   (c) Both Q & R only (d) Both P & S
4. Spingomyelin is comes under which of the following class of complex lipid? P) Phospholipid Q) Glycolipid R) Lipoprotein S) Sulpholipid. Choose the correct option.
   (a) Only P (b) Only S
   (c) Both Q & R only (d) Both P & S
5. In short hand representation of fatty acids, second digit indicates what?
   (a) Number of carbons (b) Number of double bonds
   (c) Position of double bonds (d) Number of oxygens

6. Which of the following fatty acids are known as essential fatty acids? P) Palmitic acid Q) Linoleic acid R) Oleic acid S) Linolenic acid. Choose the correct option.
   (a) Both P & Q (b) Both R & S
   (c) Both P & R (d) Both Q & S
7. Which of the following is important for the synthesis & transport of lipoproteins and reverse transport of cholesterol?
   (a) Phospholipid (b) Glycolipid
   (c) Lipoprotein (d) Sulpholipid
8. The following substance(s) is(are) ketogenic
   (a) Fatty acids (b) Leucine
   (c) Lysine (d) All of them
9. Which of the following compounds possessing characteristics of lipids? P) Carotenoids Q) Squalene R) Pentacosane S) Alkaloids. Choose the correct option.
   (a) Both P & Q (b) Both R & S
   (c) Both P, Q & R (d) Both Q, R & S
10. Which lipoprotein possess the highest quantity of phospholipid.
   (a) HDL (b) LDL
   (c) VLDL (d) Chylomicrons
11. Which of the following is not a non-drying oil?
   (a) Almond oil (b) Peanut oil
   (c) Olive oil (d) Castor oil
12. Which of the following is example for semi-drying oil?
   (a) Olive oil (b) Mustard oil
   (c) Poppy seed oil (d) Almond oil
13. Which of the following is not on drying oil?
   (a) Linseed oil (b) Poppy seed oil
   (c) Cotton seed oil (d) Hemp oil
14. Cocoa butter is an example for what type of lipids?
   (a) Simple lipid (b) Complex lipid
   (c) Derived lipid (d) Miscellaneous lipid
15. Which of the following statement is not correct with respect to lipid functions?
   (a) It is as a concentrated fuel reserve of the body
   (b) It acts as an insulating material
   (c) It serve as a source of fat-soluble vitamins
   (d) It is not responsible for the shape and smooth appearance to the body
16. Which of the following fatty acid is not an even carbon fatty acid?
   (a) Valeric acid (b) Oleic acid
   (c) Palmitic acid (d) Stearic acid
17. Which of the following fatty acids are not an essential fatty acid?
   (a) Linoleic acid (b) Linolenic acid
   (c) Palmitic acid (d) Arachidonic acid

18. Which of the following is two-carbon fragment removed during β-oxidation of fatty acids?
    - (a) Malonyl CoA
    - (b) Formyl CoA
    - (c) Acyl CoA
    - (d) Acetyl CoA
19. Which compound is the active form of fatty acid that participated in β-oxidation?
    - (a) Malonyl CoA
    - (b) Formyl CoA
    - (c) Acyl CoA
    - (d) Acetyl CoA
20. Hypercholesterolemia is observed in which of the following(s) disorder(s).
    - (a) Hypothyroidism
    - (b) Diabetes mellitus
    - (c) Nephrotic syndrome
    - (d) All of them
21. Which hormone inhibits the hormone sensitive lipase activity.
    - (a) Epinephrine
    - (b) Insulin
    - (c) Thyroxine
    - (d) Glucocorticoids
22. What are two final products obtained in the β-oxidation of odd chain fatty acids.
    - (a) Acetyl CoA & Malonyl CoA
    - (b) Acetyl CoA & Acetyl CoA
    - (c) Acetyl CoA & Propionyl CoA
    - (d) Acetyl CoA & Succinyl CoA
23. ω-Oxidation requires which of the following? P) Cytochrome P_{450} Q) NADPH R) Oxygen S) ATP. Choose the correct option.
    - (a) Both P, Q & R
    - (b) Both Q, R & S
    - (c) Both R, S & P
    - (d) Both S, P & Q
24. Zellweger syndrome is due to the accumulation of long chain fatty acids in which organ(s).
    - (a) Brain
    - (b) Liver
    - (c) Kidney
    - (d) All of the above
25. Which of the following is true in α-oxidation of fatty acids? P) Removal of one carbon atom at a time Q) Removal of two carbon atom at a time R) No energy is produced S) Fatty acid is not binded with coenzyme A. Choose the correct option.
    - (a) Both P, Q & R
    - (b) Both Q, R & S
    - (c) Both R, S & P
    - (d) Both S, P & Q
26. Complete oxidation of one mole palmitate liberates how many ATPs?
    - (a) 5
    - (b) 133
    - (c) 131
    - (d) 129
27. Carnitine transport systems is very good example for which of the following?
    - (a) Active transport
    - (b) Passive transport
    - (c) Facilitated diffusion
    - (d) Simple diffusion
28. How any ATPs are needed for the activation of fatty acid in cytosol?
    - (a) 1
    - (b) 2
    - (c) 3
    - (d) 4
29. 10 % SIDS may be due to the deficiency of which of the following enzyme?
    - (a) Thiokinase
    - (b) Enoyl CoA hydratase
    - (c) Thiolase
    - (d) Acyl CoA dehydrogenase
30. Refsum's disease is due the defect in which type of fatty acids oxidation.
    - (a) oxidation
    - (b) b oxidation
    - (c) g oxidation
    - (d) w oxidation

31. Which enzyme regulates the fatty acid synthesis?
    (a) Enoyl reductase (b) Palmityl
    (c) Acetyl transacylase (d) Acetyl CoA carboxylase
32. Which of the following is an example for multi enzyme complex?
    (a) Plamitylthioesterase (b) Ketoacyl reductase
    (c) Enoyl reductase (d) FAS
33. In which part of the cell, the enzyme machinery or fatty acid production is present.
    (a) Mitochondria (b) Cytosomal fraction
    (c) Golgi apparatus (d) Lysosome
34. Which of the following compound is not an isoprenoid derivative?
    (a) IPP (b) DPP
    (c) Squalene (d) Mevalonate
35. Which of the following enzyme regulates cholesterol biosynthesis?
    (a) Thiolase (b) HMG CoA reductase
    (c) HMG CoA synthase (d) Cis-prenyl transferase
36. Cholesterol contains how many carbons?
    (a) 27 (b) 30
    (c) 25 (d) 28
37. To synthesize one mole of cholesterol how many NADPH required?
    (a) 18 (b) 16
    (c) 36 (d) 32
38. Which ketone bodie(s) are not metabolized in biological system?
    (a) Acetone (b) Acetoacetate
    (c) β-Hydroxybutyrate (d) All of the above
39. Which of the following is not a ketone body?
    (a) Acetone (b) Cholesterol
    (c) Acetoacetate (d) β-Hydroxy butyrate
40. Which of the following substance is not an intermediate in the cholesterol biosynthesis?
    (a) HMG Co A (b) IPP
    (c) β-Hydroxy butyrate (d) Squalene
41. Which of the following is not a ketone bodies metabolic disorder?
    (a) Ketonemia (b) Ketonurea
    (c) Ketoacidosis (d) Refsum's disease
42. Which of the following are primary bile acids?
    (a) Deoxycholic acid (b) Lithocholic acid
    (c) Chenodexycholic acid (d) Taurocholic acid
43. Which of the following is not synthesized from cholesterol?
    (a) Ketone bodies (b) Bile acids
    (c) Steroid hormones (d) Vitamin D
44. Hypercholesterolemia is observed in the disorder(s)?
    (a) Hypothyroidism (b) Diabetes mellitus
    (c) Nephrotic syndrome (d) All of them

45. *Adenylate cyclase* is inhibited by which hormone?
    (a) Epinephrine (b) Insulin
    (c) Glucagon (d) Thyroxine
46. Prostaglandin-E_1 inhibits which enzyme?
    (a) *Adenylate cyclase* (b) *Phosphodiesterase*
    (c) Both a &b (d) None of the above
47. Sphingomyelin is synthesized from which compound?
    (a) Serine (b) Palmityl CoA
    (c) Both a & b (d) None of the above
48. Which of the following phospholipid is referred to as platelet activating factor (PAF)?
    (a) Plasmalogens (b) Cadiolipin
    (c) Sphingomyelin (d) Phosphatidylinositol
49. Which compound is the active form of glycerol?
    (a) Glycerol-1-phosphate (b) Glycerol-2-phosphate
    (c) Glycerol-3-phosphate (d) Dihydroxy acetone phosphate
50. Which of the following formula is used to calculate body mass index (BMI)?
    (a) Weight (in Kg) × Height (in m^2) (b) Weight (in Kg) / Height (in m^2)
    (c) Weight (in Kg) × Height (in cm^2) (d) Weight (in Kg) × Height (in cm^2)

Key for Multiple Choice Questions

1. (d)	2. (a)	3. (b)	4. (a)	5. (b)
6. (d)	7. (a)	8. (d)	9. (c)	10. (a)
11. (d)	12. (b)	13. (c)	14. (a)	15. (d)
16. (a)	17. (c)	18. (d)	19. (c)	20. (d)
21. (c)	22. (b)	23. (a)	24. (d)	25. (c)
26. (d)	27. (c)	28. (b)	29. (d)	30. (a)
31. (d)	32. (d)	33. (b)	34. (d)	35. (b)
36. (a)	37. (b)	38. (a)	39. (b)	40. (c)
41. (d)	42. (c)	43. (a)	44. (d)	45. (b)
46. (a)	47. (c)	48. (a)	49. (c)	50. (b)

PART – B: Short Answers

1. Write briefly the metabolic derangements in diabetes mellitus.
2. Explain the terms: a) Hypoglycemia; b)Fatty liver.
3. What is fatty liver? Write the different causes of fatty liver.
4. What is atherosclerosis? Explain briefly its pathogenesis.
5. Note on a) Obesity; b) Hypercholesterimia.
6. Write the few words about *fatty acid synthase* (FAS) complex.
7. Explain the terms: a) Ketosis; b)Ketonemia.
8. Define Denovo synthesis of fatty acids.
9. Sketch the biosynthesis of ketone bodies.

10. Write short notes on α-oxidation of fatty acids.
11. Write a brief note on γ-oxidation of fatty acids.
12. Explain ω-oxidation of fatty acids.
13. Note on peroxisomal oxidation of fatty acids.
14. Define and classify lipids with suitable examples.
15. Define and classify fatty acid with suitable examples.
16. List out various biological significance of cholesterol.
17. Note on biological functions of lipids.
18. Explain the various biological importance of fatty acids.
19. What is carnitine transport system?
20. Explain the conversion of cholesterol to bile acids.
21. Short notes on bile salts.
22. Write the synthesis of steroid hormones from cholesterol.
23. Write the conversion of cholesterol to vitamin-D.
24. What are phospholipids. Explain in detail.
25. Write a note on synthesis of lecithin and cephalin.

PART – C: Long Answers

1. Explain β-oxidation of saturated fatty acids and write the total energy yield from one molecule of palmitic acid.
2. Explain the hormonal regulation in lipid metabolism.
3. Explain the synthesis of bile salts from cholesterol.
4. Write the steps involved in ketogenesis and explain its regulation. Add a note on ketoacidosis.
5. Note on metabolism of cholesterol.
6. Describe the biosynthesis of fatty acids.
7. Describe cholesterol levels and atherosclerosis in human body.
8. Write a note on lipid metabolism. Explain various lipid metabolic disorders.
9. Write in detail about β-oxidation of saturated fatty acids.
10. What are ketone bodies? Explain biosynthesis of ketone bodies.
11. Write a note on ketone bodies metabolism.
12. Explain the oxidation of unsaturated fatty acids.
13. Explain the biosynthesis of triglycerides.
14. Explain β-oxidation of palmitic acids.
15. Describe the biosynthesis of saturated & unsaturated fatty acids.
16. Describe the β-oxidation of unsaturated fatty acids.
17. Add a detailed note on degradation of cholesterol.
18. Write the biosynthesis of steroid sex hormones.
19. Sketch the biosynthesis of phospholipids & explain it.
20. Discuss the mechanism of β-oxidation of a molecule of palmitic acid, its regulation & energy yield in it.
21. Sketch the Denovo synthesis of a molecule of palmitic acid and how is it regulated.
22. Sketch the complete oxidation of one molecule of palmitic acid in a mitochondrion & indicate the energy yield in this process.
23. Discuss the biosynthesis of long chain saturated fatty acids and write a note on the regulation of this phenomenon.
24. Define and classify lipid and fatty acid with suitable examples. Add a note on biological significance of lipids and fatty acids.
25. Explain the biosynthesis of cholesterol.

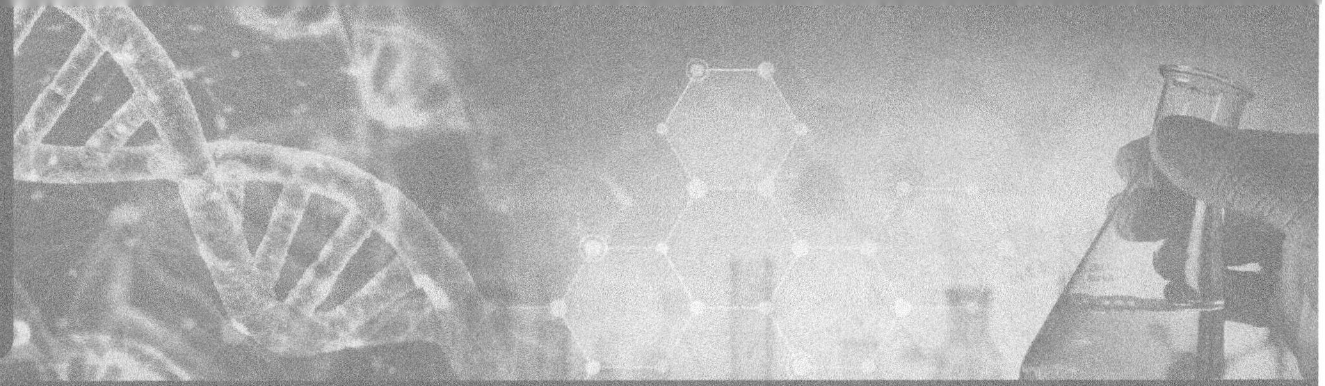

5

Protein and Amino Acid Metabolism

Proteins are the most abundant organic substances present in the living system. 50 % of the cellular dry weight is composed of proteins. Cell forms the fundamental basis of structure and functions of life. The term protein is obtained from Greek word "**proteios**" means "holding the first place (or) primary". In 1838, Dutch chemist Mulder used the term "protein" for high molecular weight nitrogen rich and most abundant substances present in plants and animals.

Proteins and peptides are polyamides composed of L-α-amino acids bonded in a head to tail manner through the carboxyl function of one amino acid with the amino function of other amino acid. The amide linkage is called a peptide bond. Hence, proteins are known as **polypeptides**. In other words, building blocks of peptides and proteins are composed of amino acids. By a variety of methods proteins undergo hydrolysis and cleaved i.e., hydrolyzed into their constituent amino acids. As proteins contain nitrogen also it acts as a major source of nitrogen to the biological system.

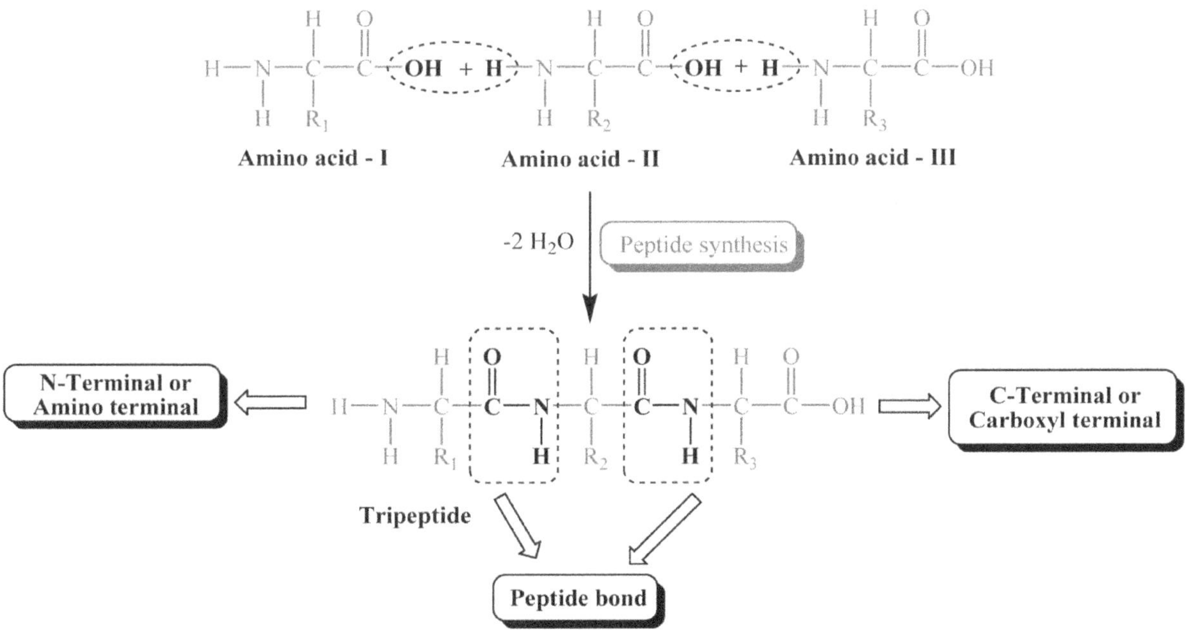

Amino acid - I   Amino acid - II   Amino acid - III

$-2\ H_2O$ Peptide synthesis

N-Terminal or Amino terminal   C-Terminal or Carboxyl terminal

Tripeptide

Peptide bond

Peptide linkage (-CO-NH-) is formed when two or more amino acids are joined together, and a chain of many amino acids is called as polypeptide. One or more polypeptide molecules are present in proteins. Peptide bonds covalently link the amino acids. Every polypeptide contains two ends, in that one end is known as amino terminal or N-terminal which has a free amino group and conventionally it is present in the left-hand amino acid. The other end is known as carboxyl terminal or C-terminal which has a free carboxyl group and conventionally it is present in the right-hand amino acid. The above figure of tripeptide shows three amino acids linked by two peptide bonds.

Elemental composition of proteins: Five major elements are predominantly present in proteins. They are, a) Carbon (50 to 55 %), b) Hydrogen (6 to 7 %), c) Oxygen (19 to 24 %), d) Nitrogen (13 to 19 %), and e) Sulphur (0 to 4 %). The other elements such as phosphorous, iron, copper, iodine, magnesium, manganese, zinc, etc. are also present in proteins. On an average about 16 % nitrogen is present in proteins. Hence, Kjeldahl's method of nitrogen estimation in laboratory is used to estimate the amount of proteins present in biological fluids and foods.

Classification of Proteins

Proteins are classified in three different ways as follows,

1. Functional classification of proteins
2. Chemical nature and solubility classification of proteins
3. Nutritional classification of proteins

1. **Functional Classification of Proteins**

   In this type of classification, proteins are broadly classified into nine different types according to its functions they perform. They are,

   1. **Structural proteins:** These proteins are basis for cellular structure. **Example:** Keratin present in hair and nail, collagen present in bones, etc.
   2. **Catalytic proteins or Enzyme proteins:** Proteins exhibit its function as enzyme comes in this category. **Example:** Almost all enzymes except ribosome, *glucokinase, pepsin,* etc.
   3. **Transport proteins:** These proteins are useful for the transport of some compounds. **Example:** Hemoglobin used for transport of oxygen, serum albumin used for the transport of bilirubin, etc.
   4. **Storage proteins:** Proteins are stored in one form in this type. **Example:** Ovalbumin is the storage form of protein in egg, glutelin is the storage form of protein in endosperm of certain seeds of the grass family, etc.
   5. **Defense proteins:** These proteins perform defense function in biological system. **Example:** Snake venom is the defense protein of snake, immunoglobulin is the defense protein of human, etc.
   6. **Hormonal proteins:** These proteins exhibit their function as hormones. **Example:** Insulin, growth hormone, etc.
   7. **Receptor proteins:** Receptors are chemically proteins. **Example:** Receptors for hormones, receptors for viruses, etc.
   8. **Genetic proteins:** These proteins involved in genetic functions. **Example:** Nucleoprotein.
   9. **Contractile proteins:** This protein plays a role in muscle contraction. **Example:** Actin, myosin, etc.

2. **Chemical Nature and Solubility Classification of Proteins**

   Proteins are classified into three major types on the basis of increasing complexity in their structure. They are,

   1. Simple proteins
   2. Conjugated or complex proteins and
   3. Derived proteins

   1. **Simple proteins:** These proteins on hydrolysis yield only α-amino acids. They are further classified into two major categories based on shape, solubility and digestion.

      A. Globular proteins

      B. Fibrous proteins

      A. **Globular proteins (Spheroproteins):** They are usually spherical or oval in shape, soluble in water and easily digestible. They are more highly branched and cross-linked condensation products of basic or acidic amino acids. As the globular proteins have diamino and

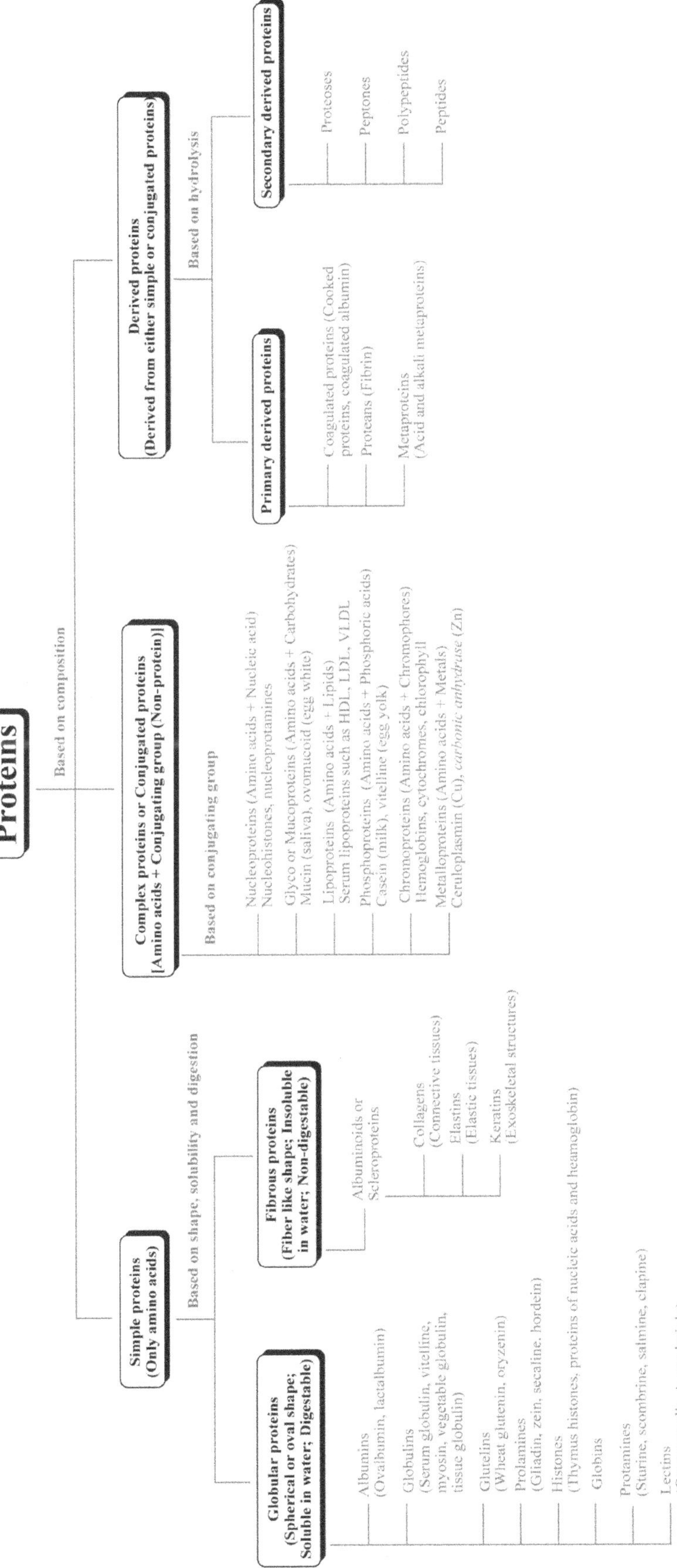
Proteins
Based on composition
Simple proteins
(Only amino acids)
Based on shape, solubility and digestion
Globular proteins
(Spherical or oval shape;
Soluble in water; Digestable)
Albumins
(Ovalbumin, lactalbumin)
Globulins
(Serum globulin, vitelline,
myosin, vegetable globulin,
tissue globulin)
Glutelins
(Wheat glutenin, oryzenin)
Prolamines
(Gliadin, zein, secaline, hordein)
Histones
(Thymus histones, proteins of nucleic acids and heamoglobin)
Globins
Protamines
(Sturine, scombrine, salmine, clapine)
Lectins
(Concanavalin-A, agglutinin)
Fibrous proteins
(Fiber like shape; Insoluble
in water; Non-digestable)
Albuminoids or
Scleroproteins
Collagens
(Connective tissues)
Elastins
(Elastic tissues)
Keratins
(Exoskeletal structures)
Complex proteins or Conjugated proteins
[Amino acids + Conjugating group (Non-protein)]
Based on conjugating group
Nucleoproteins (Amino acids + Nucleic acid)
Nucleohistones, nucleoprotamines
Glyco or Mucoproteins (Amino acids + Carbohydrates)
Mucin (saliva), ovomucoid (egg white)
Lipoproteins (Amino acids + Lipids)
Serum lipoproteins such as HDL, LDL, VLDL
Phosphoproteins (Amino acids + Phosphoric acids)
Casein (milk), vitelline (egg yolk)
Chromoproteins (Amino acids + Chromophores)
Hemoglobins, cytochromes, chlorophyll
Metalloproteins (Amino acids + Metals)
Ceruloplasmin (Cu), carbonic anhydrase (Zn)
Derived proteins
(Derived from either simple or conjugated proteins)
Based on hydrolysis
Primary derived proteins
Coagulated proteins (Cooked
proteins, coagulated albumin)
Proteans (Fibrin)
Metaproteins
(Acid and alkali metaproteins)
Secondary derived proteins
Proteoses
Peptones
Polypeptides
Peptides

dicarboxylic acids, branching and cross-linking takes place by the usual peptide linkage involving the second amino group of one amino acid and the second carboxyl group of another amino acid. The peptide chain is stabilized by intramolecular hydrogen bonds. They are further classified into several types based on their solubility.

(i) **Albumins:** They are soluble in water, acids and alkalis and are coagulated by heat and precipitated by saturated solution of ammonium sulphate. These are usually deficient in glycine. **Example:** Serum albumin (blood), ovalbumin (egg white) and lactalbumin (milk).

(ii) **Globulins:** They are insoluble in water, but soluble in dilute solutions of salt, strong inorganic acids and alkalis. They are coagulated by heat and precipitated by half saturating their solutions with ammonium sulphate. Generally, globulins contain glycine. **Example:** Serum globulin (blood), myosin (muscle), vitelline vegetable globulin and tissue globulin.

(iii) **Glutelins:** They are insoluble in water and dilute salt solution, but soluble in dilute acids and alkalis. They are coagulated by heat, and are comparatively rich in arginine, proline and glutamic acid. **Example:** Glutenin (wheat) and oryzenin (rice).

(iv) **Prolamins:** They are insoluble in water or salt solutions. But soluble in dilute acids, alkalis and 70-90 % ethyl alcohol. They contain large amounts of proline and are deficient in lysine. **Example:** Gliadin (wheat and rye), zein (corn), secaline (rye) and hordein (barley).

(v) **Histones:** They are complex chemicals in nature, soluble in water or dilute acids but insoluble in dilute ammonia. They are not coagulated by heat. These are hydrolyzed by pepsin and trypsin. **Example:** Proteins of the nucleic acids and hemoglobin and thymus histones.

(vi) **Globins:** These are also considered along with histones generally. However, globins are not basic proteins and are not precipitated by ammonium hydroxide.

(vii) **Protamines:** They are soluble in water, dilute acids and dilute ammonia. These are more basic than the histones and have a simpler structure and found in sperm cells of certain fish. **Example:** Sturine (sturgeon), scombrine (mackerel), salmine (salmon) and clapeine (herring).

(viii) **Lectins:** They are carbohydrate binding proteins and are involved in the interaction between cells and proteins. They help to maintain tissue and organ structures. In the laboratory they are used to purify carbohydrates by affinity chromatography. **Example:** Concanavalin-A and agglutinin.

B. Fibrous proteins: They are fiber like in shape, insoluble in water and resistant to digestion. They are formed by condensation of (neutral amino acids) monoamino monocarboxylic acids and there is a few or no branching. By intermolecular hydrogen bonds the linear protein chains are held together. Proteins that tend to be insoluble and strong play a structural role in organisms for support or protection. Scleroproteins or albuminoids are predominant group of fibrous proteins. They are insoluble in water and salt solution, but soluble in concentrated acids and alkalis. They are attacked by enzymes. **Example:** Keratin (from hair, nails, hooves, horns and feathers) and fibroin (silk). Albuminoids are sub-divided into three types.

(i) **Collagen:** It is the most common protein in the mammalian body. Found in skin, tendons and bones. They are attacked by pepsin and trypsin. When boiled with water, they form a water-soluble protein (gelatin).

(ii) **Elastin:** They are found in tendons, arteries and other elastic tissues. They are attacked slowly by trypsin.

(iii) **Keratins:** They are present in exoskeletal structures. **Example:** Hairs, nails and horns. Human hair contains as much as 14 % cysteine.

2. **Conjugated proteins:** Upon hydrolysis they yield α-amino acids and non-proteinous substances. They contain simple protein molecules linked with a non-protein substance. The non-proteinous moiety is referred as **prosthetic group.** On the basis of prosthetic group present in it, they are subdivided as follows.

   A. **Nucleoproteins:** The prosthetic group present in nucleoprotein is a nucleic acid. **Example:** Nucleohistones and nucleoprotamines.

   B. **Glycoproteins (mucoproteins):** They are produced by adding sugar residues through O-glycoside linkages to the hydroxyl groups of serine and threonine residues or via N -glycoside linkages to the amino group of asparagine. The prosthetic group present in glycoprotein is a carbohydrate or a derivative of carbohydrate. **Example:** Mucin of saliva and ovomucoid of egg white.

   C. **Lipoproteins:** They have the phosphorylated hydroxyl groups of serine or threonine. The prosthetic group present in lipoprotein is phospholipid (a class of fat). **Example:** Lipoproteins of serum such as HDL, LDL and VLDL.

   D. **Phosphoproteins:** The prosthetic group present in phosphoprotein is phosphoric acid. **Example:** Casein of milk and vitelline of egg yolk.

   E. **Chromoproteins:** They contain colored prosthetic group, due to the presence of a metal in their structure. **Example:** Hemoglobin (in which heme is prosthetic group and globin is the protein), chlorophyll and cytochromes.

   F. **Metalloproteins:** They contain metal ions such as Zn, Co, Fe, Mg, Cu, etc. as prosthetic group. **Example:** Copper in ceruloplasmin and zinc in *carbonic anhydrase.*

3. **Derived proteins:** These proteins are generally derived from either simple proteins or conjugated proteins. They are the products obtained by the action of heat, chemical or enzymatic agents on natural proteins. The derived proteins (intermediate hydrolysis products) are further classified on the basis of progressive cleavage into two major types.

   A. Primary derived proteins

   B. Secondary derived proteins

   A. **Primary derived proteins:** These proteins are the first hydrolyzed products of either simple proteins or conjugated proteins. They are,

      (i) **Coagulated proteins:** These are denaturated proteins. They are insoluble proteins, formed by the action of heat on proteins. **Example:** Cooked proteins and coagulated egg white albumin.

      (ii) **Proteans:** These are the earliest products of protein hydrolysis by enzymes, dilute acids, alkalis, etc. These proteins are insoluble in water. **Example:** Fibrin obtained from fibrinogen.

      (iii) **Metaproteins:** These are second stage products of protein hydrolysis obtained by treatment with slightly stronger acids and alkalis. They are insoluble in water, dilute salt solution and soluble in acids or alkalis. They are precipitated by half-saturation with ammonium sulphate. **Example:** Acid and alkali metaproteins.

   B. **Secondary derived proteins:** These proteins are the progressive hydrolytic products of protein hydrolysis. **Example:** Proteoses, peptones, polypeptides and peptides.

3. **Nutritional Classification of Proteins**

Proteins are broadly classified into three major types based on their nutritive value as follows,

1. Complete proteins
2. Partially incomplete proteins
3. Incomplete proteins

1. **Complete proteins:**

Body required proportion of all ten essential amino acids are present in complete proteins. These proteins generally promote good growth in the body. **Example:** Egg albumin and milk casein.

2. **Partially incomplete proteins:**
One or more essential amino acids are partially lacking in these proteins. These proteins generally promote moderate growth in the body. **Example:** Rice proteins and wheat proteins which are partially lacking essential amino acids such as lysine and threonine.
3. **Incomplete proteins:**
One or more essential amino acids are completely lacking in these proteins. These proteins generally do not promote growth in the body. **Example:** Gelatin which completely lacks tryptophan and zein which completely lacks tryptophan and lysine.

Structure of Proteins

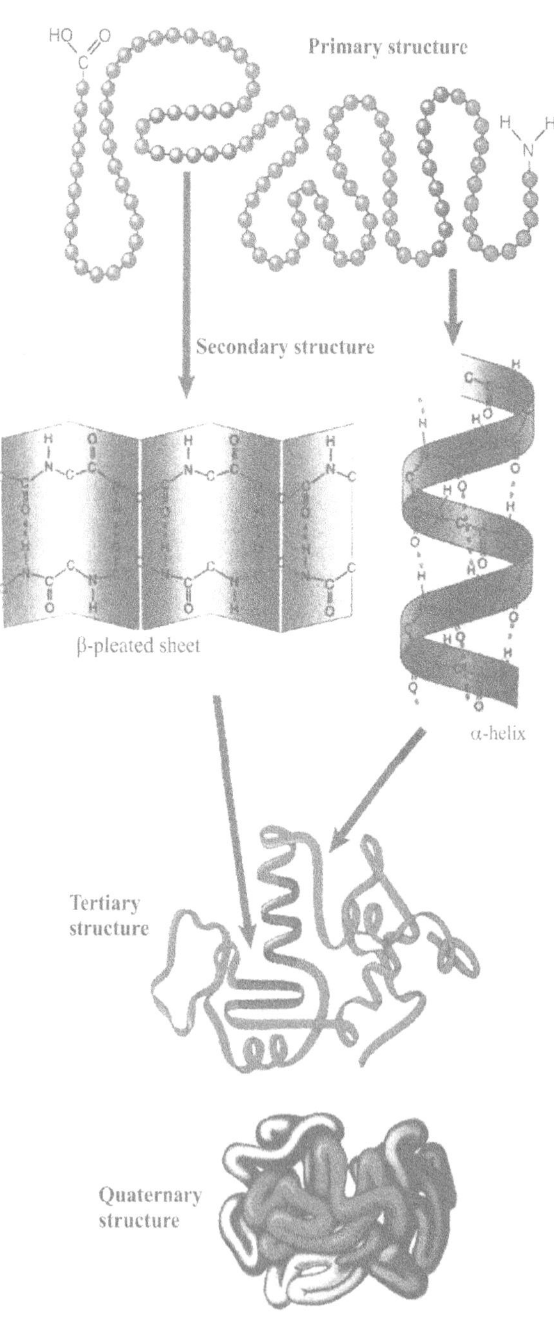

Figure 5.1 Protein structure.

Proteins are polymers of amino acids linked by peptide bonds and the various structure of proteins are presented in Figure 5.1. The following points should be addressed to establish the structure of a protein.

1. The nature of amino acids.
2. The number of such particular amino acid present in one molecule of the protein.
3. The sequence of different amino acids in which they are arranged in a protein.
   [The above three points constitute the primary structure of protein]
4. The peptide chain shape (linear, cyclic, branched or arranged in the form of helix). [This point constitutes the secondary structure of protein]
5. The forces responsible for holding the peptide together.
6. The mode in which individual peptide chains are arranged in definite manner to a macromolecule of an individual shape (folded, refolded).
   [The above two points constitute the tertiary structure of protein]
7. The number of peptide chains and arrangement in the natural proteins.
   [This point constitutes the quaternary structure of protein]

1. **Primary Structure of Proteins:**

   Simply the sequence of residues making up the protein is primary structure. Only the covalent bonds linking residues together are involved in primary structure of proteins. 50 residues or amino acids are considered as the minimum size of a protein; less than that are referred simply as peptides. Hence, a sequence of 50 residues is present in the primary structure of a small protein. Hundreds of atoms may be present in that small proteins and the molecular weights may range over 5000 Daltons (Da). So far, the largest protein discovered has about 30,000 residues but there is no theoretical maximum size. 110 Da is the average molecular weight of a residue and 3 million Da is the molecular weight of single chain. Primary structure of proteins is presented in Figure 5.2.

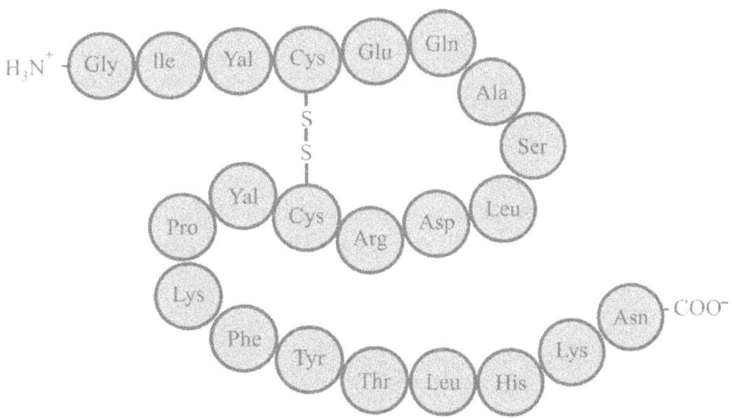

Figure 5.2 Primary structure of protein.

2. **Secondary Structure of Proteins:**

   In protein molecule, secondary structure of protein deals about peptide chain conformation. This structure clearly explains the local folding pattern of polypeptide backbone and their stabilization through hydrogen bonds between N-H and C=O groups. α-Helix is not formed by all polypeptide chains and in proteins the amount of the helix form varies ranging from 0 – 100 %. Flat nature of entire amide group is confirmed from X-ray studies of peptides. In only one plane carbonyl carbon, nitrogen and the four atoms attached are lies. Till date many types of secondary structure have been discovered, among them α-helix and β-sheet are most common because of their orderly repeating forms. The α-helical structure of protein is depicted in Figure 5.3.

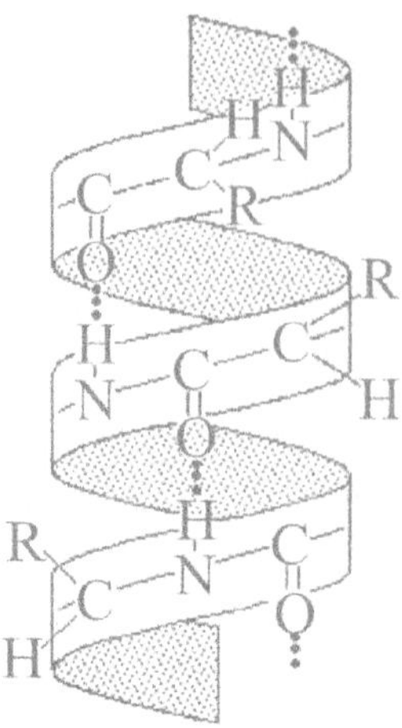

Figure 5.3 α-Helical structure of protein.

3. **Tertiary Structure of Proteins:**

   How regions of secondary structure fold together are described in this level of structure i.e. the 3D arrangement of a polypeptide chain, including α-helix, β-sheet and any other loops and folds. An interaction between side chains or between side chains and the polypeptide backbone is responsible for the tertiary structure. Usually side chains and polypeptide backbones are often distant in sequence. Particular pattern of folding is present in every protein and these are quite complex.

   Fibrous and globular are the two major molecular shapes that have been found. Large helical content is present in fibrous proteins and these proteins are essentially rigid molecules of rod like shape. Conversely, globular proteins are spherical shape due to the presence of polypeptide chain which consist partly of helical sections and folded about the random coil section to give a shape.

   Hydrogen, ionic and hydrophobic bonds are the three bonds responsible for formation of the tertiary structure of a protein. Due to number of residue hydrogen bonds between side chains may arise. Depending on the charge present in the polar group, the forces of repulsion or attraction produces electrostatic forces. Carboxylate (COO^-) and ammonium (NH_3^+) ions are the two polar groups. The protein conformation is destabilized due to repulsive forces when like charged polar groups are close together. On the other hand, the protein conformation is stabilized due to attractive forces when the polar groups have unlike charges. Ionic bonds or salt linkages are examples for the attractive forces which stabilizes the conformation.

   Hydrocarbons like side chains (between two methyl or phenyl groups) forms the hydrophobic bonds. This leads to prefer to be in the interior of the protein molecule where there is less water. Tertiary structure of proteins is presented in Figure 5.4.

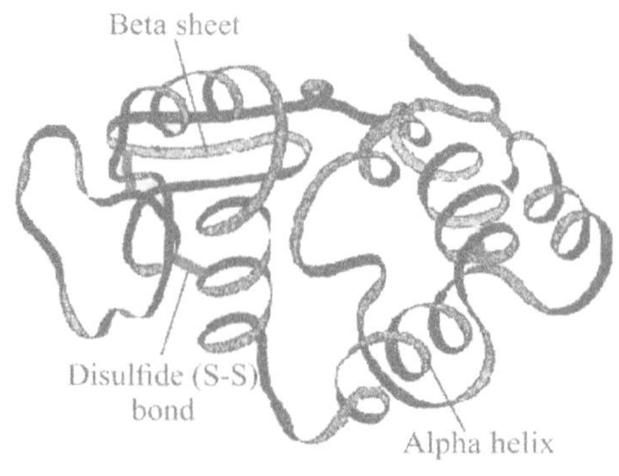

Figure 5.4 Tertiary structure of protein.

4. **Quaternary Structure of Proteins:**

   In general associations with several chains only majority of the large size and some of the medium size proteins are exist in nature. In quaternary structure, the individual chains are considered as protomers or sub-units and the protein is considered as oligomeric. Primary, secondary and tertiary structures are present in each sub-unit. Given protein contains two or more sub-units which may have identical or different above three structures. Two identical α-chains and two identical β-chains i.e., totally four sub-units are present in the hemoglobin molecule. Quaternary structure of hemoglobin resembles a sphere due to Vander Waals forces (hydrophobic forces) which held together four chains. Quaternary structure of proteins is presented in Figure 5.5.

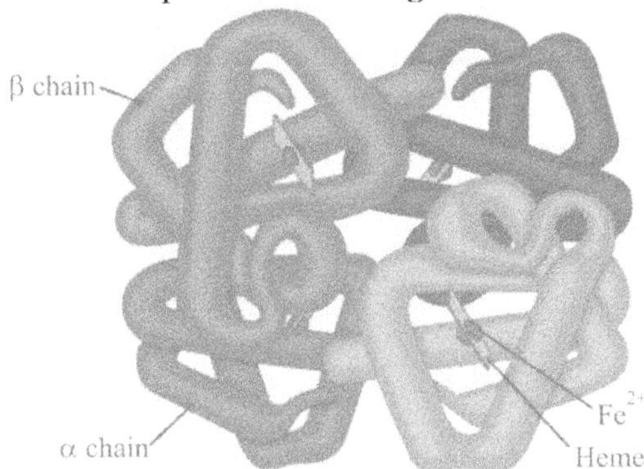

Figure 5.5 Quaternary structure of protein.

Biological Significance of Proteins

Proteins possess diverse specialized and essential biological functions. These functions are broadly categorized into two categories as,

1. Structural or static function
2. Dynamic function

1. **Structural or static functions of proteins:**

   Proteins play a major role in the structure and strength of the biological system due to their brick and mortar roles. **Example:** Some proteins like collagen and elastin in bone matrix, vascular system and other organs and keratin in epidermal tissues such as hair and nail act as biological structural materials.

2. **Dynamic functions of proteins:**

   Dynamic functions of proteins are more diversified in nature. In general, the dynamic functions of proteins are approximately regarded as the working horses of the cell. The followings are the various dynamic functions performed by proteins.

   1. Enzymes are made up of proteins, which catalyzes the biological reactions. **Example:** Almost all enzymes except ribosome, *glucokinase*, pepsin, etc.
   2. Few proteins are useful for the transport of some compounds. **Example:** Hemoglobin used for transport of oxygen, serum albumin used for the transport of bilirubin, etc.
   3. Proteins also performs storage function by stored in one form. **Example:** Ovalbumin is the storage form of protein in egg, glutelin is the storage form of protein in endosperm of certain seeds of the grass family, etc.
   4. Some of the proteins perform defense function in biological system. **Example:** Snake venom is the defense protein of snake, immunoglobulin is the defense protein of human, etc.
   5. Hormones are proteins which regulate various metabolic processes. **Example:** Insulin maintains blood sugar level and growth hormone maintains growth.
   6. Receptors are chemically proteins. **Example:** Receptors for hormone, receptors for viruses, etc.
   7. During cell division, genetic message is transmitted through nucleoproteins which is an important constituent of nucleic acids. **Example:** Nucleoproteins.

8. Some protein plays a role in muscle contraction. **Example:** Actin, myosin, etc.
9. Antibodies which makes immunity of the body for resistance to diseases are formed from blood proteins.
10. Blood clotting factors are protein in nature.
11. Immunoglobulins are also protein in nature and involved in immune functions.

Amino Acids - Introduction

Amino acid is defined as a group of organic compounds possessing two functional groups namely carboxylic acid (COOH) and amino (NH_2) group. The amino group is attached at α-position of carboxylic acid or both carboxyl group and amino groups are attached to the same carbon, hence it is known as **α-amino acids**. The carboxylic acid group is acidic in nature and the amino group is basic in nature. General structure of amino acid is given below.

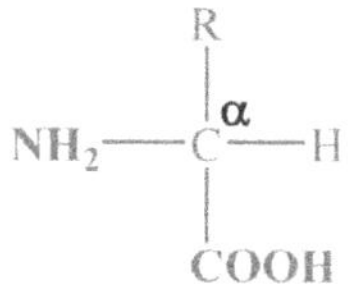

$$NH_2-\overset{\overset{R}{|}}{\underset{\underset{COOH}{|}}{C^{\alpha}}}-H \qquad \overset{\oplus}{NH_3}-\overset{\overset{R}{|}}{\underset{\underset{COO^{\ominus}}{|}}{C^{\alpha}}}-H$$

General structure of L-α-amino acid 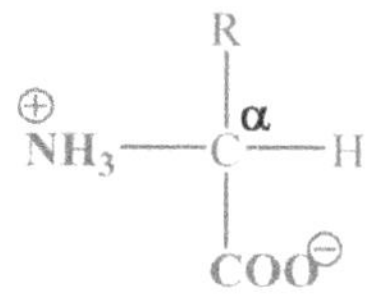 **Amino acid exist as ion**

Where α indicates position of amino group and L indicates configuration of amino acids [amino group present on left side]. If it is present on right side it is known as D-amino acid.

Classification of Amino Acids

Amino acids are classified in four different ways as follows,

1. Structural or chemical classification of amino acids
2. Nutritional classification of amino acids
3. Polarity classification of amino acids
4. Metabolic fate classification of amino acids

1. Structural or Chemical Classification of Amino Acids

It is one of the important classification method of amino acids. In this method twenty amino acids present in proteins are classified into seven different types based on its structure and chemical nature. A three letter or one letter symbol is assigned for each and every twenty amino acids present in proteins. In protein structure, these symbols are generally used to denote the amino acids.

I. **Aliphatic amino acids:** These amino acids are chemically monoamino mono carboxylic acids. They are further divided into two types based on the presence of branching as follows.

(a) **Un-branched aliphatic amino acids:** No branch is present in aliphatic chain. **Example:** Glycine and alanine.

(b) **Branched aliphatic amino acids:** These amino acids contain branches in aliphatic chain. Leucine, isoleucine, and valine are sometimes called "branched-chain amino acids" (BCAA) because human beings cannot survive unless these amino acids are present in the diet. The combination of these three amino acids makes up approximately one-third of skeletal muscle in the human body. **Example:** Valine, leucine and isoleucine.

II. **Hydroxyl group containing amino acids:** These amino acids contain hydroxyl group in their structure. **Example:** Serine, threonine and tyrosine. In general, aromatic ring is present in tyrosine. Hence tyrosine is usually considered as aromatic amino acid and not as hydroxyl group containing amino acid.

III. **Sulphur containing amino acids:** These amino acids contain sulphur atom in their structure. **Example:** Cysteine (contain sulfhydryl group), cystine (formed by condensation of two molecules of cysteine and contain disulfide group) and methionine (contain thioether group).

Table 5.1 Structural or chemical classification of amino acids.

S. No.	Name	Additional structural features present	Chemical structure	Reasoning for name	Three letters symbols	One letter symbol
I. Aliphatic amino acids						
1	Glycine	Un-branched aliphatic chain	$H-CH(NH_2)-COOH$	From the Greek word "Glukus" meaning sweet, because it was first isolated from gelatin	Gly	G
2	Alanine		$CH_3-CH(NH_2)-COOH$	"Al" is a shortening of aldehyde. The infix "an" was added to make it easier to pronounce	Ala	A
3	Valine	Branched aliphatic chain	$(CH_3)_2CH-CH(NH_2)-COOH$	Named in 1906 after a type of acid that occurs in the roots of the "valerian" plant	Val	V
4	Leucine		$(CH_3)_2CH-CH_2-CH(NH_2)-COOH$	First used in 1826 by chemist William Henry comes from the Greek word "leukos" meaning "white"	Leu	L
5	Isoleucine		$CH_3-CH_2-CH(CH_3)-CH(NH_2)-COOH$	Named in 1904 by Felix Ehrlich, who observed that it was similar but not identical to leucine	Ile	I
II. Hydroxyl group containing amino acids						
6	Serine	Hydroxyl group	$CH_2(OH)-CH(NH_2)-COOH$	From the Latin word "sericum" meaning "silk", because it was first obtained from silk protein	Ser	S
7	Threonine		$CH_3-CH(OH)-CH(NH_2)-COOH$ (printed as $CH_3-CH_2(OH)-CH(NH_2)-COOH$)	Named in 1936 after threose, a type of monosaccharide that it was thought to resemble	Thr	T
	Tyrosine		$HO-C_6H_4-CH_2-CH(NH_2)-COOH$	From Greek "tyros" meaning "cheese", because it was obtained from old cheese	Tyr	Y

Table 5.1 *Contd...*

S. No.	Name	Additional structural features present	Chemical structure	Reasoning for name	Three letters symbols	One letter symbol
III. Sulphur group containing amino acids						
8	Cysteine	Sulfhydryl group	$CH_2(SH)—CH(NH_2)—COOH$	Had an earlier spelling of cystine. That comes from the ancient Greek word for "bladder", "kustis"	Cys	C
	Cystine	Disulfide group	$CH_2(—S—S—CH_2—CH(NH_2)—COOH)—CH(NH_2)—COOH$		-	-
9	Methionine	Thioether linkage	$CH_3—S—CH_2—CH_2—CH(NH_2)—COOH$	Coined in 1926 by Barger and Coyne as a contraction of γ-methiol-α-aminobutyric acid	Met	M
IV. Acidic amino acids and their amides						
10	Aspartic acid	β-Carboxyl group	$\overset{\beta}{CH_2}(COOH)—\overset{\alpha}{CH}(NH_2)—COOH$	Named after asparagine, because it was first isolated from it by hydrolysis in 1827	Asp	D
11	Glutamic acid	γ-Carboxyl group	$\overset{\gamma}{CH_2}(COOH)—\overset{\beta}{CH_2}—\overset{\alpha}{CH}(NH_2)—COOH$	"Glut" refers how the compound was first isolated from gluten in 1866 by chemist Karl Rithausen	Glu	E
12	Asparagine	Amide group	$CH_2(CONH_2)—CH(NH_2)—COOH$	First extracted in 1806 from a sample of "asparagus" juice, after which it was named	Asn	N
13	Glutamine		$CH_2(CONH_2)—CH_2—CH(NH_2)—COOH$	Named before it was isolated, because it was hypothesized to be similar to glutamic acid	Gln	Q

Table 5.1 *Contd...*

S. No.	Name	Additional structural features present	Chemical structure	Reasoning for name	Three letters symbols	One letter symbol
V. Basic amino acids						
14	Lysine	ε-Amino group	ε CH_2—(δ, γ, β) $(CH_2)_3$—(α) CH(—NH_2)—COOH, with NH_2 on the ε-CH_2	Named in 1889 from the ancient Greek word "lusis" meaning "loosening"	Lys	K
15	Arginine	Guanidino group	NH—$(CH_2)_3$—CH(—NH_2)—COOH, with NH—C(=NH)—NH_2	From the Greek word "arginoeis" meaning "silver", due to the appearance of silver nitrate	Arg	R
16	Histidine	Imidazole ring	Imidazole ring (HN, N)—CH_2—CH(—NH_2)—COOH	From Greek "histos" meaning "tissue", because it was thought to be important to tissue function	His	H
VI. Aromatic amino acids						
17	Phenylalanine	Phenyl ring	Benzene ring—CH_2—CH(—NH_2)—COOH	Named by Erlenmeyer and Lipp in 1883 because it looks like alanine with a phenyl group	Phe	F
18	Tyrosine	Phenol analog	HO—benzene ring—CH_2—CH(—NH_2)—COOH	From Greek "tyros" meaning "cheese", because it was obtained from old cheese	Tyr	Y
19	Tryptophan	Indole ring	Indole ring (N—H)—CH_2—CH(—NH_2)—COOH	Traces to the Greek roots "tripsis" meaning "rubbing", and "phainein" meaning "to show"	Trp	W
VII. Imino acids						
20	Proline	Pyrrolidine ring	Pyrrolidine ring (N—H) with COOH	The name is a contraction of pyrrolidine, which makes up a side chain of the compound	Pro	P

IV. **Acidic amino acids and their amides:** These amino acids are generally dicarboxylic mono amino acids. They are highly acidic in character. These amino acids in general possess different codons for their incorporation into proteins. **Example:** Aspartic acid & glutamic acid are acidic amino acids and asparagine and glutamine are their corresponding amides.

V. **Basic amino acids:** These amino acids are generally dibasic monocarboxylic acids. They are highly basic in character. **Example:** Lysine and arginine (possess guanidine group) and histidine (possess imidazole ring).

VI. **Aromatic amino acids:** These amino acids are generally contains aromatic ring in their structure. **Example:** Phenylalanine and tyrosine (contain phenyl ring), tryptophan (contain indole ring) and histidine (contain imidazole ring).

IV. **Imino acids:** These amino acids generally contain imino group i.e., =NH instead of amino (NH_2) group in their structure. **Example:** Proline. Histidine, tryptophan and proline are considered as heterocyclic amino acids also as they have heterocyclic ring in their structure.

2. Nutritional Classification of Amino Acids

More than two hundred amino acids have been isolated and identified but only twenty-five are obtained from typical proteins, in turn only twenty amino acids are generally found in all proteins. Except other biological functions these twenty amino acids are needed for the synthesis of many proteins. But it is not necessary to take all these twenty amino acids in diet because some of the amino acids are biosynthesized in the biological system. Based on the dietary requirements of amino acids it is broadly classified into two major types as follows.

(a) **Essential amino acids:** Among the twenty amino acids, ten are called as essential amino acids. These amino acids **cannot be synthesized by the body** and must be supplied by dietary sources. They are also called as **indispensable amino acids.** Deficiency in any one of the essential amino acid prevents growth and may even cause death. Although there are ten essential amino acids to man, eight are more important, viz methionine, tryptophan, threonine, valine, isoleucine, leucine, phenylalanine and lysine. Two amino acids are less important namely arginine and histidine because it is partly synthesized by the body (To remember these ten essential amino acids, it can be mentioned as **MATT VIL PHLY** which corresponds to **M**ethionine, **A**rginine, **T**ryptophan, **T**heronine, **V**aline, **I**soleucine, **L**eucine, **P**henylalanine, **H**istidine and **LY**sine).

(b) **Non-essential amino acids:** The other ten amino acids are called as **non-essential amino acids** or **dispensable amino acids** and are **synthesized by the body.** Hence no need to take by dietary sources. The non-essential amino acids are alanine, asparagine, aspartic acid, cysteine, glutamine, glutamic acid, glycine, proline, serine and tyrosine.

3. Polarity Classification of Amino Acids

Based on their polarity, amino acids are broadly classified into four major types.

(a) **Non-polar amino acids:** Also known as hydrophobic amino acids because of its water hating property. These amino acids don't have any charge on "R" group. **Example:** Alanine, leucine, isoleucine, valine, methionine, phenylalanine, tryptophan and proline.

(b) **Polar amino acids with no charge on "R" group:** These amino acids don't have any charge on "R" group but having other polar groups such as hydroxyl, sulfhydryl and amide group leads to hydrogen bonding. **Example:** Glycine, serine, threonine, cysteine, glutamine, asparagine and tyrosine.

(c) **Polar amino acids with positive charge on "R" group:** These amino acids have positive charge on "R" group which makes them as polar. **Example:** Lysine, arginine and histidine.

(d) **Polar amino acids with negative charge on "R" group:** These amino acids have negative charge on "R" group which makes them as polar. **Example:** Aspartic acid and glutamic acid.

4. Fate of Metabolism of Amino Acids Classification

Amino acids are broadly classified into three types based on their fate of metabolism because the carbon skeleton of amino acids can serve as a precursor for the synthesis of carbohydrates (glucogenic) or fat (ketogenic) or both.

(a) **Glucogenic amino acids:** The amino acids serve as a precursor for the synthesis of carbohydrates such as glucose or glycogen are called as glucogenic amino acids. **Example:** Alanine, glycine, valine, serine, cysteine, methionine, arginine, threonine, histidine, aspartic acid, asparagine, glutamic acid, glutamine and proline.

(b) **Ketogenic amino acids:** The amino acids which serve especially as a precursor for the synthesis of fat are called as ketogenic amino acids. **Example:** Leucine and lysine.

(c) **Glucogenic and ketogenic amino acids:** The amino acids which serve as a precursor for the synthesis of both carbohydrates and fat are called as glucogenic and ketogenic amino acids. **Example:** Isoleucine, phenylalanine, tryptophan and tyrosine.

Nomenclature of Amino Acids

Trivial or common names are available for all the amino acids. These names are given some times based on the source from which they were first isolated. **Example:** Asparagine was first found in asparagus, glutamate in wheat gluten; tyrosine in cheese (In Greek *tyros,* means "cheese"). Sometime the names are given based on their taste. **Example:** Glycine (In Greek "*glykos*", means "sweet") was so named because of its sweet taste.

The amino acids are named in the IUPAC system, as amino derivatives of the corresponding acid with the position of the amino group defined by an appropriate number. The C-1 would be carboxyl carbon of an amino acid and the C-2 would be α-carbon, the C-3, C-4, C-5 and C-6 would be β, γ, δ and ε-carbon, respectively. The Greek lettering system is confusing in some cases, such as amino acids with heterocyclic R groups. Hence, generally the numbering system is used.

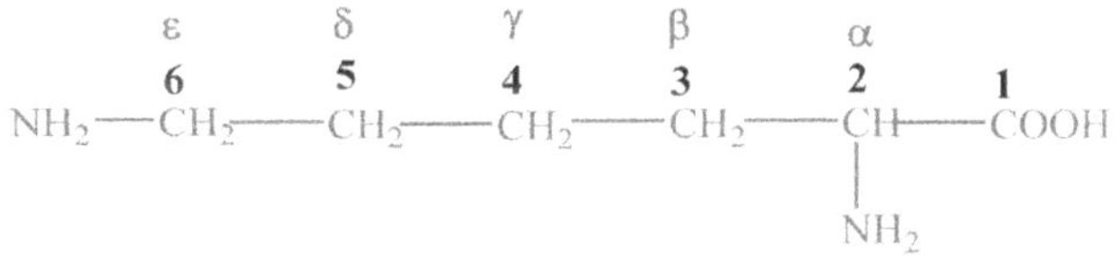

$$\overset{}{NH_2}-\overset{\varepsilon}{\overset{6}{CH_2}}-\overset{\delta}{\overset{5}{CH_2}}-\overset{\gamma}{\overset{4}{CH_2}}-\overset{\beta}{\overset{3}{CH_2}}-\overset{\alpha}{\overset{2}{\underset{NH_2}{\underset{|}{CH}}}}-\overset{1}{COOH}$$

2, 6-Diamino heptanoic acid

Biological Significance of Amino Acids

Biological significance of amino acids explained under two sub divisions as follows.

(a) **Standard amino acids:**

The 20 amino acids present in proteins are known as standard amino acids which performs several biological functions as follows.

1. 4-Hydroxyproline and 5-hydroxylysine are the major constituents of the most abundant protein in mammals i.e., collagen.
2. Many methylated or acetylated or phosphorylated amino acids are present in the histones in association with DNA.
3. γ-Carboxyglutamic acid present in certain plasma protein is participated in blood clotting process.

(b) **Non-standard amino acids:**

There are several amino acids present in nature beyond 20 standard amino acids which are present in proteins. These amino acids are commonly known as non-standard amino acids or non-protein amino acids which performs some biologically important functions. They are,

1. Creatinine is derived from muscle and excreted in urine.
2. In biological system methyl group is donated by S-adenosylmethionine (SAM).
3. Thyroxine and triiodothyronine are thyroid hormones derived from tyrosine.
4. In the metabolism of threonine, aspartate and methionine, homoserine is the intermediate.
5. DOPA is a neurotransmitter which serves as a precursor for the synthesis of melanin pigment.
6. Ornithine, citrulline and arginosuccinate are intermediates in the urea biosynthesis.

7. Ovothiol is the sulphur containing amino acids found in fertilized eggs which acts as an antioxidant.
8. In methionine metabolism, homocysteine is the intermediate which is a risk factor for coronary heart diseases.
9. Azaserine is used as anticancer agent and cycloserine is used as antitubercular drug.
10. β-Alanine is the component of vitamins such as pantothenic acid and co-enzyme A.
11. The end product of pyrimidine metabolism is β-aminoisobutyric acid.
12. Taurine is found in association with bile acids.
13. From glutamic acid the neuro transmitter GABA is biosynthesized.
14. In the synthesis of porphyrin and heme, δ-aminolevulinic acid (ALA) is the intermediate.
15. D-Penicillamine effectively chelates copper and is chemically D-dimethylglycine. It is a metabolite of penicillin and is used in the chelation therapy of Wilson's disease.
16. N-Acetylcysteine is used in cystic fibrosis and chronic renal insufficiency due to its antioxidant property.
17. Gabapentin is chemically γ-aminobutyrate linked to cyclohexane used in the treatment of convulsion.

Amino Acid Pool

The 100 g of free amino acid present in adults represents the amino acid pool of the body. Out of 100 g body amino acid pool about 50 % are glutamate and glutamine together and 10 % are essential amino acids. In general, intracellular amino acid concentration is more than extracellular amino acids. Using active transport process amino acids enter into the cell against concentration gradient. The sources that contribute (input) and the metabolic pathways that utilize amino acids (output) maintain amino acid pool. The overview of amino acid pool is presented in Figure 5.6.

Sources of amino acid pool:

Protein turnover: Protein turnover is one of the important processes which contribute for body amino acid pool. The other process that contributes for body amino acid pool is intake of dietary protein and the synthesis of non-essential amino acids. In biological system per day in normal healthy adult about 350-400 g of protein is degraded and synthesized which represents body protein turn over. But the turnover of individual amino acids varies widely. The half-life of plasma proteins and digestive enzymes are short (in hours or days), hence they degrade rapidly; whereas the half-life of structural proteins like collagen is long (in months and years), hence they degrade slowly.

Generally, many factors influence the protein turnover in body. Degradation of proteins is facilitated by a small polypeptide known as ubiquitin (Molecular weight: 8500) which tags with protein. Similarly, proteins containing sequence of amino acid like proline, glutamine (code: E), serine and threonine (PEST sequence) are rapidly degraded.

Dietary protein: Degradation of proteins leads to regular loss of nitrogen from the body. From the body everyday about 30 to 50 g of protein is lost in healthy adults. To maintain the nitrogen balance, this amount (30 to 50 g) of nitrogen must be supplied daily in the diet. Dietary proteins provide amino acids particularly essential ones for the synthesis of protein and other nitrogen compounds. Unlike carbohydrates (Storage form: glycogen) and lipids (Storage form: triacyl glycerol) there is **no special storage form for proteins**. Hence, the excess amino acids are metabolized to generate energy and utilized as a precursor for the synthesis of carbohydrates and fats. The amino groups of amino acids lost as urea. Proteolytic enzymes digest dietary proteins and produce amino acids which are absorbed in the intestine and enter into the body amino acid pool.

Synthesis of non-essential amino acids: 10 non-essential amino acids are biosynthesized in the body from essential amino acids which contribute to the body amino acid pool.

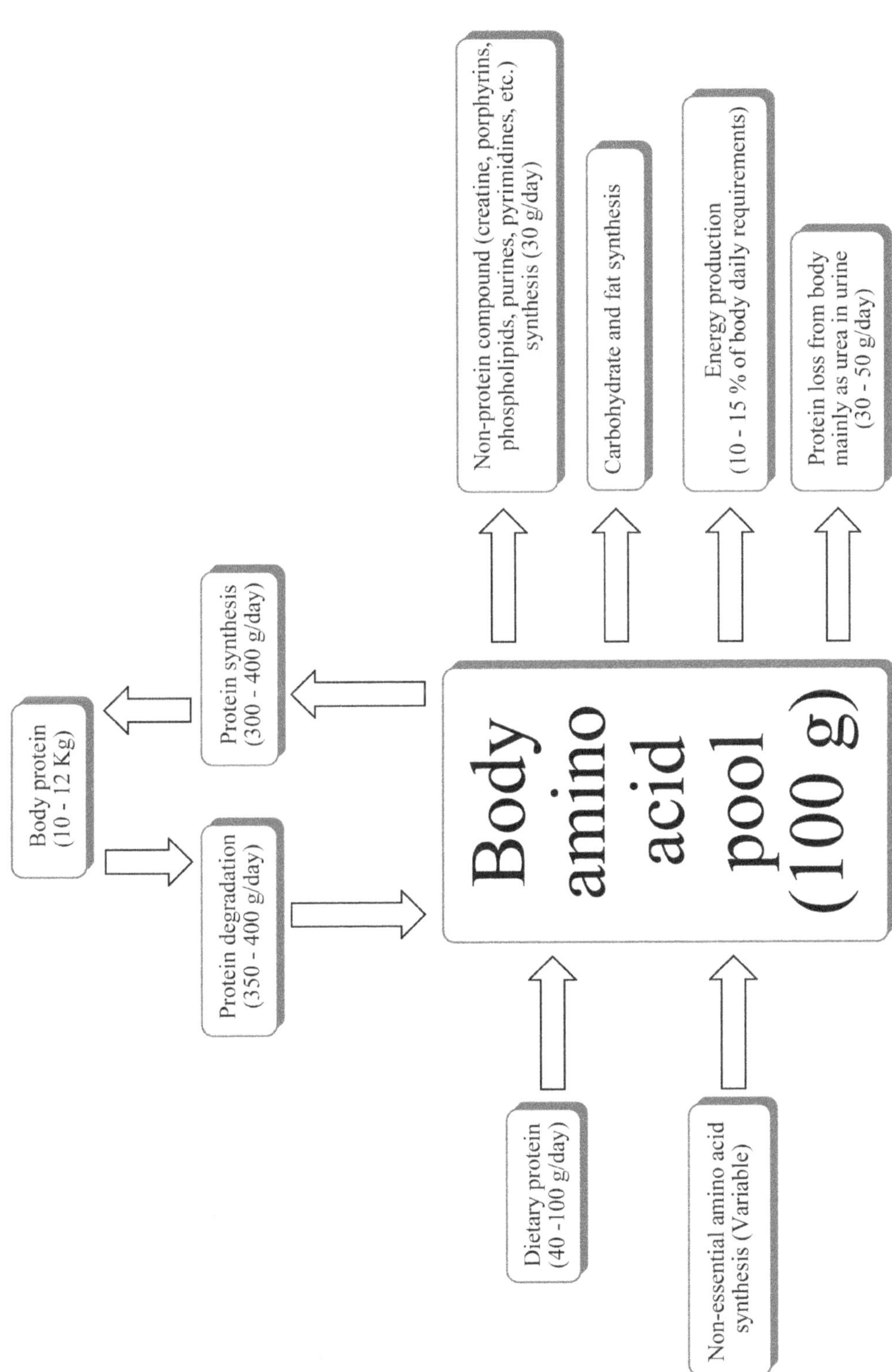

Figure 5.6 Overview of body amino acid pool.

Utilization of amino acid from body amino acid pool:

Many body proteins like enzymes, hormones, immune proteins, contractile proteins, etc. are synthesized (300 to 400 g/day) from amino acid pool. Amino acid contributes about 10 to 15 % of total body energy requirements. Amino acid is utilized as important precursor for the synthesis of many important nitrogenous compounds such as porphyrins, purines, pyrimidines, etc. When the protein consumption is more than the requirements of body then excess amino acids are predominantly converted to carbohydrates and fats.

Nitrogen Balance

Dietary protein is the major source of nitrogen to the biological system. The protein (nitrogen content: 16 %) utilization and its degradation from the body are truly represented by nitrogen balance. In general nitrogen balance is estimated by comparing the intake of nitrogen (mostly proteins) and excretion of nitrogen (mostly undigested nitrogen in feces and urea and ammonia in urine). Generally, nitrogen loss in feces, sweat, nails, etc. is represented by the term "fudge factor" (3 g approximately). In a nitrogen equilibrium, in normal healthy adult the daily dietary intake (I) is equal to loss through urine (U), feces (F) and sweat (S). The overview of nitrogen balance is depicted in Figure 5.7.

$$I = U + F + S$$

The state in which intake of nitrogen is equal to output of nitrogen is called as nitrogen balance.

Intake of nitrogen = Output of nitrogen (Nitrogen balance)

Positive nitrogen balance: The state in which intake of nitrogen is greater than output of nitrogen is called as positive nitrogen balance. The net protein in the body increases due to the retention of some amount of nitrogen. It is generally observed in growing children, pregnant women and during recovery from serious illness. Body gains weight during positive nitrogen balance.

Intake of nitrogen > Output of nitrogen (Positive nitrogen balance)

Negative nitrogen balance: The state in which output of nitrogen is greater than intake of nitrogen or intake of nitrogen is lesser than output of nitrogen is called as negative nitrogen balance. The net result leads to loss of some amount of nitrogen from the body by depleting the body protein. Even death may occur due to prolonged negative nitrogen balance. Sometimes it was observed in children suffering from kwashiorkor or marasmus. Inadequate dietary intake of protein (deficiency of even single essential amino acids), destruction of tissues and serious illness are some important reasons for negative nitrogen balance. In all these situations loss of nitrogen from the body takes place due to increased breakdown of tissue proteins because body adapts itself in these cases. Body loses weight during negative nitrogen balance.

Intake of nitrogen < Output of nitrogen (Negative nitrogen balance)

The most important factors which influence the nitrogen balance are growth, pregnancy, protein deficiency, injury and illness. Except these there are many other factors that influence the nitrogen balance. **Example:** Insulin and growth hormone promotes positive nitrogen balance; whereas corticosteroids promote negative nitrogen balance. In addition, uncontrolled diabetes mellitus and cancer produce negative nitrogen balance.

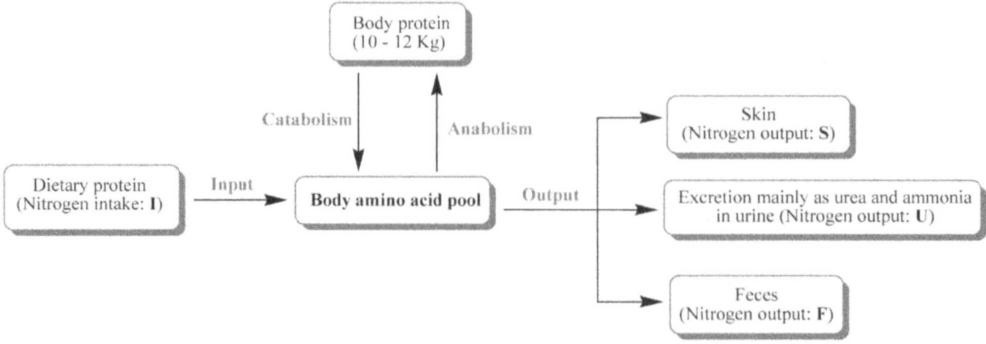

Figure 5.7 Overview of nitrogen balance.

General Aspects of Amino Acid Metabolism

Amino acid metabolism differs from other biomolecule metabolisms due to the presence of nitrogen. The nitrogen present in amino group of amino acid can be transferred from one amino acid to another keto acid [**transamination**] or removal of amino group from amino acid [**deamination**]. The carbon skeletons of amino acids are usually metabolized like carbohydrate and fat. The amino acid undergoes some common reactions like transamination followed by deamination to liberate ammonia. The liberated ammonia is utilized for the formation of **urea which is the excretory end product of protein metabolism**. The overview of amino acid metabolism is presented in Figure 5.8. Through transamination the carbon skeleton of amino acid is converted to keto acid. The produced keto acids may meet any one or more of the following fates.

1. Keto acid is used for generation of energy.
2. Keto acid is utilized for the production of glucose.
3. Keto acid is used for the synthesis of fat or ketone bodies.
4. Keto acid is involved in the synthesis of non-essential amino acid also.

The following are the three major metabolic reactions taking place in amino acid metabolism.

1. Transamination
2. Deamination
3. Decarboxylation

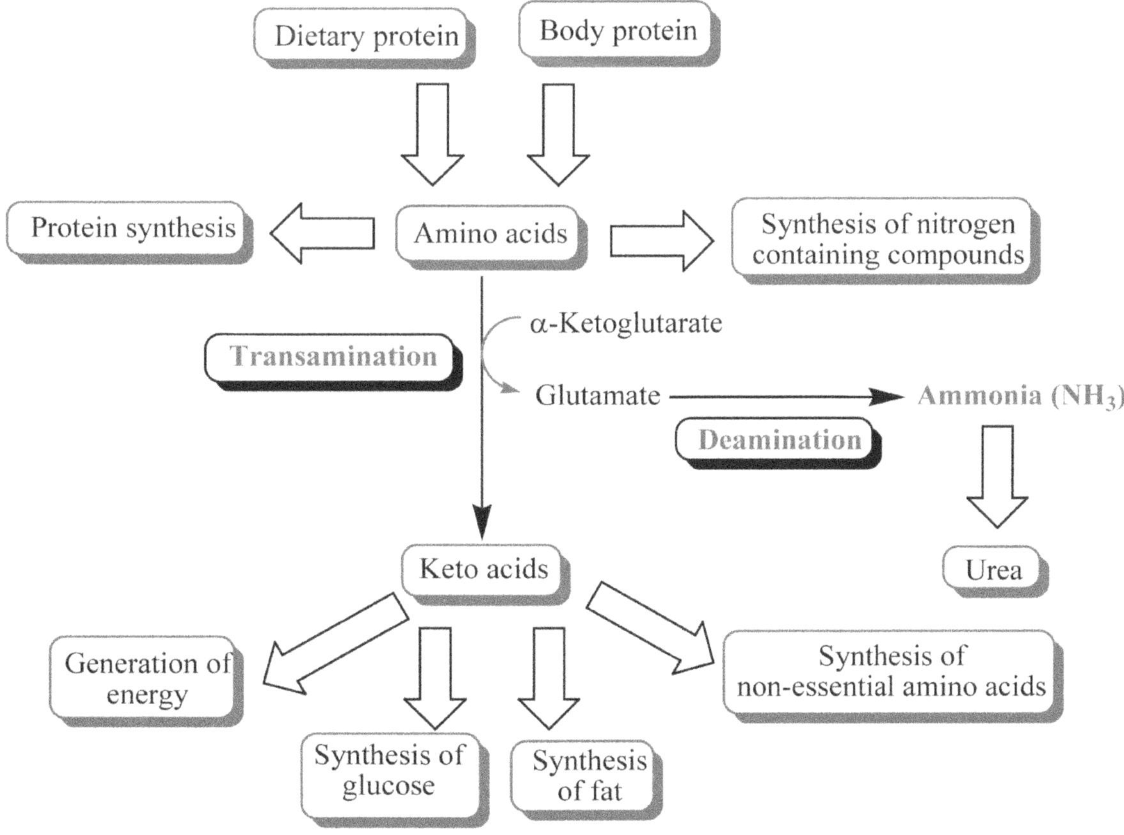

Figure 5.8 Overview of amino acid metabolism.

Transamination

Definition:

Transamination is defined as the transfer of amino (NH_2) group from amino acids to keto acids. Transamination takes place in the presence of the enzyme known as *transaminase* or *aminotransferase* (In transfer involved reactions the enzymes acted are "*transferase*" and the substrate is "amine"). *Transaminase* enzyme needs pyridoxal phosphate (PLP) as co-enzyme. Transamination involves the inter conversion of pair of amino acids and a pair of keto acids.

Transamination

Amino acid - I + Keto acid - II ⇌ Amino acid - II + Keto acid - I
(*Transaminase* or *Aminotransferase*; Pyridoxal phosphate (PLP))

$R_1-CH(NH_2)-COOH$ (**Amino acid - I**) + $R_2-C(=O)-COOH$ (**Keto acid - II**) ⇌ $R_1-C(=O)-COOH$ (**Keto acid - I**) + $R_2-CH(NH_2)-COOH$ (**Amino acid - II**)

(**Transamination**; *Transaminase*; Pyridoxal phosphate (PLP))

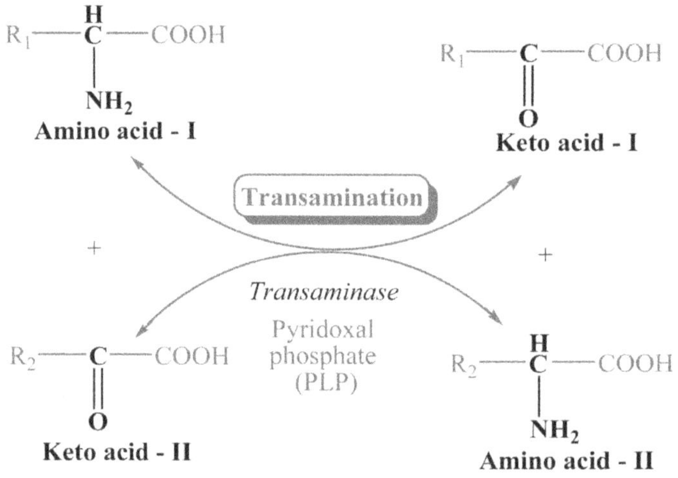

Most important features:

1. Generally, transamination reactions are reversible in nature.
2. No free ammonia (NH_3) is liberated in transamination reaction and only amino groups are transferred from one amino acid to other keto acid.
3. For each pair of amino acids and keto acids specific *transaminase* enzyme exists. Out of several *transaminase* known only two namely *aspartate transaminase (AST)* and *alanine transaminase (ALT)* made significant contribution for transamination reactions.
4. Except lysine, threonine, proline and hydroxyproline, rest all amino acids undergo transamination reaction.
5. Based on the need of cell, transamination reaction is useful for the synthesis of non-essential amino acids and for redistribution of amino groups.
6. Both synthesis (anabolism) and degradation (catabolism) of amino acids are involved in transamination reactions.
7. Some of the *transaminase* enzymes are useful clinically for the diagnosis of various diseases. **Example:** *SGPT (Serum glutamate pyruvate transaminase)* is useful for diagnosis of liver diseases and *SGOT (Serum glutamate oxaloacetate transaminase)* is useful for diagnosis of heart diseases.
8. A vitamin B_6 or pyridoxine derived co-enzyme pyridoxal phosphate (PLP) is required for the activity of all *transaminases*.
9. Excess amino acids are diverted for the production of energy by transamination reactions.

10. The nitrogen of amino acids is finally concentrated as glutamate through transamination reactions. Glutamate is the only amino acid which liberates free ammonia for the synthesis of urea by oxidative deamination reaction.
11. Transamination reactions is not only restricted for α-amino groups. δ-amino group of ornithine may also undergo transamination.

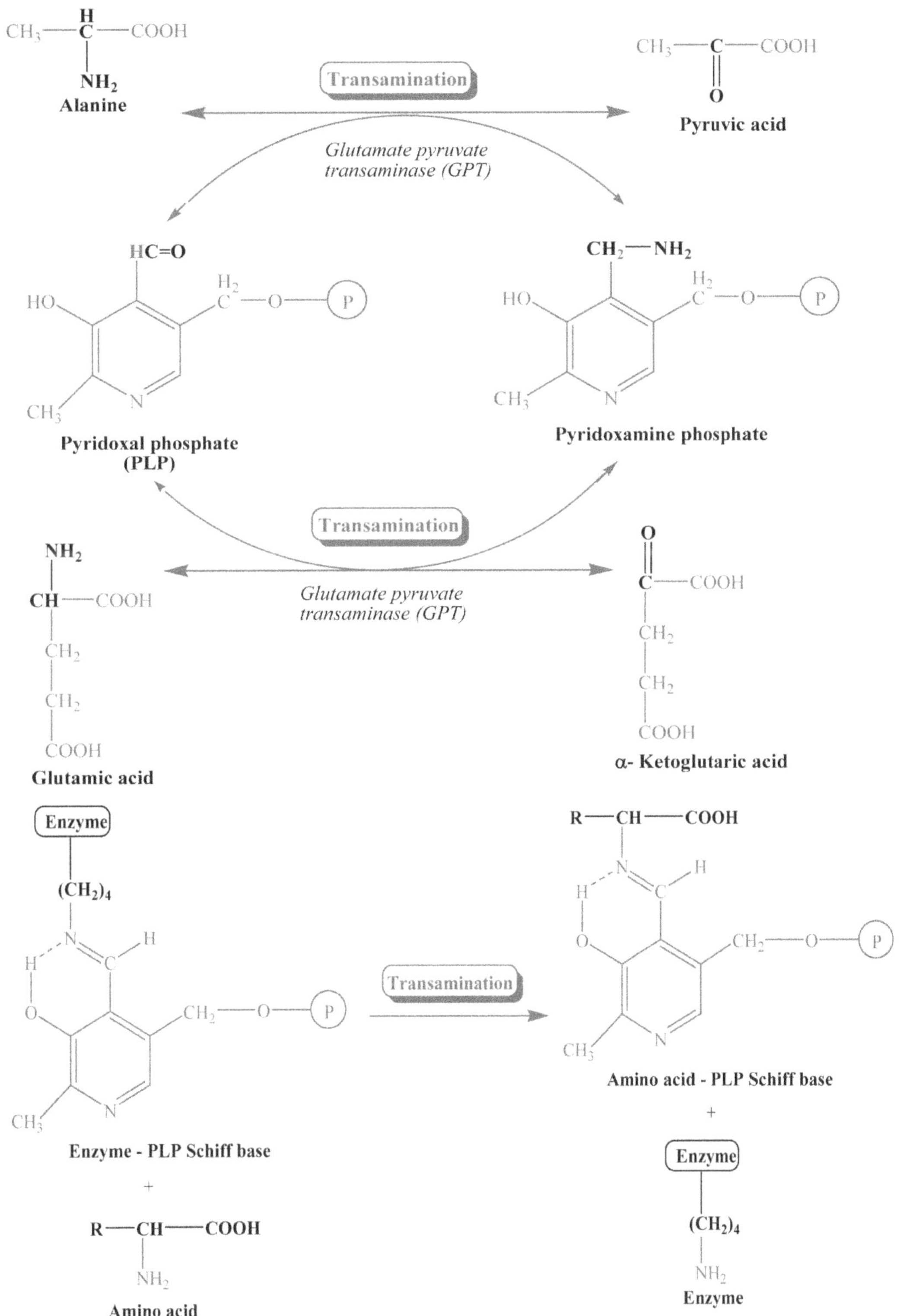

Mechanism:

Two steps are involved in the transamination.

Step 1: In the first step, pyridoxamine phosphate is formed from enzyme bounded co-enzyme pyridoxal phosphate (PLP) by transfer of amino group from amino acid.

Step 2: In second step, new amino acid is produced by transfer of amino group of pyridoxamine phosphate to a keto acid and the co-enzyme pyridoxal phosphate (PLP) is regenerated.

At the active site of *transaminase* enzyme, the aldehyde group of pyridoxal phosphate (PLP) is linked with ε-amino group of lysine residue through imine linkage (Schiff base). When amino acid (substrate) approaches the *transaminase* (enzyme) a new imine linkage (Schiff base) is formed by displacing the lysine residue. By non-covalent forces this amino acid PLP Schiff base complex tightly binds with the *transaminase* (enzyme). Later keto acid is liberated and pyridoxamine phosphate linked with enzyme is formed. From the enzyme linked pyridoxamine phosphate new amino acid is produced by reacting with keto acid in the same manner through imine linkage (Schiff base) reaction.

Deamination

Deamination is defined as removal of amino group from amino acid as ammonia and results in formation of corresponding keto acids. The enzyme responsible for deamination is *deaminase* (In removal reactions the enzymes acted are "*de*" and the substrate is "amine"). The liberated ammonia is utilized for the production of urea. Meanwhile carbon skeleton of amino acid is converted to keto acid.

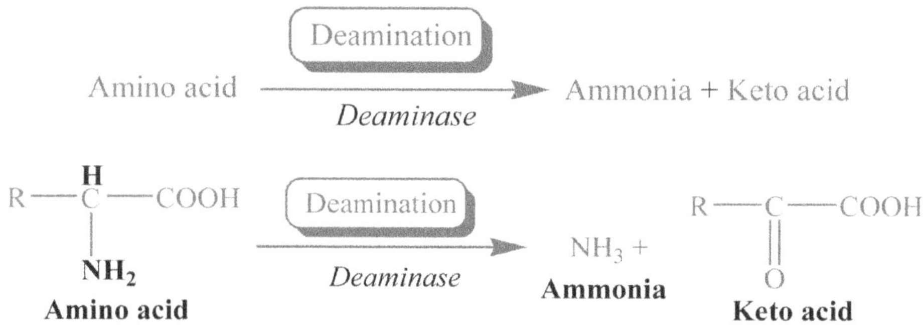

Generally, transamination and deamination occur simultaneously with glutamate as the central molecule. Hence transamination and deamination involving glutamate is commonly known as **trans deamination**. Deamination is broadly classified into two major reactions as 1) Oxidative deamination, 2) Non-oxidative deamination.

1. **Oxidative deamination:**

   In this type, the amino group of amino acid is lost as ammonia coupled with oxidation. This is a major type of deamination reaction. Glutamate is the only substrate which undergoes oxidative deamination reaction. It takes place mainly in liver and kidney and the purpose is to provide ammonia for urea synthesis and keto acids for many reactions particularly energy production.

   ***Glutamate dehydrogenase (GDH)*:** Most of amino acids transfer its amino group to α-ketoglutarate and produce glutamate through transamination. Hence in biological systems glutamate is called as collection centre for amino groups. This glutamate rapidly releases free ammonia by oxidative deamination in presence of enzyme called *glutamate dehydrogenase (GDH)* (In NAD^+ or $NADP^+$ involved reactions the enzymes acted are "*dehydrogenase*" and the substrate is "glutamate") and also produces α-ketoglutarate. The unique feature of *glutamate dehydrogenase (GDH)* is it can use either NAD^+ or $NADP^+$ as co-enzyme. The α-iminoglutarate is formed as intermediate during the conversion of glutamate to α-ketoglutarate by oxidative deamination.

The *glutamate dehydrogenase (GDH)* catalyzed reaction is reversible and it linked with TCA cycle through α-ketoglutarate. In both anabolic and catabolic reactions *glutamate dehydrogenase (GDH)* is involved. *Glutamate dehydrogenase (GDH)* is complex mitochondrial enzyme containing zinc and six identical units with 56,000 as molecular weight each. It is allosterically regulated (GTP and ATP inhibits and GDP and ADP activate). It is also inhibited by hormones like steroid and thyroid hormone. Liver glutamate level is increased after protein rich meal and it is converted to α-ketoglutarate and free ammonia. The degradation of glutamate is increased when the cellular energy is low to provide α-ketoglutarate to citric acid cycle for production of energy.

COOH–CH_2–CH_2–H–C–NH_2–COOH (**Glutamate**) ⇌ [NAD^+ or $NADP^+$ → NADH + H^+ or NADPH + H^+; Reduction; *Glutamate dehydrogenase (GDH)*] ⇌ COOH–CH_2–CH_2–C=**NH**–COOH (**α-Imino glutarate**) ⇌ [**H_2O** → NH_3; Deamination; *Glutamate dehydrogenase (GDH)*] ⇌ COOH–CH_2–CH_2–C=O–COOH (**α-Keto glutarate**)

***Amino acid oxidase (AAO)*:** FMN and FAD are present in flavoprotein namely *L-amino acid oxidase* and *D-amino acid oxidase*. These enzymes act on the corresponding amino acids and produces ammonia and α-keto acids. Oxygen is reduced in this reaction to hydrogen peroxide which is decomposed by *catalase*. Mostly in tissues like liver and kidney the activity of *D-amino acid oxidase* is high and *L-amino acid oxidase* is low. Hence *L-amino acid oxidase* do not act on dicarboxylic acid and glycine and also do not play any significant role in amino acid metabolism.

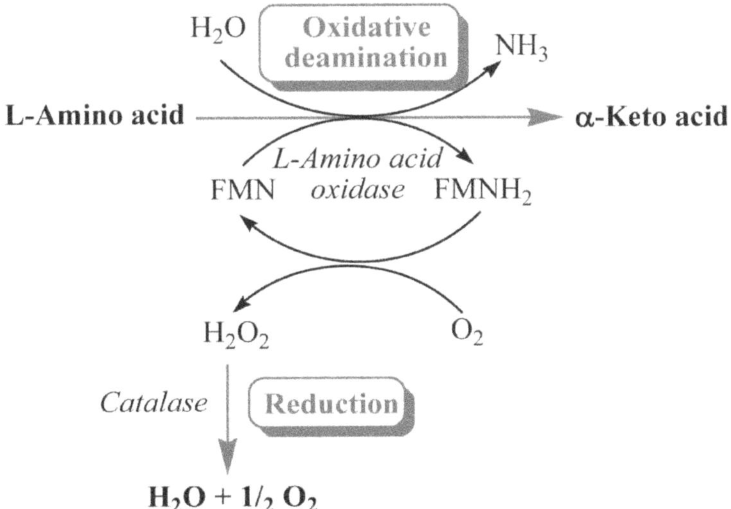

D-Amino acids are mainly present in microorganisms, plants and not present in mammalian proteins. However, D-amino acids regularly taken in the diet are metabolized by biological systems. By oxidative deamination D-amino acids are converted to corresponding α-keto acids with liberation of ammonia. This α-keto acid produces L-amino acid by transamination. The produced L-amino acid takes part in many metabolic reactions. The α-keto acid formed serves as a precursor for the synthesis of glucose and fat and also oxidized to produce energy. Hence in the body *D-amino acid oxidase* plays an important role in the conversion of unnatural D-amino acid to L-amino acid.

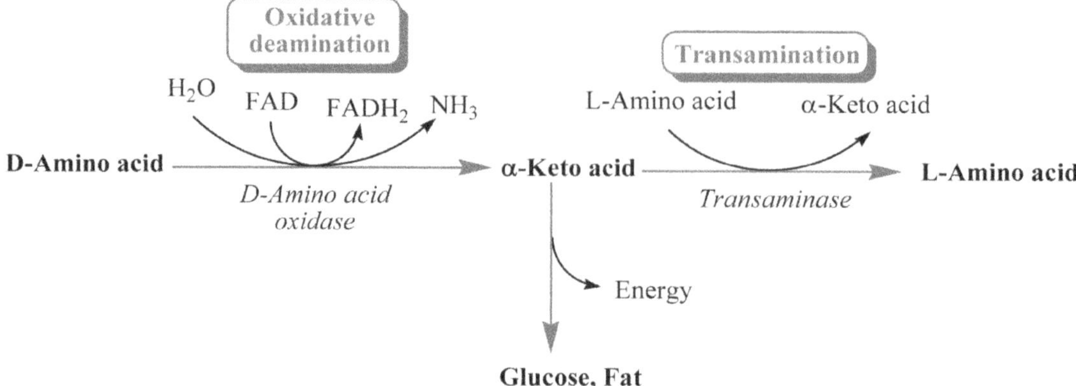

Glycine oxidase: Glycine undergoes oxidative deamination and produce glyoxylic acid in presence of *glycine oxidase* which is NADPH dependent enzyme.

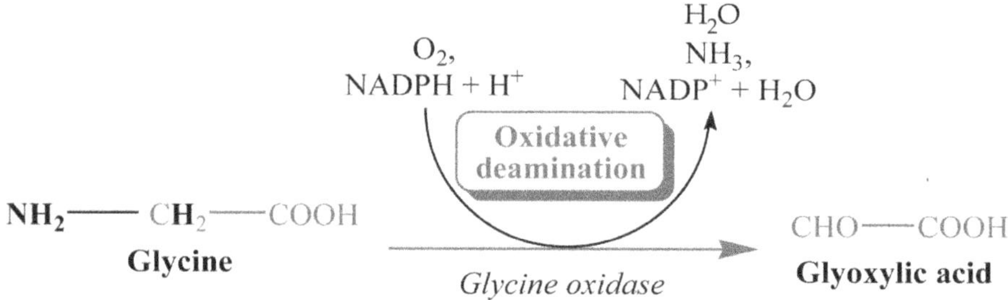

2. **Non-oxidative Deamination:** In this amino group is removed from amino acid without oxidation; hence it is known as non-oxidative deamination.

   Amino acid dehydratase: The hydroxyl (OH) group containing amino acids such as serine, homoserine and threonine undergo non-oxidative deamination in the presence of *dehydratase* enzyme (Type of reaction involved is "dehydration"). This enzyme is dependent on pyridoxal phosphate (PLP).

   Serine or Homoserine or Threonine —(Dehydration; *Dehydratase*, PLP; $-NH_3$)→ **Corresponding α-keto acids**

   Amino acid desulfhydrase: The sulphur (S) group containing amino acids such as cysteine and homocysteine undergo non-oxidative deamination coupled with desulfhydration in presence of *desulfhydrase* enzyme (Type of reaction involved is "desulfhydration").

   Desulfhydration

   SH—CH_2—**CH**(NH_2)—COOH (**Cysteine**) —(H_2O; *Desulfhydrase*; $NH_3 + H_2S$)→ CH_3—C(=O)—COOH (**Pyruvate**)

   Histidase: Histidine undergoes non-oxidative deamination in presence of *histidase* enzyme (Substrate is "histidine") and produce uroconate.

Histidine → (Non-oxidative deamination; Histidase; $-NH_3$) → Uroconate

Decarboxylation

Decarboxylation is defined as removal of carboxyl group from amino acid as carbondioxide results in formation of corresponding amines. The enzyme responsible for decarboxylation is *decarboxylase* (Type of reaction involved is "decarboxylation"). Like *transaminase, decarboxylase* also needs pyridoxal phosphate (PLP) as co-enzyme.

Amino acid → (Decarboxylation; *Decarboxylase*; Pyridoxal phosphate (PLP); $-CO_2$) → **Primary amine**

$R-CH(COOH)-NH_2$ (**Amino acid**) → (Decarboxylation; *Decarboxylase*; Pyridoxal phosphate (PLP); $-CO_2$) → $R-CH_2-NH_2$ (**Primary amine**)

Histamine: The biologically important biogenic amine "histamine" is biosynthesized in biological system by decarboxylation in presence of *histidine decarboxylase* (Substrate is "histidine" and the type of reaction involved is "decarboxylation").

Histidine → (Decarboxylation; *Histidine decarboxylase*; Pyridoxal phosphate (PLP); $-CO_2$) → **Histamine**

Tyramine: Aromatic amino acid tyrosine undergoes decarboxylation in presence of *tyrosine decarboxylase* (Substrate is "tyrosine" and the type of reaction involved is "decarboxylation") and produces tyramine.

Tyrosine → (Decarboxylation; *Tyrosine decarboxylase*; Pyridoxal phosphate (PLP); $-CO_2$) → **Tyramine**

Urea Cycle or Kreb's-Henseleit Cycle

The end excretory product of amino acid or protein metabolism is urea. The ammonia produced through transamination and oxidative deamination by nitrogen of amino acids are toxic to the biological system. Hence, it is detoxified by converting into urea. Among various nitrogen containing substances excreted in urine, 80 to 90 % are accounted by urea only. It is the first metabolic cycle discovered in the year 1932 by Hans Krebs and Kurt Henseleit.

Urea cycle is defined as a series of chemical reactions occurring in biological system to convert toxic ammonia to urea. Urea cycle is very important metabolic cycle because it directly removes the toxic ammonia into urea. Urea synthesis takes place in liver and transported to kidney for excretion in urine.

$$\underset{\textbf{Ammonia (Toxic)}}{NH_3} + \underset{\textbf{Carbondioxide}}{CO_2} \xrightarrow{\text{Liver}} \underset{\text{Urea}}{NH_2-\overset{\overset{\large O}{\|}}{C}-NH_2}$$

Pathway:

Urea contains two amino groups and one carbonyl group. The sources of two amino and carbonyl group are as follows:

1. One amino group is derived from ammonia.
2. Carbonyl group is derived from carbondioxide.
3. Another amino group is derived from amino acid aspartate.

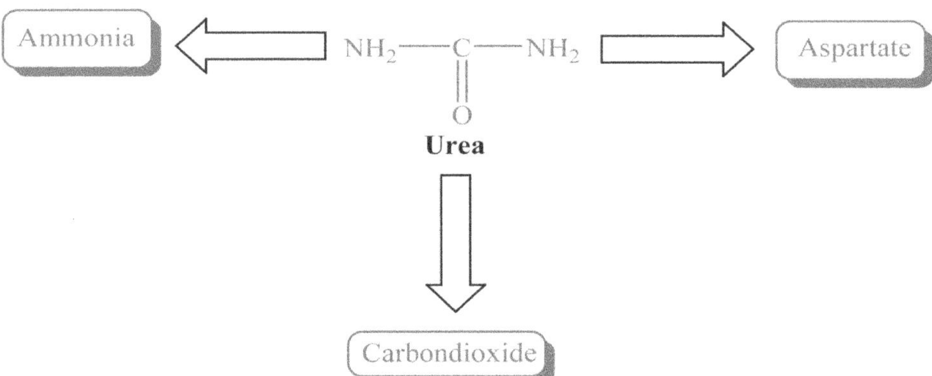

There are five important metabolic reactions in urea cycle with five distinguished enzymes. Out of that first two enzymes are present in mitochondria whereas rests of three enzymes are present in cytosol.

1. *Cabomoyl phosphate synthase – I (CPS-I)* (Product formed is "carbamoyl phosphate" and the type of reaction involved is "synthesis") present in mitochondria condense the toxic ammonia and carbon dioxide into carbamoyl phosphate. Ammonia and carbon dioxide needed for this step is obtained from trans deamination and TCA cycle, respectively. **It is a rate limiting enzyme of urea cycle** and this reaction is irreversible. Hence, ***CPS-I* regulates urea cycle**. *CPS-II* is an enzyme involved in the synthesis of pyrimidine nucleus. *CPS-I* needs N-acetylglutamate (NAG) for its activity whereas *CPS-II* doesn't need NAG for its activity. The first amino group and carboxyl group are incorporated in this step. 2 ATPs are converted into 2 ADP and one inorganic phosphate & other phosphate are taken by carbamoyl group **(2 ATP is utilized).**
2. Carbamoyl phosphate then reacts with ornithine and produce citrulline in presence of *ornithine trans carbamoylase* (Substrate is "ornithine" and the type of reaction involved is "transfer of carbamoyl group"). This reaction is similar to **aldol condensation** and takes place in mitochondria only. **Ornithine plays a catalytic role in urea cycle** as it is later regenerated (Like oxaloacetate in TCA cycle). Then,

formed citrulline is transported from mitochondria to cytosol by transporter system. Both ornithine and citrulline are basic amino acids.

3. In third step, aspartate is reacting with citrulline by dehydration condensation and produce argininosuccinate. The reaction is catalyzed by the enzyme *argininosuccinate synthase* (Product formed is "argininosuccinate" and the type of reaction involved is hydrolysis [in reverse manner]). Aspartate needed for this step is obtained from TCA cycle. In this step, the second amino group of urea is incorporated. One ATP is breakdown into AMP and pyrophosphate and the latter one is immediately breakdown into two inorganic phosphate by *pyrophosphatase* (Substrate is "pyrophosphate" and the type of reaction involved is "hydrolysis") **[2 ATP is utilized].**

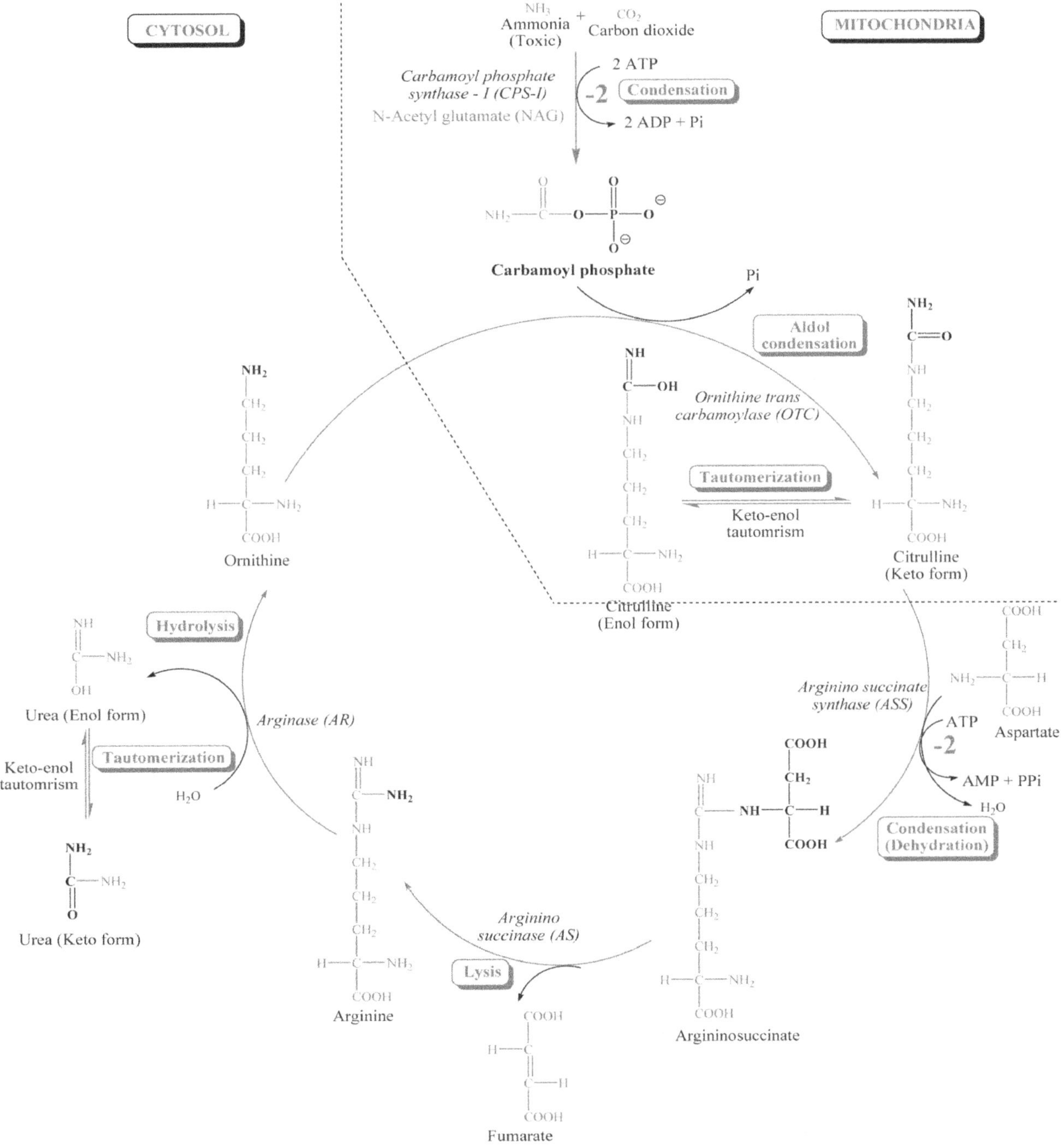

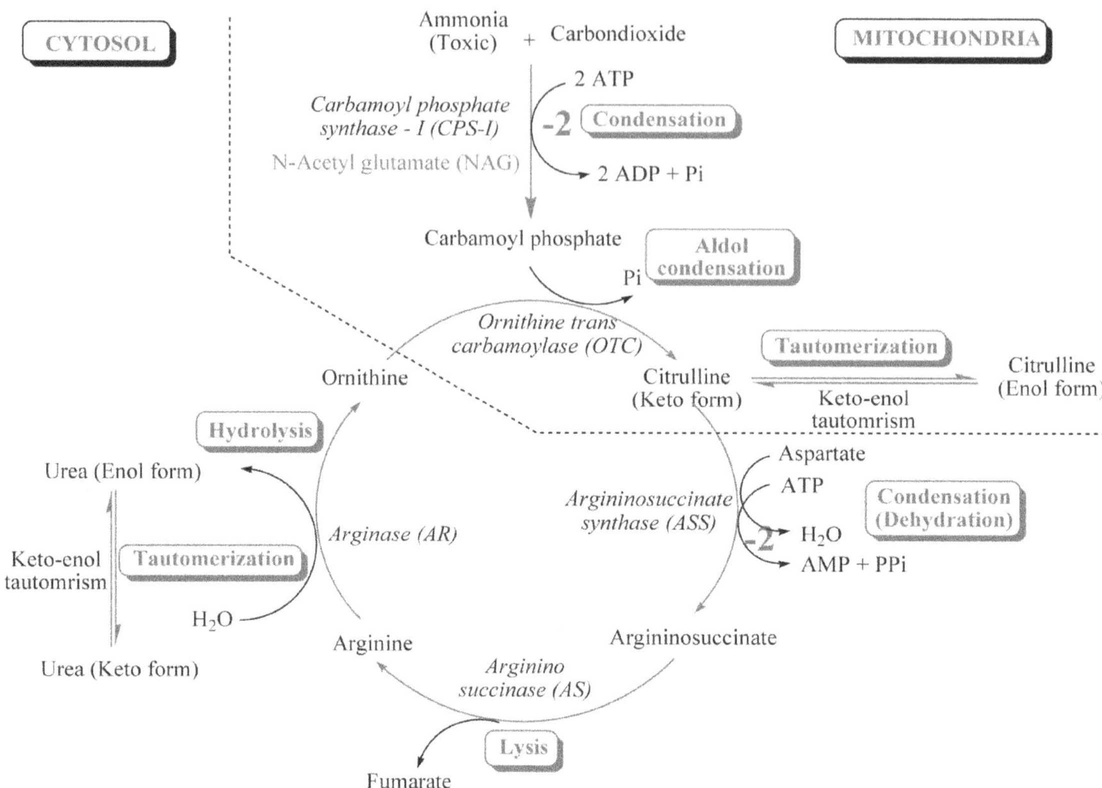

4. In the next step, argininosuccinate is cleaved into arginine and fumarate in presence of *argininosuccinase* (Substrate is "argininosuccinate" and the type of reaction involved is "lysis or cleavage"). Fumarate liberated in this step is entering into TCA cycle, gluconeogenesis, etc.
5. In last step, ornithine is regenerated with production of urea when arginine is hydrolyzed in presence of *arginase* (Substrate is "arginine" and the type of reaction involved is "hydrolysis"). Regenerated ornithine enters into mitochondria for its reuse in urea cycle. Co^{2+} and Mn^{2+} activates *arginase* enzyme.

Except *arginase* all other four enzymes of urea cycle is present in all tissues. *Arginase* is mainly present in liver only. Hence, in many tissues arginine synthesis may occur in varying degree but in liver only it can ultimately converted into urea. The first two enzymes of urea cycle are present in mitochondria whereas the rest of three enzymes are present in cytosol part of the cell. Urea cycle is irreversible in nature and totally for the synthesis of one urea molecule 4 ATPs are utilized (2 ATP in first step and another 2 ATP in third step). The overall reactions of urea cycle can be written as follows.

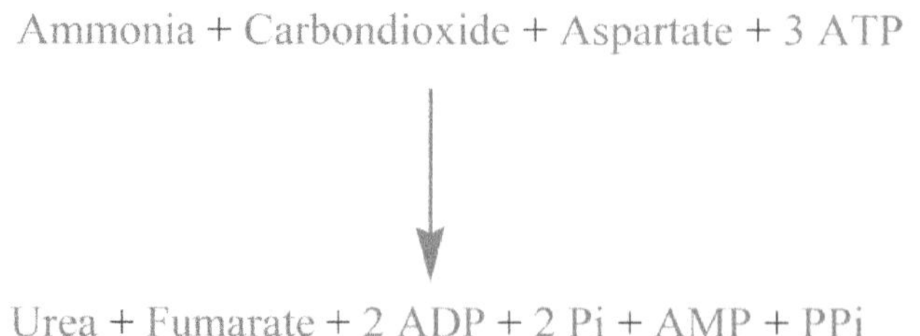

Disposal of urea: Urea synthesized in liver is freely diffused and transported in blood to kidney and excreted in urine. A small quantity of the urea may be absorbed and enter into the intestine where it is broken down into ammonia and carbondioxide by bacterial enzyme *urease* (Substrate is "urea" and the type of reaction involved is "hydrolysis"). The formed ammonia is either absorbed in the blood or excreted in feces. Uremia is a condition in which blood urea is increased due to diffusion of more urea in intestine during renal failure. Generally, kidney failure may lead to hyperammonemia. To kill the intestinal bacteria, antibiotics particularly neomycin is administered to these patients.

$$\underset{\textbf{Urea}}{NH_2-\overset{\displaystyle O}{\overset{\|}{C}}-NH_2} + H_2O \xrightarrow[\text{Urease}]{\text{Hydrolysis}} \underset{\textbf{Ammonia}}{2\,NH_3} + \underset{\textbf{Carbondioxide}}{CO_2}$$

Regulation of urea cycle:

Cabomoyl phosphate synthase – I (CPS-I) is the rate limiting enzyme in urea cycle and it is activated by N-acetyl glutamate (NAG). From glutamate and acetyl CoA, N-acetyl glutamate (NAG) is synthesized by *N-acetyl glutamate (NAG) synthase* (Substrate is "N-acetyl glutamate" and the type of reaction involved is "synthesis") and N-acetyl glutamate (NAG) is degraded by *N-acetyl glutamate (NAG) hydrolase* (Substrate is "N-acetyl glutamate" and the type of reaction involved is "hydrolysis"). Rate of urea synthesis is directly proportional to concentration of N-acetyl glutamate (NAG). Arginine and protein rich meal increases N-acetyl glutamate (NAG) in liver leads to increased synthesis of urea. *Cabomoyl phosphate synthase – I (CPS-I)* and *glutamate dehydrogenase (GDH)* are restricted in mitochondria and coordinate with each other for the synthesis of ammonia and its utilization for the production of urea. Mostly, respective substrates control the remaining four enzymes of urea cycle.

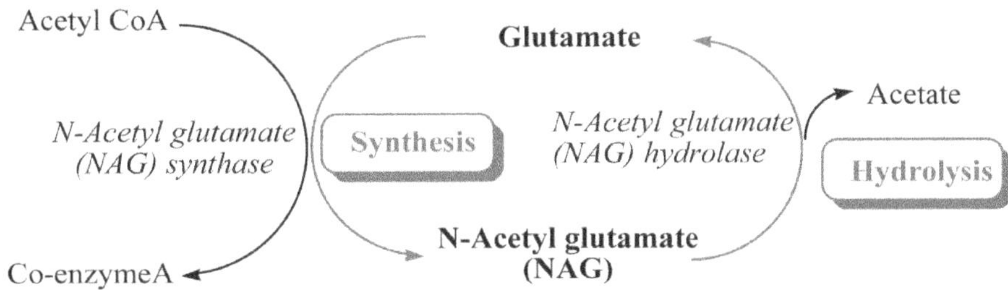

Relationship between urea cycle and TCA cycle:

In three different ways urea cycle is linked with TCA cycle. This is known as bicyclic integration between urea and TCA cycle.

1. In urea cycle the most important integrating point of TCA cycle is liberation of fumarate. Later the liberated fumarate is converted into malate followed by oxaloacetate. Aspartate is produced from oxaloacetate by transamination. Oxaloacetate is important metabolite which can combine with acetyl CoA to form citrate and oxidized finally. For the synthesis of glucose, oxaloacetate may also serve as a precursor (Gluconeogenesis). In urea cycle aspartate combines with citrulline and produce argininosuccinate.
2. In TCA cycle 12 ATPs are generated whereas in urea cycle 4 ATPs are utilized.
3. Various metabolites are completely oxidized into carbondioxide in TCA cycle. In the mitochondria carbondioxide produced in TCA cycle is utilized in urea cycle.

Metabolic disorders of urea cycle:

In the Table 5.2. metabolic disorders associated with the five enzymes of urea cycle are summarized. The clinical symptoms associated with urea cycle metabolic disorders are vomiting, lethargy, irritability, ataxia and mental retardation. Blood ammonia level is increased invariably in all the disorders which leads to toxicity. The other metabolites also accumulate depending on the specific enzyme defects.

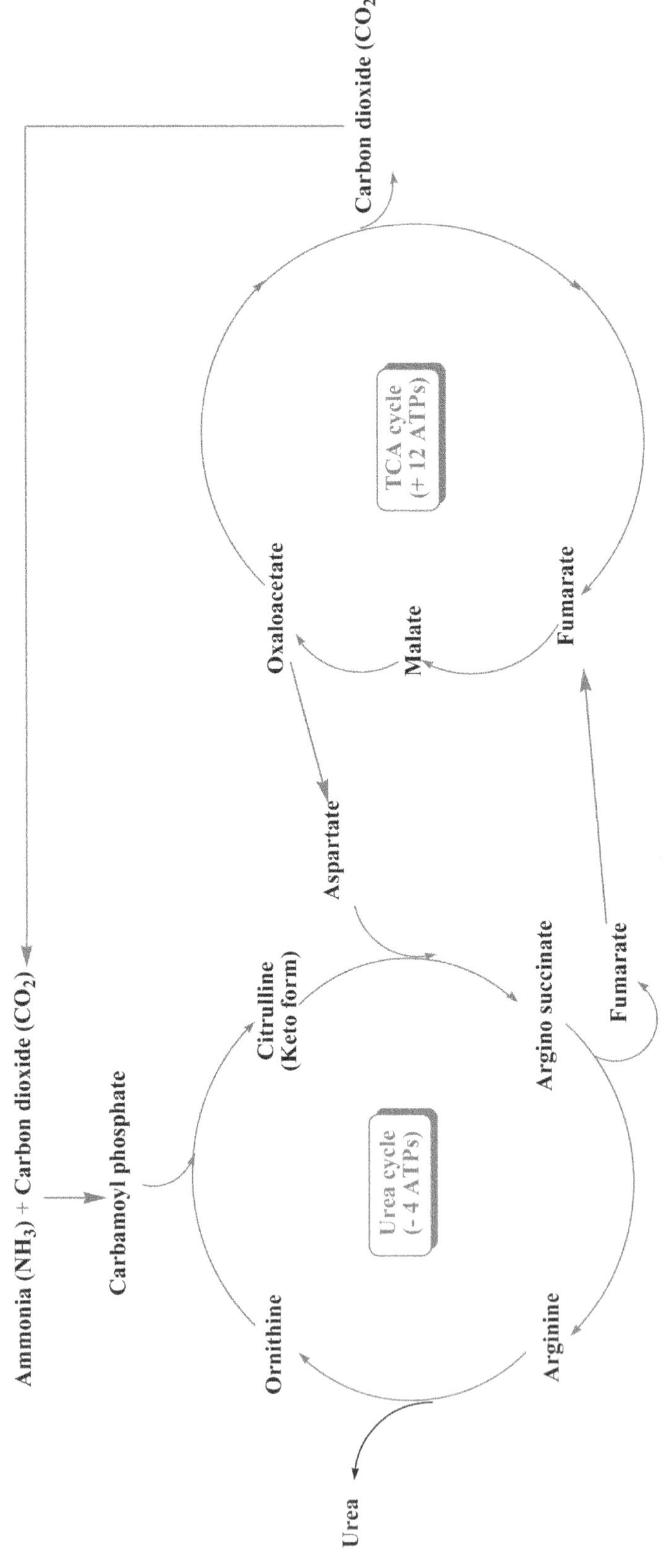
Ammonia (NH_3) + Carbon dioxide (CO_2)
Carbamoyl phosphate
Citrulline (Keto form)
Urea cycle (- 4 ATPs)
Ornithine
Urea
Arginine
Argino succinate
Fumarate
Aspartate
Oxaloacetate
Malate
Fumarate
TCA cycle (+ 12 ATPs)
Carbon dioxide (CO_2)

Table 5.2 Metabolic disorders of urea cycle.

S. No.	Metabolic disorder name	Characteristics	Enzyme responsible
1	Hyperammonemia type -I	Increased ammonia level in blood	*Carbamoyl phosphate synthase – I (CPS-I)*
2	Hyperammonemia type - II	Increased ammonia level in blood	*Ornithine trans carbamoylase (OTC)*
3	Citrullinemia	Increased citrulline level in blood	*Argininosuccinate synthase (ASS)*
4	Argininosuccinic aciduria	Increased argininosuccinate level in blood	*Argininosuccinase (AS)*
5	Hyperargininemia	Increased arginine level in blood	*Arginase (AR)*

Importance of blood urea: The normal serum urea ranges from 20 to 45 mg/100 ml and 15 to 30 g of urea (7 to 15 g of nitrogen) is excreted in urine per day. Generally, blood urea estimation is used to assess the functions of kidney. In renal failure or dysfunction, the blood urea level is elevated than the normal. The serum urea level is highly influenced by dietary protein. High protein diet increases serum urea level, whereas low protein diet decreases serum urea level. In general, serum urea level is increased in various renal diseases like glomerulonephritis, pyelonephritis, renal tuberculosis, renal carcinoma, polycystic kidneys, etc. In addition, urinary tract obstruction, dehydration, shock, hematemesis and increased tissue breakdown may also increases serum urea levels. Serum urea is decreased in acute hepatic insufficiency. During first and second trimester of pregnancy a slight decrease in serum urea occurs.

Metabolism of Phenylalanine and Tyrosine

Phenylalanine and tyrosine are aromatic amino acids which are structurally related because tyrosine is chemically *p*-hydroxyphenylalanine. Out of these two amino acids phenylalanine is essential amino acid and tyrosine is non-essential amino acid because tyrosine is biosynthesized from phenylalanine. Overview of phenylalanine and tyrosine metabolism is presented in Figure 5.9.

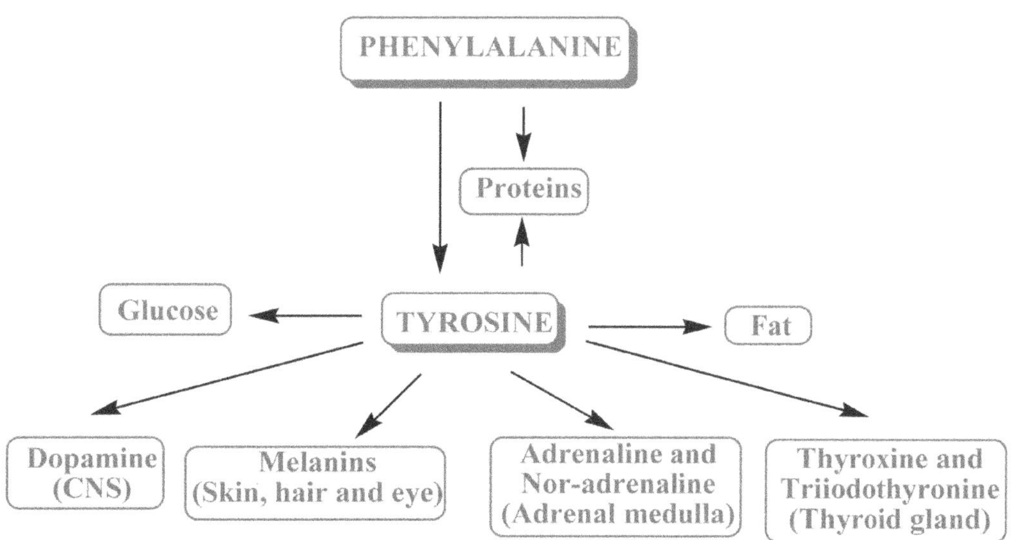

Figure 5.9 Overview of phenylalanine & tyrosine metabolism.

The major functions of phenylalanine is biosynthesis of tyrosine and incorporation into proteins. Tyrosine is involved in incorporation of proteins and synthesis of some different biologically important compounds such as a) Melanin (in skin, hair and eye), b) Dopamine (in CNS), c) Adrenaline and nor-adrenaline (in adrenal medulla), d) Thyroxine and triiodothyronine (in thyroid gland) e) Glucose & fat. Ingestion of tyrosine reduces dietary requirement of phenylalanine is referred as **sparing action of tyrosine and phenylalanine**. Tyrosine is both glucogenic and ketogenic amino acid because metabolites of tyrosine serves as a precursor for the synthesis of glucose and fat.

Degradation of Phenylalanine & Tyrosine

Phenylalanine and tyrosine metabolism are considered together. These amino acids are degraded into fumarate and acetoacetate which is a precursor for the synthesis of carbohydrates and fats, respectively. The various reactions involved in this degradation are described here.

1. Initially, phenylalanine is converted into tyrosine by hydroxylation or oxidation at aromatic carbon atom in the presence of *phenylalanine hydroxylase* (The substrate is "phenylalanine" and the type of reaction involved is "hydroxylation"). In this reaction, one mole of oxygen is involved. In that one of the oxygen atoms is incorporated in phenylalanine at *para* position and the another oxygen atom coupled with two hydrogen atoms of tetrahydrobiopterin are removed as water molecule. The tetrahydrobiopterin is converted into dihydrobiopterin as it loses two hydrogen atoms.
2. In the next step, tyrosine undergoes transamination reaction by reacting with α-ketoglutarate and produces *p*-hydroxyphenylpyruvate in presence of *tyrosine transaminase* (The substrate is "tyrosine" and the type of reaction involved is "transamination") & liberates glutamate. *Tyrosine transaminase* needs PLP (pyridoxal phosphate) as co-enzyme.
3. *p*-Hydroxyphenylpyruvate undergoes oxidative decarboxylation (oxidation at ortho position of phenyl ring and side chain) to produce homogentisate in presence of copper containing enzyme *p-hydroxyphenylpyruvate dioxygenase or p-hydroxyphenylpyruvate hydroxylase* (The substrate is "*p*-hydroxyphenylpyruvate" and the type of reaction involved is "hydroxylation"). During this reaction carboxyl group is removed as carbondioxide results in corresponding aldehyde which is further oxidized to carboxylic acid. In addition, one mole of oxygen is involved in this reaction. In that one of the oxygen atoms is incorporated in phenylalanine at *ortho* position and the other oxygen atom coupled with two hydrogen atoms of ascorbic acid and removed as water molecule. The ascorbic acid is converted into dehydroascorbic acid as it loses two hydrogen atoms. In the mean time *para* hydroxyl group of *p*-hydroxyphenylpyruvate is transferred to *meta* position (C-5) in order to get stable configuration.
4. 4-Maleylacetoacetate is produced from homogentisate by oxidative ring cleavage reaction and the reaction is catalyzed by iron containing enzyme "*homogentisate oxidase*" (The substrate is "homogentisate" and the type of reaction involved is "oxidation" with incorporation of both oxygen of molecular oxygen). The benzene ring is opened between C-1 and C-2 and produce dicarboxylic acid derivatives.
5. In the next step 4-fumarylacetoacetate is produced from 4-maleylacetoacetate by isomerization and the reaction takes place in the presence of *4-maleylacetoacetate isomerase* (The substrate is "4-maleylacetoacetate" and the type of reaction involved is "isomerization").
6. 4-Fumarylacetoacetate is hydrolyzed in the next step and produces fumarate and acetoacetate. The reaction is catalyzed by *4-fumarylacetoacetate hydroxylase* (The substrate is "4-fumarylacetoacetate" and the type of reaction involved is "hydrolysis").
7. In TCA cycle, fumarate is one of the intermediate and also it serves as a precursor for gluconeogenesis for the synthesis of glucose. The ketone body acetoacetate is used as a precursor for the synthesis of fat.

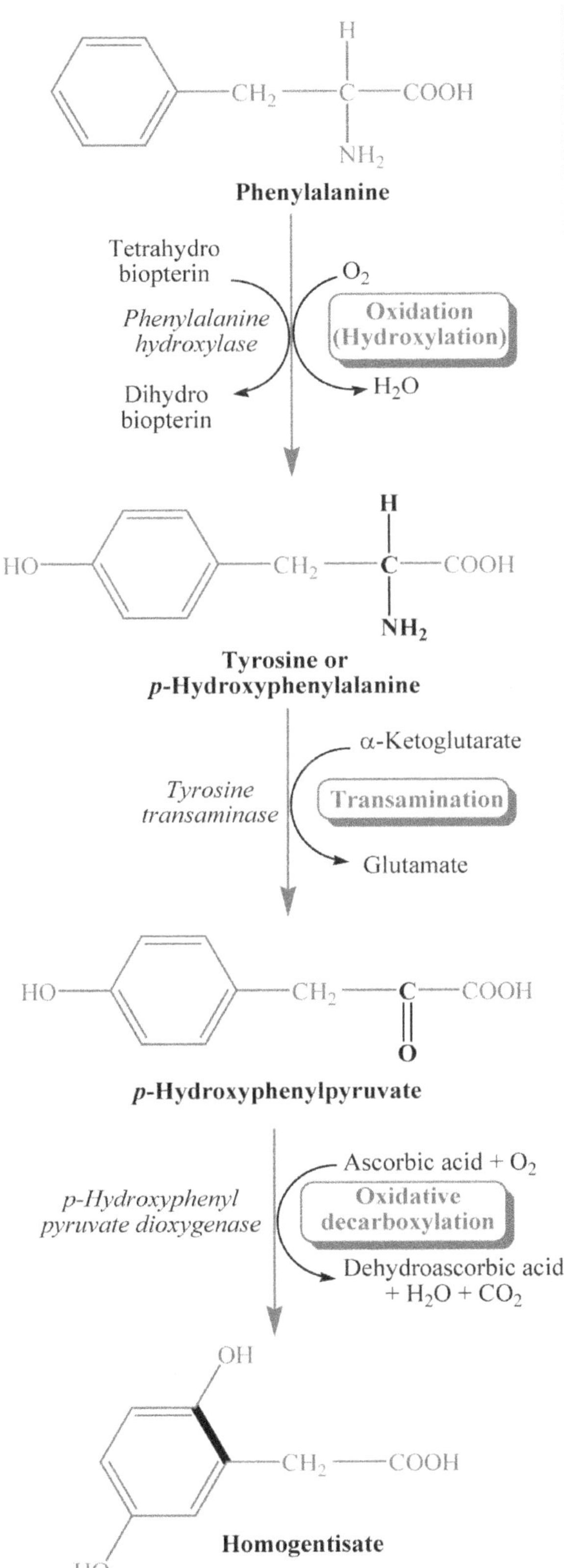
Phenylalanine
Tetrahydro biopterin
O_2
Phenylalanine hydroxylase
Oxidation (Hydroxylation)
Dihydro biopterin
H_2O
Tyrosine or p-Hydroxyphenylalanine
α-Ketoglutarate
Tyrosine transaminase
Transamination
Glutamate
p-Hydroxyphenylpyruvate
Ascorbic acid + O_2
p-Hydroxyphenyl pyruvate dioxygenase
Oxidative decarboxylation
Dehydroascorbic acid + H_2O + CO_2
Homogentisate

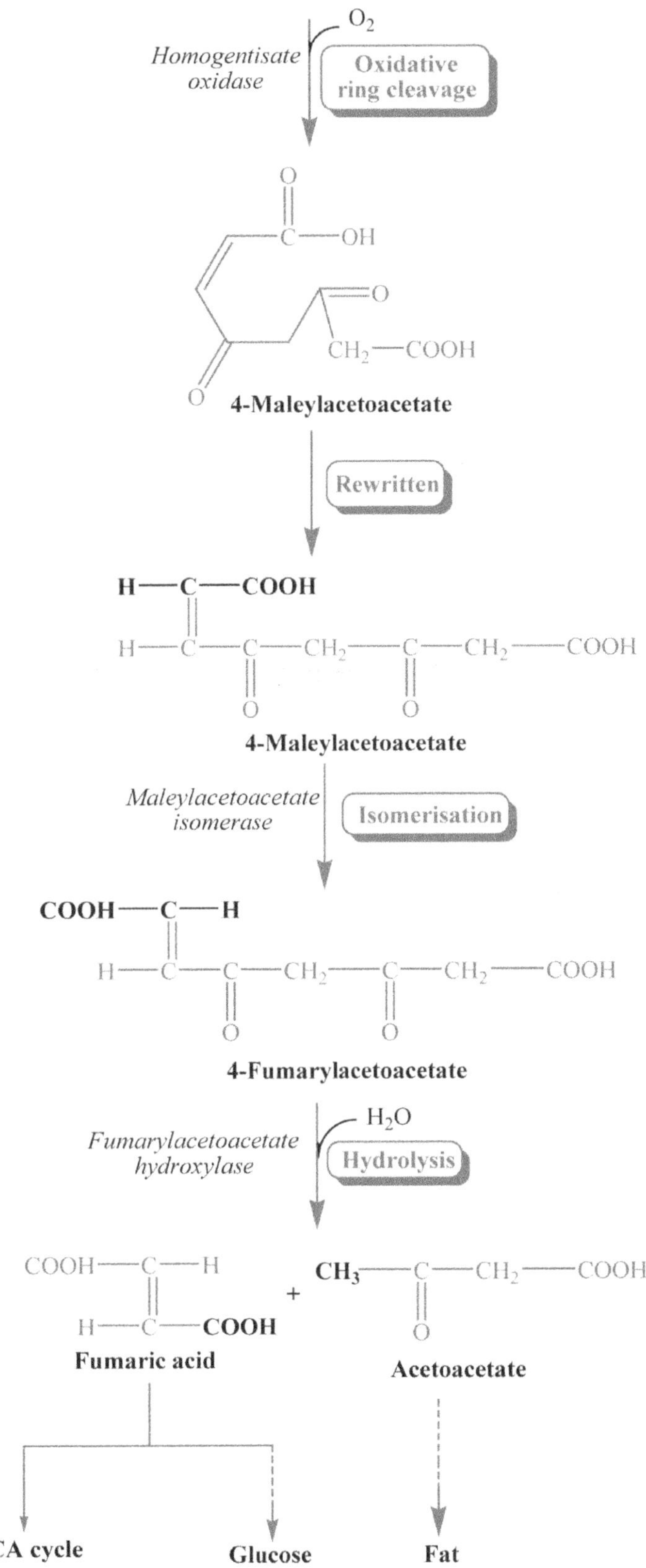
O_2
Homogentisate oxidase
Oxidative ring cleavage
4-Maleylacetoacetate
Rewritten
4-Maleylacetoacetate
Maleylacetoacetate isomerase
Isomerisation
4-Fumarylacetoacetate
H_2O
Fumarylacetoacetate hydroxylase
Hydrolysis
Fumaric acid
Acetoacetate
TCA cycle
Glucose
Fat

Phenylalanine

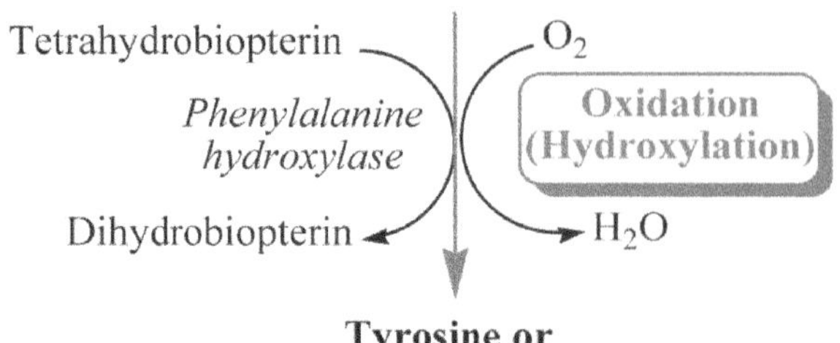

Tyrosine or *p*-Hydroxyphenylalanine

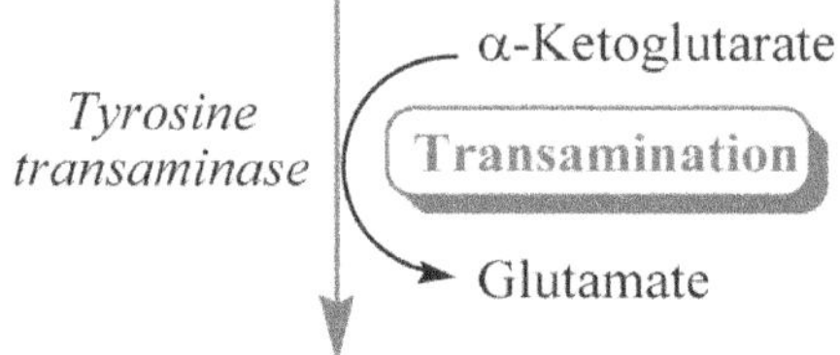

***p*-Hydroxyphenylpyruvate**

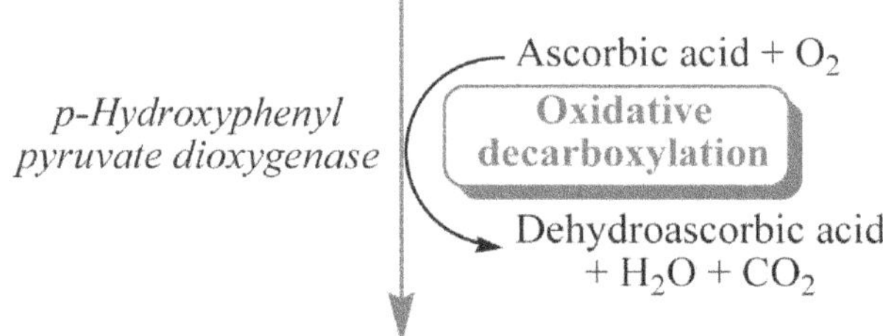

Homogentisate

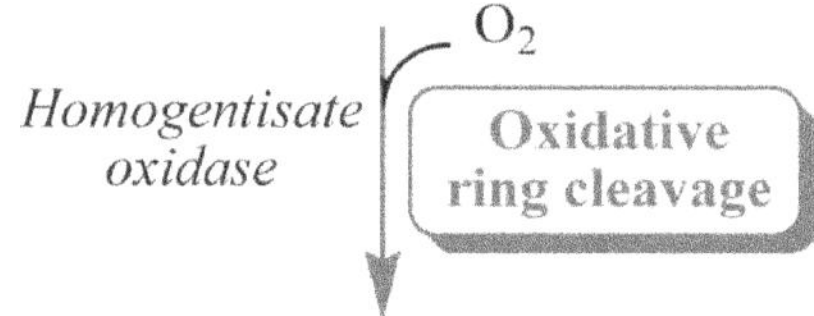

4-Maleylacetoacetate

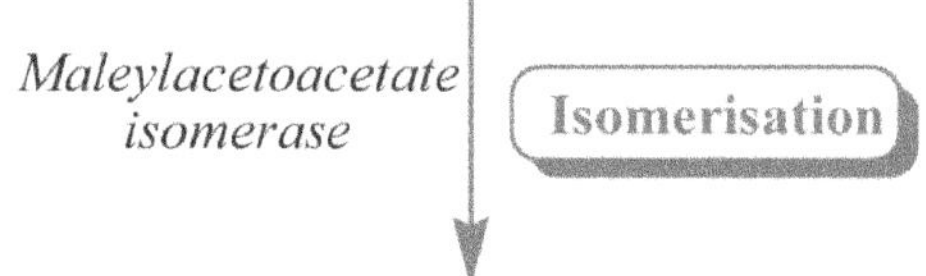

4-Fumarylacetoacetate

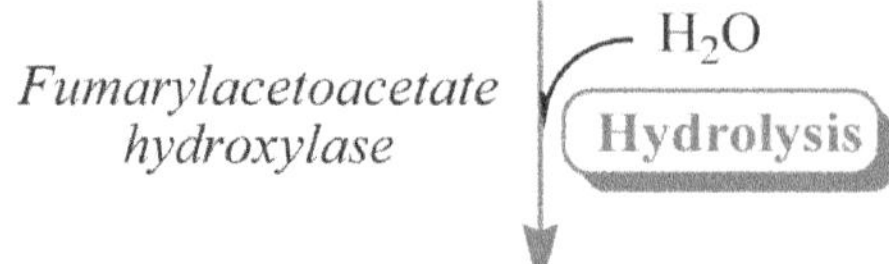

Fumaric acid + **Acetoacetate**

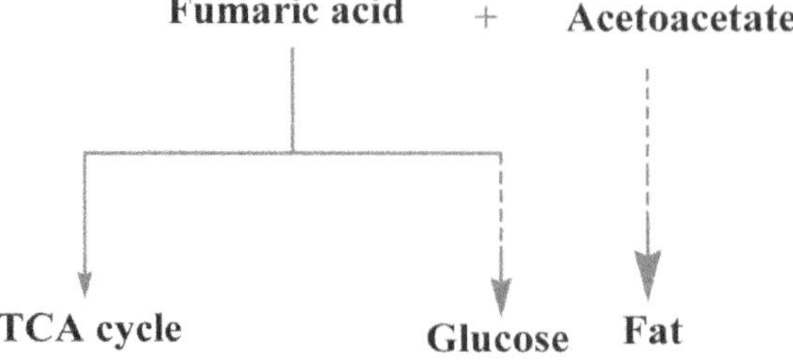

Biosynthesis of Melanin

In Greek "melan" means "black". Melanin is the pigment present in skin, hair and eye. Melanosome present in the pigment producing cell i.e., melanocytes is site of melanin synthesis. Melanin is synthesized from tyrosine in presence of one and only enzyme *tyrosinase*. It is a copper containing *oxygenase* enzyme. The various reactions involved in the synthesis of melanin are described here.

1. Tyrosine is converted into DOPA (3,4-dihydroxyphenylalanine) by hydroxylation or oxygenation at *meta* position in presence of *tyrosinase* (The substrate is "tyrosine" and the type of reaction involved is "oxygenation"). In this reaction, one mole of oxygen is involved. In that one of the oxygen atoms is incorporated in phenylalanine at *para* position and the another oxygen atom coupled with two hydrogen atoms of tetrahydrobiopterin are removed as water molecule. The tetrahydrobiopterin is converted into dihydrobiopterin as it loses two hydrogen atoms.
2. In the next step, DOPA is converted into dopaquinone in presence of the same enzyme by oxidation. In this reaction two hydrogen of DOPA and two hydrogen from tetrahydrobiopterin react with molecular oxygen and liberate two moles of water. DOPA can act as co-factor for enzyme *tyrosinase*.

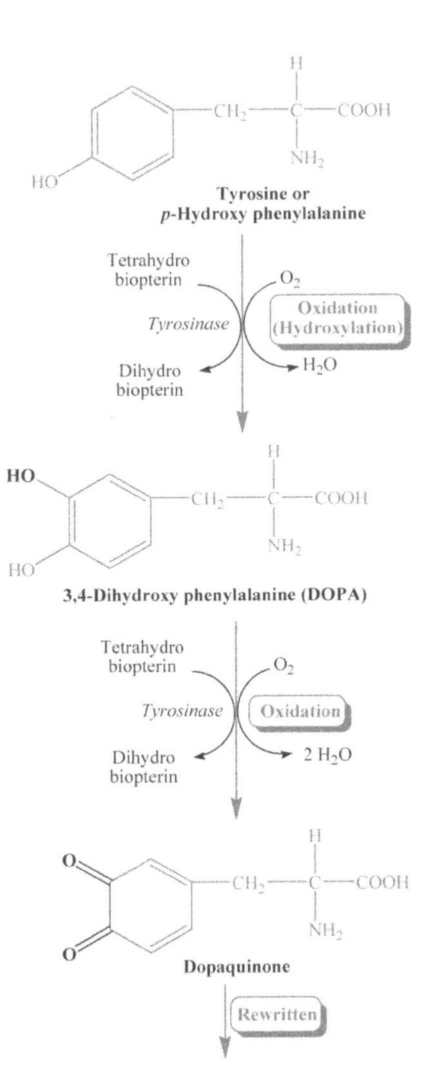

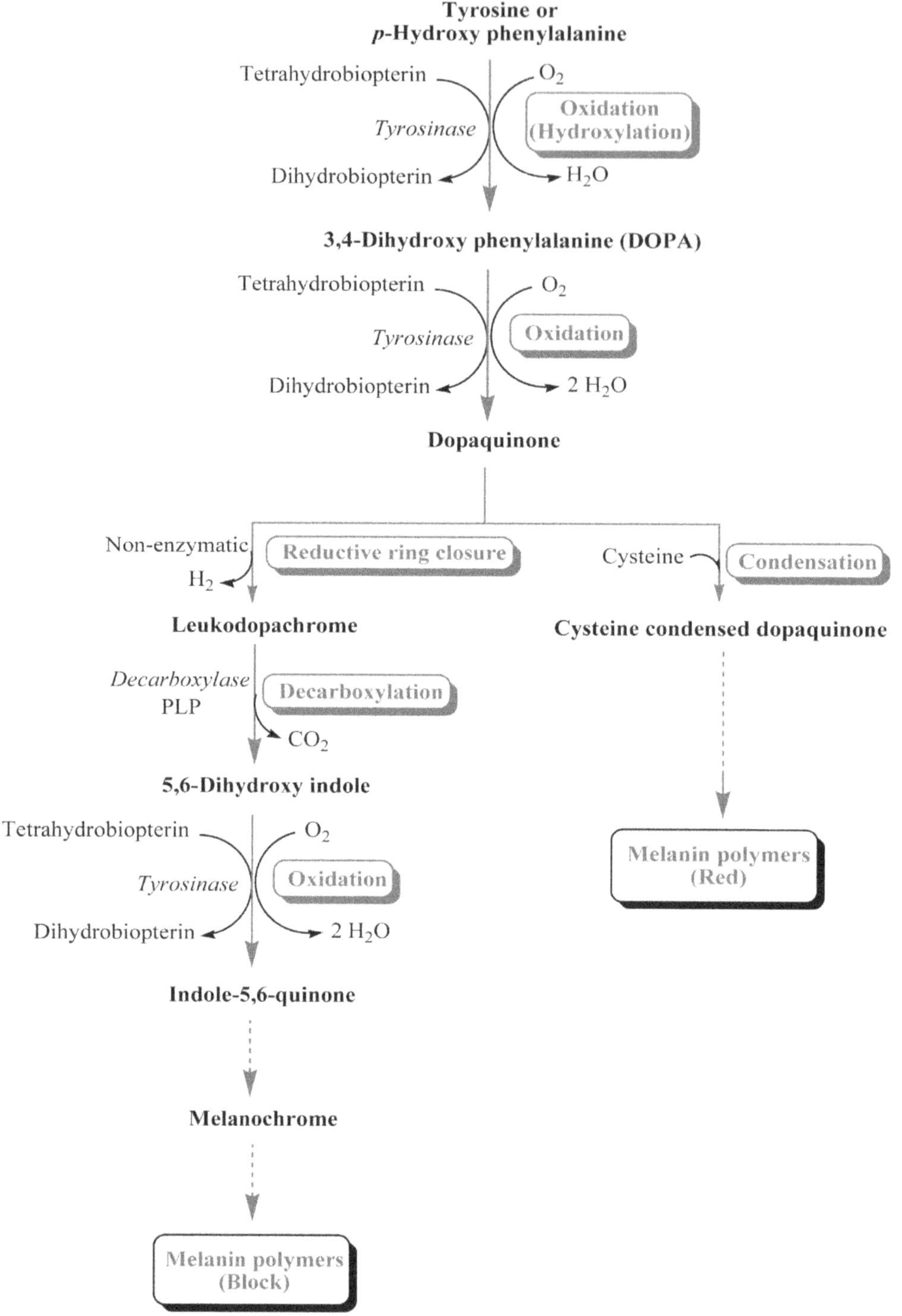

3. Dopaquinone non-enzymatically cyclizes to produce leukodopachrome.
4. The formed leukodopachrome decarboxylates (loss of carbondioxide from carboxylic acid group) and produced 5,6-dihydroxyindole.
5. In this step, 5,6-dihydroxyindole is converted into indole-5,6-quinone in presence of the same enzyme *tyrosinase* by oxidation. In this reaction two hydrogen of 5,6-dihydroxyindole and two hydrogen from tetrahydrobiopterin react with molecular oxygen and liberate two moles of water.
6. From indole-5,6-quinone, melanochromes are formed which on polymerization produces black melanin polymers.

7. Another pathway is identified from dopaquinone. In which it condenses with cysteine and in next series of reaction produces red melanin polymers.

The skin color of the individual is depends on concentration of red and black melanin which in turn depends on many factors like genetic factor, environmental factor, activity of *tyrosinase*, availability of tyrosine, density of melanocytes, etc. Hyperactivity of melanocytes leads to localized severe hyperpigmentation which is represented by presence of moles. Decreased activity of melanocytes leads to localized absence or degeneration of melanocytes results in white patches on the skin commonly known as leukoderma. Lack of melanocytes in hair root results in graying of hair.

Biosynthesis of Thyroid Hormones

Thyroid hormones such as thyroxine and triiodothyronine are biosynthesized from tyrosine in thyroid gland. The various reactions involved in the synthesis of thyroid hormones are described here.

1. Initially amino acid tyrosine is condensed with the protein thyroglobulin and produces thyroglobulin condensed tyrosine residues.

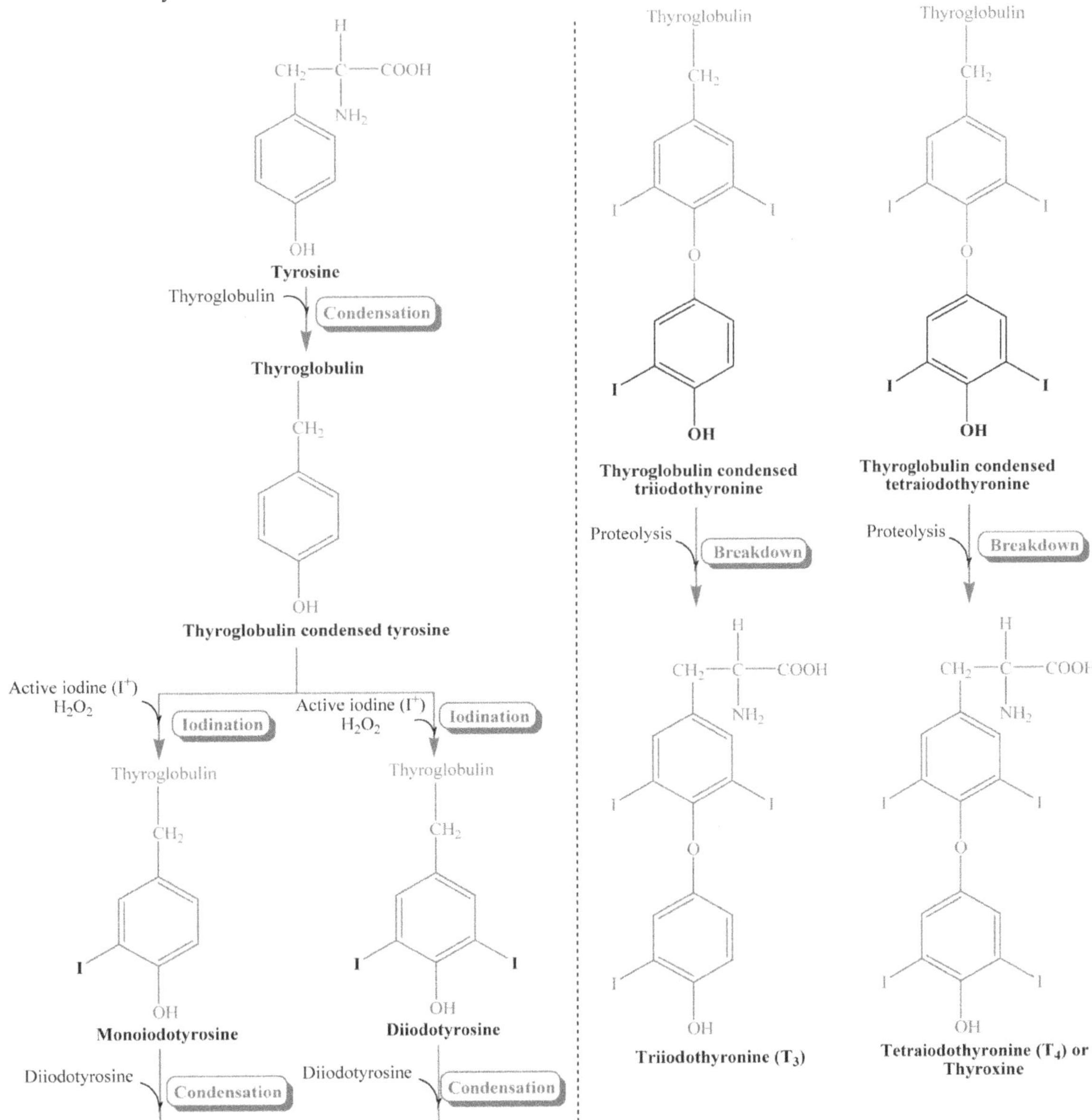

2. These thyroglobulin condensed tyrosine residues undergo iodination in presence of active iodine and hydrogen peroxide and produces monoiodotyrosine (One iodine atom is incorporated in phenyl ring of tyrosine) and diiodotyrosine (Two iodine atoms are incorporated in phenyl ring of tyrosine).
3. In the next step, synthesized monoiodotyrosine and diiodotyrosine reacts with another mole of diiodotyrosine residue and produces thyroglobulin condensed triiodothyronine and thyroglobulin condensed thyroxine, respectively.
4. Finally, thyroid hormones triiodothyronine (T_3) and thyroxine (T_4) are produced from thyroglobulin condensed triiodothyronine and thyroglobulin condensed thyroxine, respectively by proteolysis with the breakdown of protein thyroglobulin.

Biosynthesis of Catecholamines

Biologically important amines i.e., catecholamines such as dopamine, adrenaline or epinephrine and nor-adrenaline or nor-epinephrine are biosynthesized from tyrosine. Catecholamines are the amine derivatives of catechol or *o*-hydroxy phenol and its synthesis is takes place in adrenal medulla and CNS. The various reactions involved in the synthesis of catecholamines are described here.

1. Tyrosine is converted into DOPA (3,4-dihydroxyphenylalanine) by hydroxylation or oxidation at *meta* position in presence of *tyrosine hydroxylase* (The substrate is "tyrosine" and the type of reaction involved is "hydroxylation"). In this reaction, one mole of oxygen is involved. In that one of the oxygen atom is incorporated in phenylalanine at *meta* position and another oxygen atom coupled with two hydrogen atoms of tetrahydrobiopterin are removed as water molecule. The tetrahydrobiopterin is converted into dihydrobiopterin as it loses two hydrogen atoms. **It is the rate limiting step in the biosynthesis of catecholamines**. Two different enzyme systems i.e., *tyrosine hydroxylase* and *tyrosinase* exist for conversion of tyrosine to DOPA.
2. In second step, DOPA undergoes decarboxylation and produce its corresponding amine i.e., dopamine by losing carboxylic group as carbondioxide. This reaction is catalyzed by *aromatic amino acid decarboxylase* (The substrate is "DOPA" which is aromatic amino acid analog and the type of reaction involved is "decarboxylation") which requires PLP for its activity.
3. Dopamine further hydroxylated at β-position of side chain in the presence of *dopamine-β-hydroxylase* (The substrate is "dopamine" and the type of reaction involved is "β-hydroxylation") and produces nor-adrenaline or nor-epinephrine. In this reaction one mole of oxygen is involved. In that one of the oxygen atoms is incorporated in β-position of side chain in dopamine and another oxygen atom coupled with two hydrogen atoms of ascorbic acid are removed as water molecule. The ascorbic acid is converted into dehydroascorbic acid as it loses two hydrogen atoms.
4. Adrenaline or epinephrine is synthesized from nor-adrenaline or nor-epinephrine by N-methylation reaction in presence of *phenylethanolamine-N-methyl transferase* (The substrate is "nor-adrenaline or nor-epinephrine" which is phenylethanolamine derivative) and the type of reaction is "methyl group transfer"). In this reaction methyl group is donated by S-adenosyl methionine (SAM) and it is converted to S-adenosyl homocysteine after donating methyl group.

Tissue specificity exists in biosynthesis of catecholamines. Epinephrine and nor-epinephrine are prominently synthesized in adrenal medulla. In some part of the brain nor-epinephrine is synthesized but dopamine is specifically synthesized in substantia nigra and coeruleus of brain.

Biological significance of catecholamines:

1. Two catecholamines, nor-epinephrine and dopamine, act as neuromodulators in the central nervous system and as hormones in the blood circulation. The catecholamine nor-epinephrine is a neuromodulator of the peripheral sympathetic nervous system but is also present in the blood.
2. Catecholamines, including dopamine and nor-epinephrine, are the principal neurotransmitters that mediate a variety of the central nervous system functions, such as motor control, cognition, emotion, memory processing, and endocrine modulation.

3. Both epinephrine and nor-epinephrine modulate metabolism to increase blood glucose levels by stimulating glycogenolysis in the liver (via β_2 receptors), increased glucagon secretion (via β_2 receptors) and decreased insulin secretion (via α_2 receptors) from the pancreas.
4. Both epinephrine and nor-epinephrine produce lipolysis in adipose tissue (via β_3 receptors).
5. Epinephrine and nor-epinephrine increases blood pressure.
6. Decreased dopamine is linked with Parkinson's disease.
7. Epinephrine and nor-epinephrine are frequently used as vasopressor agents to treat acute hypotensive states, as well as in treatment algorithms for cardiac arrest.
8. Affinity of epinephrine and nor-epinephrine to the α-1 receptor also is used to induce localized vasoconstriction to reduce bleeding during procedures such as wound closure.
9. Catecholamine releasing agents in the form of sprays or ointments are used as nasal decongestants.
10. The pharmacodynamic inhibition of catecholamine reuptake is commonly used in the psychiatric treatment of some depressive disorders, post-traumatic stress disorder, anxiety disorders, attention deficit disorder, and panic disorders.
11. Catecholamine reuptake inhibitors may be used to treat neuropathic and chronic musculoskeletal pain.

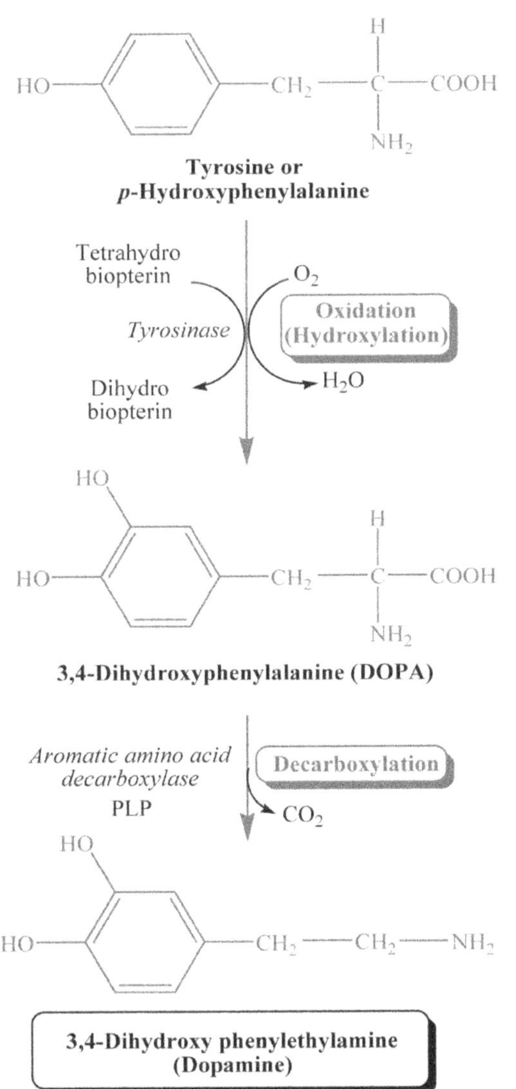

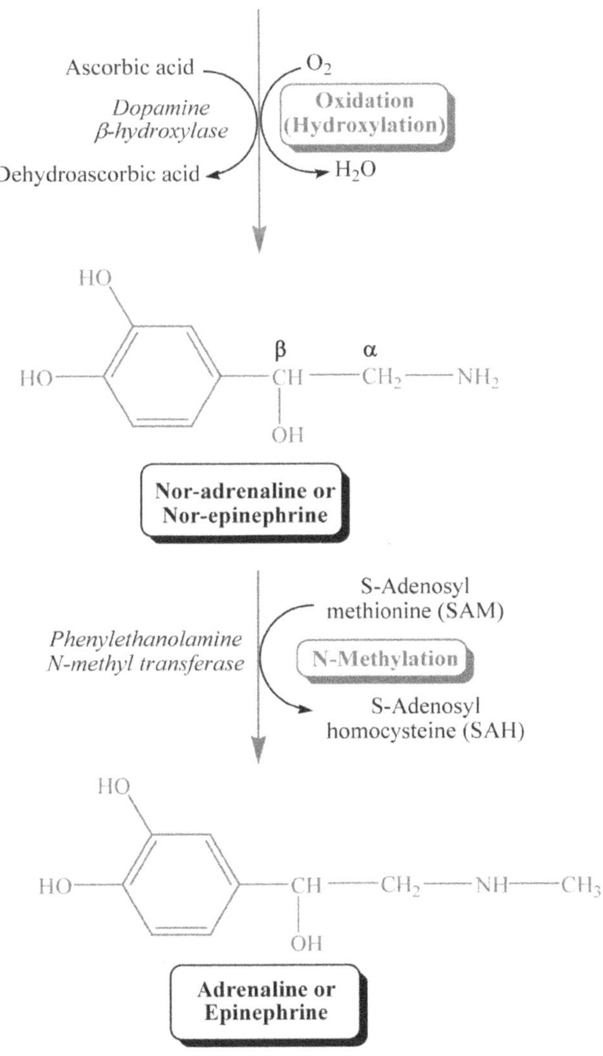

12. Epinephrine is the universal treatment for anaphylaxis and is also used to treat other causes of laryngeal edema or bronchospasm.
13. The blockage of adrenergic receptors otherwise activated by catecholamines is an integral part of the treatment of hypertension, congestive heart failure, and other cardiovascular diseases.
14. The "fight or flight" response of the sympathetic nervous system is a direct result of the multisystem action of catecholamines.
15. Epinephrine also inhibits release of mediators from mast cells and basophils in type-I hypersensitivity reactions.
16. Urine testing for catecholamine is used to detect pheochromocytoma.
17. High catecholamine levels in blood are associated with stress, which can be induced from psychological reactions or environmental stressors such as elevated sound levels, intense light, or low blood sugar levels.

Biosynthesis of 5-hydroxytryptamine (5-HT) or Serotonin and Melatonin

5-Hydroxytryptamine (5-HT) & melatonin is biosynthesized from tryptophan. 5-HT is commonly known as serotonin which is a neurotransmitter. In general, 1 % of tryptophan is utilized for the production of serotonin. In the target tissues serotonin is biosynthesized. largest amount of serotonin is biosynthesized in mammals in intestinal cells. As such platelets cannot synthesize serotonin but it contains high concentration of serotonin and the significance is not known. The serotonin synthesis is usually compared with the synthesis of catecholamines. Melatonin is a hormone biosynthesized mostly in pineal gland. Light controls the synthesis and secretion of melatonin in pineal gland. The various reactions involved in the synthesis of serotonin and melatonin are described here.

1. Tryptophan is converted into 5-hydroxytryptophan by hydroxylation or oxidation at *meta* position in presence of *tryptophan hydroxylase* (The substrate is "tryptophan" and the type of reaction is "hydroxylation"). In this reaction one mole of oxygen is involved. In that one of the oxygen atoms is incorporated in tryptophan at C-5 position and another oxygen atom is coupled with two hydrogen atoms of tetrahydrobiopterin are removed as water molecule. The tetrahydrobiopterin is converted into dihydrobiopterin as it loses two hydrogen atoms. ***Tryptophan hydroxylase* is the rate limiting enzyme of serotonin synthesis.**
2. In second step, 5-hydroxytryptophan undergoes decarboxylation and produce its corresponding amine i.e., 5-hydroxytryptamine (5-HT) or serotonin by losing carboxylic group as carbondioxide. This reaction is catalyzed by *aromatic amino acid decarboxylase* (The substrate is "5-hydroxytryptophan" which is aromatic amino acid analog and the type of reaction involved is "decarboxylation") which requires PLP for its activity.
3. Serotonin is further acetylated at amino group of side chain in presence of *serotonin-N-acetyl transferase* (The substrate is "serotonin" and the type of reaction involved is "acetyl group transfer to nitrogen") and produces N-acetylserotonin. In this reaction one mole of acetyl CoA is converted to co-enzyme A after transferring acetyl group to serotonin. ***Serotonin-N-acetyl transferase* is the rate limiting enzyme of melatonin synthesis**. In another way, serotonin is deaminated in presence of *monoamine oxidase (MAO)* (The substrate is "serotonin" which is monoamine analog and the type of reaction involved is "oxidative deamination") and produces 5-hydroxyindoleacetate which is excreted in urine. In this reaction amino group is lost as ammonia.
4. Finally, melatonin is synthesized from N-acetylserotonin by *O*-methylation reaction in presence of *N-acetylserotonin-O-methyl transferase* (The substrate is "N-acetylserotonin" and the type of reaction involved is "methyl group transfer to oxygen"). In this reaction methyl group is donated by S-adenosyl methionine (SAM) and it is converted to S-adenosyl homocysteine (SAH) after donating methyl group.
5. In other way, tryptophan is converted to indoleacetate and excreted in urine. This takes place in two different ways.

(a) In first process initially tryptophan undergoes deamination in presence of *monoamine oxidase (MAO)* (The substrate is "tryptophan" which is monoamine analog and the type of reaction involved is "oxidative deamination") and produces indole-3-pyruvate. In this reaction amino group is lost as ammonia. In the succeeding step, indole-3-pyruvate undergoes oxidative decarboxylation and produce indoleacetate by losing carboxylic group as carbondioxide. This reaction is catalyzed by *aromatic keto acid decarboxylase* (The substrate is "indole-3-pyruvate" which is aromatic keto acid analog and the type of reaction involved is "decarboxylation") which requires PLP for its activity.

(b) In second process initially tryptophan undergoes decarboxylation and produce its corresponding amine i.e., tryptamine by losing carboxylic group as carbondioxide. This reaction is catalyzed by *aromatic amino acid decarboxylase* (The substrate is "tryptophan" which is aromatic amino acid and the type of reaction involved is "decarboxylation") which requires PLP for its activity. In the next step, tryptamine undergoes deamination in presence of *monoamine oxidase (MAO)* (The substrate is "tryptamine" which is monoamine analog and the type of reaction involved is "oxidative deamination") and produces indoleacetate. In this reaction amino group is lost as ammonia.

Biological significance of serotonin:

1. Serotonin is a neurotransmitter and produces smooth muscle contraction in arterioles and bronchioles due to powerful vasoconstrictor activity.

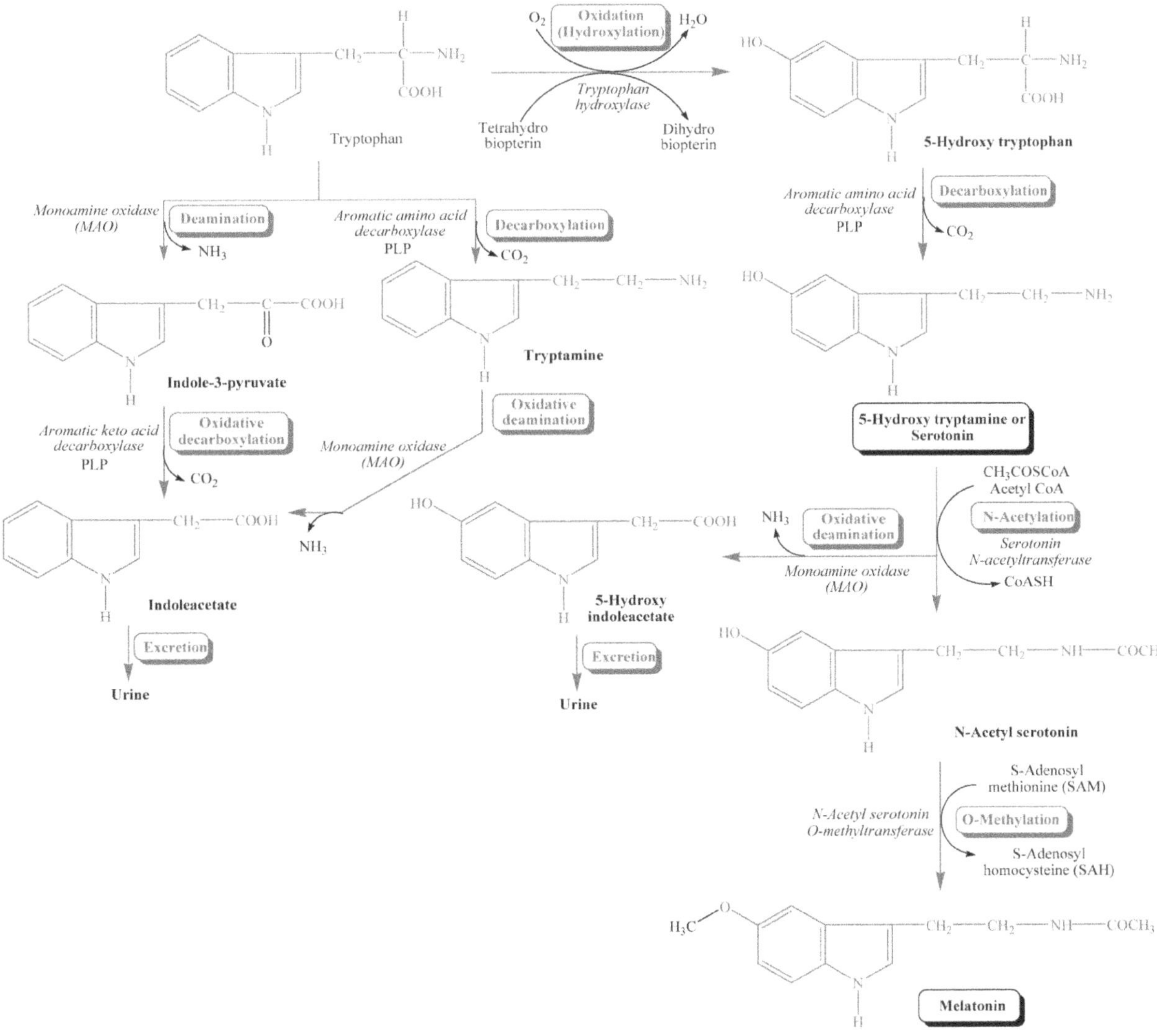

2. Cerebral activity (excitation) is closely regulated with the involvement of serotonin.
3. In psychosis patient's serotonin level is decreased in brain because serotonin is primarily stimulator of brain activity.
4. It is involved in the control of behavioral patterns, blood pressure, body temperature and sleep.
5. From gastrointestinal tract peptide hormone release is evoked by serotonin.
6. Motility of GIT or peristalsis needs serotonin.
7. Serotonin inhibitors are clinically used as depressant drugs. **Example:** Reserpine increases the degradation of serotonin, Lysergic acid diethylamide (LSD) competes with serotonin.
8. Serotonin stimulators are psychic stimulant. **Example:** Iproniazid inhibits *MAO* and elevates serotonin level.
9. Estimation of 5-hydroxyindoleacetate (5-HIA) in urine is used for the diagnosis of malignant carcinoid syndrome. 5-HIA level is increased in malignant carcinoid syndrome due to increased synthesis of serotonin.

Biological significance of melatonin:

1. Melatonin plays an important role in sleep and wake process. Because it is involved in diurnal variations or circadian rhythms.
2. It is safe and non-addictive sleep-inducing drug, which can eliminate disruptions in our circadian rhythm, in such situations as shift working, changing of time zones (during intercontinental air travelling) or insomnia.
3. Neurotransmitter function is also performed by melatonin.
4. On ovarian function melatonin exhibits some inhibitory effects.
5. Production of adrenocorticotropic hormone (ACTH) and melanocyte stimulating hormone is inhibited by melatonin.
6. Melatonin is a potent antioxidant and free radical scavenger.
7. Melatonin may be used in prophylaxis of cardiovascular system diseases, neoplastic diseases and other functional disorders of organisms.
8. Melatonin makes the immune system stronger, decreases susceptibility of the organism to stress and improves mood and general feeling.

Metabolic Disorders of Amino Acid Metabolism

Several enzyme defects in amino acid metabolism may lead to various metabolic disorders of amino acid metabolism. The following are some important metabolic disorders of amino acid metabolism.

1. Phenylketonuria
2. Albinism
3. Alkaptonuria
4. Tyrosinemia
5. Hyperbilirubinemia
6. Jaundice
7. Porphyria

1. Phenylketonuria (PKU):

Phenylketonuria is defined as increased excretion of phenyl keto-acid like phenyl pyruvate in urine due to deficiency of hepatic enzyme *phenylalanine hydroxylase*. In PKU, high concentration of other phenylalanine metabolites such as phenyl acetate, phenyl lactate and phenyl acetyl glutamine also excreted in urine.

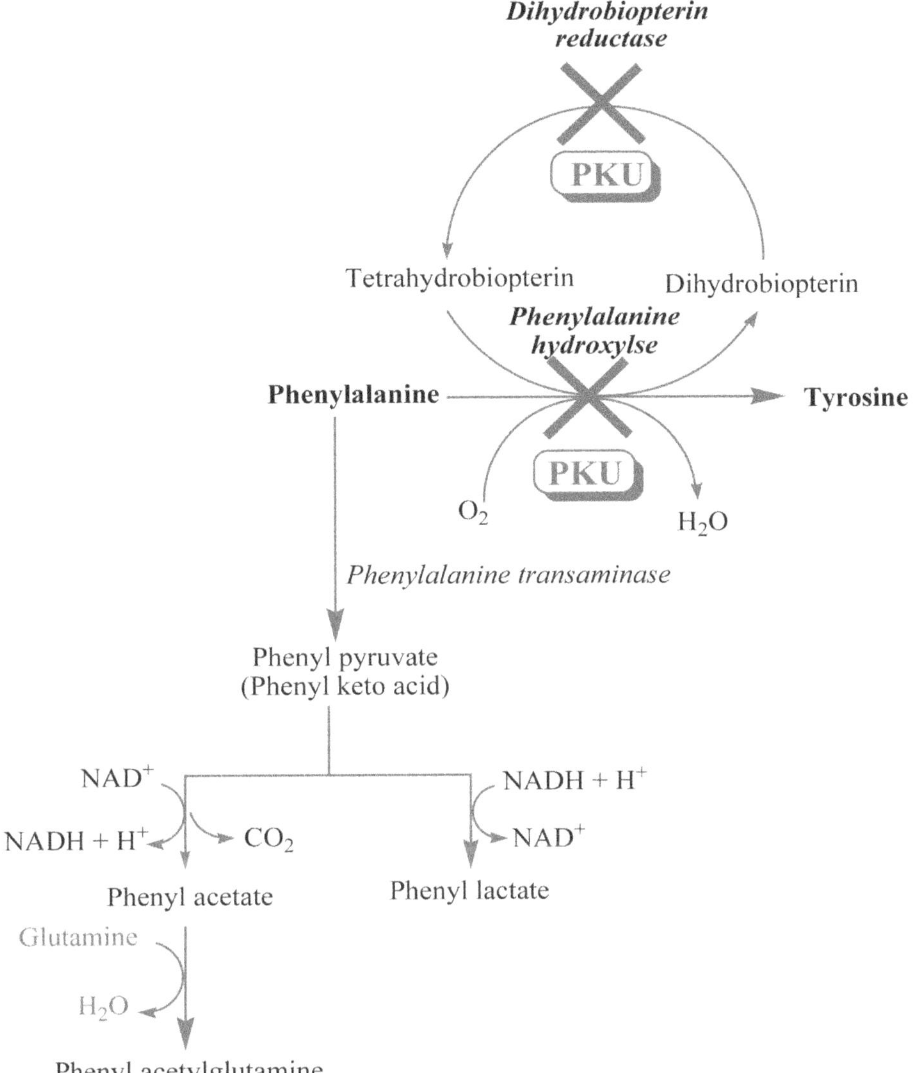

In amino acid metabolism this is the most common metabolic disorder. The prevalence of phenylketonuria is 1 in 10,000. This disorder is due to deficiency of hepatic enzyme *phenylalanine hydroxylase* (The substrate is "phenylalanine" and the type of reaction involved is "hydroxylation") caused by an autosomal recessive gene. Recently less common another type of PKU due to defect of *dihydrobiopterin reductase* is reported. This deficiency leads to impaired synthesis of tetrahydrobiopterin which is necessary for the activity of *phenylalanine hydroxylase*. Ultimately tyrosine is not produced form phenylalanine.

Primarily PKU causes increased phenylalanine concentration in blood and tissues which leads to increased excretion in urine. In PKU, conversion of phenylalanine to tyrosine is blocked, hence phenylalanine is diverted for other alternate pathways. This leads to increased production of phenyl pyruvate, phenyl acetate, phenyl lactate and phenyl acetylglutamine. Hence, high concentrations of these metabolites are excreted in urine. Mousey odor of urine is due to phenyl acetate only. The followings are the various clinical manifestation of PKU.

1. Mental retardation, failure to talk or walk, failure of growth, seizure and tremor.
2. Defect in myelin formation.
3. Impaired synthesis of serotonin due to competition of phenylalanine and its metabolite with tryptophan.

4. Hypopigmentation due to competitive inhibition of *tyrosinase* by phenylalanine causes light skin color, fair hair, blue eyes, etc.

Guthrie test (Bacterial particularly *Bacillus substilis* bioassay for phenylalanine) is used for the diagnosis of PKU. In addition, ferric chloride test is used for the detection of phenyl pyruvate in urine. PKU is treated generally by taking foods with low phenylalanine and / or feeding synthetic amino acid preparations low in phenylalanine. In serious PKU cases, 5-hydroxy tryptophan and DOPA is administered to restore the synthesis of serotonin and catecholamines. PKU with tetrahydrobiopterin deficiency needs tetrahydrobiopterin supplementation.

2. **Albinism:**

In Greek albino means "white". Albinism is also related to albinos. Albinism is due to lack of synthesis of pigment melanin and it is an inborn disorder. 1 in 20,000 is the frequency of this autosomal recessive disorder. The most common cause of albinism is defect in *tyrosinase* which is mostly responsible for the synthesis of melanin.

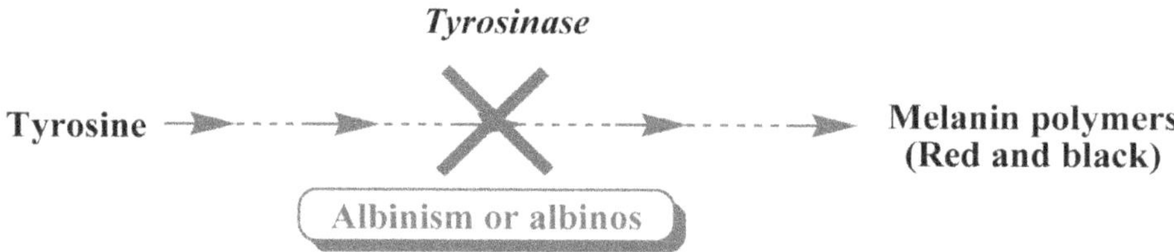

Many genes control the color of the skin and hair. Many factors influence the synthesis of melanin from tyrosine. The following are the most possible causes for albinism.

1. Lack of deficiency of enzyme "*tyrosinase*".
2. Decreased melanosomes in melanocytes.
3. Defect in melanin polymerization.
4. Protein matrix lack in melanosomes.
5. Limitation of tyrosine availability.
6. Presence of *tyrosinase* inhibitors.

Melanin protects the body from sun radiation which is the most important functions of melanin. The followings are the clinical manifestation of albinism.

1. Sensitive to sun light.
2. Increased susceptibility to carcinoma (skin cancer).
3. Photophobia (intolerance to light) is associated with lack of pigment in eyes. But there is no impairment in the eyesight.

3. **Alkaptonuria:**

It is otherwise known as **black urine disease**. The prevalence of this autosomal recessive disorder is 1 in 25,000. Alkaptonuria is defined as increased excretion of homogentisate in urine (due to lack of *homogentisate oxidase*) which on standing produces pigment alkapton in urine.

This disorder is tyrosine metabolic disorder due to lack of *homogentisate oxidase*. This is an enzyme responsible for the conversion of homogentisate into 4-maleylacetoacetate. Hence, lack of *homogentisate oxidase* increases the concentration of homogentisate in blood which accumulates and excreted in urine. On standing homogentisate undergoes oxidation and produces respective quinone derivative which further polymerized and give black or brown color. Hence alkaptonuria patient's urine looks coke in color, hence it is also known as black urine disease.

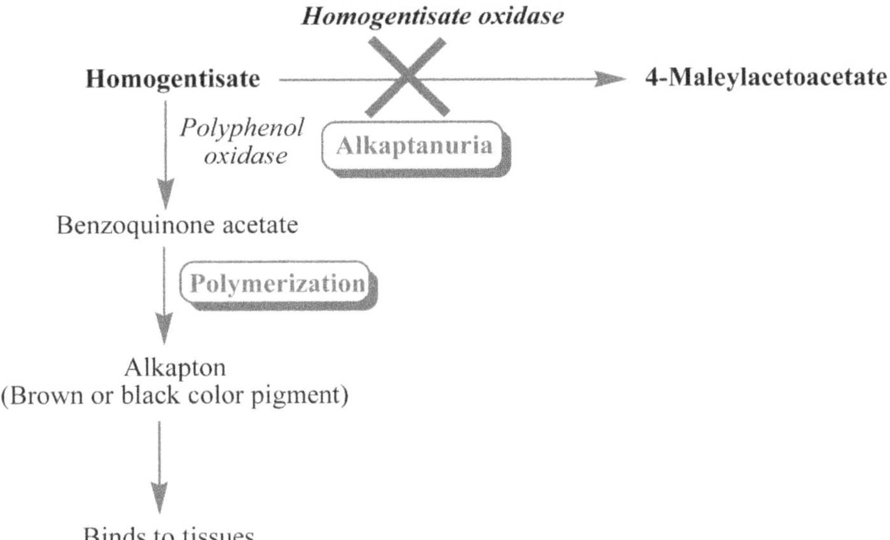

The followings are the clinical manifestation of alkaptonuria.

1. Production of pigment alkapton through benzoquinone acetate from homogentisate by oxidation in presence of *polyphenol oxidase* followed by polymerization.
2. Ochronosis is a clinical condition due to deposition of alkapton in connective tissues, bones and various organs like ear, nose, etc.
3. Arthritis in many patients due to deposition of alkapton pigment in the joints.

Alkaptonuria is easily diagnosed from urine color change on standing to brown or block. The urine gives positive test with ferric chloride, silver nitrate, Benedict's test and other reducing test due to strong reducing activity of homogentisate. No treatment is needed as it is not a dangerous disease. Even though, it is treated by consuming protein diet with relatively low phenylalanine content.

4. **Tyrosinemia:**

Tyrosinemia is defined as increased concentration of tyrosine in blood and excretion of tyrosine and its metabolic products in urine due to deficiency of enzymes involved in tyrosine degradation pathway. There are two different types of tyrosinemia. They are,

1. Tyrosinemia type – I or Tyrosinosis
2. Tyrosinemia type – II or Hanhart syndrome

Tyrosinemia type – I or Tyrosinosis: It is a rare but serious disorder due to deficiency of the enzymes *fumarylacetoacetate hydroxylase* and/or *maleylacetoacetate isomerase*. Tyrosine, its metabolites and many other amino acids are excreted in urine. Infant exhibits diarrhea, vomiting and cabbage like odor in acute tyrosinosis. Generally, tyrosinemia type – I may cause liver failure, rickets, renal tubular dysfunction and polyneuropathy. Within one-year death may occur due to liver failure. It is treated by consuming diets containing less phenylalanine, tyrosine and methionine.

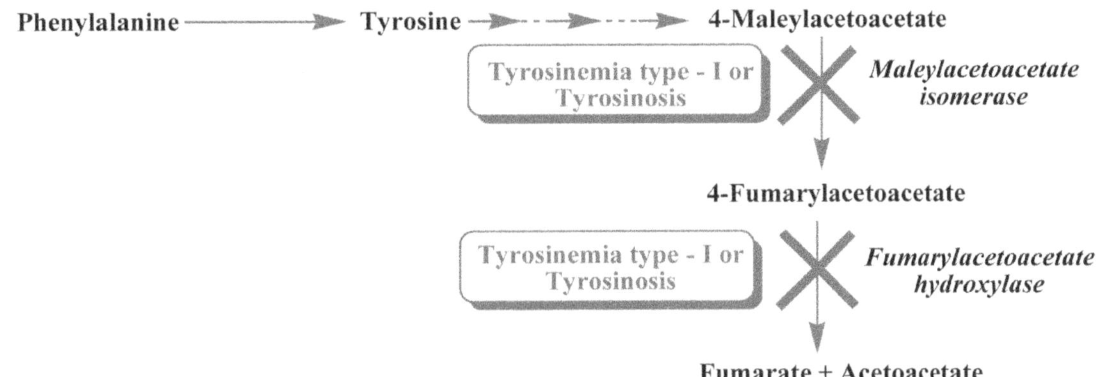

Tyrosinemia type – II or Hanhart syndrome: It is due to the deficiency of *tyrosine transaminase* which is involved in the conversion of tyrosine into *p*-hydroxyphenyl pyruvate. Hence tyrosine degradative pathway is blocked leads to accumulation and excretion of tyrosine and its metabolites such as *p*-hydroxyphenyl pyruvate, *p*-hydroxyphenyl acetate, *p*-hydroxyphenyl lactate, N-acetyl tyrosine and tyramine. In general, it is characterized by dermatitis, eye lesions and rarely mental disorder. In these patients disturbed self coordination is seen.

5. **Hyperbilirubinemia:**

Hyperbilirubinemia is defined as the increased concentration of bilirubin in blood. **Bilirubin is the excretory end product of heme metabolism** and it is a yellow color bile pigment. In liver bilirubin undergoes conjugation and produces bilirubin diglucuronide. Later, it enters in intestine where it is converted to urobilinogen further to urobilin and stercobilin (urobilin is the substances which is responsible for yellow color of urine and stercobilin is the substance which is responsible for brown color of feces).

The normal serum bilirubin levels are 0.2 to 1 mg/dl. Bilirubin can be available in both conjugated and unconjugated form in liver. The normal conjugated bilirubin serum level is 0.2 to 0.4 mg/dl. In that conjugated form 75 % are diglucuronide and 25 % are monoglucuronide. The normal unconjugated bilirubin level in serum is 0.2 to 0.6 mg/dl. Hyperbilirubinemia is characterized by increased bilirubin in the blood, increased color of urine due to more concentration of urobilin excretion and dark brown color feces due to more concentration of stercobilin excretion.

6. **Jaundice:**

When the level of bilirubin is more in blood it may leads to deposition of bile pigments in skin and white part of the eye (sclerae). Exactly speaking jaundice is not a disease; it is a symptom which denotes the increased level of bilirubin in biological system. In French, "Jaune" means "yellow". Jaundice is also known as icterus. It is a clinical condition characterized by yellow color of the white of the eyes (sclerae) and skin due to deposition of bilirubin. Jaundice is due to increased level of serum bilirubin beyond 2 mg/dl (Normal bilirubin level is < 1 mg/dl). Jaundice is caused due to multiple factors; hence it is difficult to classify jaundice. Even though for convenience jaundice are broadly classified into three major types as a) Hemolytic jaundice, b) Hepatic jaundice or hepatocellular jaundice, c) Obstructive jaundice or regurgitation jaundice.

(a) **Hemolytic jaundice:** Generally, hemolytic jaundice is associated with increased hemolysis of erythrocytes (**Example:** Malaria, sickle cell anemia and incompatible blood transfusion). If erythrocytes breakdown more it leads to more production of bilirubin. Hence, more bilirubin is excreted in bile leads to increased production of urobilinogen and stercobilinogen. Hemolytic jaundice is characterized by a) increased serum unconjugated bilirubin, b) increased excretion of urobilinogen in urine, c) dark color of feces due to high amount of stercobilinogen.

(b) **Hepatic jaundice or hepatocellular jaundice:** It is caused by liver dysfunction due to parenchymal cell damage. This may be due to presence of toxic substances such as poisons and toxins like chloroform, carbon tetrachloride, phosphorous, etc., viral infection (viral hepatitis), liver cirrhosis, heart failure, etc. The most common one is viral hepatitis. Liver damage affects bilirubin uptake and its conjugation by liver cells. Hence, hepatic jaundice is characterized by a) increased serum conjugated and unconjugated bilirubin, b) dark color urine due to increased excretion of bilirubin and urobilinogen, c) increased activity of *serum glutamate pyruvate transaminase* (*SGPT*) and *serum glutamate oxaloacetate transaminase* (*SGOT*) due to hepatocyte damage, d) pale, clay colored stools due to absence of stercobilinogen, e) nausea and anorexia (loss of appetite).

(c) **Obstructive jaundice or regurgitation jaundice:** It is due to obstruction in the bile ducts which prevents the passage of bile into the intestine. Gall stones, tumors, etc. may be the reasons for obstructions. From the liver, the conjugated bilirubin enters into the circulation due to the blockage. Obstructive jaundice is characterized by a) increased level of conjugated bilirubin in serum, b) elevated *serum alkaline phosphatase* due to release from damaged bile ducts, c) increased activity of *serum glutamate pyruvate transaminase (SGPT) and serum glutamate oxaloacetate* *transaminase* (*SGOT*) d) dark color urine due to increased excretion of bilirubin and urobilinogen, e) pale, clay colored stools due to absence of stercobilinogen, f) excess fat in feces indicates fat digestion impairments and absorption in the absence of bile particularly bile salts, g) nausea and GIT pain.

Jaundice may also cause due to some hereditary abnormalities also. The following are some type of jaundice due to genetic defects. They are,

1. Neonatal physiologic jaundice
2. Crigler-Najjar syndrome type - I
3. Crigler-Najjar syndrome type - II

7. **Porphyria:**

Porphyria are defined as a metabolic disorder of heme synthesis characterized by increased excretion of porphyrins and precursors of porphyrins. These porphyria are either inherited or acquired. Almost all porphyria are inherited as autosomal dominant disorders. Exception is congenital erythropoietic porphyria which is autosomal recessive. Acquired or toxic prophyria are acquired due to toxicity of many compounds like heavy metals (**Example:** lead, hexachlorobenzene and drugs like griseofulvin). In heme synthesis these toxic compounds inhibit many enzymes like *ALA dehydratase, uroporphyrin-I synthase* and *ferrochelatase.*

In general, porphyria are broadly classified into two major types as a) Hepatic porphyria (defect of enzyme in liver), b) Erythropoietic porphyria (defect of enzyme in erythrocyte).

Hepatic porphyria: In this type porphyria the enzyme defects lies in the liver. It was, further sub divided into four classes as a) Acute intermittent porphyria, b) Porphyria cutanea tarda, c) Hereditary coproporphyria, d) Variegate porphyria.

Acute intermittent porphyria are due to the deficiency of *uroporphyrinogen-I synthase* and are characterized by increased excretion of porphobilinogen and 8-aminolevulinate. When exposed to air the urine becomes dark due to conversion of porphobilinogen to porphobilin and porphyrin. In humansit is usually expressed after puberty. The symptom includes abdominal pain, vomiting, and cardiovascular abnormalities. In addition, neuropsychiatry symptoms also occur due to decreased activity of *tryptophan pyrrolase.* This type porphyria patient is not photosensitive because enzyme defects occur prior to the formation of uroporphyrinogen. It is treated by using hematin which is *ALA synthase* inhibitor and porphobilinogen accumulation inhibitor.

Porphyria cutanea tarda are otherwise known as cutaneous hepatic porphyria. This is most common porphyria due to the deficiency of *uroporphyrinogen decarboxylase.* Generally, it is associated with liver damage due to overconsumption of alcohol or iron overload. It is characterized by increased excretion of uroporphyrins-I and III and rarely porphobilinogen. The most important symptom is cutaneous photosensitivity. Liver exhibits fluorescence due to accumulation of high concentration of porphyrins.

Hereditary coproporphyria are due to the deficiency of *coproporphyrinogen oxidase* and are characterized by excretion of coproporphyrinogen-III and other intermediates of heme synthesis prior to the blockade in urine and feces. The various symptoms of hereditary coproporphyria are abdominal pain, photosensitivity and neuropsychiatry symptoms. It is treated by using hematin which is *ALA synthase* inhibitor and porphobilinogen accumulation inhibitor.

Variegate porphyria are due to the deficiency of *protoporphyrinogen oxidase* which blocks the formation of protoporphyrin-IX. This porphyria are characterized by accumulation and excretion of all intermediates of heme synthesis in urine and feces. The urine becomes color and symptoms are abdominal pain, photosensitivity and neuropsychiatry symptoms.

Erythropoietic porphyria: In this type porphyria the enzyme deficiency occurs in the liver. It was further sub divided into four classes as a) Congenital erythropoietic porphyria, b) Protoporphyria.

Congenital erythropoietic porphyria are due to the deficiency of *uroporphyrinogen-III co-synthase* or imbalance between activities of *uroporphyrinogen-I synthase* and *uroporphyrinogen-III co-synthase.* This porphyria is characterized by excretion of uroporphyrinogen-I and coproporphyrinogen-I which oxidize and produce red pigments uroporphyrin-I and coproporphyrin-I, respectively. The symptoms of congenital erythropoietic porphyria are photosensitivity (itching and burning sensation when exposed to light) due to accumulation of abnormal porphyrins and increased hemolysis.

Protoporphyria are otherwise known as erythropoietic protoporphyria. This class of porphyria is due to the deficiency of *ferrochelatase* and is characterized by accumulation and excretion of protoporphyrin in urine and feces. The most important symptom is photosensitivity. Reticulocytes (young RBC) and skin biopsy exhibit red fluorescence.

The various classes of porphyria are summarized along with enzyme responsible and symptoms in table 5.3.

Table 5.3 Enzyme responsible and symptoms of different porphyria.

S. No.	Type of porphyria	Enzyme responsible	Characteristics	Symptoms
1. Inherited porphyria				
a) Hepatic porphyria				
1	**Acute intermittent porphyria**	*Uroporphyrinogen-I synthase*	Increased excretion of porpho-bilinogen and 8-aminolevulinate	Abdominal pain, vomiting, cardiovascular abnormalities and neuropsychiatry symptoms
2	**Porphyria cutanea tarda or cutaneous hepatic porphyria**	*Uroporphyrinogen decarboxylase*	Increased excretion of uroporphyrins-I and III and rarely porphobilinogen	Cutaneous photosensitivity
3	**Hereditary coproporphyria**	*Coproporphyrinogen oxidase*	Excretion of coproporphyrinogen-III and other intermediates of heme synthesis prior to the blockade in urine and feces	Abdominal pain, photosensitivity and neuropsychiatry symptoms
4	**Variegate porphyria**	*Protoporphyrinogen oxidase*	Accumulation and excretion of all intermediates of heme synthesis in urine and feces. Urine becomes color	Abdominal pain, photosensitivity and neuropsychiatry symptoms
b) Erythropoietic porphyria				
5	**Congenital erythropoietic porphyria**	*Uroporphyrinogen-III co-synthase* and *uroporphyrinogen-I synthase*	Excretion of uroporphyrinogen-I and coproporphyrinogen-I which oxidize and produce red pigments uroporphyrin-I and coproporphyrin-I	Photosensitivity and increased hemolysis
6	**Protoporphyria or erythropoietic protoporphyria**	*Ferro chelatase*	Accumulation and excretion of protoporphyrin in urine and feces	Photosensitivity
2. Acquired or toxic porphyria				
7	**Acquired or toxic porphyria**	*ALA dehydratase, uroporphyrin-I synthase* and *ferro chelatase*	Toxicity of many compounds like heavy metals (**Example:** lead), hexachlorobenzene and drugs like griseofulvin	Abdominal pain, photosensitivity and neuropsychiatry symptoms

Catabolism of Heme

The life span of erythrocytes is only 120 days. After 120 days the erythrocytes are removed from the circulation and taken up by the macrophages of the reticuloendothelial (RE) system in the spleen and liver. In macrophages erythrocytes are degraded into non-protein heme and the protein part globin by cleaving. This protein part globin may be degraded into individual amino acids or as such it is reutilized for the formation of hemoglobin. The formed amino acids may undergo its own metabolism including participation in fresh globin synthesis. About 80 % of the heme subjected for degradations is obtained from erythrocytes only. The remaining 20 % are obtained from immature RBC, cytochromes and myoglobin.

Later, heme is converted into biliverdin (**Green pigment**) in the presence of enzyme *heme oxygenase* which utilizes NADPH + H^+ and oxygen and breaks the methenyl bridges present in between two pyrrole rings (A and B ring). In the mean time ferrous (Fe^{2+}) is oxidized into ferric (Fe^{3+}) ion. Carbon monoxide is also released during this reaction. In amphibian and birds, the biliverdin is excreted as such, whereas in mammals it further undergoes degradations.

In the next step, the methenyl bridge present between pyrrole ring C and D of biliverdin is reduced to methylene group and forms bilirubin (**Yellow pigment**). *Biliverdin reductase* catalyzes this reaction which is a NADPH + H^+ dependent soluble enzyme. The term bile pigments are used to collectively represent bilirubin and its derivatives like biliverdin.

Bilirubin is insoluble in aqueous solution because it is lipophilic in nature. Hence it is transported into plasma in a non-covalently bound form to albumin as bilirubin-albumin complex. Albumin has two binding sites namely high affinity site (about 25 mg of bilirubin per 100 ml of plasma tightly binds at this site) and low affinity sites (Rest of bilirubin binds loosely at this site). The later one easily detaches from the albumin and enters into the tissues. Some times bilirubin may enter into the CNS and cause damage to the neurons because certain drugs like sulfonamides and salicylates can displace the bilirubin from albumin.

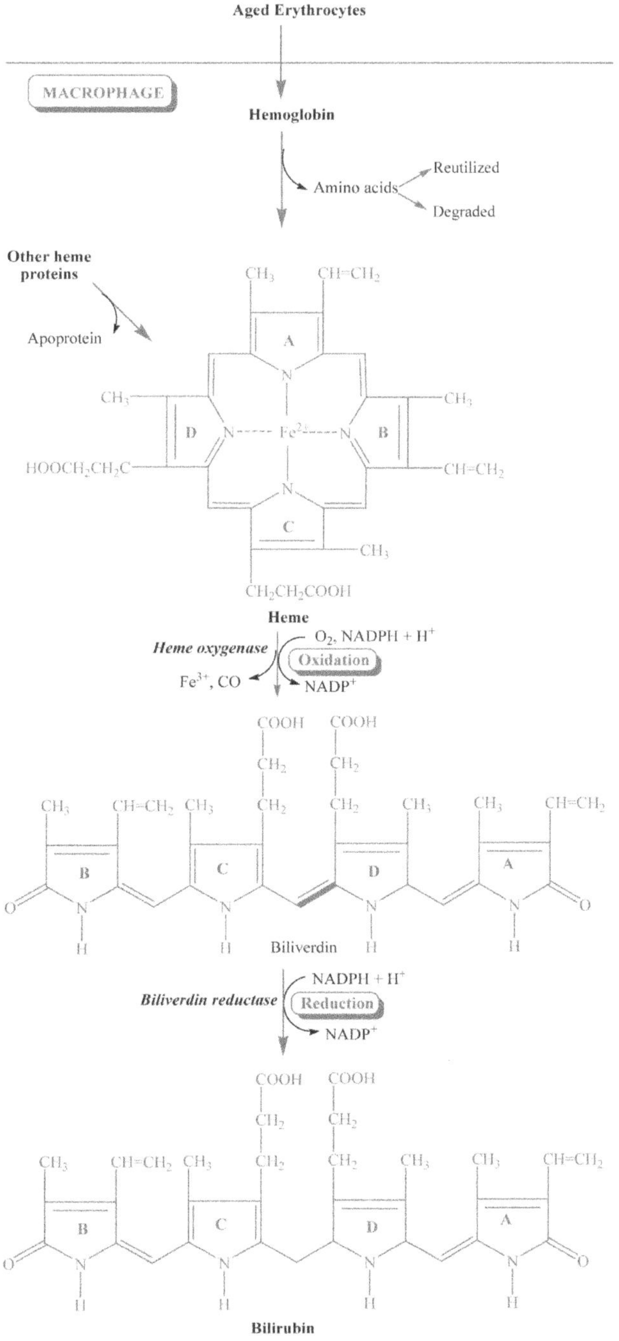

Aged Erythrocytes
MACROPHAGE
Hemoglobin
Amino acids
Reutilized
Degraded
Other heme proteins
Apoprotein
Heme
Heme oxygenase
O_2, NADPH + H^+
Oxidation
Fe^{3+}, CO
$NADP^+$
Biliverdin
Biliverdin reductase
NADPH + H^+
Reduction
$NADP^+$
Bilirubin

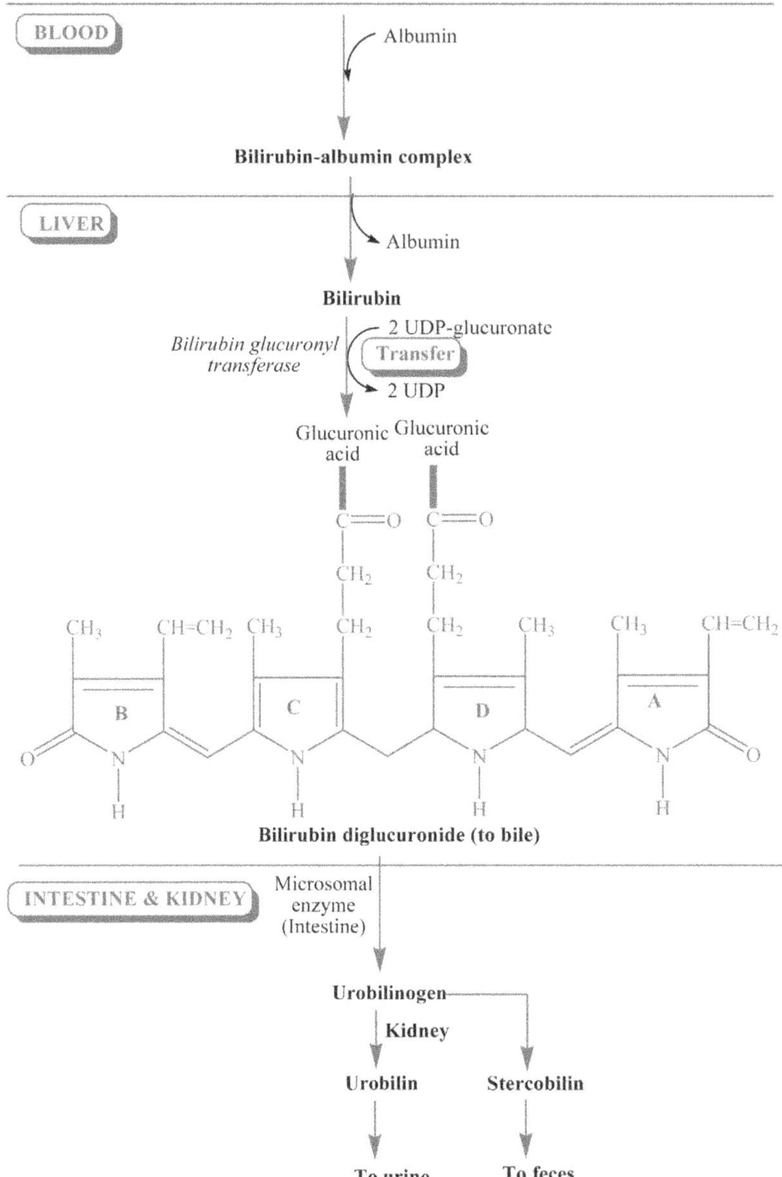

Once albumin-bilirubin complex enters into the liver, the dissociated bilirubin was taken up the sinusoidal surface of the hepatocytes through a carrier mediated active transport system. In liver, bilirubin binds with a specific intracellular protein namely ligandin. More over bilirubin in liver undergoes glucuronic acid conjugation by reacting with two moles of UDP glucuronate and produces bilirubin diglucuronide which is water soluble and liberates free UDP. This reaction is catalyzed by the enzyme called *bilirubin glucuronyl transferase* of smooth endoplasmic reticulum. This enzyme can be induced by number of drugs such as phenobarbital. When excess bilirubin is there bilirubin monoglucuronide may also accumulate in the body.

Later, conjugated bilirubin is excreted into the bile canaliculi against a concentration gradient which then enters into the bile. This transport of bilirubin diglucuronide is an energy dependent, active and rate limiting process. Almost all the bilirubin (> 98 %) enters into the bile are conjugated form only.

The specific bacterial enzymes present in the intestine namely *β-glucuronidase* hydrolyzes the bilirubin glucuronide into bilirubin. Latter, bilirubin is converted into urobilinogen which is a colorless compound and a small part of it may reabsorb into the circulation. In the kidney, urobilinogen can be converted into yellow color compound urobilin and excreted in urine. The characteristic yellow color of the urine is due to urobilin only. A major part of the urobilinogen is converted into stercobilin by the intestinal bacteria. This formed stercobilin is excreted along with feces. The characteristic brown color of the feces is due to stercobilin only.

PROBABLE QUESTIONS

PART – A: Multiple Choice Questions

1. Proteins are the polymer of which of the following?
   (P) D-α-Amino acids (Q) D-β-Amino acids
   (R) L-α-Amino acids (S) L-β-Amino acids
   Choose the correct option.
   (a) Only R (b) Only S
   (c) Both R & S (d) Both P & Q
2. Which of the following function of a protein is regarded as "The working horses" of the cell?
   (a) Structural functions (b) Dynamic functions
   (c) Both a & b (d) None of the above
3. Which of the following amino acids are essential amino acids?
   (P) Alanine (Q) Methionine
   (R) Tyrosine (S) Lysine
   Choose the correct option.
   (a) P & S (b) Q & R
   (c) P & R (d) Q & S
4. On an average how much amount of nitrogen is present in protein?
   (a) 53 % (b) 21 %
   (c) 16 % (d) 10 %
5. The term protein is generally used for polypeptide containing how many amino acids?
   (a) More than 20 amino acids (b) More than 30 amino acids
   (c) More than 40 amino acids (d) More than 50 amino acids
6. Which of the following structure of a protein is largely responsible for its function?
   (a) Quaternary structure (b) Tertiary structure
   (c) Secondary structure (d) Primary structure
7. Which of the following one is wrong with respect to peptide bond?
   (P) Rigid & planar (Q) Partial double bond character
   (R) Covalent bond (S) Weak bond.
   Choose the correct option.
   (a) P, Q & R is correct; S is wrong (b) Q, R & S is correct; P is wrong
   (c) P, Q & S is correct; R is wrong (d) P, R & S is correct; Q is wrong
8. Which of the following is true in peptide chain?
   (P) C-terminal residue at the left (Q) N-terminal residue at the left
   (R) N-terminal residue at the right (S) C-terminal residue at the right.
   Choose the correct option.
   (a) Both P & Q (b) Both P & R
   (c) Both P & S (d) Both Q & S

9. For naming peptides which of the following suffix is added by replacing existing suffix with the exception of C-terminal amino acid?
   (a) -ine (b) -yl
   (c) -ane (d) –ate
10. Which of the following bond is not present in the protein structure?
   (a) Covalent bond (b) Non-covalent bond
   (c) Hydrogen bond (d) Co-ordinate covalent bond
11. Which of the followings are not globular proteins?
   (P) Collagens (Q) Prolamines
   (R) Histones (S) Keratins
   Choose the correct option.
   (a) Both Q & R (b) Both P & S
   (c) Both R & S (d) Both P & Q
12. Casein present in milk & vitelline present in egg yolk are comes under which of the following category?
   (a) Glycoprotein (b) Nucleoprotein
   (c) Phosphoprotein (d) Lipoprotein
13. Hydroxyl group is not present in which of the following amino acid?
   (a) Proline (b) Tyrosine
   (c) Threonine (d) Serine
14. Which of the following amino acids are both glucogenic and ketogenic in nature?
   (P) Phenylalanine (Q) Isoleucine
   (R) Tryptophan (S) Tyrosine
   Choose the correct option.
   (a) P, Q & R (b) Q, R & S
   (c) P, R & S (d) P, Q, R & S
15. Which of the following amino acids is not a polar with positive R group in structure?
   (a) Arginine (b) Lysine
   (c) Alanine (d) Histidine
16. The synthesis of urea occurs in
   (a) Kidney (b) Liver
   (c) Muscle (d) Brain
17. Which of the following amino acid is not required for the formation of glutathione?
   (a) Glycine (b) Cysteine
   (c) Glutamate (d) Alanine
18. In the synthesis of cysteine, which of following compound donates the carbon skeleton?
   (a) Serine (b) Methionine
   (c) Glutamate (d) Alanine
19. In the synthesis of cysteine, which of following compound donates sulphur atom?
   (a) Serine (b) Methionine
   (c) Glutamate (d) Alanine

20. Which of the following is not true in transamination reaction?
    (P) Reversible reaction
    (Q) Requires PLP
    (R) Important for production of non-essential amino acid
    (S) Free ammonia liberated

    Choose the correct option.
    (a) P, Q & R is correct; S is wrong
    (b) Q, R & S is correct; P is wrong
    (c) P, Q & S is correct; R is wrong
    (d) P, R & S is correct; Q is wrong
21. Which of the following is obtaining when ketogenic amino acids are degraded?
    (a) Succinyl CoA
    (b) Fumarate
    (c) Acetyl CoA
    (d) Pyruvate
22. Which of the following amino acid undergoes transamination reaction?
    (a) Lysine
    (b) Alanine
    (c) Threonine
    (d) Proline
23. All *transaminase* reaction requires which coenzyme?
    (a) PLP
    (b) NAD^+
    (c) FAD
    (d) TPP
24. Which of the following reaction converts amino acids to corresponding amine?
    (P) Transamination
    (Q) Deamination
    (R) Decarboxylation
    (S) Transmethylation

    Choose the correct option.
    (a) P & Q only
    (b) R & S only
    (c) R only
    (d) S only
25. What is the other name of urea cycle?
    (a) Krebs cycle
    (b) Henseleit cycle
    (c) Krebs-Henseleit cycle
    (d) Embde-Meyerhof cycle
26. Melanin polymer is biosynthesized from which amino acid?
    (a) Glycine
    (b) Tyrosine
    (c) Alanine
    (d) Methionine
27. Which of the following amino acid was first identified as essential amino acid.
    (a) Valine
    (b) Cystine
    (c) Cysteine
    (d) Tryptophan
28. Which of the following sulphur containing amino acid is participated in transmethylation reactions?
    (a) Methionine
    (b) Cysteine
    (c) Cystine
    (d) Glutathione
29. Which of the following amino acid is not a branched chain amino acid?
    (a) Leucine
    (b) Isoleucine
    (c) Alanine
    (d) Valine
30. N-acetyl glutamate is required for the activation of which enzyme?
    (a) *CPS-I*
    (b) *CPS-II*
    (c) *Arginase*
    (d) *Arginino-succinase*

31. Which of the following enzyme is mitochondrial enzyme?
    (a) *Arginase* (b) *Arginino-succinate synthase*
    (c) *Arginino-succinase* (d) *CPS-I*
32. Which of the following compound doesn't donate any atom in the formation of urea?
    (a) CO_2 (b) Ornithine
    (c) NH_3 (d) Aspartate
33. Citrullinemia is metabolic disorder of urea cycle which is due to the defects of which enzyme?
    (a) *Arginase* (b) *Arginino-succinate synthase*
    (c) *Arginino-succinase* (d) *CPS-I*
34. Which of the following compound serves as a collection center for amino groups in the biological system?
    (a) Glycine (b) Alanine
    (c) Aspartate (d) Glutamate
35. Which enzyme regulates urea cycle?
    (a) *Arginase* (b) *Arginino-succinate synthase*
    (c) *Arginino-succinase* (d) *CPS-I*
36. How many ATPs are utilized in urea cycle?
    (a) Two (b) Three
    (c) Four (d) Five
37. Which of the following products are not biosynthesized from tyrosine?
    (a) Dopamine (b) Choline
    (c) Thyroxine (d) Melanin
38. Kynurenine and serotonin pathway are metabolic pathways of which amino acid?
    (a) Phenylalanine (b) Methionine
    (c) Tryptophan (d) Valine
39. Maple syrup urine disease is a metabolic disorder of which amino acid?
    (a) Branched chain (b) Sulphur containing
    (c) Aromatic (d) Heterocyclic
40. Among the known mammalian enzymes, which enzyme possessing shortest half-life?
    (a) *Ornithine trans carbamoylase* (b) *Ornithine decarboxylase*
    (c) *NAG synthase* (d) *NAG hydrolase*
41. Which of the following amino acid is the substrate for the production of nitric oxide?
    (a) Arginine (b) Histidine
    (c) Threonine (d) Alanine
42. Primary hyperoxaluria is due to defect in which of the following enzyme?
    (a) *Glycine synthase* (b) *Glycine oxidase*
    (c) *Serine dehydratase* (d) *Glycine transaminase*
43. Glutamate is metabolically converted to α-ketoglutarate and NH_4^+ by a process __________
    (a) Oxidative deamination (b) Transamination
    (c) Reductive deamination (d) Deamination

44. Free ammonia combined with glutamate to yield glutamine by the action of ___________
    (a) *Glutaminase* (b) *Glutamine synthase*
    (c) *Glutamate dehydrogenase* (d) *Amino transferase*
45. Pyridoxal phosphate and its aminate form, pyridoxamine phosphate are tightly bound co-enzymes of ___________
    (a) *Amino transferase* (b) *Glutaminase*
    (c) *Glutamine synthase* (d) *Glutamate dehydrogenase*
46. Which is the first step in the catabolism of most L-amino acids once they have reached the liver is promoted?
    (a) *Amino transferase* (b) *Glutaminase*
    (c) *Glutamine synthase* (d) *Glutamate dehydrogenase*
47. The combined action of *aminotransferase* and *glutamate dehydrogenase* is referred as ___________
    (a) Oxidative deamination (b) Transamination
    (c) Reductive deamination (d) Transdeamination
48. Urea cycle converts ___________
    (a) Keto acids into amino acids (b) Amino acids into keto acids
    (c) Ammonia into a less toxic form (d) Ammonia into a more toxic form
49. Which is the end product of heme metabolism?
    (a) Urea (b) Uric acid
    (c) Bilirubin (d) Amino acid
50. Which of the following is a metabolic disorder of heme synthesis characterized by increased excretion of porphyrins and precursors of porphyrins?
    (a) Porphyria (b) Jaundice
    (c) Alkaptonuria (d) Hyperbilirubinemia

Key for Multiple Choice Questions

1. (a)	2. (b)	3. (d)	4. (c)	5. (d)
6. (d)	7. (a)	8. (d)	9. (b)	10. (d)
11. (b)	12. (c)	13. (a)	14. (d)	15. (c)
16. (b)	17. (d)	18. (a)	19. (b)	20. (a)
21. (c)	22. (b)	23. (a)	24. (c)	25. (c)
26. (b)	27. (d)	28. (a)	29. (c)	30. (a)
31. (d)	32. (b)	33. (b)	34. (d)	35. (d)
36. (c)	37. (b)	38. (c)	39. (a)	40. (b)
41. (a)	42. (d)	43. (a)	44. (b)	45. (a)
46. (a)	47. (d)	48. (c)	49. (c)	50. (a)

PART – B: Short Answers

1. What is hemolytic jaundice? How is it diagnosed?
2. Explain briefly about the different states of nitrogen balance.
3. What are transamination reactions? Give one example.
4. How urea cycle is regulated?
5. Write the elemental composition of proteins.
6. Give an account of nitrogen balance.
7. Define porphyria.
8. Explain the term "oxidative deamination".
9. What is non-oxidative deamination.
10. What are decarboxylation reactions? Give one example.
11. Define essential and non-essential amino acids with example.
12. What is the difference between glucogenic and ketogenic amino acids?
13. Define and list out various types of jaundice?
14. What is the relationship between hyperbilirubinemia and jaundice?
15. Write a note on urea cycle metabolic disorders.
16. Write a note on phenylketonuria.
17. What is albinism?
18. Explain alkaptonuria.
19. Define and explain tyrosinemia.
20. List out the biological significance of catecholamines.
21. What is the importance of melatonin?
22. Explain about complete proteins.
23. What is conjugated protein?
24. List out the biological importance of amino acids.
25. What is the relationship between urea cycle and citric acid cycle?

PART – C: Long Answers

1. Define and list out various types of protein classification. Explain any one classification in detail with suitable examples?
2. Write a detailed note on chemical nature and solubility classification of proteins.
3. Write a note on structures of protein.
4. Explain the biological significance of proteins.
5. Define and list out various types of amino acid classification. Explain any one classification in detail with suitable examples?
6. How amino acids are classified based on their chemical structure? Explain with suitable structure of amino acids.
7. Explain the biological significance of amino acids.
8. Explain the term "amino acid pool" and add a note on "nitrogen balance".
9. Write in detail about the general aspects of amino acid metabolism.
10. Explain in detail about three major metabolic reactions taking place in amino acid metabolism.
11. Write a note on transamination & deamination of amino acid metabolism.
12. Write about catabolism of amino acids.
13. Explain urea cycle and its metabolic disorders.
14. Write about the urea cycle. Discuss about transamination and decarboxylation.

15. Describe the general metabolic pathways of amino acids.
16. Note on Kreb's-Henseleit cycle.
17. Detailed note on metabolism of phenylalanine.
18. Write about biosynthesis of melanin and thyroid hormones.
19. How catecholamines are biosynthesized in biological system. Add a note on biological significance of catecholamines.
20. Explain the metabolism of tryptophan.
21. How serotonin and melatonin is biosynthesized? Explain their biological significance also.
22. Write a detailed note on metabolic disorders of amino acid metabolism.
23. Explain a) Jaundice b) Tyrosinemia?
24. Write about hyperbilirubinemia & phenylketonuria.
25. Write a note on metabolism of heme.

6

Nucleic Acid & Its Metabolism

Nucleic acids are the polynucleotides and nucleotides are composed of nitrogen base, pentose sugar and phosphate group. Nucleic acids primarily serve as repositories and transmitters of genetic information. The pentose sugar present in RNA and DNA is ribose and 2-deoxyribose, respectively. Either directly or indirectly, nucleotides participate in almost all biochemical processes. Nucleotides are the structural components of nucleic acids such as DNA and RNA and co-enzymes. In addition, several metabolic reactions are also regulated by nucleotides.

Classification or Types of Nucleic Acids

Nucleic acids are broadly classified into two major types based on the sugar molecules present in them. They are,

1. Deoxyribonucleic acid or DNA
2. Ribonucleic acid or RNA

Deoxyribonucleic acid or DNA: It is a polymer of deoxyribonucleotides composed of deoxyribose sugar, nitrogen bases such as purines (adenine & guanine), pyrimidines (thymine and cytosine) and phosphate group.

Ribonucleic acid or RNA: It is a polymer of ribonucleotides composed of ribose sugar, nitrogen base such as purines (adenine & guanine), pyrimidines (uracil and cytosine), and phosphate group.

Composition of Nucleic Acid

Nucleic acids are chemically polynucleotides held by 3′- and 5′-phosphate bridges or nucleic acids are built up by the monomeric units known as nucleotides. Upon hydrolysis, nucleic acids produce nucleotides. Further, the hydrolysis of nucleotides produces nucleosides and phosphoric acid. Hence, **nucleotides are defined as phosphate esters of nucleosides**. Hydrolysis of nucleoside produces nitrogen base and sugar. Nucleosides are chemically composed of nitrogen base and sugars. In nucleic acids, there are two different types of nitrogen bases such as purines and pyrimidines are present. Adenine and guanine are two purine nitrogen bases and thymine, cytosine and uracil are three pyrimidine nitrogen bases present in nucleic acid. Out of three pyrimidine nitrogen bases, thymine and cytosine is present in DNA and cytosine and uracil is present in RNA. In nucleic acids, two different types of sugar molecules such as ribose and deoxyribose are present. In that, deoxyribose sugar is present in DNA and ribose sugar is present in RNA.

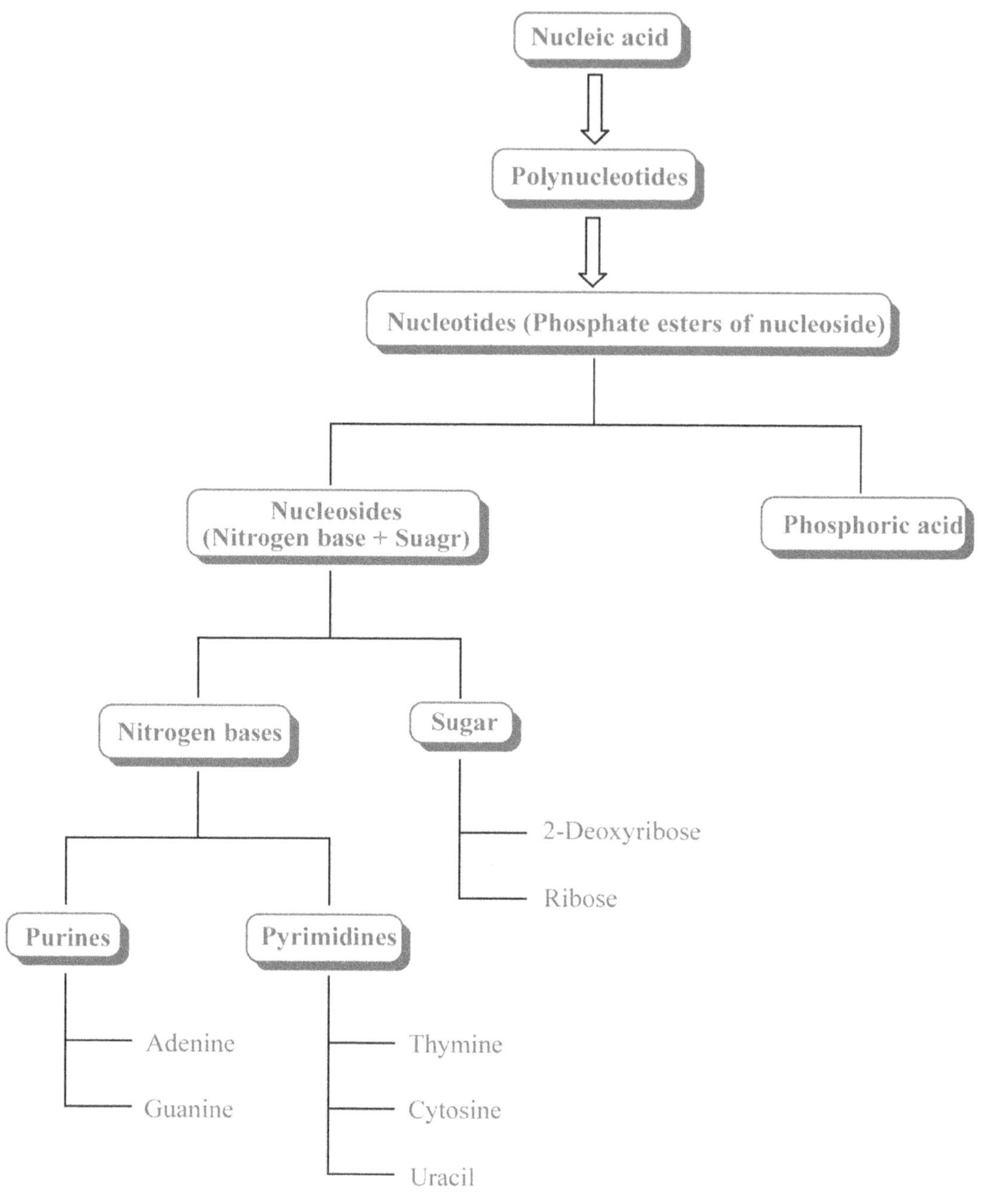

Nitrogen Bases

Nitrogen bases are chemically aromatic heterocyclic compounds. Two types of nitrogen bases present in nucleic acid are mentioned below.

1. Purines
2. Pyrimidines

In general, purines are numbered in anti-clockwise direction whereas pyrimidines are numbered in clockwise direction. The general structures of purines and pyrimidines are represented in the below structures.

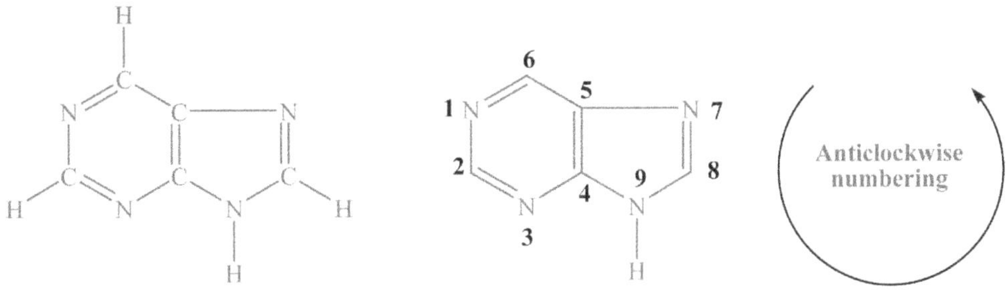

General structure of purine nitrogen base

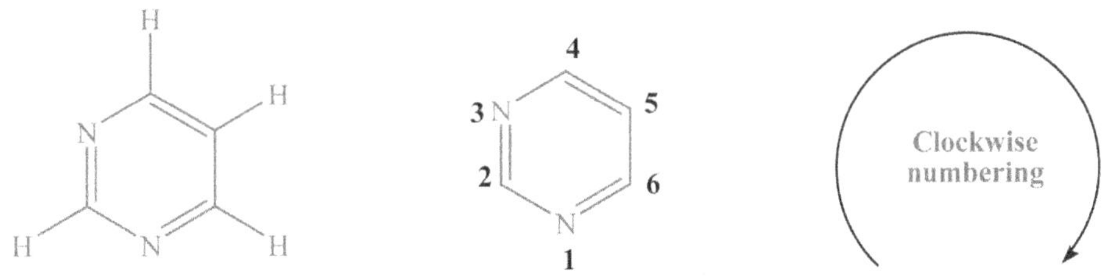

General structure of pyrimidine nitrogen base

Purines: Adenine and guanine are the two purine bases present in the nucleic acids. Both adenine and guanine are present in DNA and RNA. Existence of molecules in a lactam (keto) form and lactim (enol) form is known as tautomerism. Purine with an oxo (C=O) functional group exhibits tautomeric forms as follows.

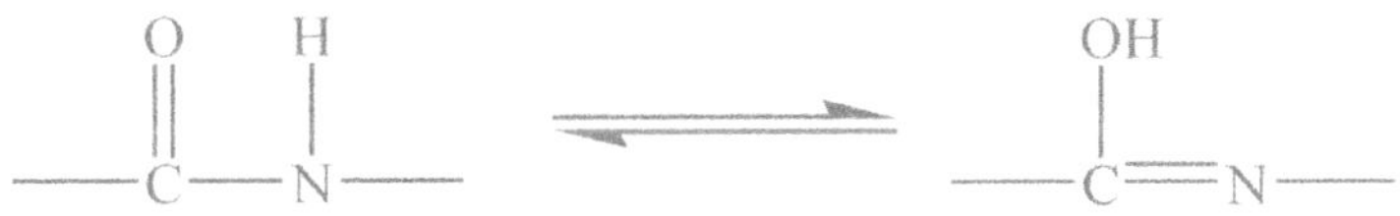

Lactam form or Keto form ⇌ **Lactim form or Enol form**

Table 6.1 Chemical structures of nitrogen bases.

S. No.	Name of base	Chemical name	Lactam form or Keto form	Lactim form or Enol form
A. Purine bases				
1	Adenine	6-Aminopurine (or) 9H-Purin-6-amine	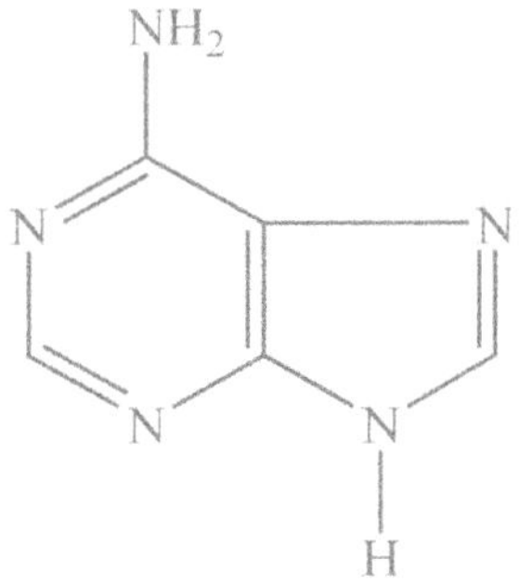	----
2	Guanine	2-Amino-6-oxopurine (or) 2-Amino-1H-purin-6(9H)-one	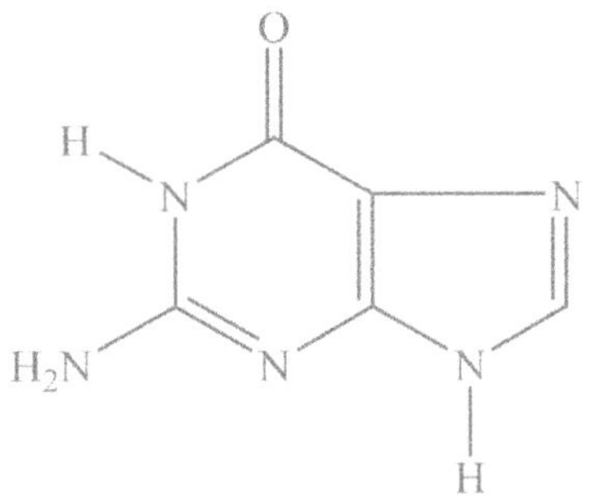	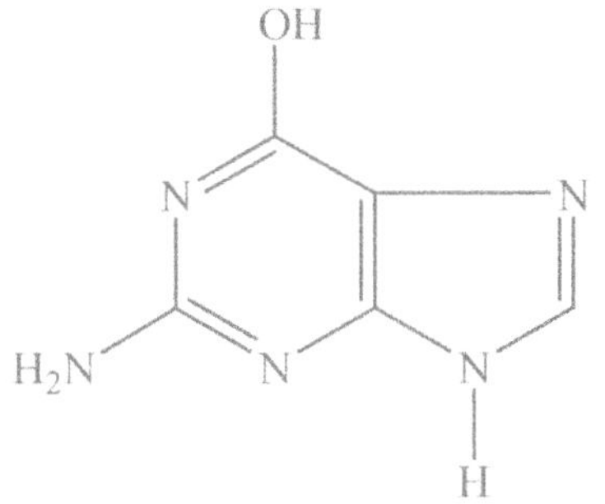

Table 6.1 Contd...

S. No.	Name of base	Chemical name	Lactam form or Keto form	Lactim form or Enol form
B. Pyrimidine bases				
3	Thymine	2,4-Dioxy-5-methylpyrimidine or 5-Methyluracil	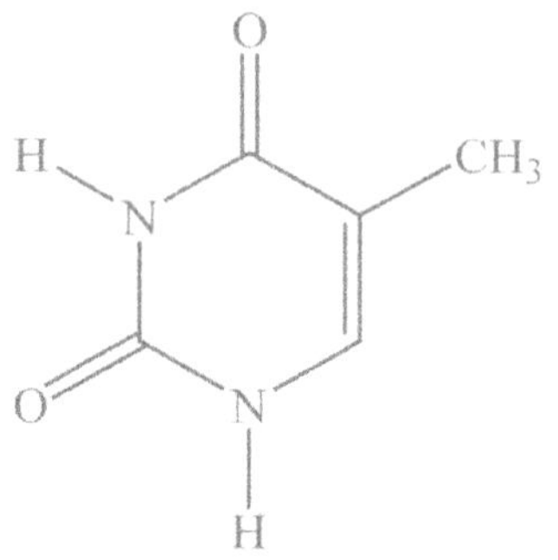	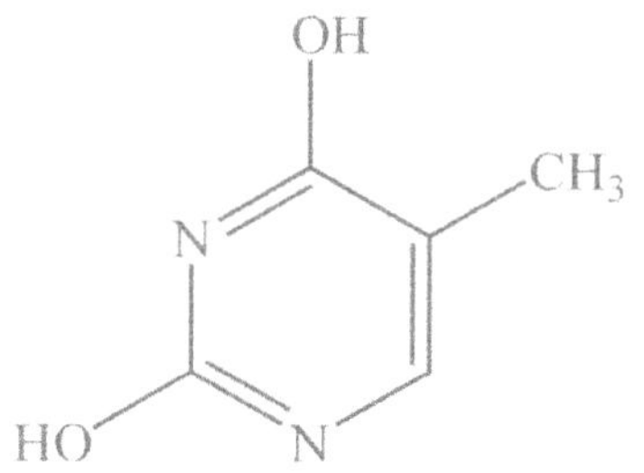
4	Cytosine	2-Oxo-4-aminopyrimidine	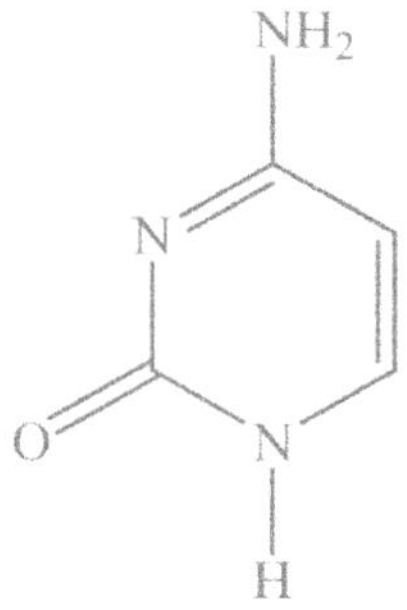	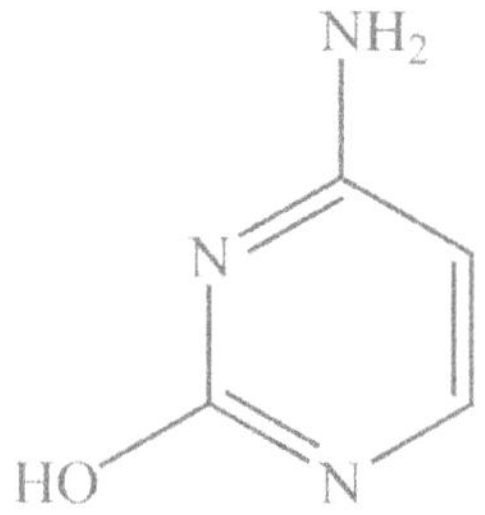
5	Uracil	2,4-Dioxypyrimidine (or) Pyrimidine – 2, 4 (1H, 3H) - dione	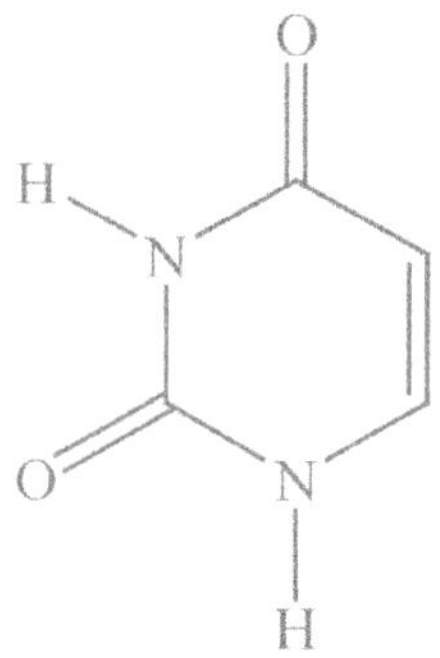	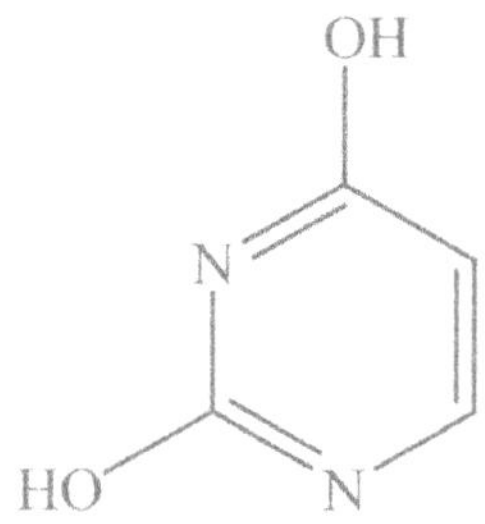

Pyrimidines: Thymine, cytosine and uracil are the three pyrimidine bases present in the nucleic acids. Thymine is present only in DNA and uracil is present only in RNA. Cytosine is present in both DNA and RNA. Like purines, pyrimidines with oxo (C=O) functional groups exhibit tautomeric forms. At physiological pH lactam forms are predominantly present. Chemical structures of various purine and pyrimidine nitrogen bases are listed in Table 6.1.

Minor bases: Many minor and unusual bases other than the bases described above are also present in nucleic acid. They are 5-methylcytosine, N^4-acetylcytosine, N^6-methyladenine, N^6, N^6-dimethyladenine, pseudo uracil, etc. These unusual bases present in nucleic acids are helpful in the recognition of specific enzymes.

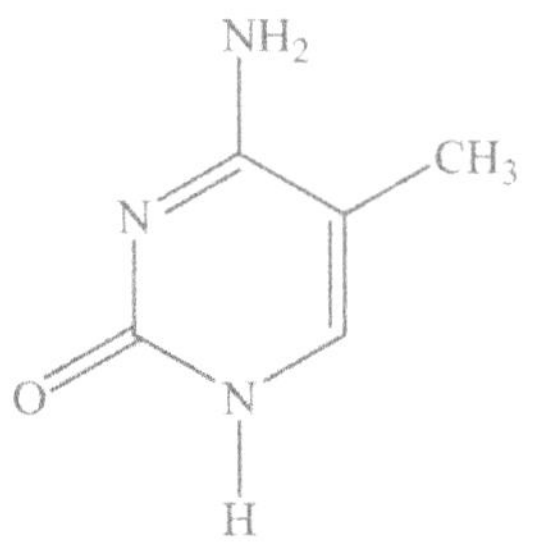

5-Methylcytosine 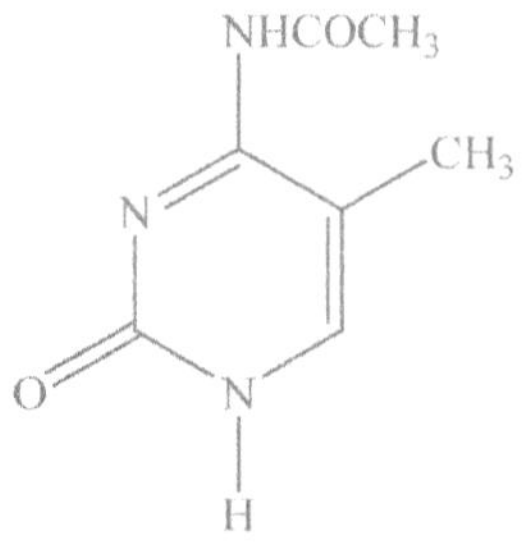 **N^4-Acetylcytosine** 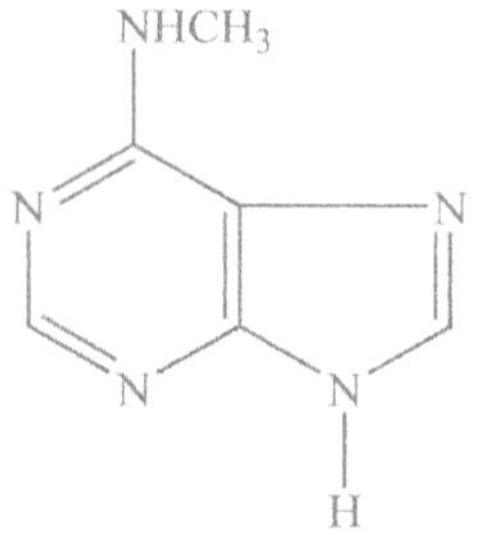 **N^6-Methyladenine**

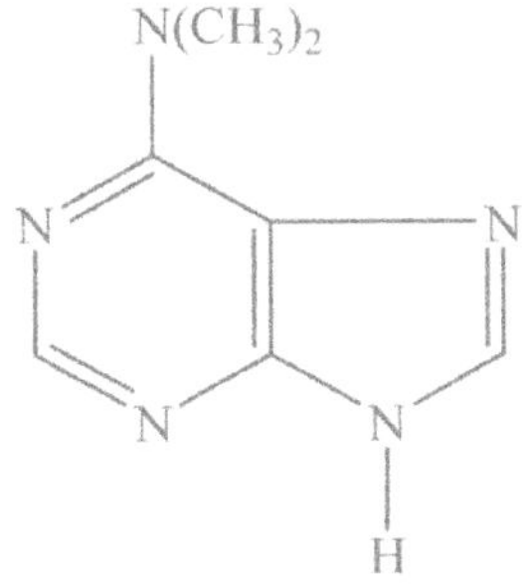

N(CH3)2 N N N N H

N^6, N^6-Dimethyladenine

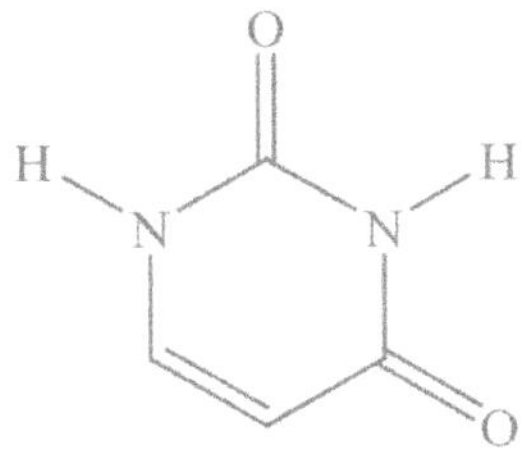

O H N N H O

Pseudo uracil

Other biologically important bases: In cells, other biologically important nitrogen bases such as hypoxanthine, xanthine and uric acid are present in free state. Uric acid is the end product of purine degradation and hypoxanthine and xanthine are intermediates in purine synthesis.

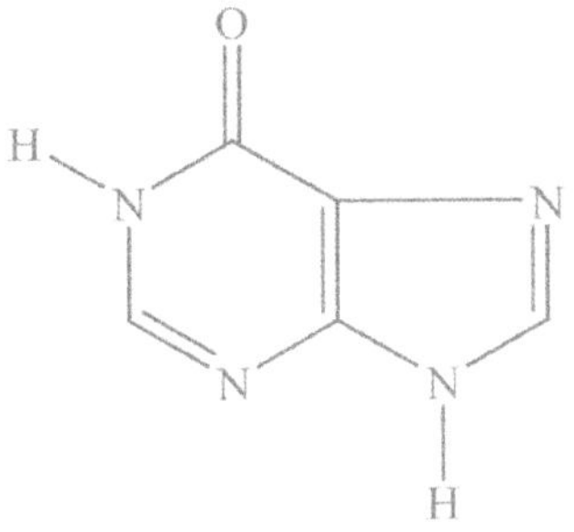

Hypoxanthine

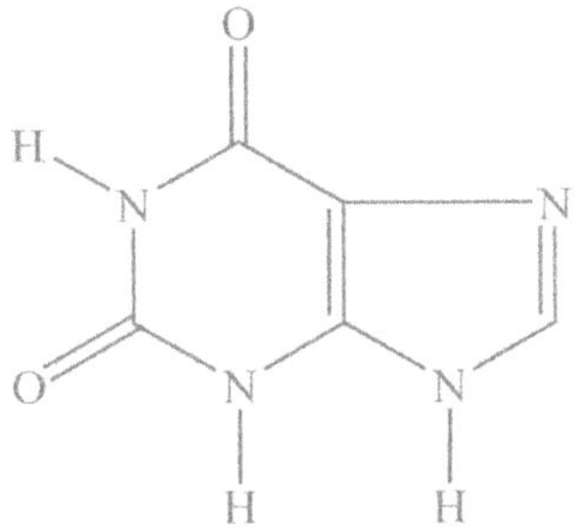

Xanthine

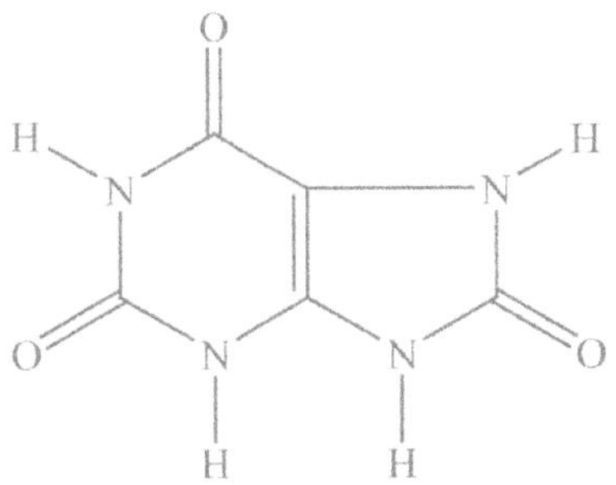

Uric acid

Important plant bases: Caffeine (from coffee), theophylline (from tea) and theobromine (from cocoa) are methylated purines present in plants that possess some important pharmacological activities.

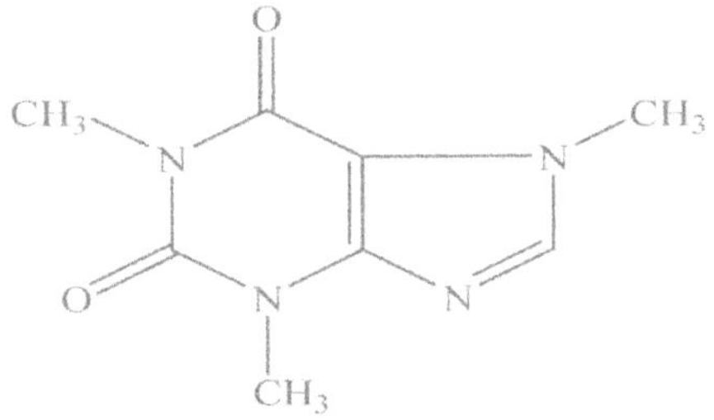

Caffeine (or) 1,3,7-Trimethylxanthine

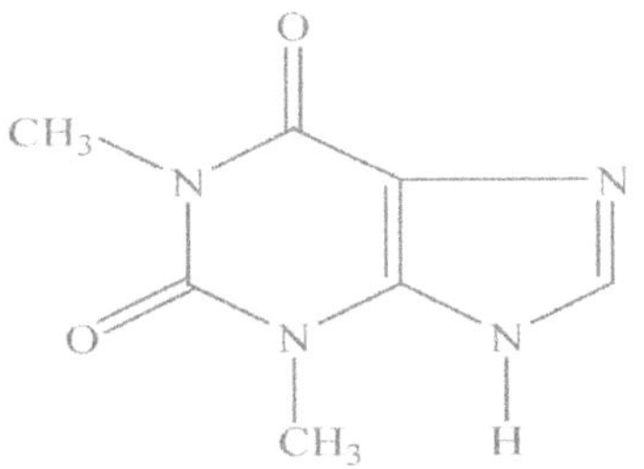

Theophylline (or) 1,3-Dimethylxanthine

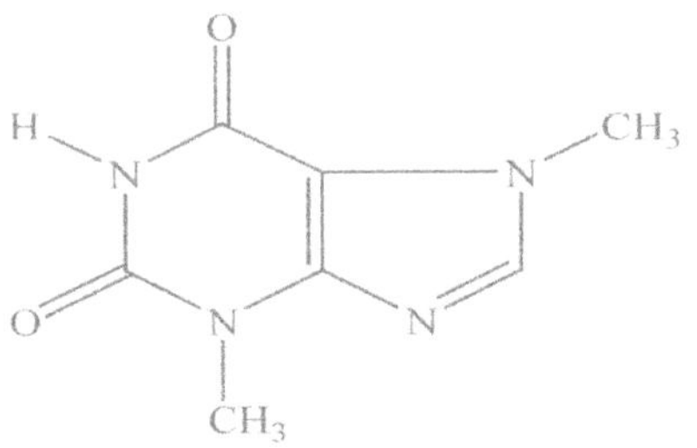

Theobromine (or) Xantheose (or) 3,7-Dimethylxanthine

Sugars: Nucleic acid contains pentose sugars (five carbon monosaccharides) such as ribose and 2′-deoxyribose. For differentiation from nitrogen base numbering, sugar molecule numbers are represented with an associated prime (′). The two sugars mentioned above are differing in their structure at C-2′ only. Deoxyribose possess one less oxygen at C-2′ compared to ribose. DNA contains 2′-deoxyribose and RNA contains ribose sugar.

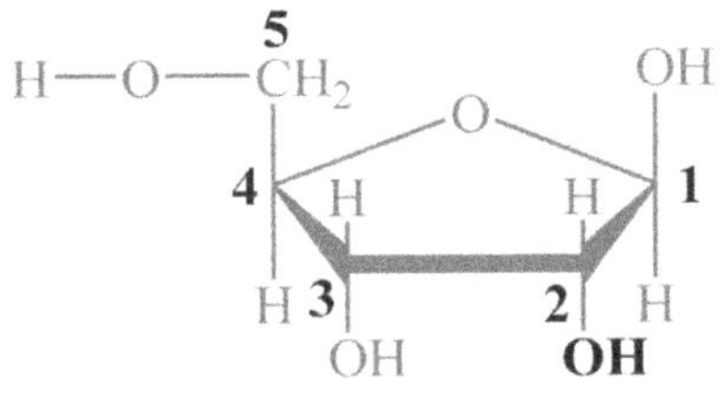

β-D-Ribose

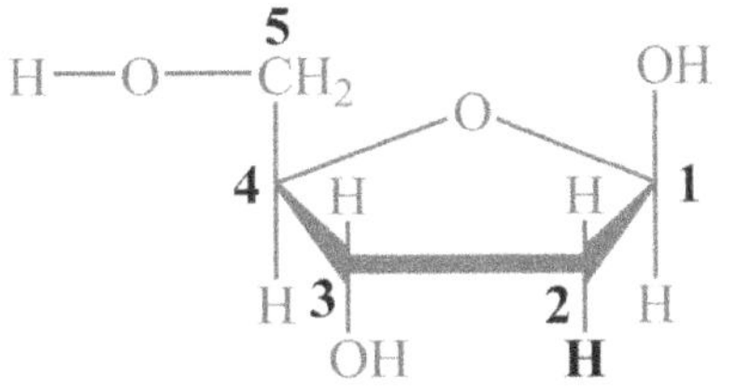

β-D-2-Deoxyribose

Nomenclature of Nucleotides

Nucleosides are formed when pentose sugars are added to the nitrogen bases. If the sugar attached is ribose it is called ribonucleoside. The ribonucleosides of bases adenine, guanine, cytosine and uracil are adenosine, guanosine, cytidine and uridine, respectively. If the sugar attached is 2-deoxyribose then it is called deoxyribonucleoside. The prefix deoxy is added to the corresponding ribonucleoside name to get the deoxyribonucleoside name. The deoxyribonucleosides of bases adenine, guanine, cytosine and thymine are deoxyadenosine, deoxyguanosine, deoxycytidine and deoxythymidine, respectively.

When a nucleoside is attached to a single phosphate moiety, the term mononucleotide is used. For example, adenosine attached to single phosphate moiety is named as adenosine monophosphate (AMP) which is composed of adenine, ribose and phosphate moiety. The various bases present in the nucleic acid and their corresponding nucleoside, mononucleotides and abbreviations are listed in the Table 6.2.

Table 6.2 Various bases, nucleoside, mononucleotides present in nucleic acid.

S. No.	Nitrogen base	Nucleoside	Mononucleotide	Abbreviation
A. Ribonucleotide				
1	Adenine (A)	Adenosine (Adenine + Ribose)	Adenosine-5'-monophosphate or adenylate (Adenosine + Phosphate)	AMP
2	Guanine (G)	Guanosine (Guanine + Ribose)	Guanosine-5'-monophosphate or guanylate (Guanosine + Phosphate)	GMP
3	Cytosine (C)	Cytidine (Cytosine + Ribose)	Cytidine-5'-monophosphate or cytidylate (Cytidine + Phosphate)	CMP
4	Uracil (U)	Uridine (Uracil + Ribose)	Uridine-5'-monophosphate or uridylate (Uridine + Phosphate)	UMP
B. Deoxyribonucleotide				
5	Adenine (A)	Deoxyadenosine (Adenine + 2-Deoxyibose)	Deoxyadenosine-5'-monophosphate or Deoxyadenylate (Deoxyadenosine + Phosphate)	dAMP
6	Guanine (G)	Deoxyguanosine (Guanine + 2-Deoxyibose)	Deoxyguanosine-5'-monophosphate or Deoxyguanylate (Deoxyguanosine + Phosphate)	dGMP
7	Cytosine (C)	Deoxycytidine (Cytosine + 2-Deoxyibose)	Deoxycytidine-5'-monophosphate or Deoxycytidylate (Deoxycytidine + Phosphate)	dCMP
8	Thymine (T)	Deoxythymidine (Thymine + 2-Deoxyibose)	Deoxythymidine-5'-monophosphate or Deoxythymidylate (Deoxythymidine + Phosphate)	dTMP

Binding of nucleotide components: The pentose sugars are bonded to nitrogen bases by N-glycosidic bonds. C-1′ of sugars are covalently attached to the N-9 of purine bases or N-1 of pyrimidine bases to form corresponding nucleosides. In nucleosides, the hydroxyl group present at C-5′ or C-3′ of sugar molecules is esterified with phosphates to produce corresponding 5′- or 3′- monophosphates (i.e., nucleotide). Generally, esterification takes place at C-5′, hence 5′ is usually omitted while writing names of nucleotides. In case if esterification takes place at C-3′ then 3′ is included while writing names of nucleotides. The structures of some nucleotides such as AMP & dTMP are given below.

Nucleoside di and triphosphates: Only one phosphate moiety is present in nucleoside monophosphates like AMP, GMP, CMP, UMP, dAMP, dGMP, dCMP and dTMP. When second or third phosphates are attached to nucleoside it produced nucleoside diphosphates like ADP, GDP, CDP, UDP, dADP, dGDP, dCDP and dTDP or nucleoside triphosphates like ATP, GTP, CTP, UTP, dATP, dGTP, dCTP and dTTP, respectively. The negative charges of the phosphate groups are responsible for anionic properties of nucleotides and nucleic acids.

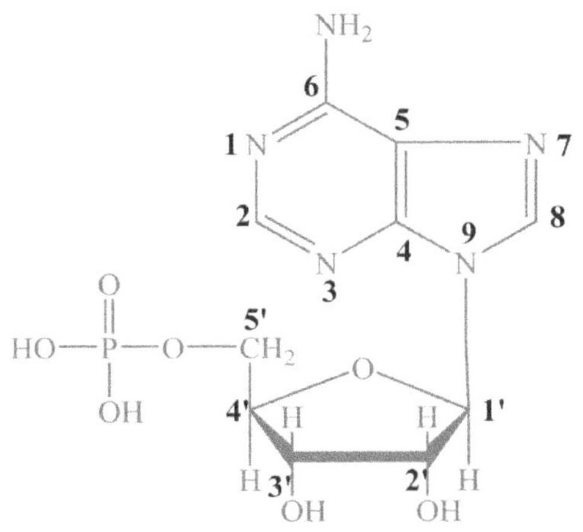

Adenosine monophosphate (AMP)

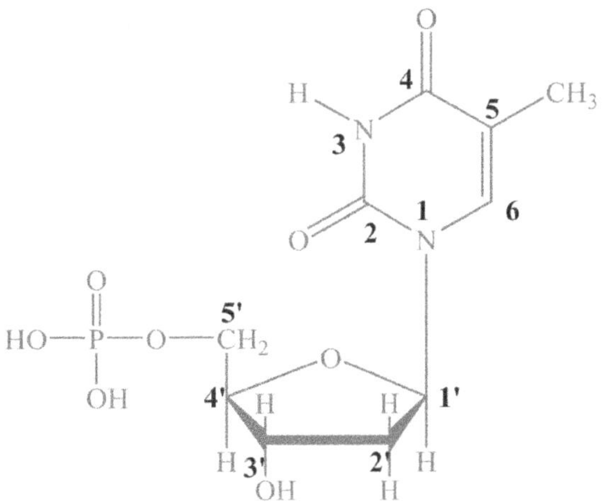

Deoxythymidine monophosphate (dTMP)

Biological Significance of Nucleic Acids

The various biological significance of nucleic acids are given under the following different headings.

(a) DNA

1. DNA is the chemical basis of heredity organized into genes. The fundamental unit of genetic information is gene.
2. DNA is regarded as the reserve bank of genetic information.
3. Over millions of years, identities of different species are maintained by DNA only.
4. In addition, DNA controls every aspect of cellular functions.
5. Through RNA mediation, gene controls the synthesis of proteins.
6. DNA is the precursor for the synthesis of RNA by a process called transcription.

(b) RNA

1. RNA is useful for the synthesis of protein by a process called translation.
2. To synthesize proteins, mRNA transfers genetic information from genes to ribosomes.
3. For protein synthesis, tRNA transfers amino acids to mRNA.
4. rRNA provides a structural framework for ribosomes.
5. hnRNA serves as a precursor for the synthesis of all RNAs including mRNA.
6. snRNA is involved in processing of mRNA.
7. snoRNA plays a major role in processing of rRNA.
8. scRNA is involved in the secretion of proteins for export.
9. In bacteria, tmRNA is mostly present and it facilitates the degradation of incorrectly synthesized proteins by adding short peptide tags to proteins.

(c) Ribozymes

Ribozymes are types of RNA which act as enzymes. Before the occurrence of protein enzymes during evolution, ribozymes were probably functioning as a catalyst. The following are the selected list of ribozymes and their corresponding biochemical reactions.

1. In protein synthesis rRNA is involved in peptide bond formation.
2. *Ribonuclease P (RNase P)* is a component of RNA and is a ribozyme containing protein. It is involved in cleavage of RNA particularly tRNA precursors to generate mature tRNA molecules. It is also involved in ligation.
3. Self-splicing RNA is involved in cleavage of DNA.

4. RNAs of spliceosome is involved in splicing of RNA.
5. *In vitro* selected RNAs are involved in RNA polymerization, RNA aminoacylation, RNA phosphorylation, redox reactions, glycoside bond formation and disulfide exchange.

(d) Nucleotides

1. Nucleotides are the monomeric unit or building blocks of nucleic acid.
2. Nucleotides are the structural components of some B-complex vitamin co-enzymes like FAD, NAD^+, etc.
3. ATP is one of the important nucleotides which is energy currency of the cell involved in energy reactions.
4. In addition, nucleotides also regulate the metabolic reactions.
5. Clinically some nucleotide analogs are used due to its pharmacological properties. They are,
   (a) Allopurinol is used in the treatment of gout and hyperuricemia.
   (b) Many nucleotide analogs are used in the treatment of cancers. **Example:** 6-Mercaptopurine, 5-fluorouracil, 3-deoxyuridine, 5-iodouracil, 5- or 6-azauridine, 5- or 6-azacytidine and arabinosylcytosine.
   (c) During transplantation azathioprine is used to suppress the immunological rejection of transplanted organs.
   (d) Neurological disease and viral encephalitis are treated by using arabinosyladenine.
   (e) Drugs like zidovudine, 3-azido-2′,3′-dideoxythymidine and didanosine are used in the treatment of AIDS.

Biosynthesis of Purine Nucleotides

Purine rings of the nucleotides are contributed by many compounds. Sources of individual atoms in purine ring are presented in Figure 6.1. They are,

1. N_1 of purine is derived from the amino group of aspartate.
2. C_2 and C_8 of purine are derived from N^{10}-formyl THF.
3. N_3 and N_9 of purine are derived from the amide group of glutamine.
4. C_4, C_5 and N_7 of purine are derived from glycine.
5. C_6 of purine is derived from carbondioxide.

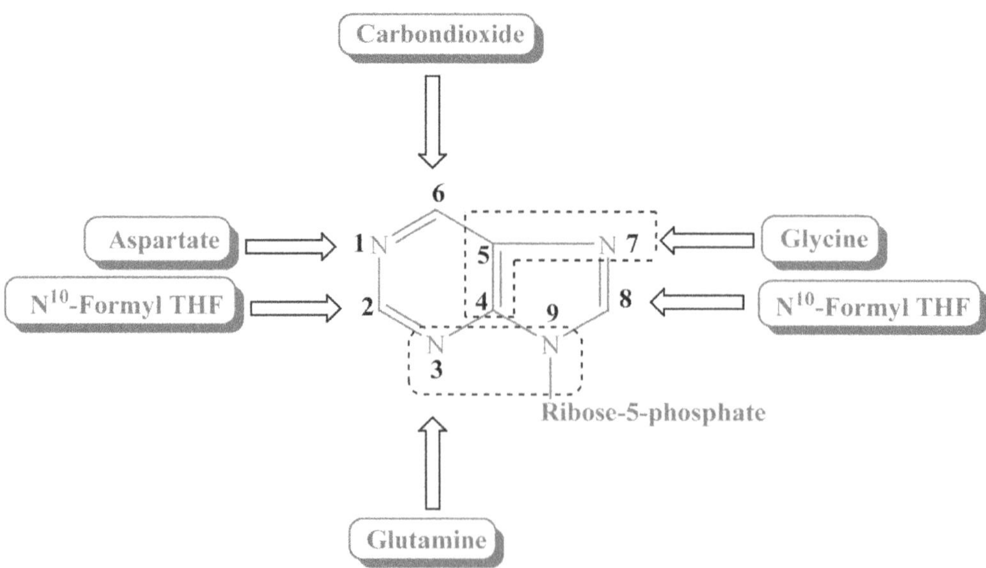

Figure 6.1 Sources of individual atoms in purine ring.

Pathway:

Purine bases are synthesized as ribonucleotides and not as a free base. Hence, biosynthesis of purine nucleotides in the body is a complex process. In the pre-existing ribose-5-phosphate, purines are built and synthesized. Purine nucleotides are mainly synthesized in the liver. Purine nucleotides are not synthesized in erythrocytes, polymorphonuclear leukocytes and the brain. The parent purine nucleotide is inosine monophosphate (IMP) and is synthesized by the following ways from α-D-ribose-5-phosphate.

1. The HMP shunt pathway of carbohydrate metabolism produces pentose sugar ribose-5-phosphate which acts as a precursor for the synthesis of purine nucleotides. In the first step, ribose-5-phosphate is reacted with ATP in presence of *phosphoribosyl pyrophosphate (PRPP) synthetase* (Product formed is "phosphoribosyl pyrophosphate (PRPP)"and the type of reaction involved is "synthesis") and produces 5-phosphoribosyl-α-pyrophosphate (PRPP) with liberation of AMP by simple pyro phosphorylation reaction. In this reaction, one ATP is converted to AMP **(2 ATP is utilized)**.
2. In the next step, PRPP initially undergoes hydrolysis followed by reaction with glutamine and gains amide nitrogen by replacing with pyrophosphate at C-1 of ribose sugar results in formation of β-5-phosphoribosylamine. The reaction is catalyzed by *PRPP glutamyl amido transferase* (Substrate is "PRPP" and the type of reaction involved is "amide transfer") and **it is a committed step (rate limiting step) of purine nucleotide biosynthesis**. By feedback inhibition of nucleotides such as IMP, AMP and GMP, the enzyme *PRPP glutamyl amido transferase* is controlled.
3. Later, the formed β-5-phosphoribosylamine undergoes amidation by reacting with glycine and produces glycinamide ribosyl-5-phosphate with one water molecule in the presence of *synthetase* (The type of reaction involved is "synthesis"). During this reaction, the energy needed is provided by breakdown of ATP into ADP and inorganic phosphate **(1 ATP is utilized)**.
4. In the succeeding step, formyl group from N^{10}-formyl THF is transferred to glycinamide ribosyl-5-phosphate by formylation reaction in presence of *formyl transferase* (Group transferred is "formyl" and the type of reaction involved is "transfer") produces formylglycinamide ribosyl-5- phosphate.
5. Then, obtained formylglycinamide ribosyl-5- phosphate reacts with glutamine and gains amide nitrogen to produce formylglycinamidine ribosyl-5-phosphate with a loss of water molecule in presence of *synthetase* (The type of reaction involved is "synthesis"). The energy needed by this reaction is provided by breakdown of ATP into ADP and inorganic phosphate **(1 ATP is utilized)**.
6. In the next step, formylglycinamidine ribosyl-5-phosphate in enol form undergoes cyclization with a loss of water molecule to produce 5-aminoimidazole ribosyl-5- phosphate in presence of *synthetase* (The type of reaction involved is "synthesis"). The energy needed for this reaction is obtained from the breakdown of ATP into ADP and inorganic phosphate **(1 ATP is utilized)**.
7. Through carboxylation, 5-aminoimidazole ribosyl-5-phosphate is converted to 5-aminoimidazole carboxylate ribosyl-5-phosphate by reacting with carbondioxide in the presence of *carboxylase* enzyme (The type of reaction involved is "carboxylation"). Unlike other carboxylation reactions, this carboxylation doesn't need biotin and / or ATP.
8. In this step, aspartate is condensed with the formed 5-aminoimidazole carboxylate ribosyl-5-phosphate to produce 5-aminoimidazole-4-succinyl carboxamide ribosyl-5-phosphate with loss of water molecule. *Synthetase* enzyme (The type of reaction involved is "synthesis") catalyzes this reaction and it needs energy which is derived from breakdown of ATP into ADP and inorganic phosphate **(1 ATP is utilized)**.
9. Later, the obtained 5-aminoimidazole-4-succinyl carboxamide ribosyl-5-phosphate undergoes lysis reaction with the removal of fumarate and produces 5-aminoimidazole-4-carboxamide ribosyl-5-phosphate. *Adenosuccinate lyase* (Substrate is "5-aminoimidazole-4-succinyl carboxamide ribosyl-5-phosphate" which is adenosuccinate derivative and the type of reaction involved is "lysis") is an enzyme responsible for this reaction.

α-D-Ribose 5-phosphate

PRPP synthetase — ATP → AMP (Phosphorylation)

5- Phosphoribosyl-α-pyrophosphate (PRPP)

PRPP glutamyl amido transferase — Glutamine + H_2O → Glutamate + PPi (Hydrolysis followed by amination)

Configuration inverted

β-5-Phosphoribosylamine

Synthetase — NH_2CH_2COOH (Glycine) + ATP → H_2O + ADP + Pi (Amidation or Condensation)

Glycinamide ribosyl-5-phosphate

Formyl transferase — N^{10}- Formyl THF → THF (Formylation)

Ribose-5-phosphate

Formylglycinamide ribosyl-5-phosphate

Synthetase — Glutamine + ATP → Glutamate + H_2O + ADP + Pi (Amidation)

Ribose-5-phosphate

Formylglycinamidine ribosyl-5-phosphate (Keto form)

Keto-enol tautomerism (Tautomerization)

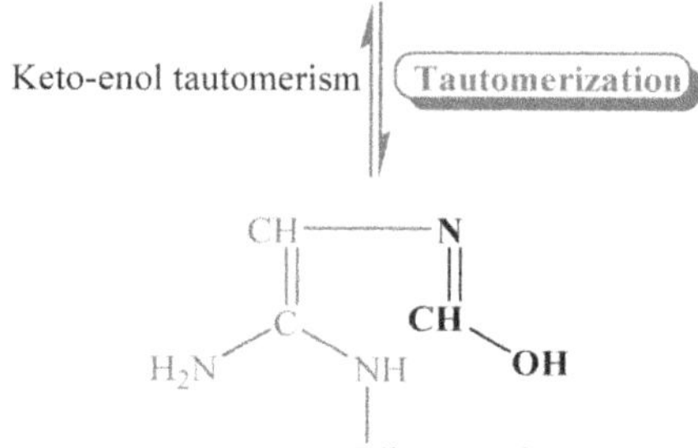

Formylglycinamidine ribosyl-5-phosphate (Enol form)

Synthetase — ATP → ADP + Pi + H_2O (Cyclization)

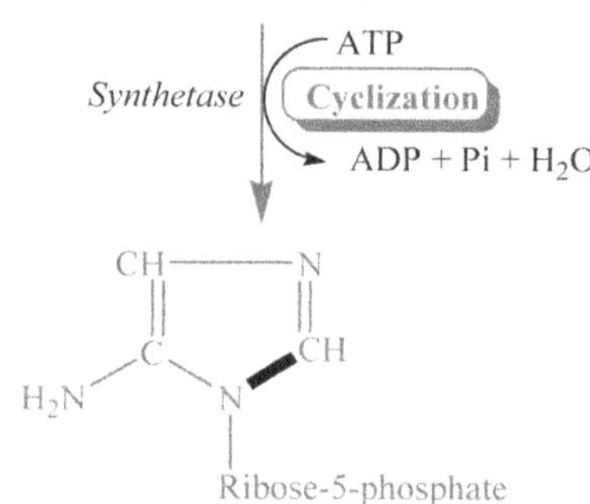

5- Aminoimidazole ribosyl-5-phosphate

Carboxylase — CO_2 (Carboxylation)

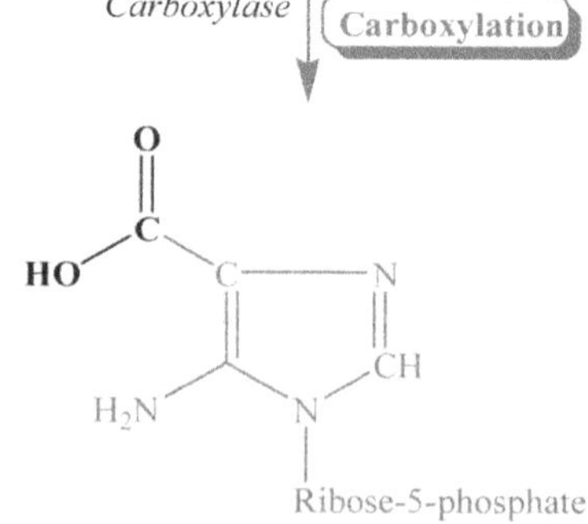

5- Aminoimidazole carboxylate ribosyl-5-phosphate

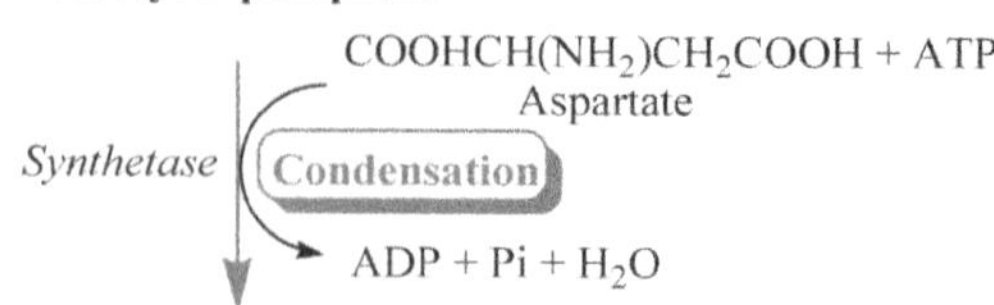

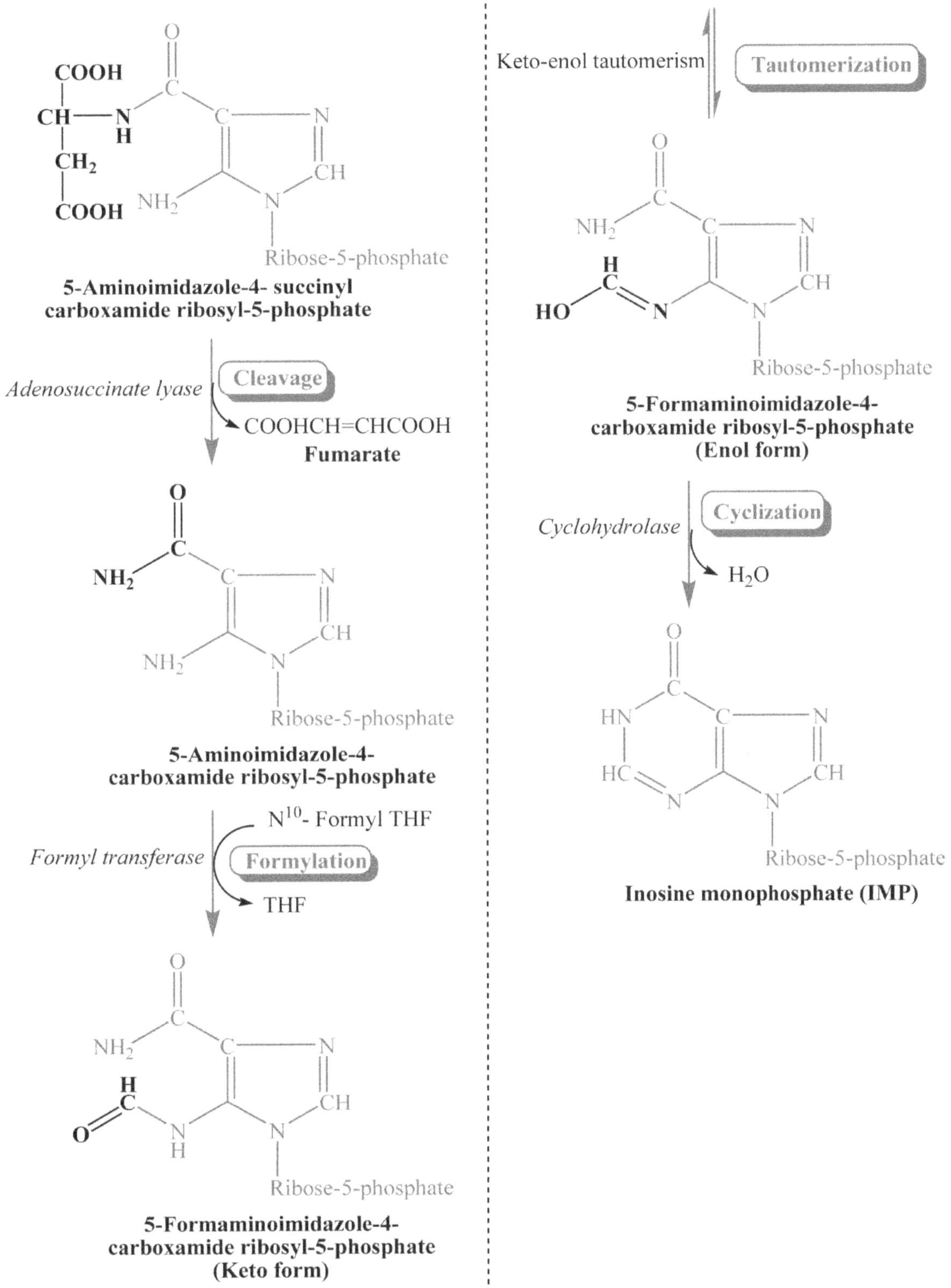

5-Aminoimidazole-4- succinyl carboxamide ribosyl-5-phosphate

Adenosuccinate lyase — Cleavage → COOHCH=CHCOOH (Fumarate)

5-Aminoimidazole-4-carboxamide ribosyl-5-phosphate

Formyl transferase — Formylation: N^{10}- Formyl THF → THF

5-Formaminoimidazole-4-carboxamide ribosyl-5-phosphate (Keto form)

Keto-enol tautomerism — Tautomerization

5-Formaminoimidazole-4-carboxamide ribosyl-5-phosphate (Enol form)

Cyclohydrolase — Cyclization → H_2O

Inosine monophosphate (IMP)

α-D-Ribose 5-phosphate

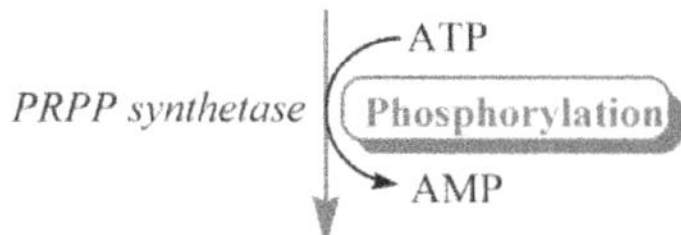

5- Phosphoribosyl-α-pyrophosphate (PRPP)

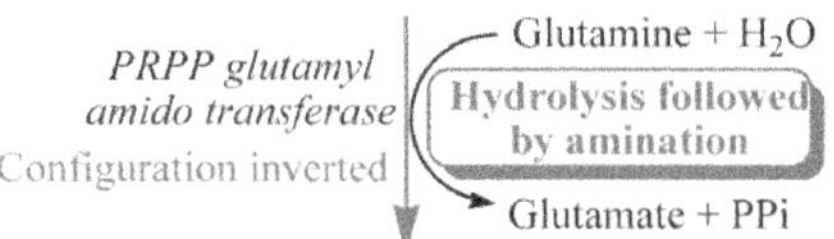

β-5-Phosphoribosylamine

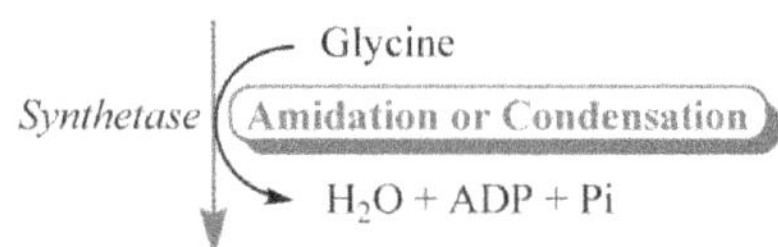

Glycinamide ribosyl-5-phosphate

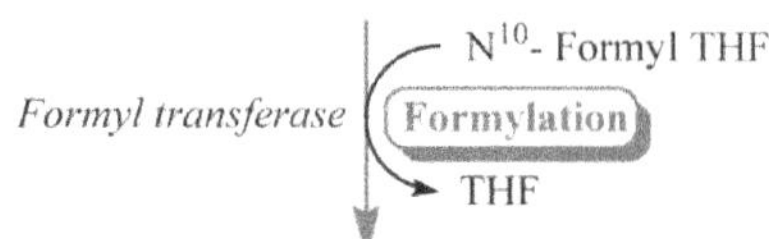

Formylglycinamide ribosyl-5-phosphate

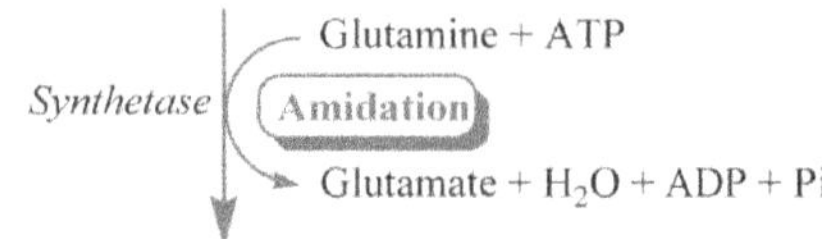

Formylglycinamidine ribosyl-5-phosphate (Keto form)

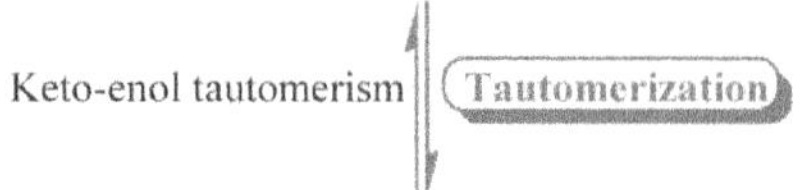

Formylglycinamidine ribosyl-5-phosphate (Enol form)

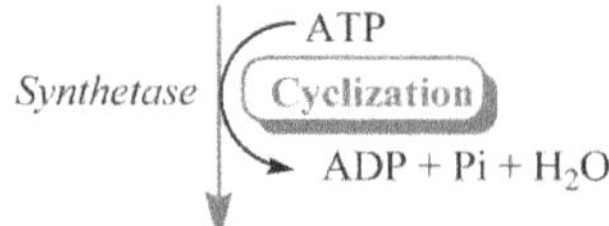

5- Aminoimidazole ribosyl-5-phosphate

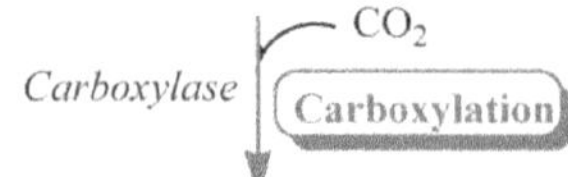

5- Aminoimidazole carboxylate ribosyl-5-phosphate

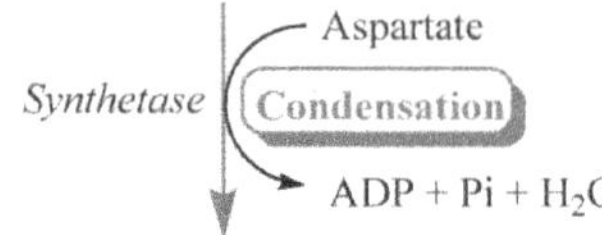

5-Aminoimidazole-4- succinyl carboxamide ribosyl-5-phosphate

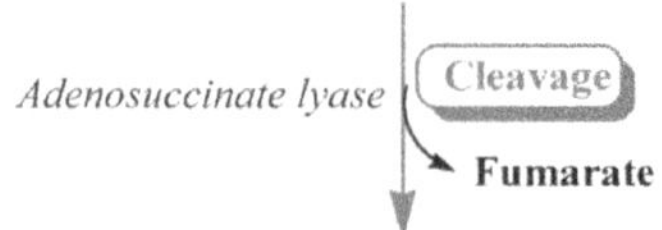

5-Aminoimidazole-4-carboxamide ribosyl-5-phosphate

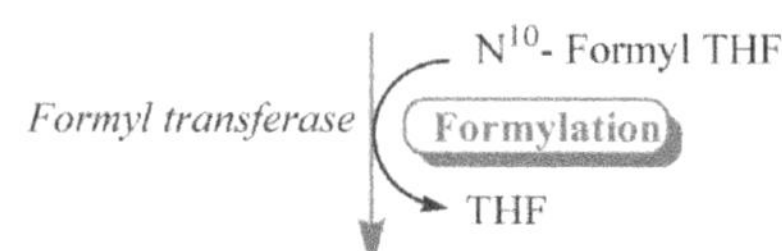

5-Formaminoimidazole-4-carboxamide ribosyl-5-phosphate (Keto form)

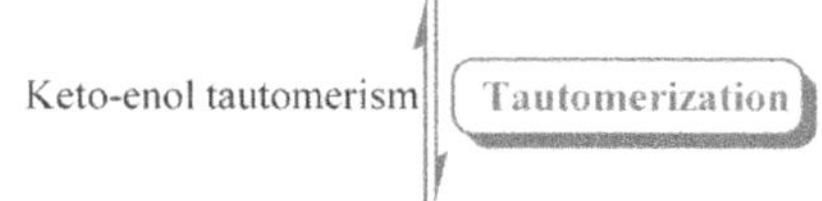

5-Formaminoimidazole-4-carboxamide ribosyl-5-phosphate (Enol form)

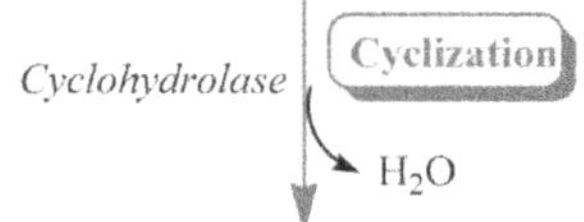

Inosine monophosphate (IMP) (Keto form)

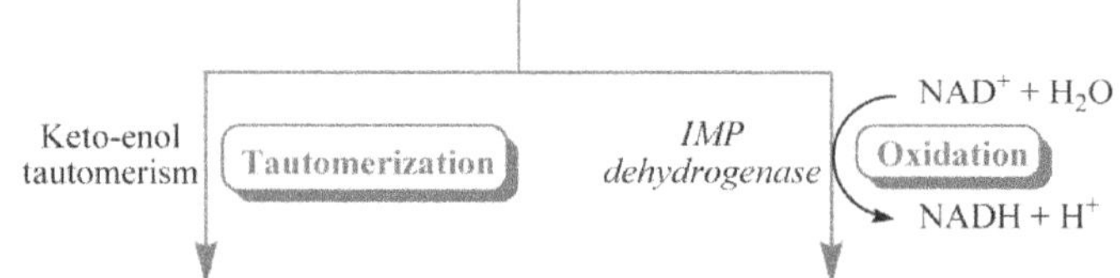

Inosine monophosphate (IMP) (Enol form)

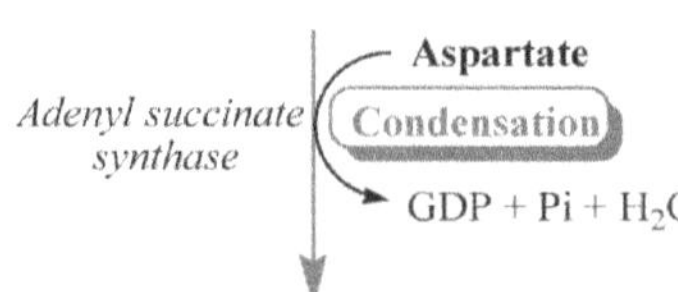

Adenyl succinate

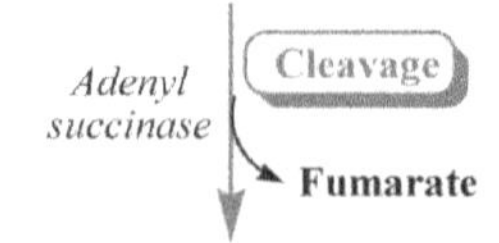

Adenosine monophosphate (AMP)

Xanthosine monophosphate (XMP) (Keto form)

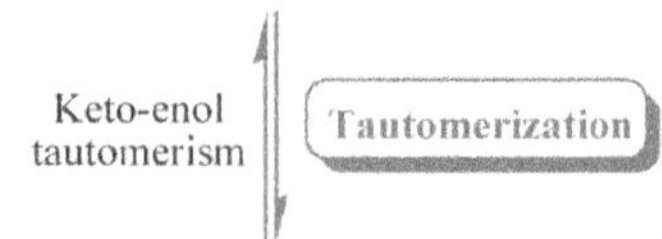

Xanthosine monophosphate (XMP) (Enol form)

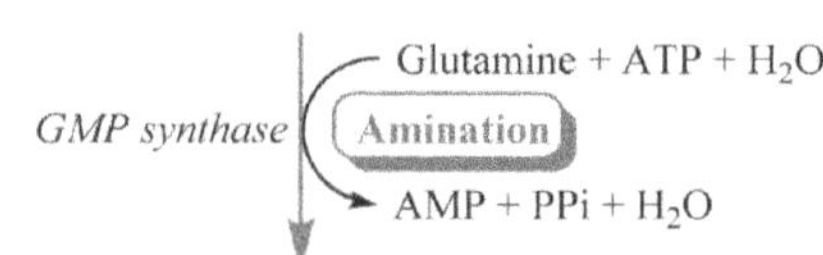

Guanosine monophosphate (GMP)

10. In the pre final step, 5-aminoimidazole-4-carboxamide ribosyl-5-phosphate undergoes formylation reaction by reacting with N^{10}-formyl THF in presence of *formyl transferase* (Group transferred is "formyl" and the type of reaction involved is "transfer") to produce 5-formaminoimidazole-4-carboxamide ribosyl-5-phosphate. All the carbon and nitrogen atoms of purine rings are contributed by the respective sources with this step.
11. Finally, 5-formaminoimidazole-4-carboxamide ribosyl-5-phosphate in enol form undergoes cyclization in presence of *cyclohydrolase* (The type of reaction involved is "cyclization with removal of water molecule") produces parent purine ribonucleotide i.e., inosine monophosphate (IMP) with loss of water molecule. The other purine ribonucleotides are synthesized from this inosine monophosphate (IMP).

Inhibitors of purine nucleotide synthesis

For the synthesis of purine nucleotides, folic acid is necessary. Sulfonamides are the drugs which inhibit the synthesis of folic acid in microorganisms due to structural similarities with *p*-aminobenzoic acid (PABA). Hence, indirectly, sulfonamides inhibit the synthesis of purine nucleotides there by synthesis of nucleic acid such as DNA and RNA. The sulfonamide is not producing any effect in the human because folic acid is not synthesized in humans and is supplied through diet.

Methotrexate is the analog of folic acid and it is used to control the cancer. Methotrexate inhibit *formyl transferase* (the steps in which N^{10}-formyl THF is involved) leads to inhibition of purine nucleotide synthesis there by synthesis of nucleic acid. In this reaction one carbon moiety (formyl group) is transferred. Proliferations of normal growing cells are also affected by these inhibitors which lead to several side effects such as anemia, baldness, scaly skin, etc.

Synthesis of AMP and GMP from IMP

The immediate precursor for the production of adenosine monophosphate (AMP) and guanosine monophosphate (GMP) is inosine monophosphate (IMP).

1. In the enol form IMP reacts with aspartate to produce adenyl succinate or adenylosuccinate with loss of water molecule by condensation in presence of *adenyl succinate synthase* or *adenylosuccinate synthase* (The product formed is "adenyl succinate" and the type of reaction involved is "synthesis"). The energy needed for this reaction is derived from breakdown of GTP into GDP and inorganic phosphate **(1 ATP is utilized)**.
2. Later, the obtained adenyl succinate breakdown with the removal of fumarate and produces adenosine monophosphate (AMP). *Adenyl succinase* (The substrate is "adenyl succinate" and the type of reaction involved is "lysis") is an enzyme responsible for this reaction.
3. In other ways, inosine monophosphate (IMP) undergoes oxidation by reacting with reducing equivalent NAD^+ and water molecules produce xanthosine monophosphate (XMP) and the reaction is catalyzed by *IMP dehydrogenase* (In NAD^+ / $NADP^+$ / FAD involved reactions, the enzymes acted are "*dehydrogenase*" and the substrate is "IMP").
4. Finally, xanthosine monophosphate (XMP) in enol form reacts with glutamine and gains amide nitrogen to produce guanosine monophosphate (GMP) with a loss of water molecule in presence of *GMP synthetase* (The product formed is "GMP" and the type of reaction involved is "synthesis"). The energy needed by this reaction is provided by breakdown of ATP into AMP and pyrophosphate **(2 ATP is utilized).**

Drugs such as 6-mercaptopurine acts on *adenyl succinase* of AMP pathway and *IMP dehydrogenase* of IMP pathway leads to inhibition of AMP and GMP synthesis. Hence, 6-mercaptopurine is considered as AMP and GMP synthesis inhibitors.

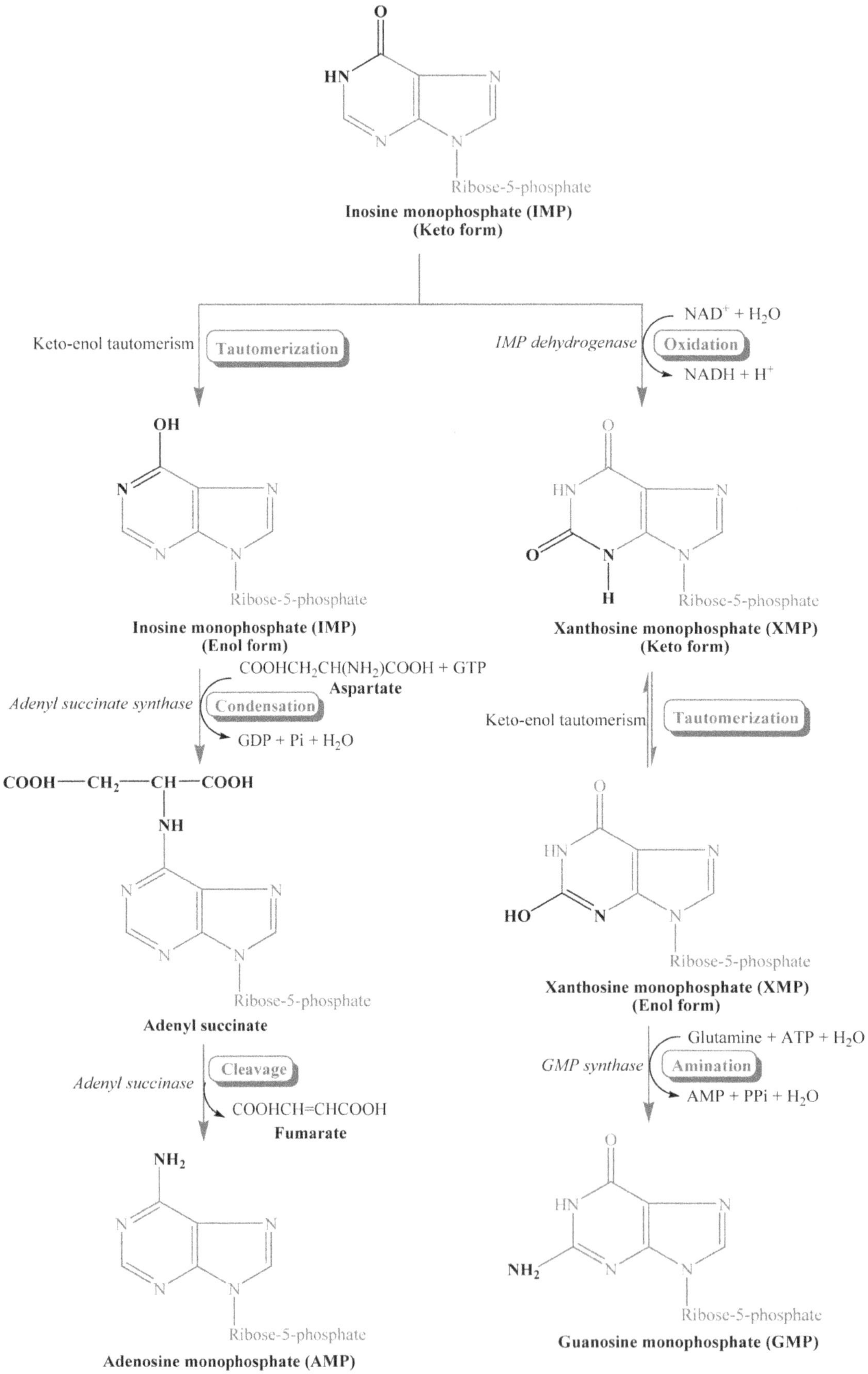

Inosine monophosphate (IMP)
(Keto form)

Keto-enol tautomerism — Tautomerization

IMP dehydrogenase — Oxidation ($NAD^+ + H_2O$ → $NADH + H^+$)

Inosine monophosphate (IMP)
(Enol form)

Adenyl succinate synthase — Condensation ($COOHCH_2CH(NH_2)COOH$ + GTP, Aspartate → GDP + Pi + H_2O)

$COOH—CH_2—CH—COOH$ / NH

Adenyl succinate

Adenyl succinase — Cleavage (→ COOHCH=CHCOOH, Fumarate)

Adenosine monophosphate (AMP)

Xanthosine monophosphate (XMP)
(Keto form)

Keto-enol tautomerism — Tautomerization

Xanthosine monophosphate (XMP)
(Enol form)

GMP synthase — Amination (Glutamine + ATP + H_2O → AMP + PPi + H_2O)

Guanosine monophosphate (GMP)

Synthesis of purine nucleoside diphosphate and purine nucleoside triphosphate

In most of the metabolic reactions, nucleoside diphosphate (NDP) and nucleoside triphosphate (NTP) are participating. These NDP and NTP are produced from nucleoside monophosphate (NMP) by reacting with ATP in presence of *NMP kinase* (In ATP / GTP involved reactions, the enzymes acted are "*kinase*" and the substrate is "NMP") and *NDP kinase* (In ATP / GTP involved reactions, the enzymes acted are "*kinase*" and the substrate is "NDP"), respectively.

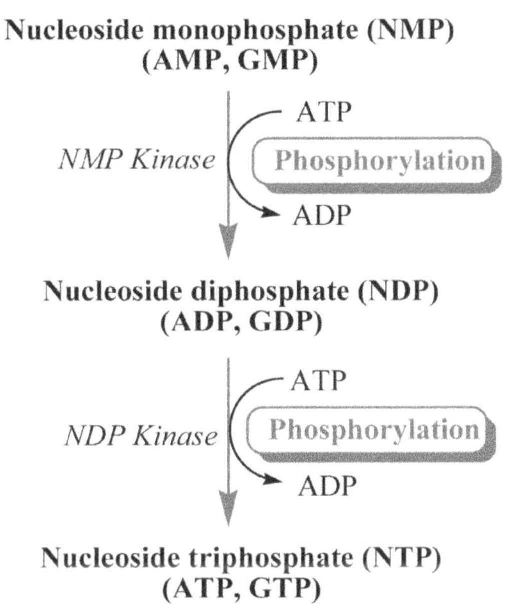

Salvage pathway for purine nucleotide synthesis

From the dietary source and normal turnover of nucleic acid particularly RNA, free purines such as adenine, guanine and hypoxanthine are formed. The direct conversion of these purine bases into their corresponding purine nucleotide is known as salvage pathway. AMP is obtained from adenine by reacting with PRPP by removal of pyrophosphate in presence of *adenine phosphoribosyl transferase* (*APRT*) (The substrate is "adenine" and the type of reaction involved is "transfer of ribose-5-phosphate"). Similarly, GMP is obtained from guanine by reacting with PRPP by removal of pyrophosphate in presence of *hypoxanthine-guanine phosphoribosyl transferase (HGPRT)* (The substrate is "guanine" and the type of reaction involved is "transfer of ribose-5-phosphate") and IMP is obtained from hypoxanthine by reacting with PRPP with removal of pyrophosphate in presence of *hypoxanthine-guanine phosphoribosyl transferase (HGPRT)* (The substrate is "hypoxanthine" and the type of reaction involved is "transfer of ribose-5-phosphate"). In these reactions PRPP acts as a donor of ribose-5-phosphate to the purine nitrogen base to produce its corresponding purine nucleotides.

In tissues like erythrocytes and brain, *De nova* synthesis of purines (normal direct purine nucleotide synthesis) does not occur. Hence, in these tissues, the salvage pathway is more important for the supply of nucleotides. Lesch-Nyhan syndrome is caused due to the deficiency of *hypoxanthine-guanine phosphoribosyl transferase (HGPRT)*.

Transfer of ribose-5-phosphate

Phosphoribosyl pyrophosphate (PRPP) → PPi

Adenine phosphoribosyl transferase (APRT)

Adenine → **Adenosine monophosphate (AMP)** (Ribose-5-phosphate)

Transfer of ribose-5-phosphate

Phosphoribosyl pyrophosphate (PRPP) → PPi

Hypoxanthine-guanine phosphoribosyl transferase (HGPRT)

Guanine → **Guanosine monophosphate (GMP)** (Ribose-5-phosphate)

Transfer of ribose-5-phosphate

Phosphoribosyl pyrophosphate (PRPP) → PPi

Hypoxanthine-guanine phosphoribosyl transferase (HGPRT)

Hypoxanthine → **Inosine monophosphate (IMP)** (Ribose-5-phosphate)

Regulation of purine nucleotide biosynthesis

Depending on the cellular demands the purine nucleotides are biosynthesized. The biosynthesis of purine nucleotides is regulated mainly by the following three ways.

1. To a large extent, purine nucleotides biosynthesis is regulated by intracellular concentration of PRPP. Availability of ribose-5-phosphate and *PRPP synthetase* maintains the concentration of PRPP.
2. Purine nucleotides control the *PRPP glutamyl amido transferase* by a feedback mechanism. To meet the cellular requirements if sufficient amount of AMP and GMP is present in the body then their synthesis is inhibited at *amido transferase* reaction.
3. In addition, *adenyl succinate synthetase* and *IMP dehydrogenase* is inhibited by AMP and GMP, respectively. Thus, by a feedback mechanism the respective synthesis of AMP and GMP from IMP is controlled by themselves.

Biosynthesis of deoxyribonucleotides from ribonucleotides:

Reduction at C-2 of ribose moiety present in purine and pyrimidine ribonucleotides generally produces corresponding purine and pyrimidine deoxyribonucleotides in the presence of *ribonucleotide reductase* (The substrate is "ribonucleotide" and the type of reaction involved is "reduction"). This enzyme contains multi subunits such as two B_1 and two B_2 subunits in their structure. The hydrogen atom needed for this above-mentioned reduction is provided by the sulfhydryl groups present in the reduced form of thioredoxin which is a monomeric protein with two cysteine residues. At the end of reduction, thioredoxin is converted to its oxidized form. This oxidized form of thioredoxin is converted back to their reduced form by *thioredoxin reductase* (The substrate is "thioredoxin" and the type of reaction involved is "reduction") which are dependent on NADPH + H^+. The formed reduced form of thioredoxin is utilized again and again. Hence, thioredoxin serves as a co-factor in an enzymatic reaction.

Regulation: Deoxyribonucleotides are mainly needed for the synthesis of DNA and their synthesis and adequate supply is regulated by the enzyme *ribonucleotide reductase*. This *ribonucleotide reductase* is inhibited by the drug hydroxyurea by destroying the free radicals needed by this enzyme. Hence, hydroxyurea is used in the treatment of cancers such as chronic myelogenous leukemia.

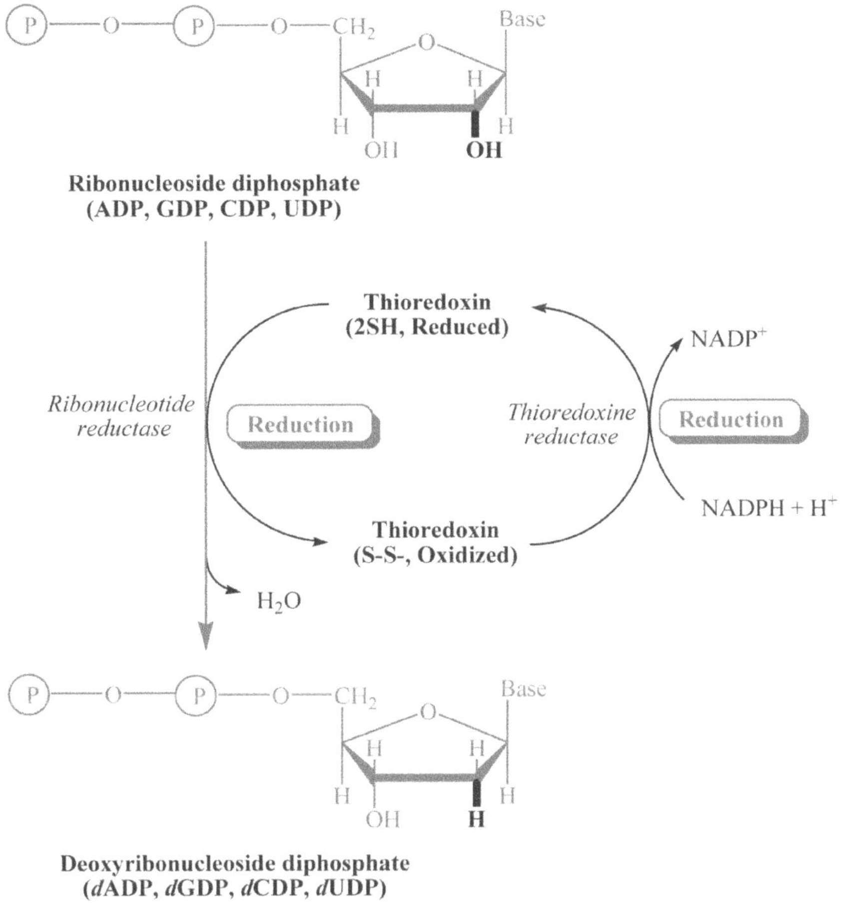

P—O—P—O—CH_2 Base O H H H OH **OH** H

Ribonucleoside diphosphate
(ADP, GDP, CDP, UDP)

Ribonucleotide reductase

Reduction

Thioredoxin
(2SH, Reduced)

$NADP^+$

Thioredoxine reductase

Reduction

$NADPH + H^+$

Thioredoxin
(S-S-, Oxidized)

H_2O

P—O—P—O—CH_2 Base O H H H OH **H** H

Deoxyribonucleoside diphosphate
(*d*ADP, *d*GDP, *d*CDP, *d*UDP)

Degradation of Purine Nucleotides

Uric acid is the end product of purine metabolism. The various reactions involved in the degradation of purine nucleotides are as follows.

1. Firstly, all the purine nucleotides (AMP, IMP and GMP) are converted to their corresponding purine nucleoside (adenosine, inosine and guanosine) by simple hydrolysis with the loss of inorganic phosphate in presence of *nucleotidase* (The substrate is "nucleotide" and the type of reaction involved is "hydrolysis").
2. AMP and adenosine undergo deamination by reacting with water in presence of *AMP deaminase* (The substrate is "AMP" and the type of reaction involved is "deamination") and *adenosine deaminase* (The substrate is "adenosine and the type of reaction involved is "deamination") and produced IMP and inosine, respectively with a loss of ammonia.
3. In the presence of *purine nucleoside phosphorylase* (The substrate is "purine nucleoside" and the type of reaction involved is "phosphorylation"), inosine and guanosine undergoes phosphorylation reaction by reacting with inorganic phosphate to produce their corresponding nitrogen base such as hypoxanthine and guanine, respectively. During this reaction, sugar molecule ribose is removed as ribose-1-phosphate. Adenosine is not degraded by this *purine nucleoside phosphorylase*, hence, it is converted to inosine by the above-mentioned deamination reaction.

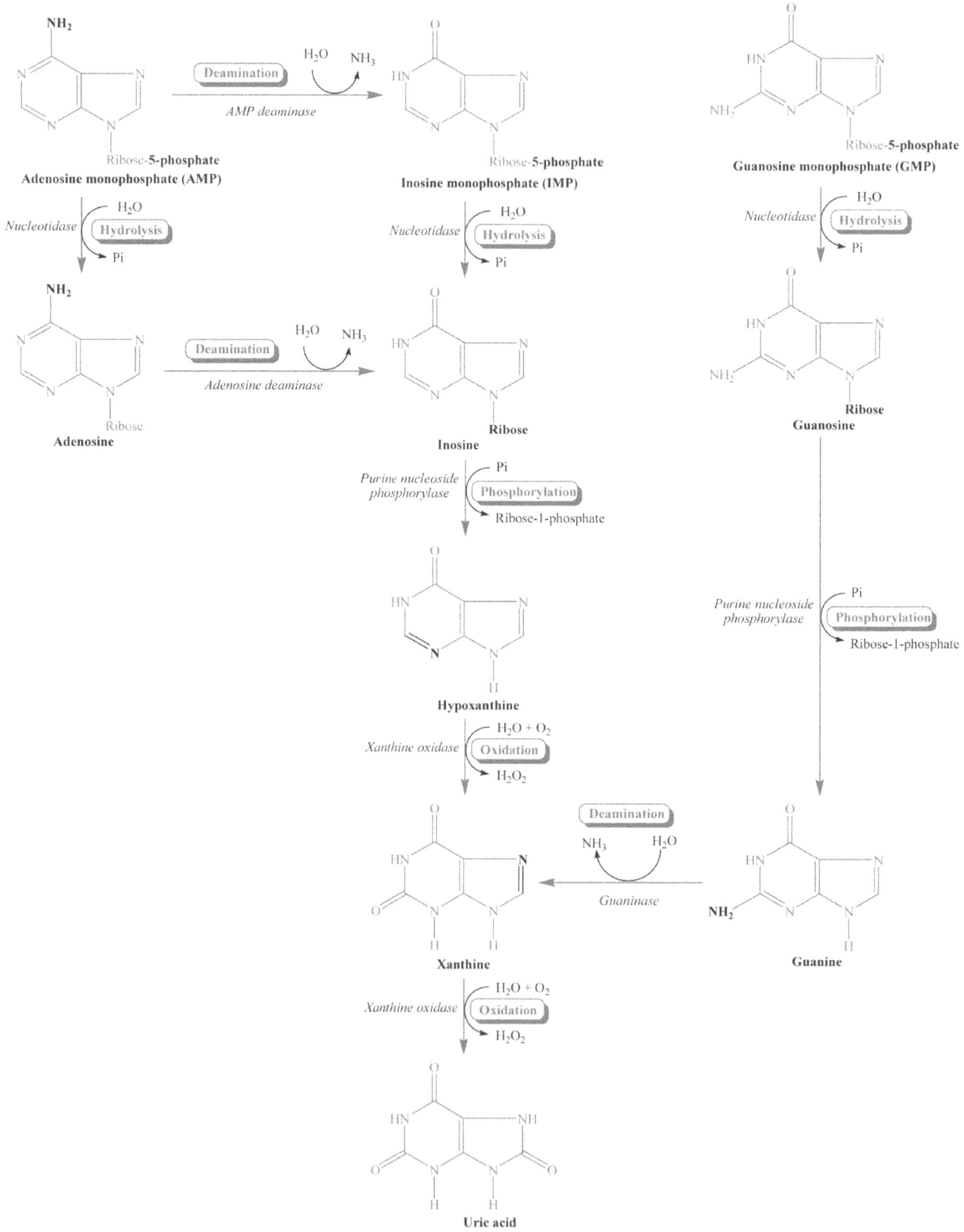

NH2
N
N
N
N
Ribose-5-phosphate
Adenosine monophosphate (AMP)
Deamination
H_2O
NH_3
AMP deaminase
O
HN
N
N
N
Ribose-5-phosphate
Inosine monophosphate (IMP)
O
HN
N
NH2
N
N
Ribose-5-phosphate
Guanosine monophosphate (GMP)
Nucleotidase
H_2O
Hydrolysis
Pi
Nucleotidase
H_2O
Hydrolysis
Pi
Nucleotidase
H_2O
Hydrolysis
Pi
NH2
Ribose
Adenosine
Deamination
H_2O
NH_3
Adenosine deaminase
Ribose
Inosine
Ribose
Guanosine
Purine nucleoside phosphorylase
Pi
Phosphorylation
Ribose-1-phosphate
Hypoxanthine
Purine nucleoside phosphorylase
Pi
Phosphorylation
Ribose-1-phosphate
Xanthine oxidase
$H_2O + O_2$
Oxidation
H_2O_2
Deamination
NH_3
H_2O
Guaninase
Xanthine
Guanine
Xanthine oxidase
$H_2O + O_2$
Oxidation
H_2O_2
NH
Uric acid

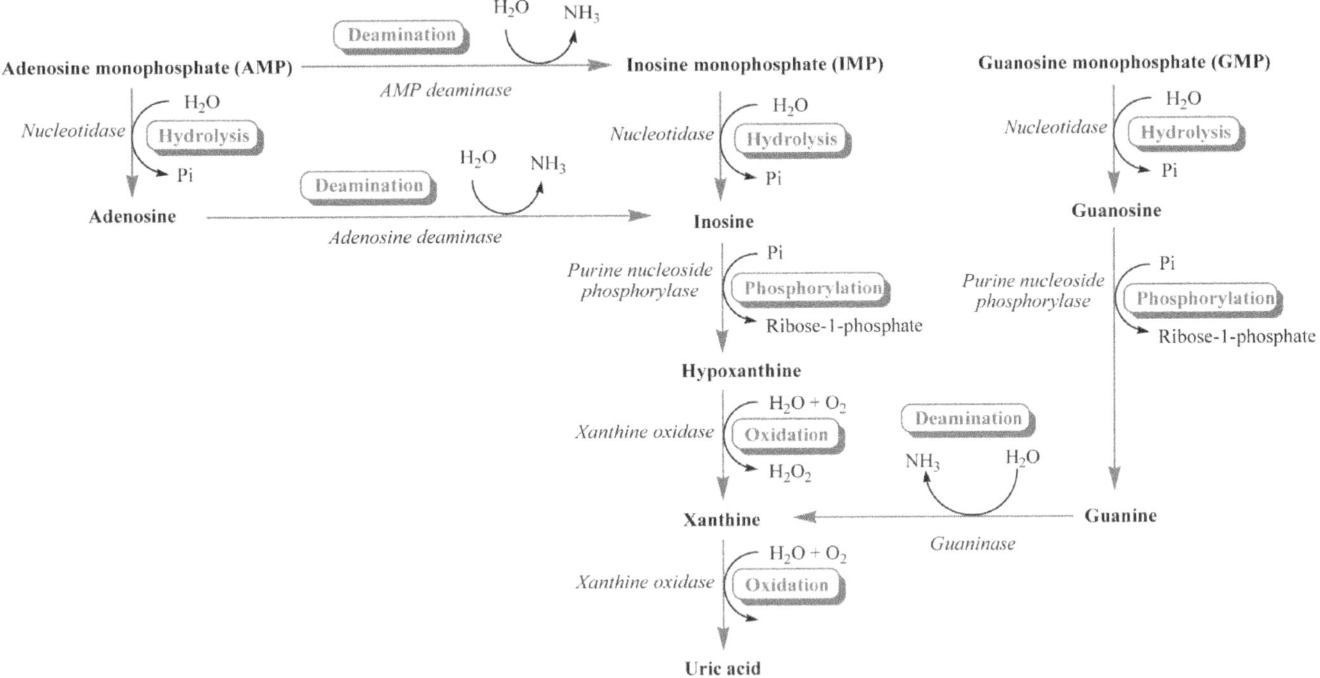

4. Guanine undergoes deamination by reacting with water in the presence of *guanine deaminase* (The substrate is "guanine" and the type of reaction involved is "deamination") and produces xanthine with a loss of ammonia.
5. Finally, hypoxanthine is reacted with water and oxygen to produce xanthine with the liberation of hydrogen peroxide in the presence of *xanthine oxidase* (The product formed is "xanthine" and the type of reaction involved is "oxidation"). The reaction involved in this process is simple oxidation. In a similar manner, xanthine is reacted with water and oxygen to produce uric acid with the liberation of hydrogen peroxide in the presence of *xanthine oxidase* (The substrate is "xanthine" and the type of reaction involved is "oxidation"). *Xanthine oxidase* is exclusively found in the liver and small intestine and it contains FAD, molybdenum and iron. The hydrogen peroxide liberated in this reaction is very harmful to the tissues because it is capable to produce free radicals. *Catalase* is an enzyme which cleaves hydrogen peroxide into water and oxygen.

Uric acid is chemically 2,6,8-trioxypurine and is the end product of purine metabolism excreted through urine in humans. Non-enzymatically, uric acid gets itself converted to allantoin and serves as an important antioxidant. In primates, the antioxidant role of ascorbic acid is replaced by uric acid because ascorbic acid is not synthesized in primates due to lack of enzyme responsible for the synthesis of ascorbic acid i.e., *gulonolactone oxidase.*

Other than primates, in most animals, uric acid is further degraded. Initially, in the presence of *uricase* (The substrate is "uric acid" and the type of reaction involved is "oxidation"), uric acid is converted to allantoin by oxidative ring cleavage. In the next step, allantoin is further converted to allantoic acid in presence of *allantoinase* (The substrate is "allantoin" and the type of reaction involved is "oxidation") by oxidative ring cleavage. In some fishes, this allantoic acid is excreted. In most fishes, amphibians and some molluscs, allantoic acid further degraded to urea with the liberation of glyoxylic acid in the presence of *allantoicase* (The substrate is "allantoic acid" and the type of reaction involved is "oxidation") by oxidative cleavage; whereas in marine invertebrates, urea is further hydrolyzed to produce ammonia and carbondioxide in the presence of *urease* (The substrate is "urea" and the type of reaction involved is "hydrolysis").

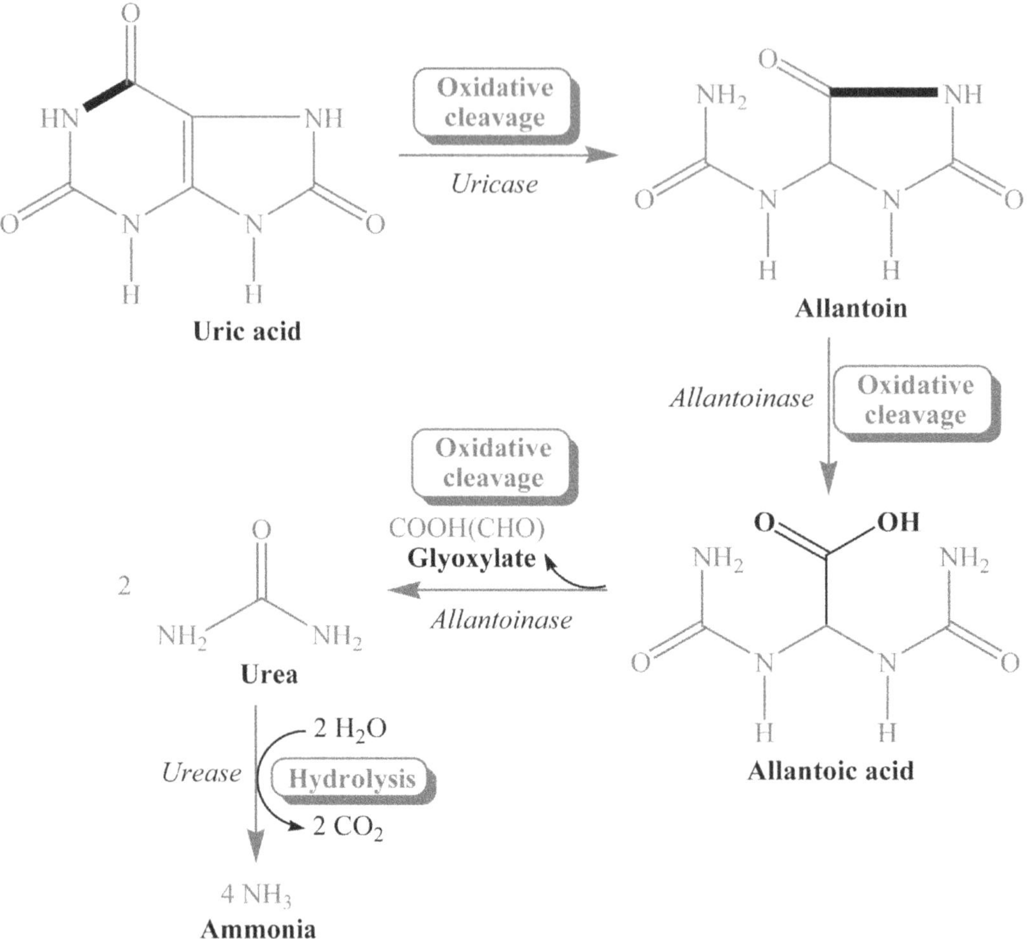

Figure 6.2 Degradation of uric acid in animals other than man.

Metabolic Disorders of Purine Metabolism

The following are some important metabolic disorders of purine metabolism. They are,

1. Hyperuricemia
2. Uricosuria
3. Gout
   (a) Primary gout
   (b) Secondary gout
4. Pseudogout
5. Lesch-Nyhan syndrome
6. Severe combined immune deficiency (SCID)
   (a) B-cell dysfunction
   (b) T-cell dysfunction
7. Hypouricemia

Hyperuricemia:

In humans, the end excretory product of purine metabolism is uric acid. In adults, the normal serum concentration of uric acid is 3 to 7 mg/dl. Compared to men, in women, it is slightly lower by about 1 mg/dl. Per day about 500 to 700 mg of uric acid is excreted in the body through urine.

Hyperuricemia is defined as the increased concentration of uric acid in serum. Sometimes hyperuricemia is associated with uricosuria.

Uricosuria:

Uricosuria is defined as the increased excretion of uric acid in urine and it is sometimes associated with hyperuricemia.

Gout:

It is a metabolic disorder of purine metabolism and is associated with the overproduction of uric acid. Sodium urate is the more soluble form of uric acid at physiological pH. In severe hyperuricemia, the sodium urate crystals are deposited in the soft tissues, particularly in joints. Tophi are the common name for such deposition in the body. A painful gouty arthritis is produced due to the inflammation in the joints because of sodium urate crystals deposition. In the kidney, and ureter also, uric acid and / or sodium urate may precipitate which leads to stone formation and renal damage. Gout is most common in alcohol consumption, over eating and high living. In the previous centuries, during the manufacture and storage, lead contaminates alcohol. This lead poisoning leads to kidney damage and the decreased uric acid excretion causes gout. In general, the risk of gout is increased with consumption of a diet rich in meat and sea foods. Mostly, it affects males and the prevalence is 3 in 1000 people. Like men, post-menopausal women are susceptible for this disorder. Gout is broadly classified into two major types as,

(a) Primary gout
(b) Secondary gout

Primary gout: This type of gout is an inborn error of metabolism due to overproduction of uric acid. The reason behind over production of uric acid is increased synthesis of purine nucleotides. The following are the major metabolic defects associated with primary gout.

1. Elevation of *phosphoribosyl pyrophosphate (PRPP) synthetase*
2. Elevation of *PRPP glutamyl amidotransferase*
3. Deficiency of *hypoxanthine-guanine phospho ribosyl transferase (HGPRT)*
4. Deficiency of *glucose-6-phosphatase*
5. Elevation of *glutathione reductase*

Elevation of *phosphoribosyl pyrophosphate (PRPP) synthetase*: Purine nucleotides such as ADP and GDP, control the *PRPP synthetase* in normal circumstances by feedback regulation. Even though the variant forms of *PRPP synthetase* are not controlled by feedback regulation. Hence, the increased production of *PRPP synthetase* ultimately leads to over synthesis of purine nucleotides.

Elevation of *PRPP glutamyl amidotransferase*: Like *PRPP synthetase*, lack of feedback regulation by purine nucleotides results in the increased production of *PRPP glutamyl amidotransferase* leads to over synthesis of purine nucleotides.

Deficiency of *hypoxanthine-guanine phospho ribosyl transferase (HGPRT)*: *HGPRT* is an enzyme involved in the salvage pathway of purine nucleotide synthesis. The deficiency of *HGPRT* produces Lesch-Nyhan syndrome. In general, this disorder is associated with increased production of purine nucleotides by two fold mechanism. In one way, *PRPP* is accumulated in the salvage pathway due to decreased utilization of purines such as hypoxanthine and guanine; hence, *PRPP* is diverted for purine nucleotide synthesis. In other ways, IMP and GMP levels are decreased due to defects in salvage pathway leads to impairment in the tightly controlled feedback regulation of their products.

Deficiency of *glucose-6-phosphatase*: Glucose-6-phosphate cannot be converted to glucose in Von Gierke's disease or type - I glycogen storage disease due to *glucose-6-phosphatase* deficiency. Hence, glucose-6-phosphate is more utilized by HMP shunt results in increased production of ribose-5-phosphate which, in turn, increases the synthesis of phosphoribosyl pyrophosphate (PRPP) leads to overproduction of purine nucleotides. In other ways in Von Gierke's disease, glucose-6-phosphate is diverted to glycolysis which leads to the overproduction of lactic acid. The accumulation lactic acid in the body interferes with uric acid excretion through renal tubules.

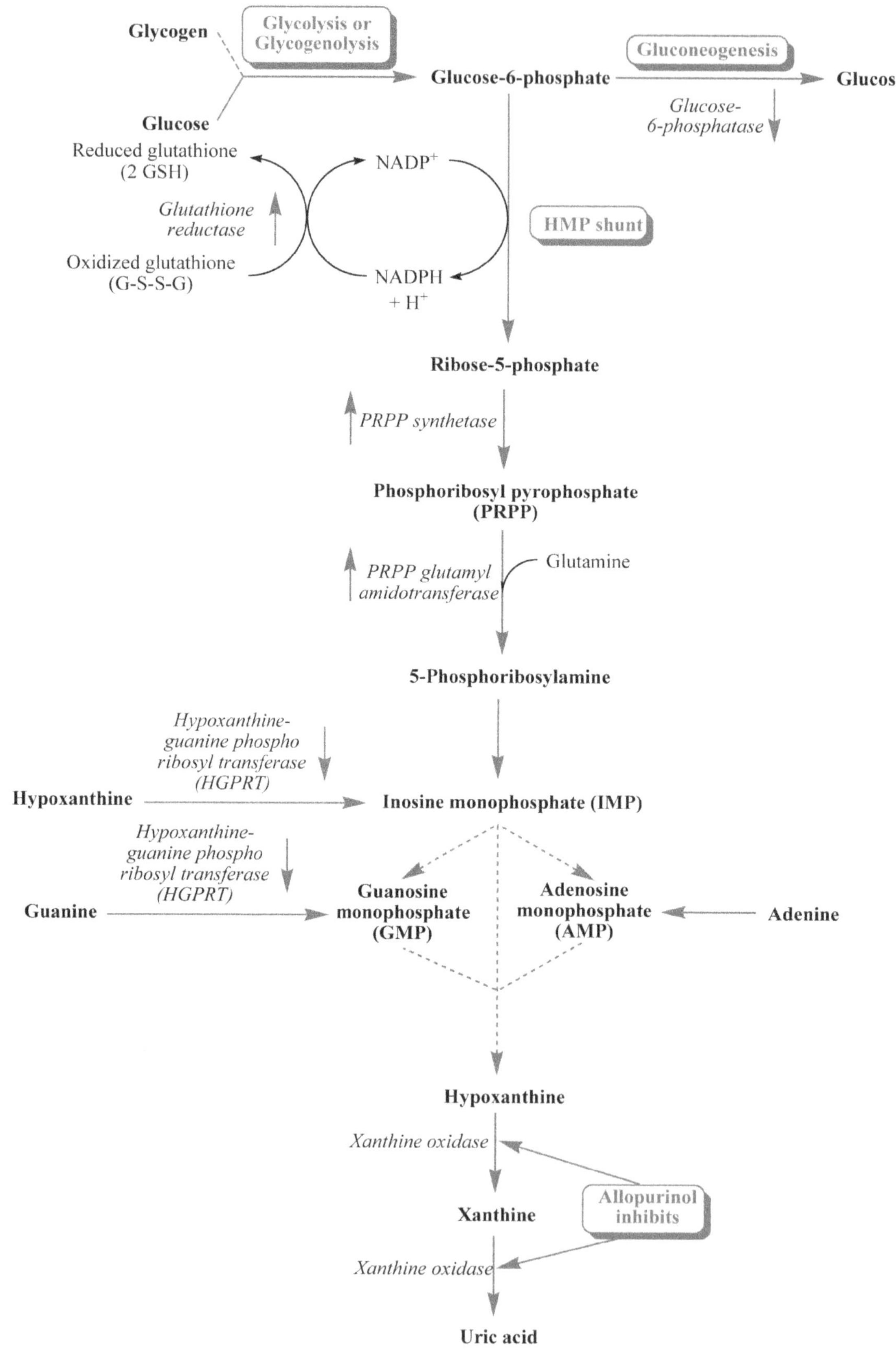

Figure 6.3 Summary of possible enzyme alterations causing gout.

Elevation of *glutathione reductase*: More $NADP^+$ is generated by increased *glutathione reductase.* The increased $NADP^+$ is utilized by HMP shunt results in increased ribose-5-phosphate which, in turn, increases the synthesis of phosphoribosyl pyrophosphate (PRPP) leads to overproduction of purine nucleotides.

This metabolic disorder is a very good example to prove how an abnormality in one metabolic pathway influences the other. Among these five enzymes mentioned, the first three enzymes are directly involved in the synthesis of purine nucleotides; whereas the last two enzymes indirectly regulate the synthesis of purine nucleotides.

Secondary gout or secondary hyperuricemia: This type of gout is due to various diseases causing increased production or decreased excretion of uric acid. In various cancers such as leukemia, polycythemia, lymphomas, etc., psoriasis and increased tissue breakdown conditions such as trauma, starvation, etc. nucleic acid degradation is increased leads to increased production of uric acid. In case of renal function impairment, excretion of uric acid is decreased leading to accumulation of uric acid, resulting in gout.

Diagnosis of gout: The miscible uric acid pool in the body can be calculated by administering the uric acid isotope (N^{15}). The normal value of miscible uric acid pool is 1200 mg and this value is greatly increased to 3000 mg or more in gout patients.

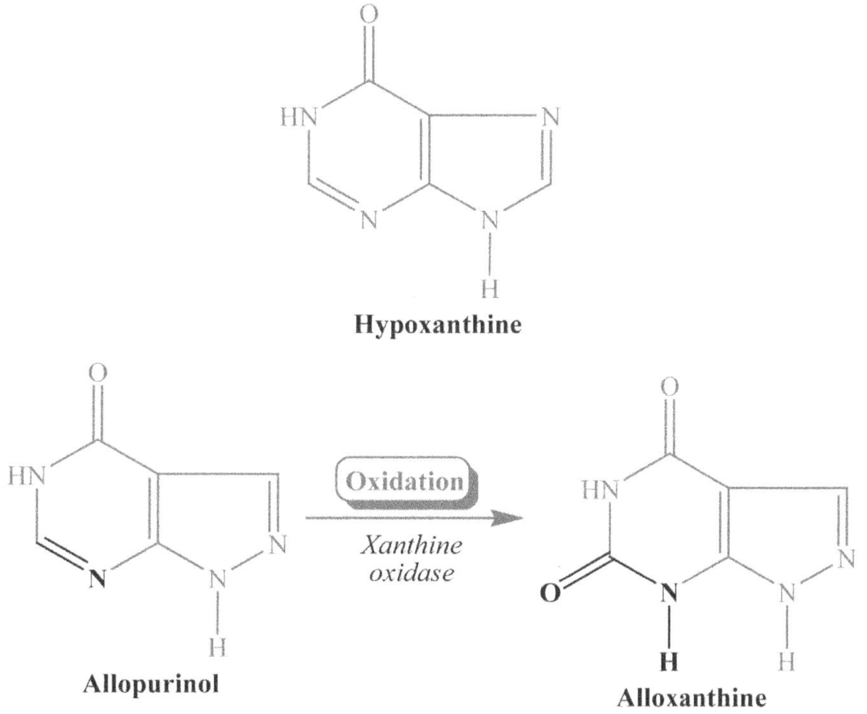

Figure 6.4 Structure of hypoxanthine and its structural analogs.

Treatment: Allopurinol is the drug used for the treatment of primary gout. Allopurinol competitively inhibits the *xanthine oxidase* enzyme because it is chemically a structural analog of hypoxanthine. In addition, alloxanthine is produced by allopurinol by simple oxidation in presence of *xanthine oxidase*. Alloxanthine is a more powerful *xanthine oxidase* inhibitor than allopurinol. This type of enzyme inhibition is known as suicide inhibition. Hypoxanthine and xanthine are accumulated in the body due to inhibition of *xanthine oxidase* by allopurinol. Compared to uric acid, hypoxanthine and xanthine are more soluble in water, hence, it is easily excreted in urine.

Restriction of dietary intake of purines and alcohol is also advised besides the drug therapy. In addition, drinking more water is also very useful.

In general, for the treatment of gouty arthritis, anti-inflammatory drug colchicine is used. Other anti-inflammatory drugs such as indomethacin, phenylbutazone, oxyphenbutazone and corticosteroids are also used for the treatment of gouty arthritis.

Pseudogout: It is similar to gout by clinical manifestation but it is caused by deposition of calcium pyrophosphate crystals in joints. In addition, serum uric acid level is normal in pseudogout.

Biosynthesis of Pyrimidine Nucleotides

Pyrimidine biosynthesis process is much simpler than that of the purine biosynthesis process. First, pyrimidine nitrogen base is synthesized and then sugar molecule i.e., ribose-5-phosphate is attached to the pyrimidine nitrogen base to synthesize pyrimidine nucleotide. In case of purine nucleotide synthesis purine nitrogen base is synthesized in a pre-existing ribose-5-phosphate. Pyrimidine rings of the nucleotides are contributed by many compounds. They are,

1. N_1, C_4, C_5 and C_6 of pyrimidine are derived from aspartate.
2. C_2 of pyrimidine is derived from carbon dioxide.
3. N_3 of pyrimidine is derived from the amide group of glutamine.

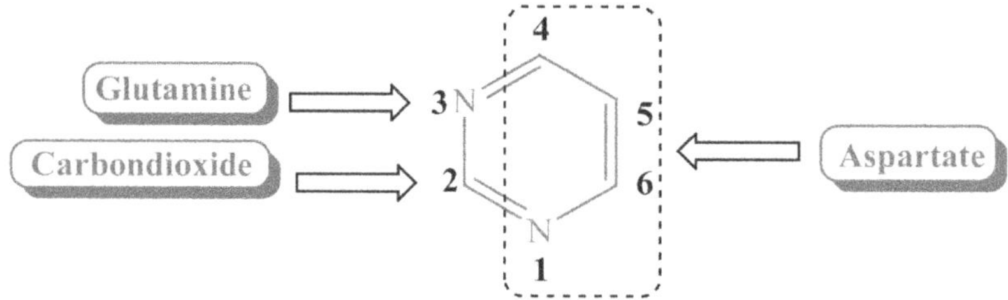

Figure 6.5 Sources of individual atoms in pyrimidine ring.

Pathway:

1. At first, carbondioxide reacts with glutamine and ATP to produce carbamoyl phosphate in presence of cytosomal enzyme *carbamoyl phosphate synthetase – II (CPS – II)* (The product formed is "carbamoyl phosphate" and the type of reaction involved is "synthesis") by simple condensation. In this reaction, energy needed by the reaction is provided by the breakdown of ATP and glutamate is liberated after donating the amine group of glutamines. Two ATP is used in this reaction. One for phosphorylation and the another one for energy purpose **(2 ATP is utilized)**.

   ATP and phosphoribosyl pyrophosphate (PRPP) activate *carbamoyl phosphate synthetase – II (CPS – II)*; whereas UTP inhibits *CPS – II*. In urea biosynthesis, carbamoyl phosphate is synthesized from ammonia and carbondioxide in presence of microsomal enzyme *carbamoyl phosphate synthetase – I (CPS – I)* which needs N-acetyl glutamate (NAG) for its activity. Only one *carbamoyl phosphate synthetase* is present in eukaryotes for the biosynthesis of pyrimidines and arginine.
2. In the next step, carbamoyl phosphate is reacted with aspartate by simple condensation and produces carbamoyl aspartate with a loss of inorganic phosphate in the presence of *aspartate transcarbamoylase* (The substrate is "aspartate" and the type of reaction involved is "transfer of carbamoyl group").
3. Later, in presence of *dihydroorotase* (The product formed is "dihydroorotate" and the type of reaction involved is "hydrolysis" in reverse manner), carbamoyl aspartate undergoes ring closure reaction with a loss of water molecule produces dihydroorotate. Enzymes such as *CPS – II*, *aspartate transcarbamoylase* and *dihydroorotase* are the functional units of the same protein. Hence, it is also a very good example for a **multi-functional enzyme**.
4. Orotate is synthesized from dihydroorotate by dehydrogenation i.e., oxidation reaction which are dependent on NAD^+ in presence of *dihydroorotate dehydrogenase* (In NAD^+ / $NADP^+$ / FAD involved reactions, the enzymes acted are "*dehydrogenase*" and the substrate is "dihydroorotate"). In this reaction one NAD^+ is converted to NADH + H^+. In ETC, one NADH + H^+ produces 3 ATP **(3 ATP is generated).**
5. In this step, phosphoribosyl pyrophosphate (PRPP) donates ribose-5-phosphate to orotate in order to synthesize orotidine monophosphate (OMP) with the liberation of pyrophosphate. This reaction is

catalyzed by *orotate phospho ribosyl transferase* (The substrate is "orotate" and the type of reaction involved is "transfer of ribose-5-phosphate group"). This enzyme is usually compared with *hypoxanthine-guanine phosphoribosyl transferase (HGPRT)* in its function.

CO_2 + NH_2—C(=O)—CH_2—CH_2—CH(NH_2)—COOH

Glutamine

Carbamoyl phosphate synthetase-II (CPS-II) — 2 ATP + H_2O → 2 ADP +Pi — Condensation or Amide transfer

HO—C(=O)—CH_2—CH_2—CH(NH_2)—COOH

Glutamate

NH_2—C(=O)—O—(P)

Carbamoyl phosphate

Aspartate transcarbamoylase — HO—C(=O)—CH_2—CH(NH_2)—COOH (**Aspartate**) → Pi — Condensation or Amidation

Carbamoyl aspartate

Dihydroorotase — Cyclization or Ring closure → H_2O

Dihydroorotate

Dihydroorotate dehydrogenase — NAD^+ → NADH + H^+ — Oxidation

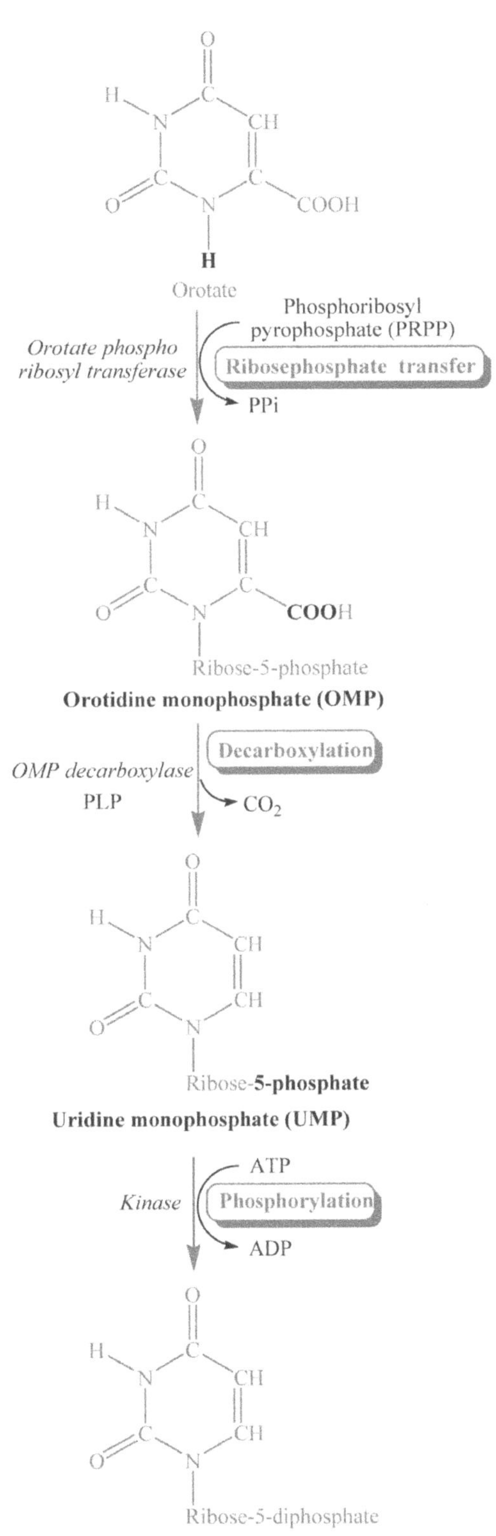

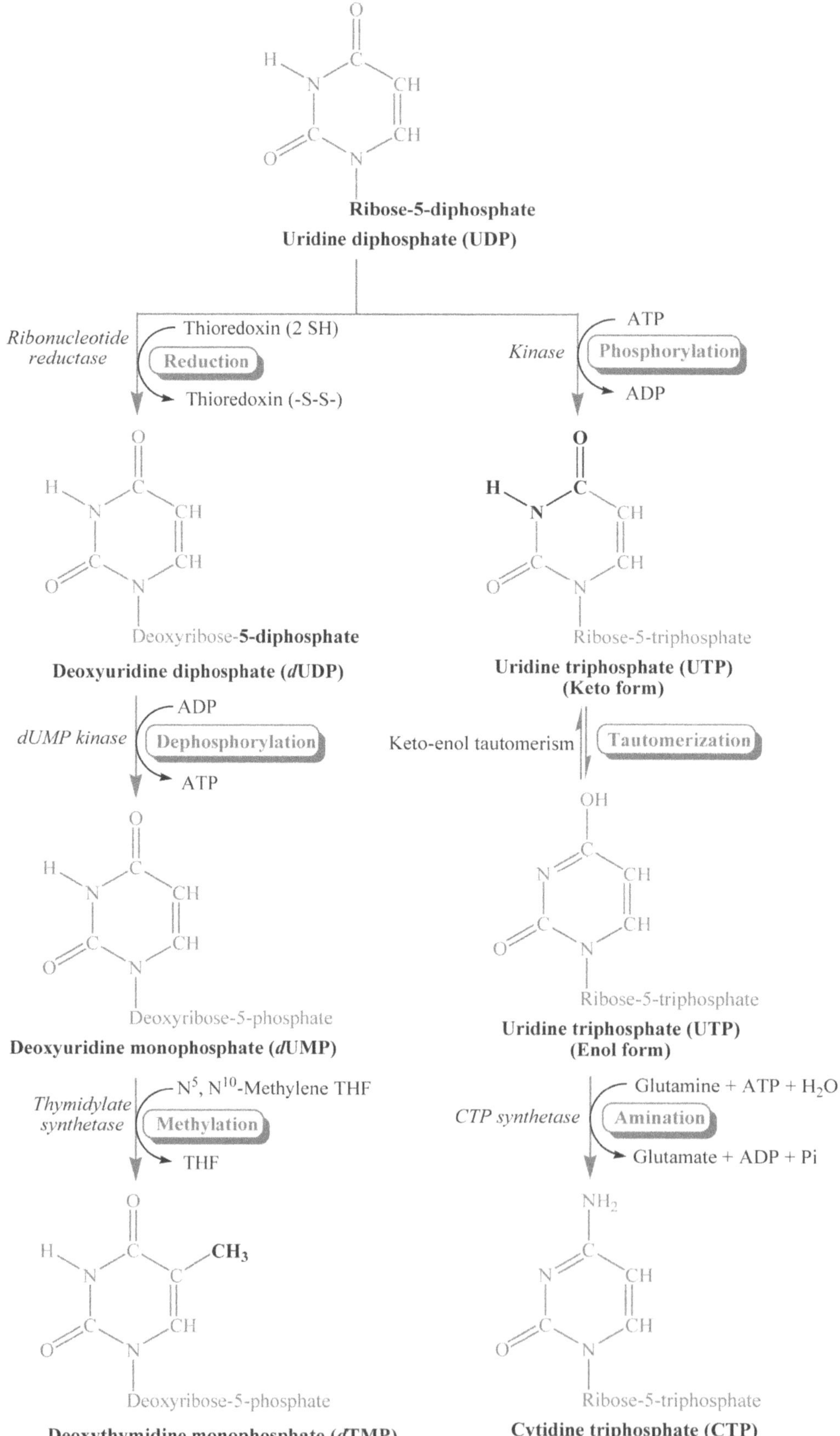

Ribose-5-diphosphate
Uridine diphosphate (UDP)
Ribonucleotide reductase
Thioredoxin (2 SH)
Reduction
Thioredoxin (-S-S-)
Kinase
ATP
Phosphorylation
ADP
Deoxyribose-5-diphosphate
Deoxyuridine diphosphate (dUDP)
Ribose-5-triphosphate
Uridine triphosphate (UTP)
(Keto form)
dUMP kinase
ADP
Dephosphorylation
ATP
Keto-enol tautomerism
Tautomerization
Deoxyribose-5-phosphate
Deoxyuridine monophosphate (dUMP)
Ribose-5-triphosphate
Uridine triphosphate (UTP)
(Enol form)
Thymidylate synthetase
N5, N10-Methylene THF
Methylation
THF
CTP synthetase
Glutamine + ATP + H2O
Amination
Glutamate + ADP + Pi
CH3
NH2
Deoxyribose-5-phosphate
Deoxythymidine monophosphate (dTMP)
Ribose-5-triphosphate
Cytidine triphosphate (CTP)

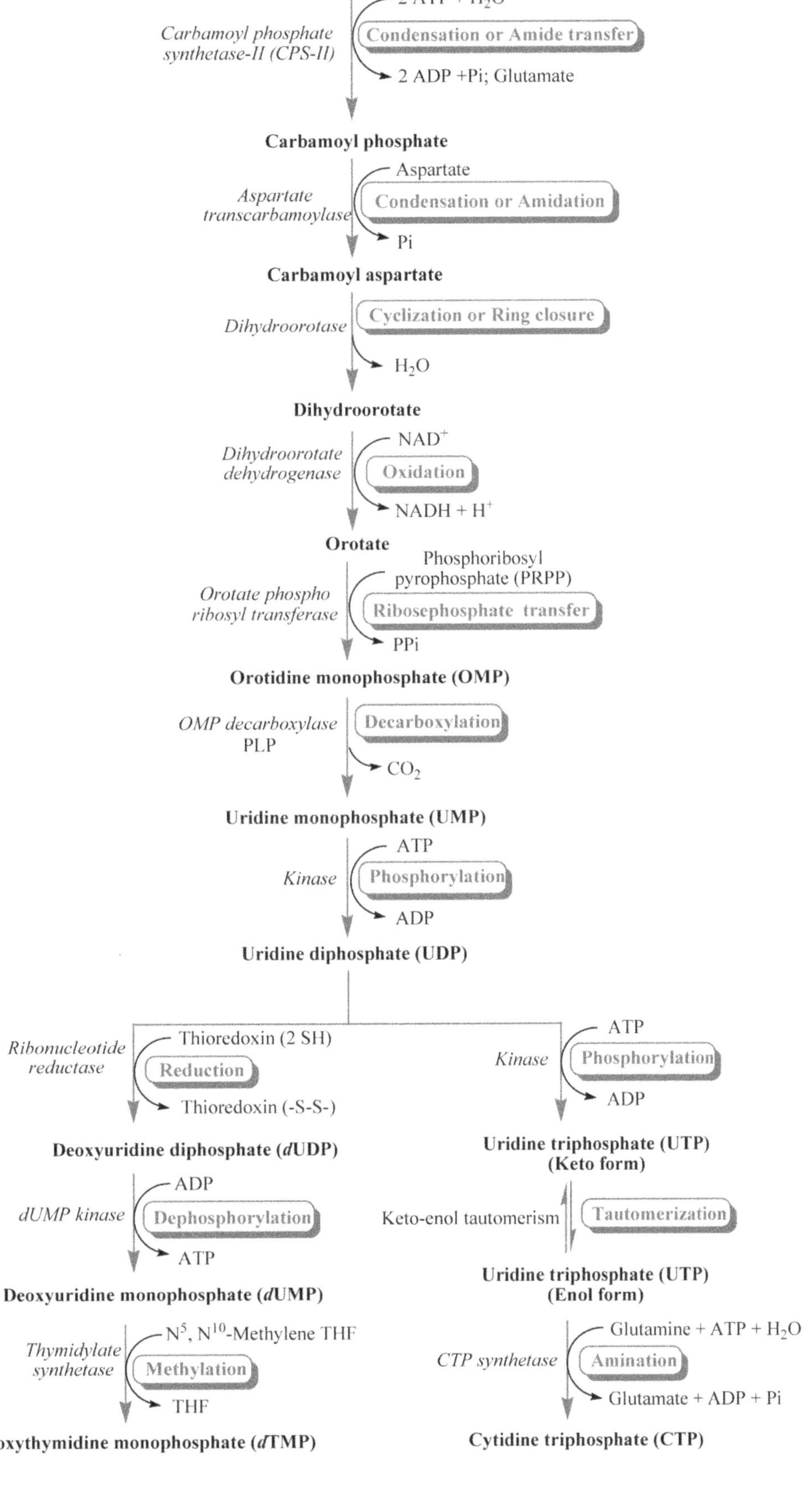

CO_2 + Glutamine
2 ATP + H_2O
Carbamoyl phosphate synthetase-II (CPS-II)
Condensation or Amide transfer
2 ADP +Pi; Glutamate
Carbamoyl phosphate
Aspartate
Aspartate transcarbamoylase
Condensation or Amidation
Pi
Carbamoyl aspartate
Dihydroorotase
Cyclization or Ring closure
H_2O
Dihydroorotate
NAD^+
Dihydroorotate dehydrogenase
Oxidation
$NADH + H^+$
Orotate
Phosphoribosyl pyrophosphate (PRPP)
Orotate phospho ribosyl transferase
Ribosephosphate transfer
PPi
Orotidine monophosphate (OMP)
OMP decarboxylase PLP
Decarboxylation
CO_2
Uridine monophosphate (UMP)
ATP
Kinase
Phosphorylation
ADP
Uridine diphosphate (UDP)
Ribonucleotide reductase
Thioredoxin (2 SH)
Reduction
Thioredoxin (-S-S-)
Deoxyuridine diphosphate (dUDP)
ADP
dUMP kinase
Dephosphorylation
ATP
Deoxyuridine monophosphate (dUMP)
N^5, N^{10}-Methylene THF
Thymidylate synthetase
Methylation
THF
Deoxythymidine monophosphate (dTMP)
ATP
Kinase
Phosphorylation
ADP
Uridine triphosphate (UTP) (Keto form)
Keto-enol tautomerism
Tautomerization
Uridine triphosphate (UTP) (Enol form)
Glutamine + ATP + H_2O
CTP synthetase
Amination
Glutamate + ADP + Pi
Cytidine triphosphate (CTP)

6. In the succeeding step, OMP loss its carboxyl group present in C-6 as carbondioxide by simple decarboxylation in presence of *OMP decarboxylase* (The substrate is "OMP" and the type of reaction involved is "decarboxylation") to produce uridine monophosphate (UMP). *Orotate phospho ribosyl transferase* and *OMP decarboxylase* is the functional unit of the same protein. Hence, it is also a very good example for a bifunctional enzyme and the deficiency of this bifunctional enzyme causes orotic aciduria.
7. Later, UMP is converted into uridine diphosphate (UDP) by simple phosphorylation reaction by reacting with ATP with liberation of ADP in the presence of *kinase* (In ATP / GTP involves reaction the enzyme acted are "*kinase*"). In this reaction, one ATP is converted to ADP **(1 ATP is utilized)**. UDP acts as a precursor for the synthesis of deoxyuridine diphosphate (*d*UDP), deoxyuridine monophosphate (*d*UMP), deoxythymidine monophosphate (*d*TMP), uridine triphosphate (UTP), and cytidine triphosphate (CTP).
8. UDP undergoes two different types of reactions. In first reaction, UDP reacts with the reduced form of thioredoxin (2 SH) to produce *d*UDP by simple reduction reaction in the presence of *ribonucleotide reductase* (The substrate is "UDP which is ribonucleotide" and the type of reaction involved is "reduction"). After the reaction, oxidized form of thioredoxin (S-S) is liberated. Later, *d*UDP undergoes a dephosphorylation reaction to produce *d*UMP and the liberated inorganic phosphate is taken by ADP and converted to ATP. The reaction is catalyzed by *kinase* enzyme (In ATP / GTP involved reaction the enzyme acted are "*kinase*"). Finally, *d*UMP is converted to *d*TMP by the transfer of the methyl group from N^5, N^{10}-methylene THF in the presence of *thymidylate synthetase* (The product formed is "*d*TMP which is a thymidine analog" and the type of reaction involved is "synthesis") with the liberation of THF.
9. In another way, UDP is converted into uridine triphosphate (UTP) by simple phosphorylation reaction by reacting with ATP with the liberation of ADP in the presence of *kinase* (In ATP / GTP involved reaction the enzyme acted are "*kinase*"). In this reaction, one ATP is converted to ADP **(1 ATP is utilized)**. Later, in enol form, UTP reacts with glutamine and produces CTP with the liberation of glutamate after removing the amine group. This reaction is a simple amination reaction and is anabolic in nature. The energy is obtained from the breakdown of ATP into ADP. In this reaction, one ATP is converted to ADP **(1 ATP is utilized)**.

Regulation:

***Aspartate transcarbamoylase* (*ATCase*) is a rate limiting enzyme involved in the biosynthesis of pyrimidines in bacteria**. The end product CTP controls the *aspartate transcarbamoylase (ATCase)* by a feedback mechanism. In addition, UTP also inhibits *aspartate transcarbamoylase (ATCase)*; whereas ATP stimulates the activity of *aspartate transcarbamoylase (ATCase)*.

In animals, *carbamoyl phosphate synthetase – II (CPS – II)* is the regulatory enzyme that is involved in the biosynthesis of pyrimidine nucleotides. PRPP and ATP activate *CPS – II*; whereas, UDP and UTP inhibit *CPS – II*. In addition, *OMP decarboxylase* also controls the biosynthesis of pyrimidine nucleotides. UMP and CMP inhibit the enzyme *OMP decarboxylase*.

Degradation:

Like purine nucleotides, pyrimidine nucleotides also undergoe a similar type of degradation by reactions involving dephosphorylation, deamination and breakage of glycosidic bonds to produce nitrogen bases such as uracil, cytosine and thymine. Later, highly soluble amino acids such as β-alanine and β-aminoisobutyrate are produced from degradation of nitrogen bases such as uracil, cytosine and thymine. Finally, the obtained amino acids such as β-alanine and β-aminoisobutyrate produced acetyl CoA and succinyl CoA, respectively through transamination and other reactions.

Salvage pathway:

In the salvage pathway, pyrimidines can serve as a precursor for the synthesis of corresponding pyrimidine nucleotides like purines. In this reaction, PRPP acts as a donor of ribose-5-phosphate to the pyrimidine nitrogen base to produce their corresponding pyrimidine nucleotides. The enzyme involved in this reaction is *phosphoribosyl transferase*.

Metabolic disorders:

1. **Orotic aciduria:** Excretion of orotic acid in urine, retardation of growth and severe anemia are the characterization of this rare metabolic disorder. The bifunctional enzyme *orotate phosphoribosyl transferase* and *OMP decarboxylase* is responsible for this metabolic disorder. The effective treatment for orotic aciduria is feeding a diet rich in uridine and/or cytidine because by phosphorylation these compounds synthesize pyrimidine nucleotides needed for the synthesis of DNA and RNA. In addition, *carbamoyl phosphate synthetase – II (CPS – II)* is inhibited by UTP results in blocking of orotic acid synthesis.
2. **Rey's syndrome:** This disorder is due to the deficiency of *ornithine transcarbamoylase* of urea cycle results in accumulation of carbamoyl phosphate. The accumulated carbamoyl phosphate is diverted for the increased synthesis and degradation of orotic acid. Hence, Rey's syndrome is considered as secondary orotic aciduria.

Structure of DNA

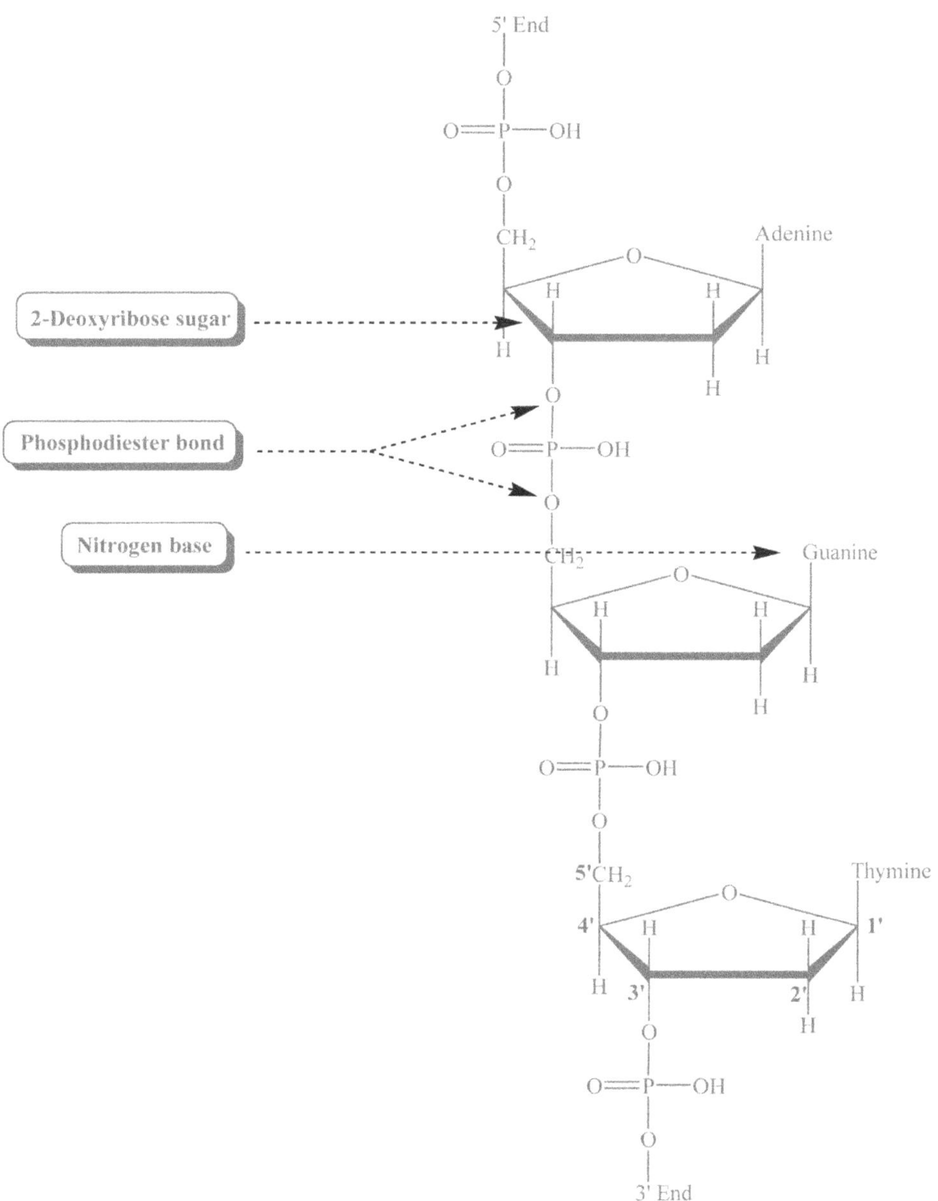

Figure 6.6 Structure of polydeoxyribonucleotide.

Composition:

DNA is a polymer of deoxyribonucleotides or simply deoxynucleotides. The various monomeric units present in DNA are as follows,

1. Deoxyadenylate (*d*AMP)
2. Deoxyguanylate (*d*GMP)
3. Deoxycytidylate (*d*CMP) and
4. Deoxythymidylate (*d*TMP)

The DNA contains,

1. **Nitrogen base:** Purine (Adenine & guanine) and pyrimidine (Cytosine & thymine)
2. **Sugar:** 2-Deoxyribose and
3. Phosphate group.

Schematic representation:

In DNA, the monomeric deoxyribonucleotides are attached together by 3′,5′-phosphodiester bridges. It is often observed that the structure of nucleic acid such as DNA and RNA is represented by a shorthand form. The carbon chains of sugars are usually indicated by a horizontal line; the base attached at C-1 is represented at the right hand side corner of the horizontal line and the phosphate linkage is present between C-3 of one sugar which is mentioned near the middle of the horizontal line and the C-5 of another sugar which is mentioned in next horizontal line left hand side corner.

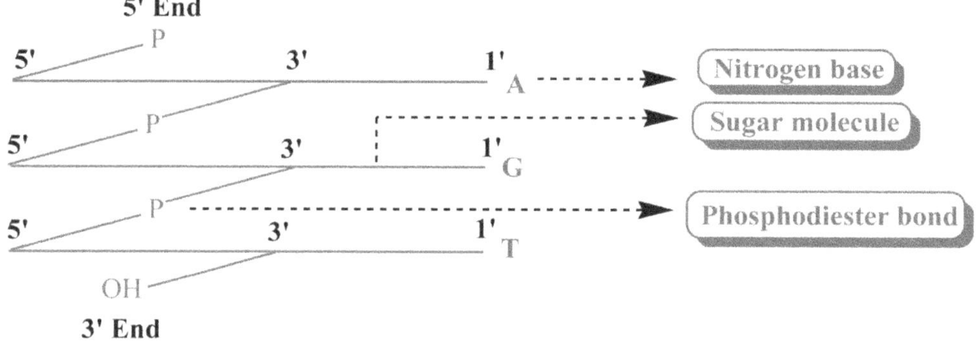

Figure 6.7 Shorthand form of oligonucleotides.

Chargaff's rule:

In the year 1940, from the different species, Erwin Chargaff quantitatively analyzed DNA hydrolysis and observed that in all the species the number of adenine and thymine residue (A = T) are equal in DNA and similarly, guanine and cytosine residue (G = C) are equal in the DNA. This concept is known as Chargaff's rule of molecular equivalence between the purines and pyrimidines in DNA structure. This rule gives

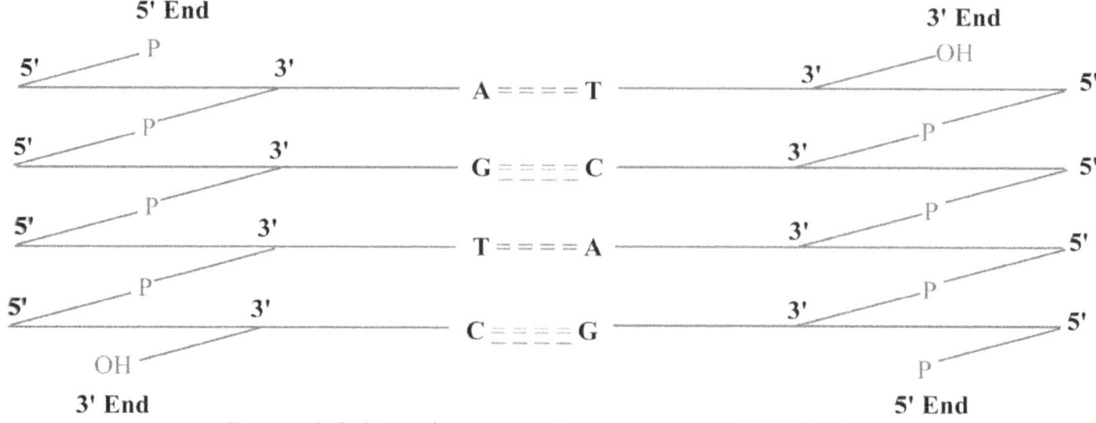

Figure 6.8 Complementary base pairing in DNA helix.

strength to the double helical structure of DNA. This Chargaff's rule is not obeyed by single stranded DNA and RNA (usually single stranded). In certain viruses, as a genetic material, RNA is present in a double stranded form which obeys the Chargaff's rule.

DNA double helix:

In the year 1953, James Watson and Francis Crick proposed the double helical structure of DNA. In modern biology, the DNA structure elucidation is considered as a milestone. Usually, the twisted ladder was used to compare the DNA double helix. Now, the Watson-Crick model of DNA is known as B-DNA and its various salient features are as follows.

1. DNA is the right-handed double helix composed of two strands i.e., polydeoxyribo nucleotide chains twisted around a common axis.
2. Out of these two strands, one strand runs in 5′ to 3′ direction; whereas the other strand runs in the opposite direction i.e., 3′ to 5′ direction. Hence, the two strands of DNA are antiparallel to each other and are usually compared with two parallel roads carrying traffic in opposite directions.
3. 20 A° or 2 nm is the width or diameter of the double helix.

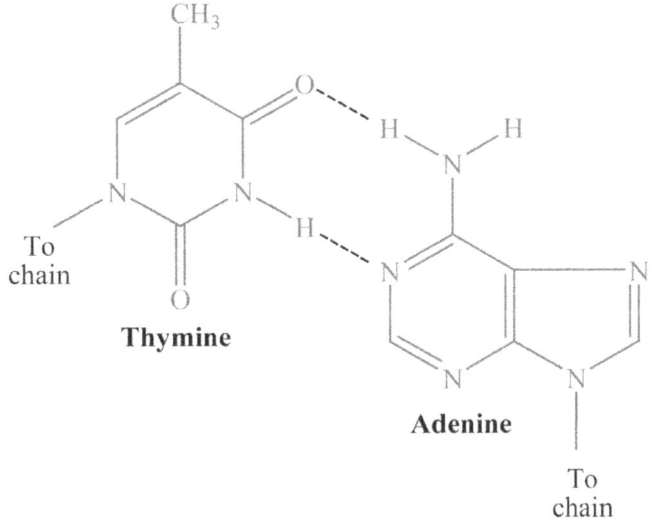

(A) Thymine pairs with adenine by 2 hydrogen bonds

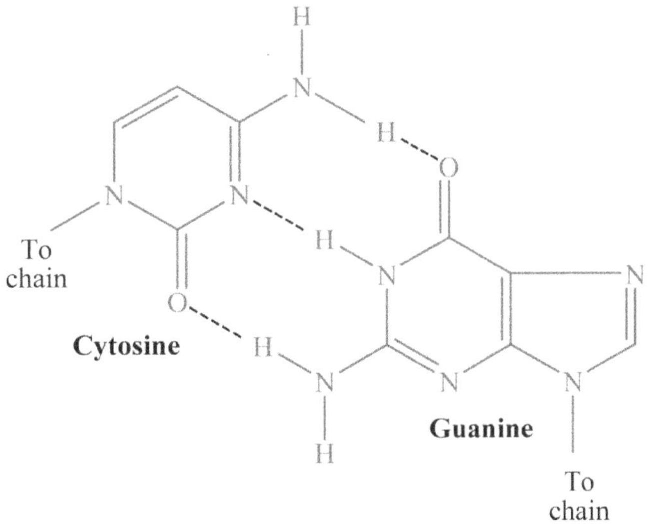

(B) Cytosine pairs with guanine by 3 hydrogen bonds

Figure 6.9 Complementary base pairing in DNA.

4. 34 A° or 3.4 nm is the size of each pitch or turn of the helix. Each turn contains ten pairs of nucleotides and each pair is placed at 3.4 A° or 0.34 nm distance.
5. The periphery or outside of each strand contains hydrophilic deoxyribose phosphate backbone (3′-5′ phosphodiester bonds) and inside or core the hydrophobic bases are stacked.
6. Due to base pairing, the two strands or polydeoxyribonucleotide chains of DNA are complementary to each other and are not identical.
7. Complementary base pairs form hydrogen bonds which are used to hold together the two strands. Two hydrogen bonds are formed between adenine and thymine (A = T) and three hydrogen bonds are formed between guanine and cytosine (G ≡ C). In addition, guanine-cytosine hydrogen bond (G ≡ C) is 50 % stronger than adenine-thymine hydrogen bond (A = T).
8. In general, the hydrogen bond is formed between purine base with pyrimidine base only. If two purines are facing each other, it will not fit in the allowable space. Similarly, if two pyrimidine bases face each other it will be too far to form the hydrogen bonds. In DNA, only the following four base arrangements are possible due to spatial consideration. They are, A-T, G-C, T-A and C-G.
9. The Chargaff's rule is proved by the complementary base pairing in the DNA helix. In general, in the DNA, the content of adenine is equal to thymine and the content of guanine is equal to cytosine.
10. Out of two strands, the genetic information resides in only one strand which is known as the sense strand or the template strand. The other strand is known as the anti-sense strand. Along the phosphodiester backbone, the double helix has major groove (wide) and minor groove (narrow). In these grooves without disturbing the base pairs and double helix, proteins interact with DNA.

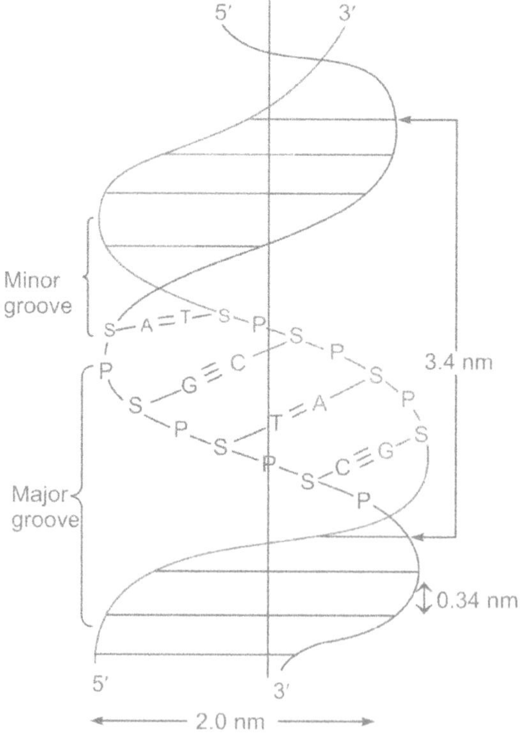

Figure 6.10 Right-handed double helical structure of DNA.

Conformations of DNA double helix:

In nucleotides of DNA, the conformation variation is associated with conformational variants of DNA. At least six different forms of DNA double helical structures such as A to E and Z exist in nature. B, A and Z forms are important among these six forms. Under physiological conditions, the most predominant form is B-form of DNA double helix described by Watson and Crick model. The width of the B-form is 2 nm and ten base pairs are present in each turn, spanning a distance of 3.4 nm. The A-form is also a right-handed helix and it contains eleven base pairs in each turn. From the central axis the base pairs are tilted by 20 °C away. The Z-form is a left-handed helix and it contains twelve base pairs in each turn. In zig-zag fashion, the polynucleotide strands of DNA are moving; hence, this form is named as Z-form. In regulation of gene expression, the transition between different helical forms of DNA plays a significant role. The right-handed double helical structure of DNA is depicted in Figure 6.10.

Other types of DNA structure:

DNA also exists in other unusual structures. It is believed that for molecular recognition of DNA by proteins and enzymes, these structures are important. In addition, for DNA to exhibit its function in an appropriate manner, it needs these structures. The following are the various important unusual structures of DNA.

1. Bent DNA
2. Triple stranded DNA and
3. Four stranded DNA

Bent DNA: Generally, DNA tracts are rigid and straight when they possess adenine base. When other bases replace A-tracts or into the minor groove of A-tract collapse of the helix leads to occurrence of bent conformation of DNA. The photochemical damage or mispairing of bases also report to produce bending in DNA structure. In DNA, bent structure is produced by some anticancer agents like cisplatin. This may lead to DNA damage by taking up proteins due to structure changes.

Triple stranded DNA: Generally, this type of DNA is formed due to additional hydrogen bonds between the bases. Two Hoogsteen hydrogen bonds are selectively formed by thymine to the adenine of the A-T pair to form T-A-T. Similarly, two hydrogen bonds formed by protonated cytosine with guanine of G-C pair result in C-G-C. Compared to double helical structure, triple helical structure is less stable because in triple helix electrostatic repulsion is increased due to three negatively charged backbone strands. The Hoogsteen triple helical structure of DNA is presented in Figure 6.11.

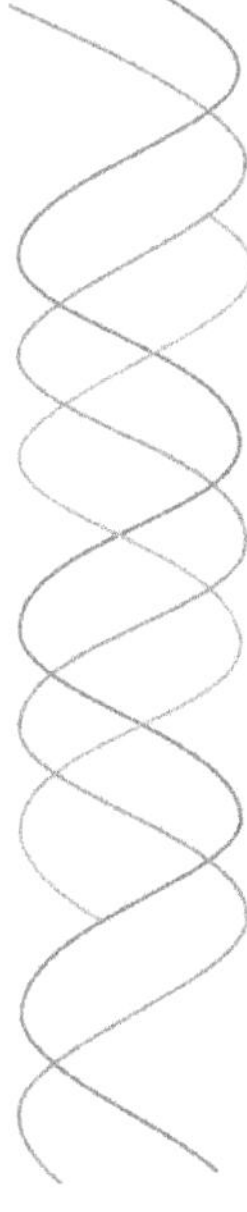

Figure 6.11 Hoogsteen triple helical structure of DNA.

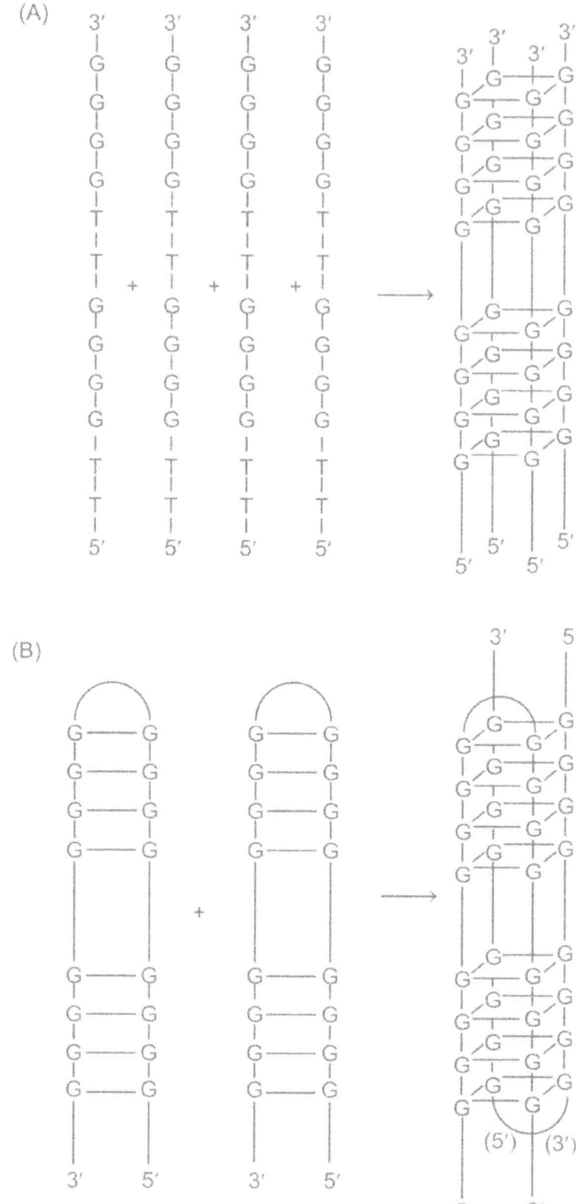

Figure 6.12 Four stranded DNA structure; A) Parallel G-quartets; B) Anti-parallel G-tetraplex.

Four stranded DNA: G-quartets are the novel tetrameric structure formed by the polynucleotides with very high contents of guanine. These structures are connected by Hoogsteen hydrogen bonds and are planar in nature. G-Tetraplexes are the antiparallel four stranded DNA which is also reported. G-Tetraplexes are formed by telomeres (ends of eukaryotic chromosomes) which are rich in guanine. In anticancer therapies, now a days telomers becomes the target. In the dimerization of double stranded genomic, RNA of the human immuno deficiency virus (HIV) and recombination of immunoglobulin genes G-tetraplexes are implicated. The four stranded DNA structure is presented in Figure 6.12.

Denaturation of DNA strands:

Hydrogen bonds hold together the two strands of DNA helix. Polynucleotide strands are separated due to the disruption of hydrogen bonds by pH changes or increased temperature. Denaturation is the phenomenon of loss of helical structure of DNA. Generally, denaturation does not break phosphodiester bond. Using spectrophotometer helical structure loss i.e., denaturation is measured by increase in absorbance at 260 nm. Hyperchromicity is the phenomenon of increase in the absorbance of purines and pyrimidines following denaturation.

The temperature at which half of the helical structure of DNA is lost is known as the melting temperature and is denoted by Tm. DNA with higher G-C content poses greater melting temperature (Tm) because G-C base pairs containing three hydrogen bonds are more stable than A-T base pairs with two hydrogen bonds. Hence, for 35 % G-C content the Tm is 65 °C; whereas for 50 % G-C content the Tm is 70 °C. Melting temperature (Tm) is lowered by formamide because it destabilizes hydrogen bonds of base pairs. Hence, in recombinant DNA experiment formamide is effectively used.

The process of forming a double helix from the separated complementary DNA strand is known as "renaturation". Denaturation and renaturation of DNA is diagrammatically represented in Figure 6.13.

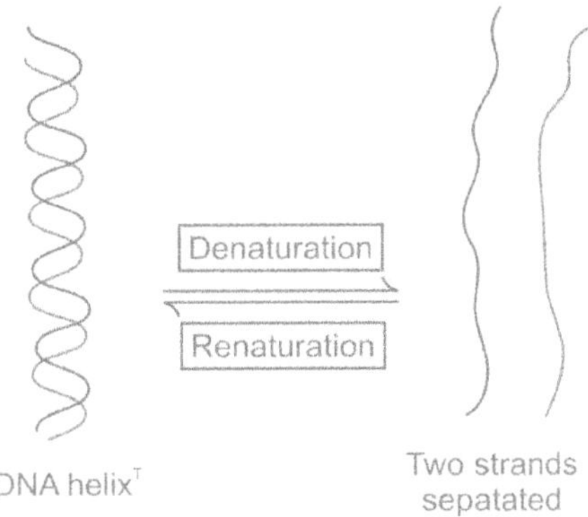

Figure 6.13 Denaturation and renaturation of DNA.

Organization of Mammalian Genome or Organization of DNA in the Cell

In each chromosome, the length of double stranded DNA is thousand times of its diameter of the nucleus. In humans, 2 meter long DNA is packed in 10 μm diameter of the nucleus. It is possible inside the cell due to the excellent and compact organization and packing of DNA.

Organization of prokaryotic DNA:

In the form of a double stranded circle, DNA is organized in prokaryotic cells as a single chromosome. By interacting with proteins and certain cations like polyamines, in the form of nucleoids these bacterial enzymes are packed.

Organization of eukaryotic DNA:

Naked DNA double helix (**2 nm**)

⇩

Beads on a string which is a form of chromatin (**10 nm**)

⇩

30 nm chromatin fiber composed of nucleosomes (**30 nm**)

⇩

Chromosomes in an extended form (non-condensed loops; **300 nm**)

⇩

Condensed form of chromosome (**700 nm**)

⇩

Metaphase chromosome (**1400 nm**)

In eukaryotic cells, to form chromatin the DNA is associated with various proteins. Later, chromatin is getting organized into compact structures known as chromosomes. The basic histones are the core proteins which wrapped the double helix of DNA. Two molecules of histones (H2A, H2B, H3 and H4) compose the core proteins. The basic unit of chromatin is nucleosome which wraps round each core with two turns of DNA (approximately with 150 base pairs). Spacer DNA separates the nucleosomes in which histones are attached. 10 nm fibers are the continuous string of nucleosomes representing beads on a string form of chromatin. This 10 nm fibers formation considerably reduces the length of DNA. Further, 30 nm fiber is formed from 10 nm fiber by coiling. 30 nm fibers have a solenoid structure with six nucleosomes in every turn. Further, by anchoring the fiber these 30 nm fibers are organized into loops at A/T rich regions namely scaffold associated regions (SARS) to a protein scaffold. The loops are further coiled and the chromosomes are condensed and become visible during the process of mitosis. Organization of eukaryotic DNA structure in the form of chromatin and chromosomes is presented in Figure 6.14 and the structure of nucleosome is presented in Figure 6.15.

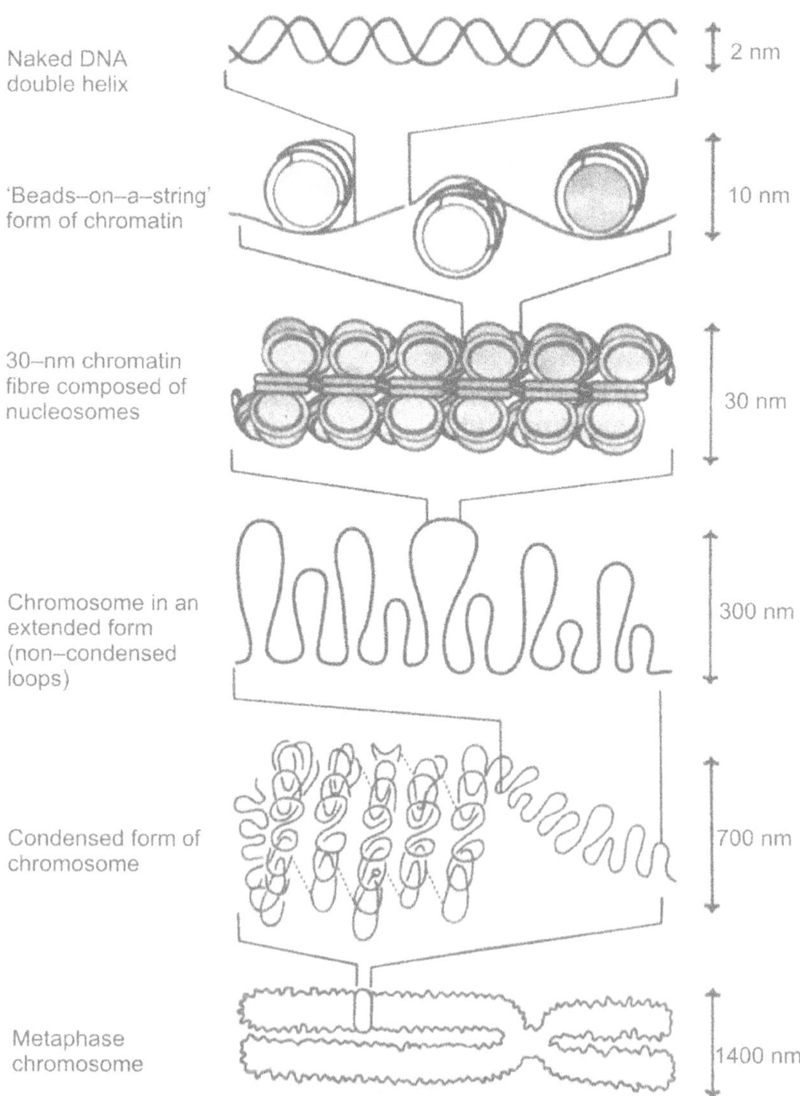

Figure 6.14 Organization of eukaryotic DNA structure in the form of chromatin and chromosomes.

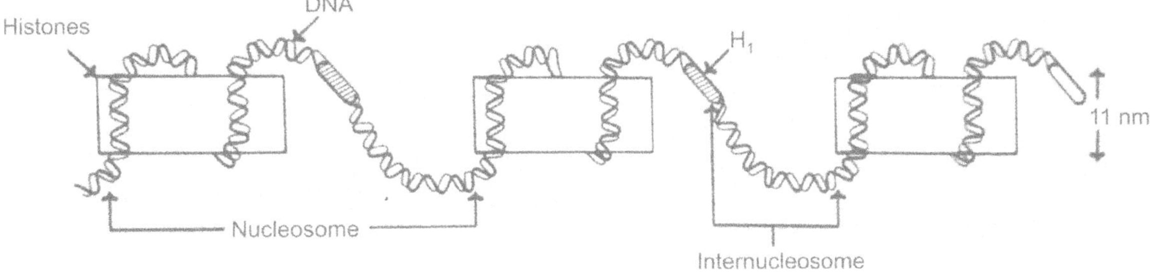

Figure 6.15 Structure of nucleosome.

Structure of RNA

Composition:

RNA is a polymer of ribonucleotides and is linked by 3′,5′-phosphodiester bridges. The various monomeric units present in RNA are as follows,

1. Adenosine monophosphate (AMP)
2. Guanosine monophosphate (GMP)
3. Cytidine monophosphate (CMP) and
4. Uridine monophosphate (UMP)

The RNA contains,

1. **Nitrogen base:** Purine (Adenine & guanine) and pyrimidine (Cytosine &uracil)
2. **Sugar:** Ribose and
3. Phosphate group.

Comparison between DNA and RNA:

The following are the differences between RNA and DNA even though they have certain similarities.

1. **Pentose sugar:** Ribose is present in RNA in contrast to deoxyribose in DNA.
2. **Pyrimidine base:** In place of thymine in DNA, RNA contains uracil.
3. **Single strand:** In general RNA is single stranded polynucleotide whereas DNA is double stranded polynucleotide. Even though in RNA at certain places if complementary base pairs are in close proximity this single strand may fold to give a double stranded structure.
4. **Chargaff's rule:** In RNA there is no specific relationship between purine and pyrimidine contents due to the single stranded nature. That means content of cytosine is not equal to content of guanine (C # G).
5. **Alkali hydrolysis susceptibility:** Due to the presence of hydroxyl group at C-2 of ribose, RNA undergoes alkali hydrolysis and produces 2′,3′-cyclic diesters. Whereas DNA is not hydrolyzed by alkali due to lack of hydroxyl group at C-2 of sugar molecules.
6. **Orcinol color reaction:** RNA contains ribose in its structure, hence historically it gives orcinol color reactions; whereas DNA not due to lack of ribose sugar.

   The various similarities and differences between the DNA and RNA are summarized in the Table 6.3.

Table 6.3 Comparison between DNA and RNA.

S. No.	Parameter	DNA	RNA
Differences			
1	Nucleotide	Deoxyribonucleotide	Ribonucleotide
2	Pentose sugar	2-Deoxyribose	Ribose
3	Pyrimidine base	Cytosine & thymine	Cytosine & uracil
4	Structure	Double helix	Single strand
5	Chargaff's rule	Obey	Not obey
6	Alkali hydrolysis	Not susceptible	Susceptible
7	Orcinol color reaction	No characteristic reaction (Negative)	Characteristic reaction (Positive)
8	Types	No types	mRNA, tRNA, rRNA, hnRNA, snRNA, snoRNA, scRNA, tmRNA
9	Other forms	Bent DNA, triple stranded DNA and four stranded DNA	No other forms
10	Function	Hereditary function or genetic information	Biosynthesis of protein
11	Enzyme function	Not act as enzyme	Certain RNA like ribozymes act as enzyme
12	Biosynthesis	From parent DNA by replication	From DNA by transcription
Similarities			
13	Purine base	Adenine & guanine	Adenine & guanine
14	Linkage or bridges	3',5'-phosphodiester bridges	3',5'-phosphodiester bridges
15	Composition	Nitrogen base, sugar and phosphate	Nitrogen base, sugar and phosphate

Types of RNA:

RNAs are primarily involved in the process of protein biosynthesis and are synthesized from DNA. RNAs vary in their structure and functions. Based on the cellular composition there are many different types of RNAs that exist. Among them the first three types are major. They are,

1. **Messenger RNA (mRNA):** 5-10 % mRNA is present in total RNA. To synthesize proteins mRNA transfers genetic information from genes to ribosomes.
2. **Transfer RNA (tRNA):** 10-20 % tRNA is present in total RNA. For protein synthesis it transfers amino acids to mRNA.
3. **Ribosomal RNA (rRNA):** 50-80 % rRNA is present in total RNA. It provides a structural framework for ribosomes.
4. **Heterogenous nuclear RNA (hnRNA):** It serves as a precursor for the synthesis of all RNAs including mRNA.
5. **Small nuclear RNA (snRNA):** It is involved in the processing of mRNA.
6. **Small nucleolar RNA (snoRNA):** It plays a major role in processing of rRNA.
7. **Small cytoplasmic RNA (scRNA):** It is involved in the secretion of proteins for export.
8. **Transfer messenger RNA (tmRNA):** In bacteria it is mostly present and it facilitates the degradation of incorrectly synthesized proteins by adding short peptide tags to proteins.

Messenger RNA (mRNA):

In the nucleus of eukaryotes messenger RNA (mRNA) is synthesized as heterogenous nuclear RNA (hnRNA). The functional mRNA is liberated from hnRNA on processing and this functional mRNA enters into cytoplasm to participate in protein biosynthesis. The half-life of mRNA is short and it has high molecular weight. Compared to prokaryotes mRNA, eukaryotes mRNA is more stable and possess long half-life. 7-Methylguanosine triphosphate capped the 5′-terminal end of eukaryotic mRNA. Hydrolysis of mRNA is prevented by this cap form *5′-exonucleases.* In addition, for protein synthesis this cap is involved in recognition of mRNA. Poly (A) tail is the 3′-terminal ends of mRNA composed of 20 to 250 adenylate residues. This tail prevents mRNA from the attack of 3′-exonuclease and also provides stability to mRNA. Often in the internal structures of mRNA 6-methyl adenylates which are modified bases are present.

Transfer RNA (tRNA):

It is otherwise known as soluble RNA made up of mostly 75 (71 to 80) nucleotides with 25,000 molecular weight. Corresponding to 20 amino acids present in protein there are at least 20 different species of tRNAs present. Holley first elucidated the structure of tRNA for alanine. The structure of tRNA resembles clover leaf and contains four arms. Due to the existence of complementary base pairs in the arms of tRNA, the structure of tRNA is maintained. Base paired stem is present in each arm. Structure of tRNA is presented in Figure 6.16. The following are the five arms of tRNA.

1. **The acceptor arm:** To the acceptor arm amino acid is attached and is capped in 5′ to 3′ direction with a sequence of CCA. Seven base pairs are present in this arm.
2. **The anticodon arm:** Triplet codon of mRNA is recognized by this anticodon arm only. Three specific nucleotide bases are present in this arm. The codon and anticodon are complementary to each other. In this arm five base pairs are present.
3. **The D-arm:** Dihydrouridine is present in this arm; hence, it is named as D-arm. Four base pairs are present in this arm.
4. **The TΨC-arm:** This arm contains a sequence of T, pseudo define (represented by psi, ø) and C. In this arm five base pairs are present.
5. **The variable arm:** In tRNA this arm is most variable. tRNAs are classified into two major categories based on this variability as follows,
   (a) **Class – I tRNA:** The length of this class tRNA is 3 to 5 base pair length and is the most predominant one with around 75 %.
   (b) **Class – II tRNA:** The length of this class tRNA is 13 to 20 base pair length and is less common with around 25 %.

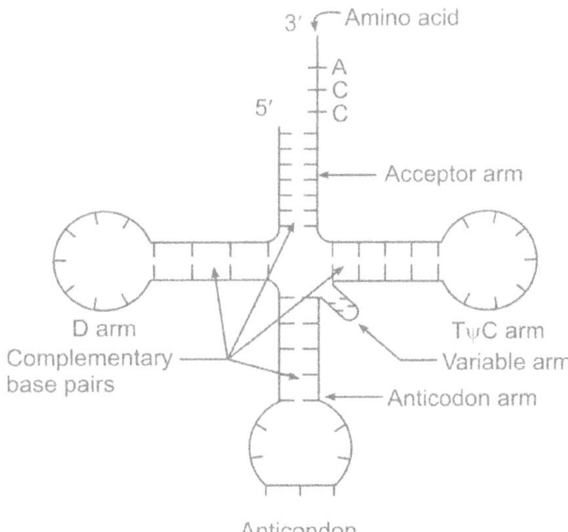

Figure 6.16 Structure of tRNA.

Ribosomal RNA (rRNA):

The protein synthesis factories are ribosomes. Two major nucleoprotein complexes such as 60S subunit and 80S subunit are present in eukaryotic ribosomes. 28S rRNA, 5S rRNA and 5.8S rRNA are present in 60S subunit and 18S rRNA is present in 40S subunit. In ribosomes the function of rRNA is not clearly known. It is believed that they play a significant role in the binding of mRNA to ribosomes and protein synthesis.

Ribozymes (Catalytic RNAs):

Ribonucleoproteins (protein associated RNA) of RNA is catalytically active in certain instances and such RNAs are known as ribozymes. Just like proteins i.e., enzymes, RNA molecules adapt tertiary structures.

The reason behind the biocatalyst functions of RNA is its specific conformation. During the course of evolution before the occurrence of protein enzymes, ribozymes were functioning as catalysts. The following are some important ribozymes.

(a) **rRNA:** In protein synthesis it is involved in peptide bond formation.

(b) ***Ribonuclease P (RNase P)*:** It is a component of RNA and is a ribozyme containing protein. It is involved in cleavage of RNA particularly tRNA precursors to generate mature tRNA molecules. It is also involved in the ligation.

(c) **Self-splicing RNA:** It is involved in the cleavage of DNA.

(d) **RNAs of spliceosome:** It is involved in splicing of RNA.

(e) ***In vitro* selected RNAs:** It is involved in RNA polymerization, RNA aminoacylation, RNA phosphorylation, redox reactions, glycoside bond formation and disulfide exchange.

Recombinant ribozymes (rRibozymes): Any RNA can be cleaved by designing recombinant ribozymes. At present for curing diseases these recombinant ribozymes are considered as therapeutic agents. Theoretically in disease, recombinant ribozymes selectively degrades faulty RNAs such as mutated or inappropriately expressed RNAs. From the cells the specific RNAs can be eliminated by this way which will help to inhibit the disease process.

The Central Dogma of Life

The central dogma of life is flowing of biological information from DNA to RNA and from there to proteins. Through protein synthesis DNA ultimately controls every function of the cell.

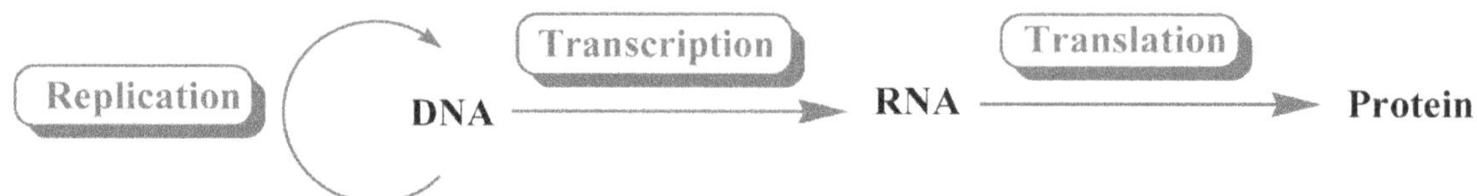

In the cell as a carrier of genetic information, DNA must be replicated (duplicated), maintained and passed down accurately to the daughter cells. For this purpose, three Rs of DNA such as replication, recombination and repair are specifically designed. The following are the common features of these three Rs of DNA.

1. They act on DNA (Same substrate)
2. The backbone of DNA structure is phosphodiester bonds. These three Rs are primarily concerned with the making and breaking of these phosphodiester bonds.
3. In these three processes, the enzymes used are similar or comparable.

DNA Replication

Definition

From the parent cell, the daughter cells receive identical copies of genetic information when the cell divides. **The replication is defined as a process in which DNA copies itself to produce identical daughter molecules of DNA.** For the survival of species DNA is essential, hence, with high loyalty replication is carried out. Replication process is a complex one involving a series of steps.

Replication in prokaryotes:

Semi-conservative replication: Two strands which are complementary to each other are present in parent DNA. Two daughter molecules are produced by simultaneous replication of both two strands. In a newly synthesized DNA, one half is original i.e., one strand from parent DNA and the other half is duplicate i.e., another strand is newly synthesized or copied. Since, half of the original DNA is conserved in the daughter DNA this type of replication is called a semi-conservative model. In 1958, Meselson and Stahl provided the first experimental evidence for this semi-conservative DNA replication. In Figure 6.17, semi-conservative DNA replication is presented.

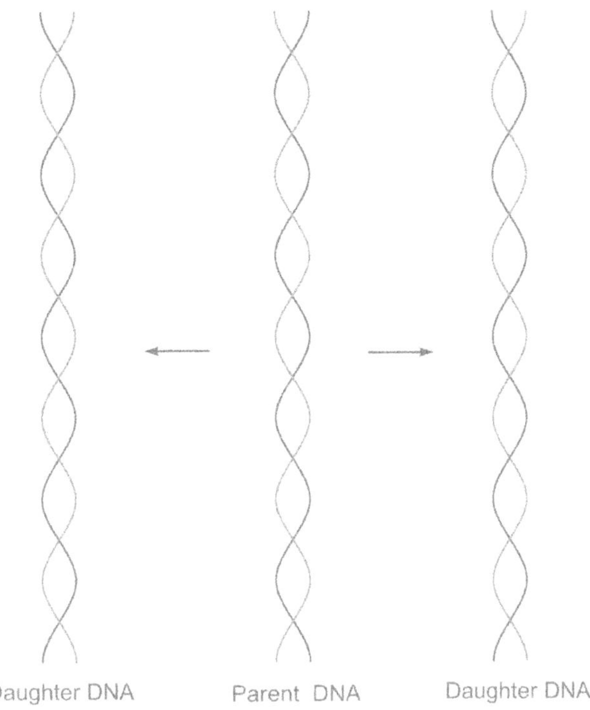

Figure 6.17 Semi-conservative DNA replication.

Initiation of replication: Origin of replication is the site for DNA synthesis initiation. There are multiple sites of origin in eukaryotes whereas in prokaryotes only a single site of origin. Mostly in these sites, a short sequence of A-T base pairs is present. For replication, dna A is a specific protein containing 20 to 50 monomers bound with the site of origin leads to separation of double stranded DNA.

Replication bubble: To form a replication bubble, at the site of replication two complementary strands of DNA are separated. For a rapid replication process in eukaryotic DNA, multiple replication bubbles are formed. Multiple replication bubbles formed in DNA replication is schematically presented in Figure 6.18.

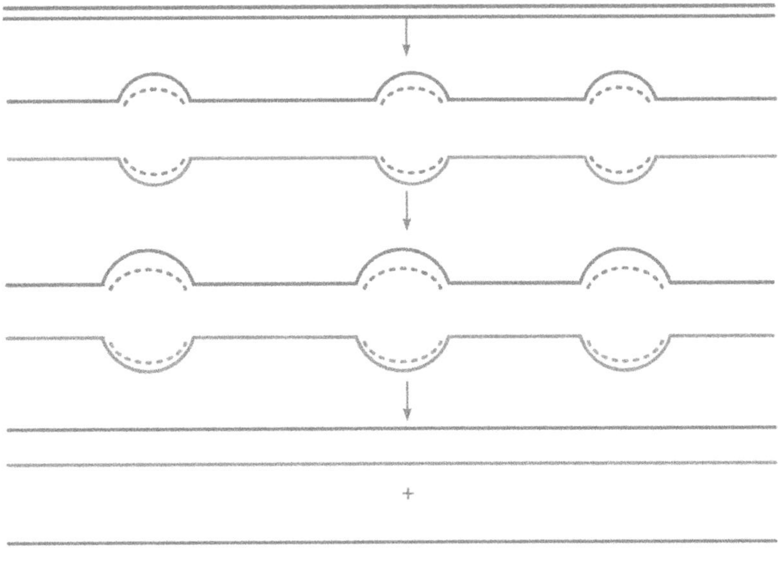

Figure 6.18 Multiple replication bubbles in DNA replication (Schematic representation).

RNA primer: RNA primer is a short fragment of RNA (contains 5 to 50 nucleotides which is variable with species) needed for the synthesis of new DNA. Primosome is a complex formed by a specific *RNA polymerase* enzyme i.e., *primase* in association with single stranded DNA binding protein (SSBP). RNA primers are produced by *primase*. On the lagging strand of DNA, RNA primer synthesis and supply should occur constantly. In the case of leading strands, almost a single RNA primer is occurring.

Semi discontinuous and bidirectional synthesis of DNA: On both strands of DNA, replication simultaneously occurs in 5′ to 3′ direction. The DNA synthesis is continuous in one strand and that strand is called a leading or continuous or forward strand. In the other strand, DNA synthesis is discontinuous and that strand is known as lagging or discontinuous or retrograde strand. In the latter strand i.e., lagging strand, short pieces of DNA possessing 15 to 250 nucleotides are produced. From the point of origin of replication bubble, DNA synthesis occurs in both the directions.

Replication fork: Replication fork is formed as a result of separation of two strands of parent DNA. In this region, only active synthesis of DNA takes place. As the daughter DNA molecules are synthesized, the replication fork moves along the parent DNA.

***DNA helicase*:** At the replication fork the enzyme *DNA helicase* binds to both DNA strands. Two strands of DNA are separated when a *DNA helicase* moves along the DNA helix. The function of *DNA helicase* is usually compared with a zip opener and is dependent on ATP for supply of energy.

Single stranded DNA binding protein (SSBP): DNA helix destabilizing protein is the other name of single stranded DNA binding protein (SSBP). Only to a single stranded DNA separated by *DNA helicase,* single stranded DNA binding protein (SSBP) bounds and keep the two strands separate. The template for new DNA synthesis is provided by single stranded DNA binding protein (SSBP). In addition, degradation of single stranded DNA by *nuclease* is also protected by a single stranded DNA binding protein (SSBP).

***DNA polymerase – III*:** In 5′ to 3′ direction new strands of DNA is synthesized and this reaction is catalyzed by *DNA polymerase – III.* To the parent template DNA strand this synthesis is antiparallel. The essential prerequisite for the replication is the presence of all four deoxyribonucleotide such as *d*ATP, *d*GTP, *d*CTP and *d*TTP. Simultaneously two new DNA strands are synthesized but in the opposite direction (One is in 5′ to 3′ direction which is continuous towards the replication fork and another one in 3′ to 5′ direction which is discontinuous away from the replication fork). To the 3′ end of the growing DNA chain one after another the incoming deoxyribonucleotides are added. For addition of each nucleotide one mole of pyrophosphate is removed. The base sequence of the newly synthesized complementary DNA is determined by the parent template DNA strand.

Polarity problem: By sequential addition of new nucleotides, the DNA leading strand with its 3′ end oriented towards the fork can be elongated. In case of DNA lagging strand with 5′ end present some problem due to lack of *DNA polymerase* enzyme which catalyze the addition of nucleotide to the 5′ end i.e., 3′ to 5′ direction of the growing chain. A series of small fragments are synthesized in these strands to solve this problem. In this small fragment synthesis takes place in a normal 5′ to 3′ direction and later joined together. Overview of DNA replication is presented in Figure 6.19.

Okazaki fragments: The small fragments of the discontinuously synthesized DNA are known as Okazaki fragments or pieces. In the parent DNA Okazaki fragments are produced on the lagging DNA strand and are later joined together to form a continuous strand of DNA in presence of *DNA polymerase – I* and *DNA ligase*.

***DNA polymerase – III*:** For the very existence of an organism, fidelity of replication is most important. *DNA polymerase – III* also performs proof reading activity along with 5′to 3′ directed catalytic activity. To the growing DNA strand, it allows only the correct complementary base by checking the incoming nucleotides. In addition, it removes the wrongly placed nucleotide base and edits its mistakes, if any.

RNA primer replacement: Till close proximity to RNA primer, the synthesis of DNA strand continues. *DNA polymerase – I* takes its position by removing the RNA primer. Generally, RNA primer is replaced by a small fragment of DNA synthesized in 5′ to 3′ direction catalyzed by *DNA polymerase – I.*

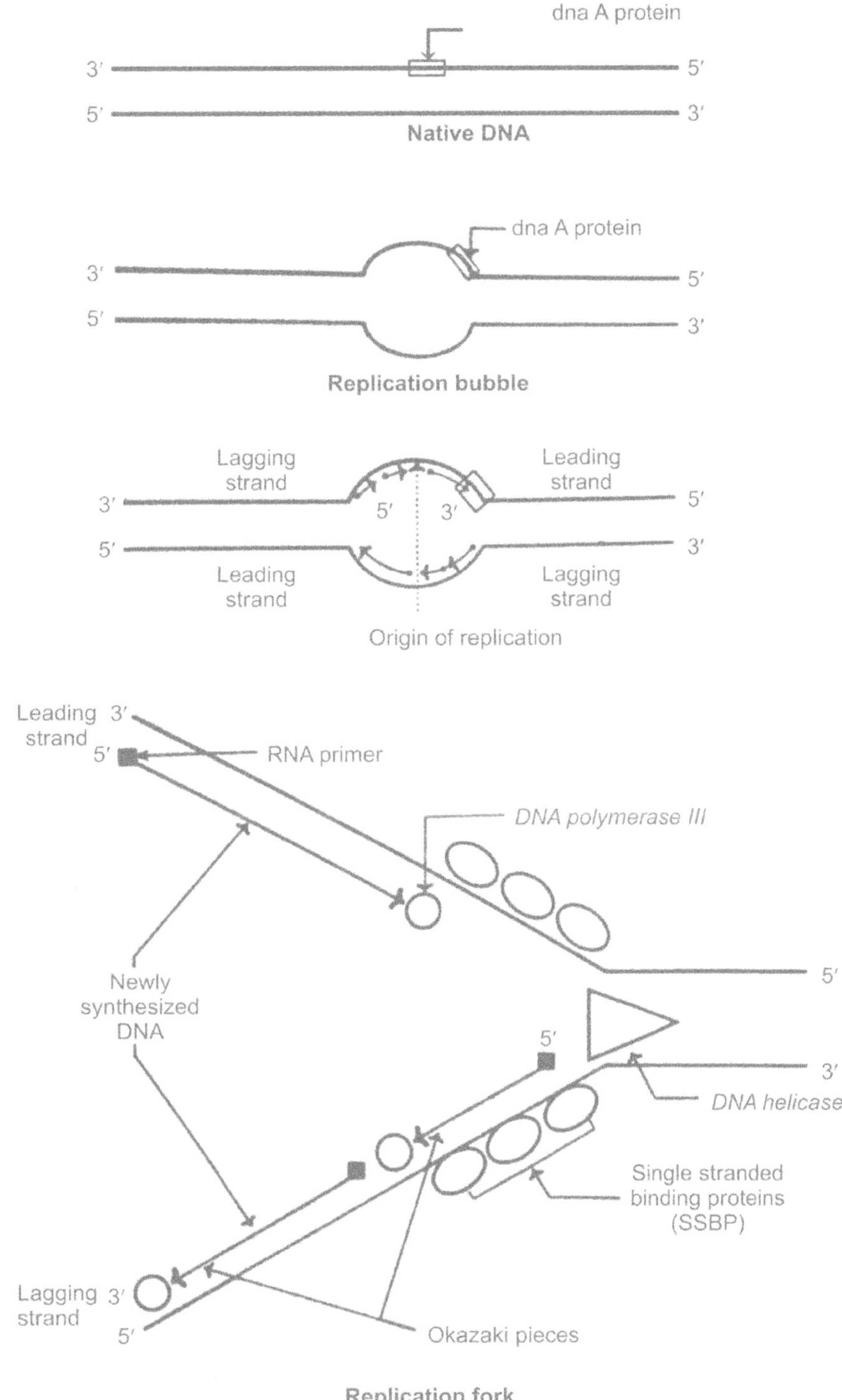

Figure 6.19 Overview of DNA replication.

***DNA ligase*:** DNA synthesized by *DNA polymerase – III* and the small fragment of DNA synthesized by *DNA polymerase – I* are linked by phosphodiester linkage in which the reaction is catalyzed by *DNA ligase*. This process is called nick sealing and it needs energy which is provided by the breakdown of ATP into AMP and pyrophosphate. Overview of *DNA polymerase* & *DNA ligase* action is presented in Figure 6.21.

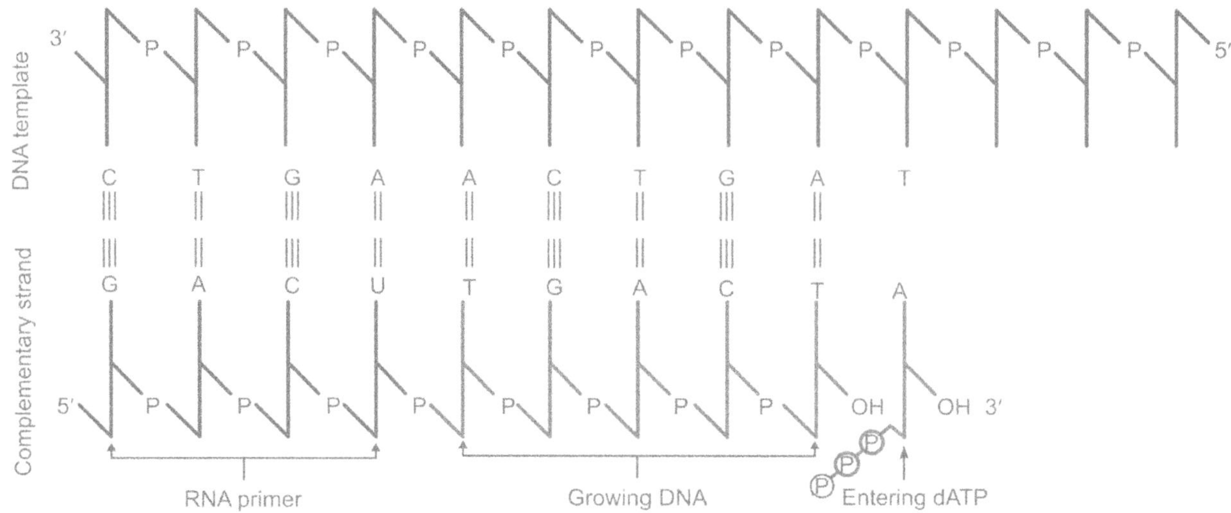

Figure 6.20 Growing complementary strand in DNA replication.

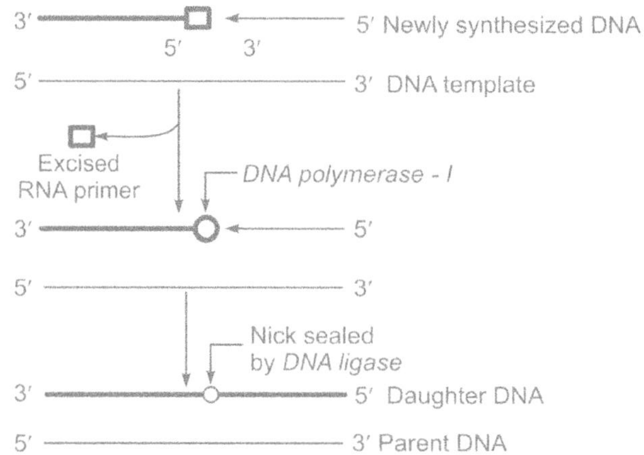

Figure 6.21 Overview of *DNA polymerase* & *DNA ligase* action.

DNA polymerase* – *II: In the DNA repair process, this enzyme participates.

DNA topoisomerase: From one side DNA double helix separates and on the other side, the replication proceeds and super coils form. One end tied two twisted ropes are generally used for the comparison of DNA helix to understand the formation of super coils. The formation of the super coil is clearly observed by holding the rope at the tied end in a fixed position and letting your friend pulls the ropes apart from the other side. There are two *DNA topoisomerase i.e., DNA topoisomerase – I* and *DNA topoisomerase –II*. Among these two, *DNA topoisomerase – I* exhibited *nuclease* activity to overcome the super coils problem by cutting the single DNA strand and then resealed by *DNA ligase*. *DNA topoisomerase – II* is otherwise known as *DNA gyrase* which cuts both strands and reseals them to overcome the super coil problem. In the cancer treatment many drugs target *DNA topoisomerases* only. **Example**: Camptothecin targets *DNA topoisomerase –I* and amsacrine and etoposide targets *DNA topoisomerase – II*.

Replication in eukaryotes:

It closely resembles prokaryotes replication with existence of certain differences. In eukaryotic cells, the characteristic feature is multiple origin of replication. In addition, in eukaryotes five distinct *DNA polymerase* are known and to number these enzymes Greek letters are used. The five distinct *DNA polymerase* of eukaryotic replication are,

1. ***DNA polymerase* – α:** In both leading and lagging strand *DNA polymerase* – α is responsible for the synthesis of RNA primer.

2. ***DNA polymerase* – β:** In prokaryotes replication the function of *DNA polymerase* – β is compared with *DNA polymerase – I*. It is mainly involved in the DNA repairs.
3. ***DNA polymerase* – γ:** In the replication of mitochondrial DNA it participates.
4. ***DNA polymerase* – δ:** It also possess proofreading activity along with leading strand DNA replication.
5. ***DNA polymerase* – ε:** It also possess proofreading activity along with lagging strand DNA replication.

In antibacterial therapy, the difference in the DNA replication between bacteria and human cells attributed by the enzymes are successfully used to target pathogens (bacteria) replication and sparing the host (human) cell.

DNA polymerase – δ and sliding clamp known as proliferating cell nuclear antigen (PCNA) makes the DNA leading or continuous strand replication rather simple. In the nuclei of replicating cells as an antigen, PCNA was first detected; hence, it is named as proliferating cell nuclear antigen (PCNA). Around DNA, a ring is formed by PCNA in which *DNA polymerase* – δ binds. Replication factor – C (RFC) is the other factor needed for the formation of the above-mentioned ring.

Compared to prokaryotes DNA replication, lagging or discontinuous strand DNA replication of eukaryotes is more complex. Even the leading or continuous strand DNA replication of eukaryotes is also complex when compared to prokaryotes DNA replication.

The *helicase* enzyme separates the parental strands of the DNA. Replication protein-A (RPA) is a single stranded binding protein (SSBP) binds to the exposed single stranded template. Replication fork (RNA primer with a previously formed Okazaki fragment) opened up this stand. The Okazaki fragment synthesis is initiated by the enzyme complex made of *primase* and *polymerase CC*. 10 base pair RNA primer is capably produced by *primase* activity of pol α-primase complex. Later, the activity is switched to *DNA polymerase* – α which adds 20 to 30 deoxyribonucleotides and elongates the primer. A short stretch of DNA attached RNA is formed by the action of pol α-primase complex. From the DNA now complex dissociates.

In the succeeding step, the short RNA-DNA (elongated primer) replication factor – C (RFC) is bonded. This RFC catalyzes the assembly of proliferating cell nuclear antigen (PCNA) molecules by serving as a clamp loader. To a final length of around 150 to 200 base pairs,the Okazaki fragment is elongated by *DNA polymerase* – δ when binding to the sliding clamp. RNA primer of the previous Okazaki fragment is approached by the replication complex by this elongation. Pair of enzymes namely *RNase H* and *flap endonuclease – I (FENI)* performs the removal of RNA primer. Continued elongation of the new Okazaki fragment by *DNA polymerase* – δ fills the gap created by RNA removal. *DNA ligase* finally seals the remaining small nick.

In eukaryotic DNA, nucleosomes are formed by tight binding of basic protein known as histones. Later, these nucleosomes are organized into chromosomes. The chromosomes are relaxed and the nucleosomes are loosened during the process of DNA replication. For replication the DNA strands separate and the parental histones associate with one of the parental DNA strands. On the parent strands histones are produced simultaneously when the synthesis of new DNA strands proceeds. Two daughters chromosomal DNA is produced at the end of replication. Parental histones are present among the one daughter chromosomal DNA; whereas newly synthesized histones are present in the other daughter chromosomal DNA. DNA replication on the lagging strand in eukaryotes are outlined in Figure 6.22.

Inhibitors of DNA replication:

DNA topoisomerase – II is otherwise known as *DNA gyrase* is a specific enzyme present in bacteria which cuts and reseals the circular DNA of bacteria to overcome the super coil problem. Antibiotics such as ciprofloxacin, novobiocin and nalidixic acid exhibit its activity by inhibiting this *DNA gyrase* enzyme. These antibiotics effectively block the DNA replication and multiplication of cells; hence they are widely used as antibacterial agents. On human enzymes, these antibiotics have almost no effect.

Anticancer agents such as etoposide, and doxorubicin inhibit human *topoisomerase*. In addition, nucleotide derivatives such as 6-mercptopurine and 5-fluorouracil which inhibit DNA replication are also used as anticancer agents.

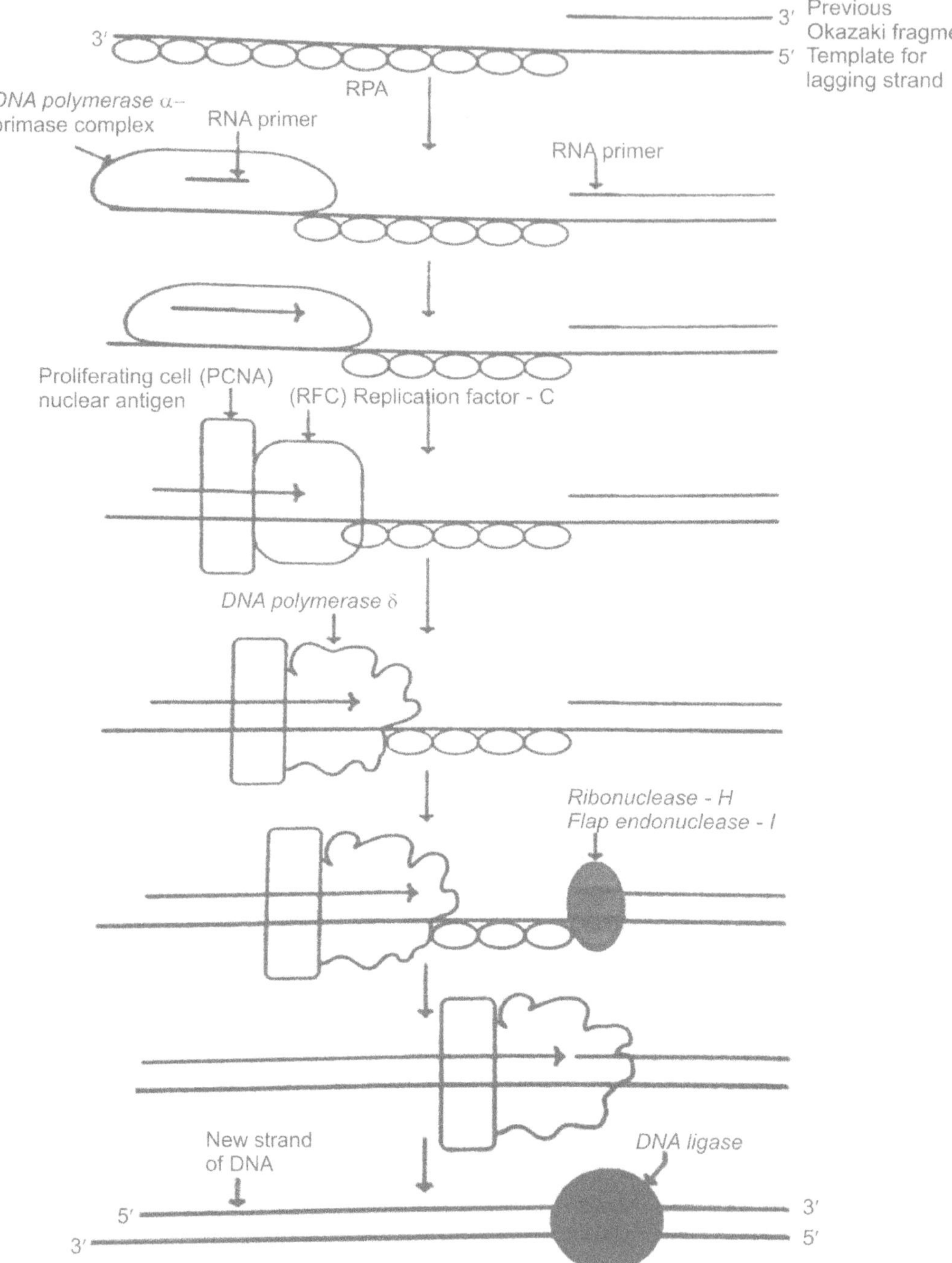

Figure 6.22 DNA replication on the lagging strand in eukaryotes – An outline.

DNA Recombination

Basically, the exchange of genetic information is involved in the recombination and they are classified into two major types.

1. **Homologous recombination:** It is otherwise known as general recombination. In this type, genetic information is exchanged between identical or nearly identical chromosomes i.e., DNA sequences. **Example:** Recombination between the paternal and maternal chromosomal pairs.

2. **Non-homologous recombination:** It is otherwise known as illegitimate recombination. In this type, no need of special homologous sequences of DNA for exchange of genetic information. **Example:** Transposition (movement of specific pieces of DNA in the genome) and random integration of outside genes into mammalian chromosomes.

DNA Repair

Replication errors or mutations cause damage to DNA which results in serious consequences. The damaged DNA is repaired by inbuilt systems present in the cell. By four different mechanisms this repair may be achieved. They are,

1. Base excision repair
2. Nucleotide excision repair
3. Mismatch repair
4. Double strand break repair.

Transcription

Molecular biology is oversimplified by the concept of central dogma of life. In conventional concepts, central dogma of life is represented by "DNA makes RNA makes protein". Currently, the central dogma of life is represented by the terms genome, transcriptome and proteome due to the advancement in cell biology and rapid developments in bioinformatics. Molecular biology or central dogma of life is schematically represented in Figure 6.23.

Genome: Genome represents the total genetic information (DNA) present in an organism or cell. The storehouse of the biological information is known as the genome which includes DNA in mitochondria and chloroplast and chromosomes in the nucleus. Genomics is the study of the structure and function of the genome.

Transcriptome: Transcriptome represents the RNA copies of the active protein coding genes. It is the initial product of gene expression which directs the synthesis of proteins. Transcriptomics is the study of transcriptome that involves all the RNA molecules made by a cell, tissue or an organism.

Proteome: Proteome is the cell's repertoire (Storehouse / repository) of proteins with their nature and biological functions. In a cell, a proteome represents the entire range of proteins and their biological functions. Proteomics is the study of the proteome.

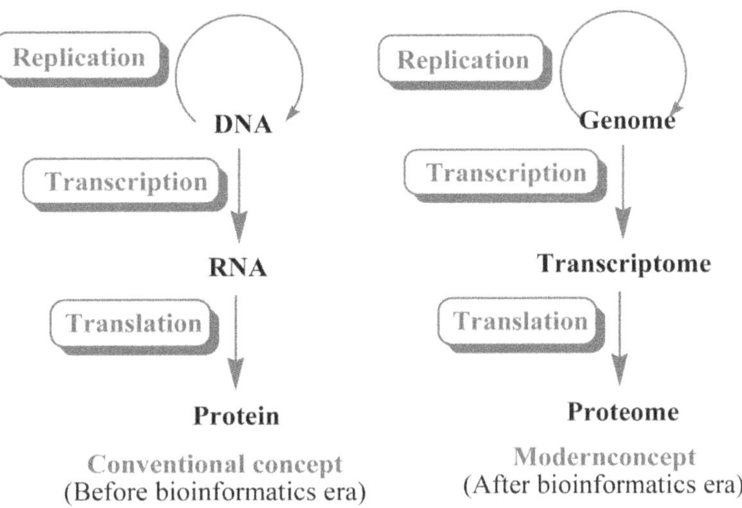

Figure 6.23 Molecular biology or Central dogma of life.

Metabolomics: Metabolomics represents the synthesis of small molecules or metabolites using genome sequence analysis for determining the capability of a cell, tissue or an organism.

Replication, transcription and translation are the key or core processes which ultimately control life whether the central dogma of life is represented either by conventional or recent form.

Definition:

The process of synthesizing ribonucleic acid (RNA) from deoxyribonucleic acid (DNA) is known as transcription. The functional unit of the DNA that can be transcribed is called a gene. Hence, through RNA, DNA expresses the genetic information stored in it. The working copies of RNA molecules produced from antisense or non-coding or template strand which is one of the two strands of DNA. Another one strand is represented as a sense or coding or non-template strand which does not participate in the process of transcription.

Transcription is selective because the entire molecule of DNA is not expressed in transcription. In some selected regions of DNA only RNA is synthesized. In other regions of DNA, there is no transcription at all. In DNA molecules, some inbuilt signals are present which may be responsible for this selectiveness but the exact reasons not known. The primary RNA transcript is the product formed in the transcription and is generally inactive. The functionally active RNA is produced from the primary RNA transcript by some alterations such as splicing, terminal addition, base modification, etc. Some differences are observed between prokaryotes transcription and eukaryotes transcription.

Transcription in Prokaryotes

In prokaryotes, *RNA polymerase* or *DNA dependent RNA polymerase* is the single enzyme involved in the synthesis of all RNAs. Five polypeptide units (Molecular weight: 465 kDa) such as two α, one β, one β′ and one σ is present in the *RNA polymerase* which is a complex holoenzyme of *Escherichia Coli (E. coli)*. *RNA polymerase* of *E. coli* & overview of transcription is presented in Figure 6.24 & Figure 6.25, respectively. Without sigma factor or subunits, the enzyme is referred as core enzyme i.e., $\alpha_2\beta\beta'$. Three different stages are involved in the transcription. They are,

1. Stage - 1 or Initiation stage
2. Stage - 2 or Elongation stage
3. Stage - 3 or Termination stage

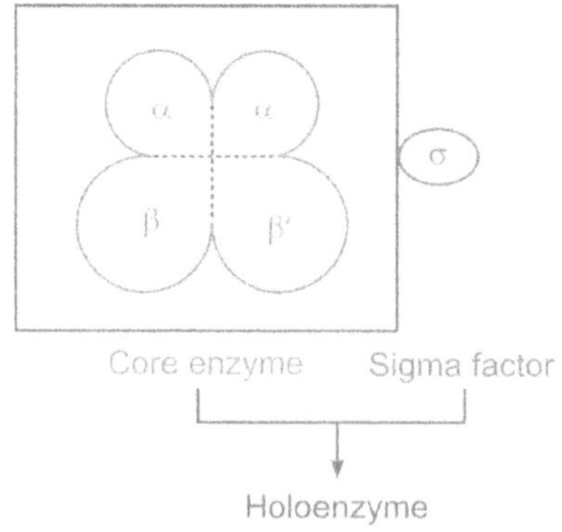

Figure 6.24 *RNA polymerase of E. coli.*

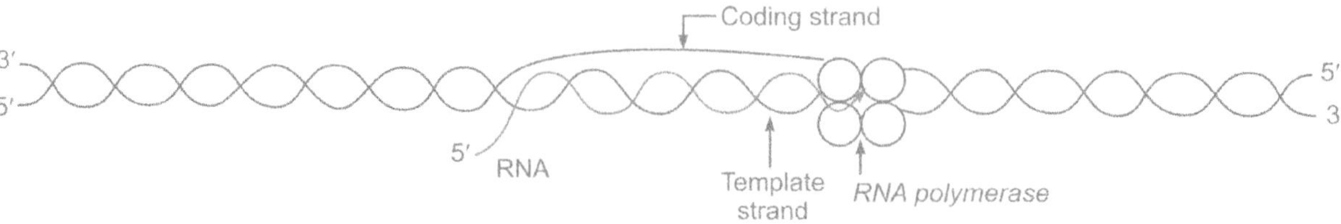

Figure 6.25 Overview of transcription.

Stage - 1 or Initiation Stage

For the starting of transcription, the prerequisite needed is the binding of *RNA polymerase* to DNA. Promoter region is the specific region of the DNA where the enzyme binds. The transcription initiation is recognized by *RNA polymerase* through two base sequences present on the coding strand. The two base sequences are,

1. **TATA box or Pribnow box:** In the promoter region of DNA this is the first recognition site. From the starting point of transcription, the TATA box is located about 10 bases away (upstream) on the left side and consists of six nucleotide bases such as TATAAT.
2. **The -35 sequence:** In the promoter region of DNA, this is the second recognition site. From the starting point of transcription, the -35 sequence is located about 35 bases away (upstream) on the left side and consists of six nucleotide bases such as TTGACA.

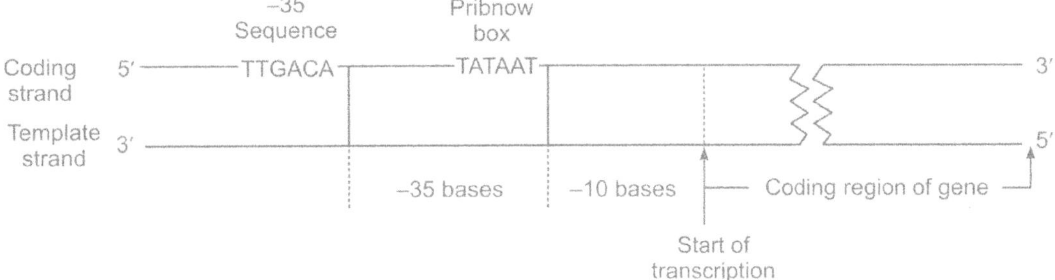

Figure 6.26 Promoter regions of DNA in prokaryotes.

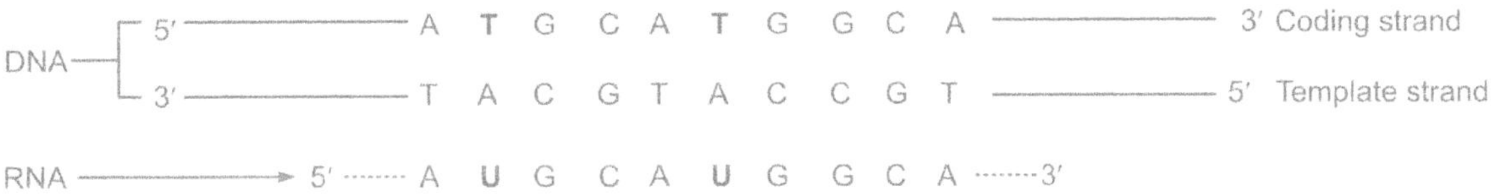

Figure 6.27 Complementary base pair relationship in transcription.

Stage - 2 or Elongation stage:

The sigma factor is released and the transcription proceeds when the *RNA polymerase* recognizes the promoter region as holoenzyme. To the DNA template, RNA is synthesized antiparallelly i.e., 5′ end to 3′ end. RNA is formed using ribonucleotide triphosphate such as ATP, GTP, CTP and UTP by *RNA polymerase.* A pyrophosphate moiety is released for addition of each nucleotide to the growing chain. In mRNA, nucleotide base sequence is complementary to the template DNA strand. However, it is identical to that of coding strand except that RNA contains U in place of T in DNA. In two aspects *RNA polymerase* is differ from *DNA polymerase.* They are,

1. *RNA polymerase* does not require primer for its activity, whereas *DNA polymerase* requires primer for its activity.
2. *RNA polymerase* does not possess *endonuclease* and *exonuclease* activity whereas *DNA polymerase* possesses *endonuclease* and *exonuclease* activity.

Mistakes in the synthesized RNA cannot be repaired i.e., proofreading activity by *RNA polymerase* due to lack of *endonuclease* and *exonuclease* activity. In the case of DNA, the replication process is carried out with high fidelity; even though mistakes in RNA synthesis are less dangerous because it is not transmitted to the daughter cells. In addition, super coiling problems in DNA replication due to double helical structure of DNA is overcome by *topoisomerase.*

Stage - 3 or Termination stage:

Termination signals stop the process of transcription. Two different terminations are identified. They are,

1. **Rho (ρ) dependent termination:** To the growing RNA (not to *RNA polymerase*) or weakly to DNA, a specific protein namely ρ factor is bound. This ρ factor terminates transcription and releases RNA by

acting as *ATPase* in bound state. In addition, for dissociation of *RNA polymerase* from DNA, this ρ factor is also responsible.

2. **Rho (ρ) independent termination:** In this case, termination is brought by hairpins formation in the newly synthesized RNA due to palindromes presence. Palindrome is a word that reads alike forward and backward (**Example:** Madam and rotor). The termination region is known by the presence of palindromes (same when read in opposite directions also) in the base sequence of DNA template. Hence, hairpins are formed by the newly synthesized RNA by folding due to complementary base pairing. This may lead to termination of transcription. The various stages involved in the process of prokaryotes transcription is presented in Figure 6.28.

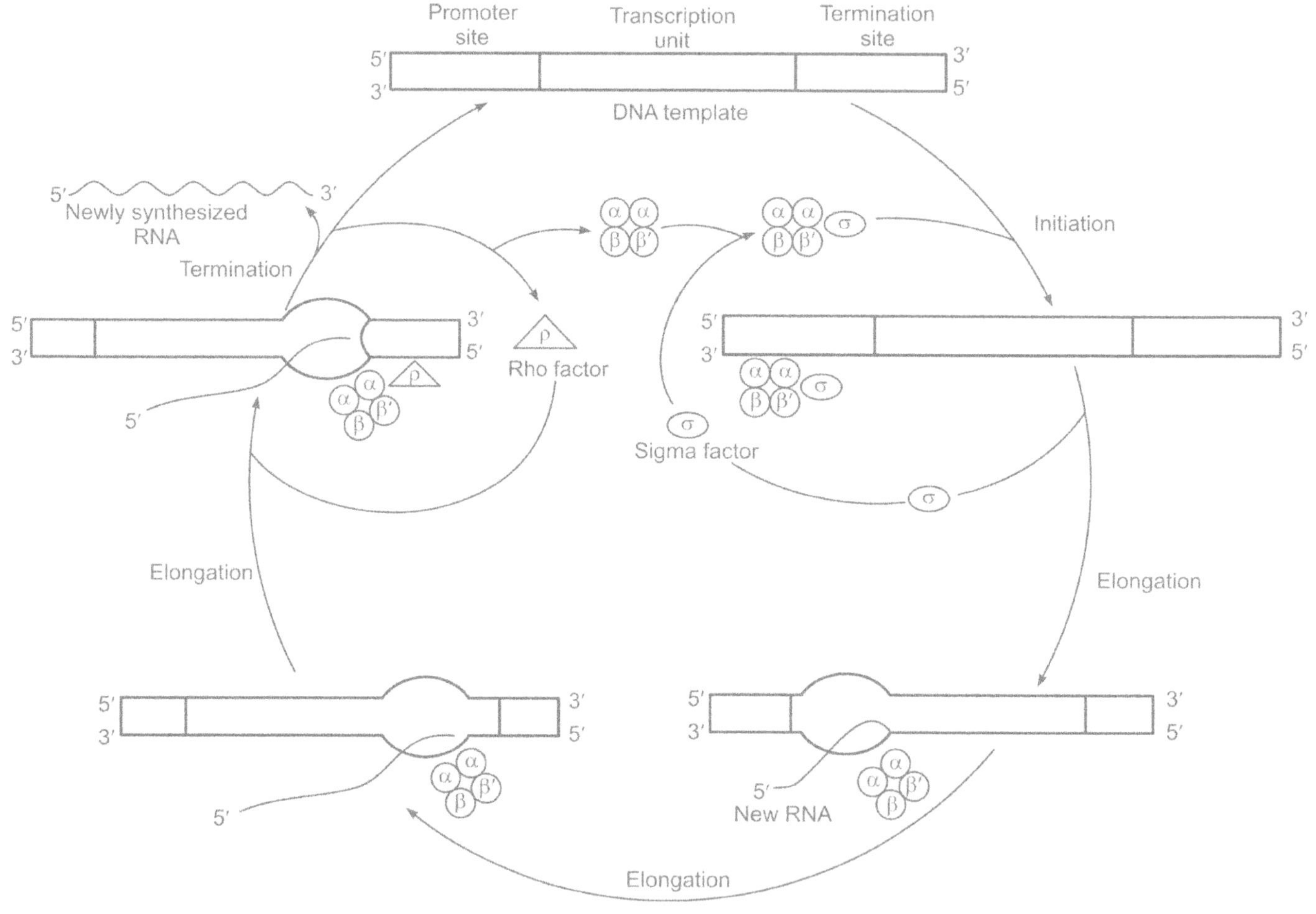

Figure 6.28 Stages involved in prokaryotes transcription.

Transcription in Eukaryotes

The process of synthesizing RNA (transcription) is much more complex in eukaryotes compared to prokaryotes. All details particularly termination of transcription in eukaryotes are not clearly known. Hereby, the available information is discussed below and the overview of transcription in eukaryotes is presented in Figure 6.29.

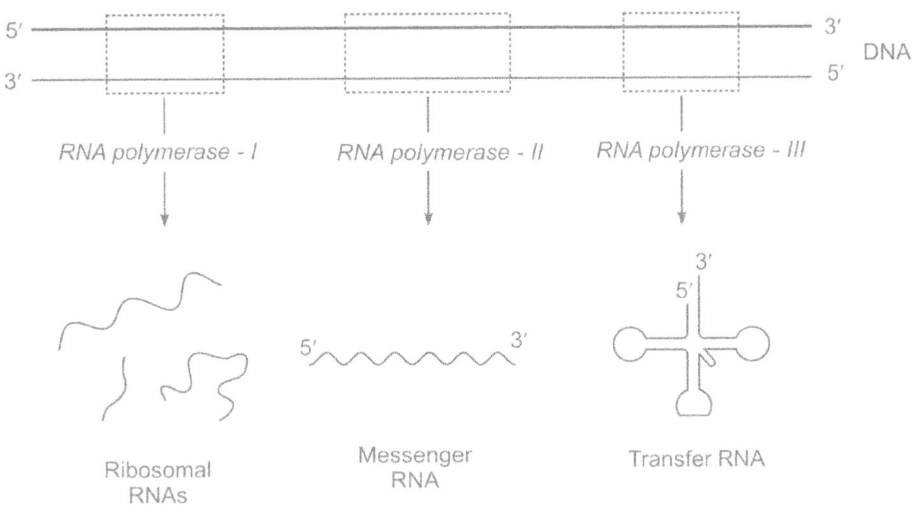

Figure 6.29 Overview of transcription in eukaryotes.

RNA polymerase:

Three different *RNA polymerases* are found in the nuclei of eukaryotic cells and one *RNA polymerase* is found in mitochondria. The first three *RNA polymerases are* present in nuclei and the last one is present in mitochondria. They various *RNA polymerases* are,

1. ***RNA polymerase – I:*** This enzyme is responsible for the synthesis of precursors for the large rRNAs.
2. ***RNA polymerase – II:*** This enzyme is responsible for the synthesis of precursors for mRNAs and snRNAs.
3. ***RNA polymerase – III:*** This enzyme participates in the formation of tRNAs and small rRNAs.
4. ***Mitochondrial RNA polymerase:*** The structure and functions of this *RNA polymerase* resembles prokaryotic *RNA polymerase*.

Promoter sites:

The sequence of DNA bases which are almost identical to the pribnow box or TATA box of prokaryotes is identified in eukaryotes. This base sequence is known as Hogness box or TATA box and is located from the starting site of mRNA synthesis on the left side about 25 nucleotides away (upstream). Another site of recognition also exists between 70 and 80 nucleotides away (upstream) from the start of transcription. This second promoter region is known as CAAT box. One of these promoter sites or sometimes both helps to recognize the requisite sequence on DNA for transcription by *RNA polymerase – II*. Promoter regions of DNA in eukaryotes is presented in Figure 6.30.

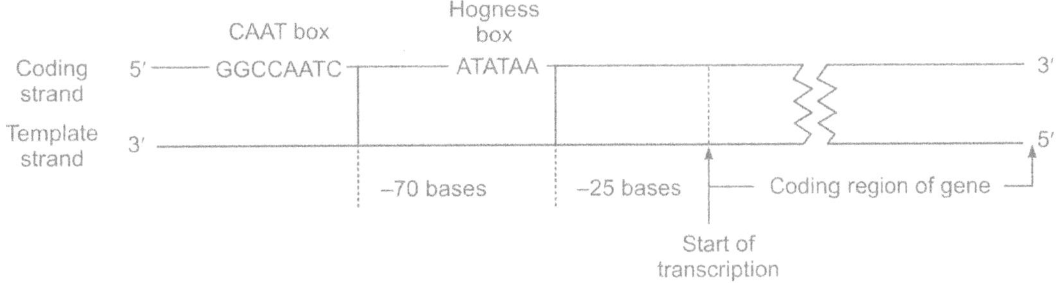

Figure 6.30 Promoter regions of DNA in eukaryotes.

Initiation of transcription:

In eukaryotes the initiation process of transcription is more complex and involves three stages.

1. **Stage – 1:** In this stage, transcription machinery is made accessible to the promoter sequence present in chromatin.

2. **Stage - 2:** In the promoter region transcription factors (TFs) are bonded to DNA sequences. In eukaryotic promoter regions large numbers of transcription factors (TFs) are interacting. About 6 TFs such as TFIIA, TFIIB, TFIID, TFIIE, TFIIF and TFIIH are identified in humans. These TFs are bound to each other as well as to *RNA polymerase*.
3. **Stage - 3:** In this stage enhancers stimulate the transcription. About 100 folds gene expression is increased by enhancers because it binds with TFs to form activators. To facilitate transcription the chromatin forms a loop that allows the promoter and enhancer to be close together in space.

In eukaryotes the *RNA polymerase* produced primary mRNA transcript which is usually referred as heterogeneous nuclear RNA (hnRNA). Later, mRNA needed for protein synthesis is produced from hnRNA.

Post transcriptional modifications:

Primary transcript is RNA synthesized during transcription. This primary transcript which undergoes post transcriptional modifications such as terminal base addition, base modification, splicing, etc. The active form of RNA is needed for this post transcriptional modification. *Ribonucleases* are the group of enzymes responsible for the processing of tRNAs and rRNAs of both prokaryotes and eukaryotes. In prokaryotes, the functional mRNA is almost similar to the mRNA synthesized in transcription; whereas in eukaryotes hnRNA undergoes extensive post transcriptional changes & is outlined in Figure 6.31.

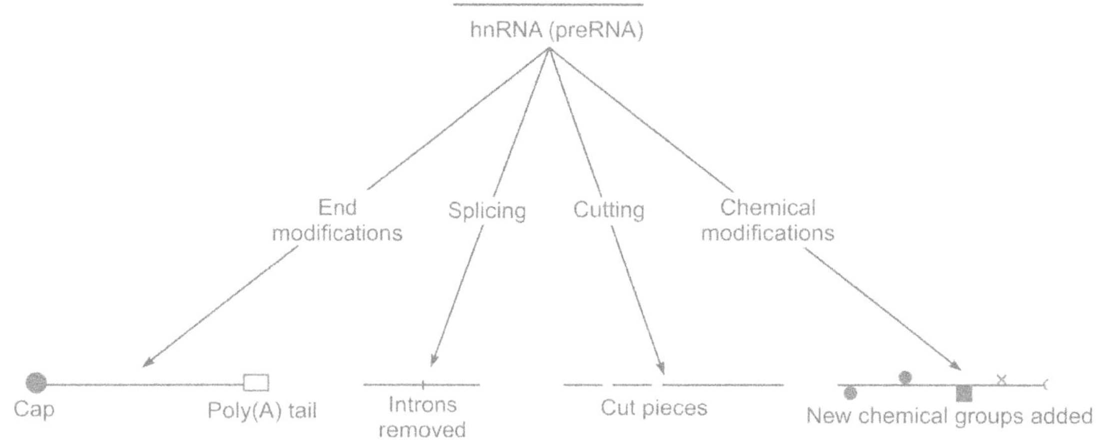

Figure 6.31 Post transcriptional changes of RNA.

Messenger RNA (mRNA):

In eukaryotes, mRNA is synthesized from heterogeneous nuclear RNA (hnRNA) through many modifications. They are,

1. **The 5′ capping:** By usual 5′ to 5′ triphosphate linkage, the 5′ end of mRNA is capped with 7-methylguanosine. The methyl group is donated by S-adenosyl methionine (SAM). This cap is needed for the stability of mRNA structure and translation.
2. **Poly - A tail:** At 3′ end, adenine nucleotide chain is present in a large number of eukaryotic mRNAs. During transcription this poly - A tail is as such not produced. To stabilize mRNA it is added later. However, when the mRNA enters cytosol, poly - A chain gets reduced.
3. **Introns and their removal:** In mRNA, introns are the intervening nucleotide sequences which do not code for proteins. Genetic code is present in the exons of mRNA and is responsible for synthesis of protein. Small nuclear ribonucleo protein particles (snRNPs) promote the removal of introns. When small nuclear RNA (snRNA) is associated with proteins, snRNPs (pronounced as snurps) will form.

Spliceosome is a term used to represent the association of snRNP with hnRNA at exon - intron junction. In the nucleus post transcriptional modifications of mRNAs take place. Later, to perform its function i.e. translation the mature RNA enters into cytosol. Figure 6.32 represents the formation of mature RNA from eukaryotic mRNA. Relationship between eukaryotic chromosomal DNA & mRNA is schematically represented in Figure 6.33.

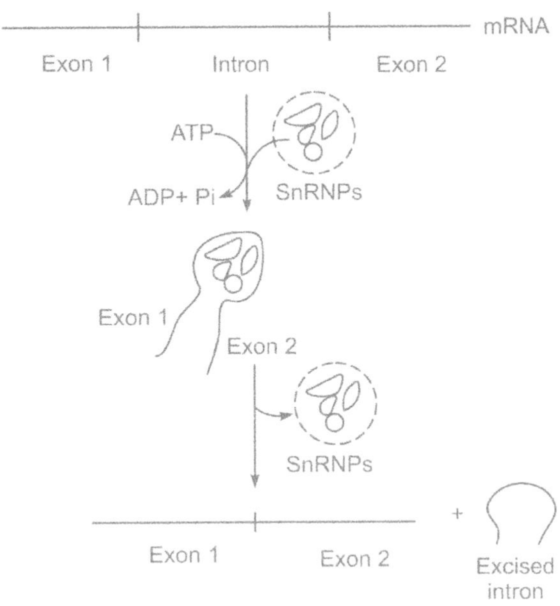

Figure 6.32 Formation of mature RNA from eukaryotic mRNA.

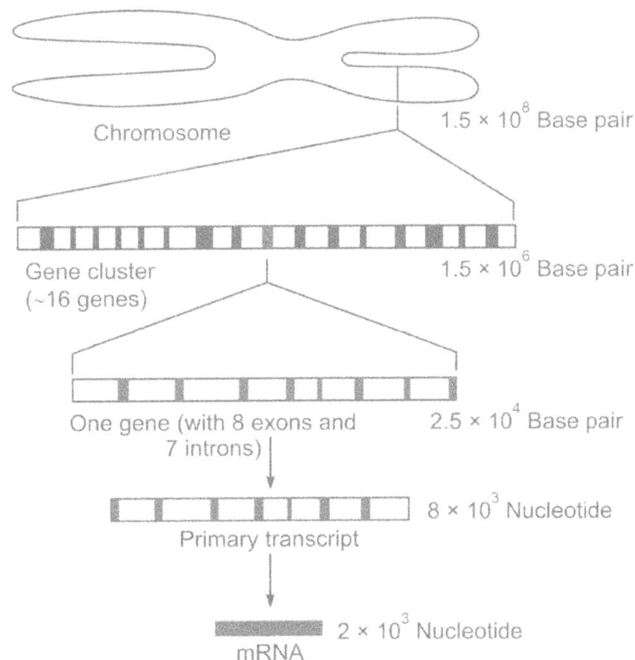

Figure 6.33 Relationship between eukaryotic chromosomal DNA & mRNA.

Inhibitors of transcription:

Certain toxins and antibiotics inhibit the synthesis of RNA.

1. **α-Amanitin:** *Amanita phalloide* is a delicious mushroom in taste but it produces a toxin called α-amanitin. This α-amanitin inhibits transcription by binding with *RNA polymerase – II* of eukaryotes. Hence, *Amanita phalloide* mushroom is a poisonous one.
2. **Actinomycin-D or Dactinomycin:** *Streptomyces* species synthesize dactinomycin. It blocks the movement of *RNA polymerase* by binding with DNA template strand. For the treatment of cancer this was the very first antibiotic used.
3. **Rifampin:** For the treatment of tuberculosis and leprosy, the antibiotic rifampin is widely used. It inhibits the activity of prokaryotic *RNA polymerase* by binding with their β-subunit.

Translation

In DNA, the stored genetic information is passed to RNA through transcription and in the language of proteins through translation it is ultimately expressed. Translation is defined as the process of biosynthesizing protein or polypeptide in a living cell. The biochemical translation of four-letter language information from nucleic acid to 20 letter language of proteins is represented by the term translation. Nucleotide base sequence of mRNA determines the sequence of amino acids in the protein synthesis.

Variability of cells in translation:

With respect to the quality and quantity of proteins synthesized, there are wide variations in the cells and mainly it depends on the need and ability of the cells. Erythrocytes cannot synthesize proteins because it lacks the machinery for translation. Generally large quantities of proteins are synthesized by growing and dividing cells. Continuous synthesis of proteins is taking place in some cells for export (**Example:** Albumin and blood clotting factors are continuously synthesized in liver cells for export into the blood for circulation). In the human body, the liver is considered as a protein factory because liver cells are very rich in protein biosynthetic machinery.

Genetic code:

Genetic code is simply known as codons. Genetic code is constituted by triplet (three nucleotides) base sequences in mRNA that act as code words for amino acids in protein. In protein the sequence of amino acids is determined by genetic code and this genetic code is considered as a dictionary of nucleotide bases (A, G, C and U). Generally, codons consist of four nucleotide bases such as purine bases [adenine (A) and guanine (G)] and pyrimidine base [cytosine (C) and uracil (U)]. 64 (4^3) combinations of three base codons are produced by these four bases. In mRNA, from 5′ to 3′ direction, the nucleotide sequence of codons is written. For the twenty different amino acids in protein sixty-one codons are available. The remaining three codons such as UAA, UAG and UGA do not code for amino acids. In protein synthesis, these three codons stop the signals, hence they are termed as termination codons or non-sense codons. The codons UAA, UAG and UGA are often referred to as ochre, amber and opal codons, respectively. In addition, codons AUG and sometimes GUG act as initiating codons.

The following are some other characteristics of genetic code.

1. **Universal:** In all the living organisms, for the same amino acids, same codons are used. Thus, during the course of evolution, the genetic code has been conserved. Hence, the genetic code is regarded as universal, approximately. Even though there are few exceptions. **Example:** In mitochondria for methionine the codon is AUA, whereas in cytoplasm the same codon codes for isoleucine. Therefore, the genetic code is universal with some exceptions.
2. **Specific:** Same amino acid is always coded by a particular codon only. Hence, genetic code is highly specific or unambiguous. **Example:** For tryptophan the codon is UGG.
3. **Non overlapping:** As a continuous base sequence the genetic code is read from a fixed point. It is usually non overlapping, comma less and without any punctuations. **Example:** UUUCUUAGAGGG is read as UUU / CUU / AGA / GGG. In mRNA the message sequence is radically changed due to addition or deletion of one or two bases. Such mRNA will produce protein which is totally different. This is encountered in the frame shift mutations which cause an alteration in the reading frame of mRNA.
4. **Degenerate:** More than one codon is available for most of the amino acids. For twenty amino acids there are sixty-one codons available, hence, the codon is redundant or degenerate. **Example:** Four codons available for glycine. The codons that designate the same amino acids are called synonyms and differ only in the third base (3′ end) of the codon.

Codon-anticodon recognition:

Anticodon of tRNA recognizes the codon of the mRNA. In antiparallel direction (5′ to 3′ of mRNA with 3′ to 5′ of tRNA), they pair with each other. Between the first two bases of codon and last two bases of anticodon, the usual conventional complementary base pairing (A=U, C=G) occurs. With regard to the complementary base, the third base of the codon is rather lenient or flexible. Seven nucleotides are present in the anticodon region of tRNA. and, in mRNA, it recognizes the three letter codon.

Wobble hypothesis:

More than one codon can be recognized by a single tRNA and this phenomenon is known as the Wobble hypothesis which is put forth by Crick. In the anticodon (5′ base), the specific complementary base is not recognized by the third base (3′ base) present in the codon. This is the reason behind this hypothesis. The difference in the spatial arrangement of the 5′ end of the anticodon is attributed by the wobbling. The possible pairing of 5′ end base of anticodon of tRNA with 3′ end base of codon mRNA is given below.

Anticodon		Codon	
C	-	G	} Conventional base pairing
A	-	U	
U	-	G or A	} Non-conventional base (bolded) pairing
G	-	U or C	

The degeneracy of the genetic code is explained by Wobble hypothesis (Multiple codon existence for single amino acids). Only around forty tRNA is available for 61 codons for amino acid due to wobbling.

Codon bias: Even though multiple codons are available for many amino acids; the organism preferably uses one or two codons only and not all of them. This phenomenon is known as codon bias. Depends on the organism the codon bias is variable. For the rarely used codons only low amounts of tRNA is used due to codon bias. The various genetic code along with their respective amino acids are tabulated in Table 6.4.

Table 6.4 Genetic code along with respective amino acids.

First base 5' end	Second base (Middle one)				Third base 3' end
	U	C	A	G	
U	UUU Phe UUC UUA Leu UUG	UCU UCC Ser UCA UCG	UAU Try UAC UAA Stop UAG Stop	UGU Cys UGC UGA Stop UGG Trp	U C A G
C	CUU CUC Leu CUA CUG	CCU CCC Pro CCA CCG	CAU His CAC CAA Gin CAG	CGU CGC Arg CGA CGG	U C A G
A	AUU AUC Ile AUA AUG Met (initiation)	ACU ACC Thr ACA ACG	AAU Asn AAC AAA Lys AAG	AGU Ser AGC AGA Arg AGG	U C A G
G	GUU GUC Val GUA GUG	GCU GCC Ala GCA GCG	GAU Asp GAC GAA Glu GAG	GGU GGC Gly GGA GGG	U C A G

Protein Biosynthesis

The following are the five different stages involved in the synthesis of proteins which involves the translation of nucleotide base sequence of mRNA into the language of amino acid sequences.

1. Components requirement
2. Amino acids activation

3. Proper protein synthesis
4. Chaperones and protein folding
5. Post-translational modifications of proteins

1. Components requirement:

Protein synthesis needs many components such as amino acids, ribosomes, messenger RNA (mRNA), transfer RNA (tRNA), energy sources like ATP and GTP and protein factors.

Amino acids: Proteins are the polymer of amino acids. Hence, amino acid presence is the primary requirement for protein synthesis. Protein present in nature only twenty amino acids are repeatedly present. Among these, the body is able to synthesize ten amino acids which are known as non-essential amino acids and hence these amino acids are not necessary to take through dietary sources. The remaining ten amino acids are not synthesized in the body which are known as essential amino acids and hence, these amino acids are necessary to be taken through dietary sources. When all the amino acids needed for the synthesis of protein are available, then only the protein synthesis takes place. Even deficiency of one essential amino acid in dietary sources leads to stopping of translation. Hence, the dietary source must contain all essential amino acids in sufficient quantities to maintain protein synthesis as amino acids are pre-requisite for synthesis of proteins. In case of prokaryotes from inorganic components, all twenty amino acids are synthesized, hence, no amino acid is required.

Ribosomes: The center or factories for protein synthesis are ribosomes. In translation, ribosomes are considered as workbenches. Ribosomes are the huge complex structure (70S for prokaryotes and 80S for eukaryotes) of proteins and ribosomal RNAs. One big and one small sub units are present in each ribosome. A-site and P-site are the two sites of functional ribosomes. Both the sub units are covered by each site. During the course of translation, A-site is considered as acceptor site and aminoacyl tRNA binds in it; whereas P-site is considered as donor site and peptidyl tRNA binds in it. In case of eukaryotes, a third site is present which is commonly known as E-site or exit site. In the cytosomal fraction of the cell, ribosomes are present.

In general, ribosomes are found in association with rough endoplasmic reticulum (RER) to form RER-ribosomes in which synthesis of protein takes place. On a single mRNA, if many ribosomes simultaneously translate then the ribosome is known as polysome or polyribosome.

Messenger RNA (mRNA): For the synthesis of a given protein, the specific information required is present on the mRNA. In the form of codons, the genetic information is passed from DNA to mRNA to translate into a protein sequence.

Transfer RNA (tRNA): To the growing polypeptide chain, the amino acids are carried and handed over by tRNA. At 3′-end amino acids are covalently bonded to tRNA. Anticodon is the three-nucleotide base sequence present in each tRNA which is responsible to recognize the codon (complementary bases) of mRNA for protein synthesis. In a bacteria, forty different tRNAs and in a man fifty different tRNAs are found. Amino acids with multiple codons have more than one tRNA.

Energy sources: During protein synthesis, energy is supplied by both ATP and GTP. In general, energy is obtained by the breakdown of ATP and GTP into AMP and GMP, respectively with liberation of pyrophosphate. Two high energy phosphates equivalent to two ATP is consumed by each one of these reactions.

Protein factors: There are a number of protein factors involved in the process of translation. In the translation process, these protein factors are needed for initiation, elongation and termination. Compared to prokaryotes, the protein factors are complex in eukaryotes.

2. Amino acids activation:

In a two-step reaction, the amino acids are activated and attached to tRNAs. *Aminoacyl tRNA synthetases* are a group of enzymes needed for this process. For the amino acids and their corresponding tRNAs these enzymes are highly specific. First, to the enzyme utilizing ATP, amino acids are attached to form enzyme-AMP-amino acid complex. Later, to form aminoacyl tRNA, the amino acid is transferred to the 3′ end of the tRNA.

3. **Proper protein synthesis**

Rather polyribosomes, the polypeptide or protein synthesis is occurring on ribosomes only. The polypeptide synthesis proceeds from N-terminal end to C-terminal end by mRNA reading in the 5′ to 3′ direction. Translation is directional and collinear with mRNA. Eukaryotic mRNA codes for a single polypeptide, hence termed as monocistronic and in contrast prokaryotic mRNA codes for a multiple polypeptide due to presence of many coding regions in mRNA, hence termed as polycistronic.

In prokaryotes, both transcription and translation take place simultaneously because before transcription of gene is completed translation commences. In case eukaryotes, it is not possible because in nucleus transcription occurs and in cytosol translation occurs. In addition, to generate functional mRNA, the hnRNA (primary transcript synthesized from DNA) undergoes several modifications. Compared to eukaryotes in prokaryotes, the protein synthesis is comparatively simple. Earlier in eukaryotic translation, many steps were not understood but now it is better understood due to advancement in molecular biology.

Eukaryotic translation is divided into three different stages as initiation, elongation and termination.

(a) **Initiation:**

In eukaryotes, at least ten different eukaryotic initiation factors (eIFs) are involved in initiation of translation, hence it is complex. Multiple (3 to 8) sub-units are present in some of eIFs. Four steps are involved in the initiation process. They are,

1. Dissociation of ribosomes
2. 43S pre-initiation complex formation
3. 48S initiation complex formation
4. 80S initiation complex formation

1. **Dissociation of ribosomes:** 40S and 60S subunits are formed by dissociation of 80S ribosomes. To the newly formed 40S subunit eIF-1A and eIF-3 are binds and blocks the re-association of eIF-1A and eIF-3 with 60S subunit. Hence these initiating factors are also known as anti-association factors.
2. **43S pre-initiation complex formation:** 43S pre-initiation complex is formed by attaching GTP bound a ternary complex possessing met-rRNA′ (Superscript ′ is used in met-tRNA because it is specifically involved in binding to the initiation codon AUGs) and elf-2 to 40S ribosomal subunit. This complex is stabilized by the presence of elf-3 and elf-1A.
3. **48S initiation complex formation:** This complex is formed by binding of mRNA to 43S pre-initiation complex through the intermediate 43S initiation complex. In this interaction between elFs and activation of mRNA is involved.
4. **80S initiation complex formation:** This complex is formed by binding of 48S initiation complex with 60S ribosomal subunit. Hydrolysis of elF bound GTP is involved in the binding. elF-5 is involved in the facilitation of this step.

Recognition and regulation of initiation: The initiation codon is 5′-AUG and the specific nucleotides surrounding it facilitates its recognition. Identification of AUG by this marker sequence is known as Kozak consensus sequences. In case of prokaryotes, Shine – Dalgarno sequence recognizes initiation codon sequence. The initiation and thus translation are controlled by elF-4F complex formation by the assembly of three initiation factors. The rate limiting step in the translation is recognition of mRNA cap by the elF-4F complex in which elF-4E is the primary component involved in this. To some extent, protein synthesis is also controlled by elF-2 involved in the formation of 43S pre-initiation complex.

Initiation of translation in prokaryotes: Compared to eukaryotes the initiation of translation in prokaryotes is a simple process and less complicated. IF-3 is bound to the 30S ribosomal subunit and attached to the ternary complex of IF-2, formyl met-tRNA and GTP. In the formation of pre-initiation complex IF-1 also participates. Shine – Dalgarno sequence recognizes initiation codon AUG sequence. In prokaryotes 70S initiation complex is produced by binding of a 50S ribosome unit with 30S unit.

(b) Elongation:

Polypeptide chain is elongated by ribosomes through a sequential addition of amino acids. In the specific mRNA the order of codons determines the amino acid sequence. Certain elongation factor is involved in the cyclic process of elongation. This cyclic process involves three steps as follows,

1. Binding of aminoacyl tRNA to A-site
2. Formation of peptide bond
3. Translocation

Binding of aminoacyl tRNA to A-site: A-site is free and in the P-site met-tRNA′ is present in the 80S initiation complex. In the A-site another aminoacyl tRNA is placed. Energy supply by CTP, involvement of EF-1a (elongation factor 1a) and mRNA proper codon recognition is required for this process. Another aminoacyl tRNA is brought by recycled EF-1a and GDP because in the A-site, aminoacyl tRNA is placed.

Formation of peptide bond: Peptide bond formation is catalyzed by the enzyme *peptidyl transferase*. On 28S RNA of 60S ribosomal subunit the activity of *peptidyl transferase* lies. Hence, the peptide bond formation is catalyzed by rRNA (and not protein) referred to as ribozyme. For peptide bond formation there is no need for additional energy because in the aminoacyl tRNA, amino acid is already activated. In the A-site, a growing peptide chain is attached as the net result of peptide bond formation.

Translocation: Towards 3′-end, ribosomes are moved to the next codon of the mRNA as the peptide bond formation occurs. In the basic process of translocation from A-site growing peptide chain is moved to P-site. EF-2 and CTP are required for translocation and the energy for mRNA movement is provided by the hydrolysis of GTP. For translocation EF-2 and GTP complex recycles. In eukaryotes recently E-site i.e., exit site is identified. Into the E-site the deacylated tRNA moves from where it leaves the ribosome. The elongation factors are different in case of prokaryotes and they are, EF-Tu and EF-Ts in place of EF-1a and EF-G in place of EF-2.

In eukaryotes during the course of translocation, per second about six amino acids are incorporated; whereas in prokaryotes it is twenty amino acids. Hence with a great speed and accuracy in translation the protein or polypeptide synthesis occurs.

(c) Termination:

Compared to initiation and elongation, the process of termination is simple. The growing polypeptide chain is terminated by one of the termination codons i.e., UAA, UAG and UCA after the several cycles of elongation. No specific tRNA is available to bind for the termination codons. A-site of the ribosome is occupied by termination codon and the stop signal is recognized by the release factor namely eRF. In the P-site the peptide bond formed between the polypeptide and tRNA is cleaved by eRF-GTP complex in association with enzyme *peptidyl transferase*. Instead of amino acid, water molecules are added in this step. From the P-site, protein and tRNA is released by this hydrolysis. 40S and 60S subunits (obtained from dissociation of 80S ribosome) are recycled and the mRNA is also released.

4. Chaperones and protein folding:

Chaperones are the heat shock proteins which facilitate and favor the interactions on the polypeptide surfaces to finally give the specific conformation of a protein. One major function of chaperones is to prevent both newly synthesized polypeptide chains and assembled subunits from aggregating into nonfunctional structures. Chaperones are found mainly in the endoplasmic reticulum (ER), since protein synthesis often occurs in this area. Human chaperones are broadly classified into four major types. They are,

1. General chaperones: GRP78/BiP, GRP94, GRP170
2. Lectin chaperones: Calnexin and calreticulin
3. Non-classical molecular chaperones: HSP47 and ERp29
4. Folding chaperones: *Protein disulfide isomerase (PDI), Peptidyl prolyl cis-trans-isomerase (PPI),* ERp57

5. **Post-translational modifications of proteins:**
   As such the protein synthesized in the translation is not functional. In the polypeptides many changes are takes place after initiation of protein synthesis or mostly after the completion of protein synthesis. The following processes are collectively known as post-translational modifications. They are,
   1. Protein folding
   2. Trimming by proteolytic degradation
   3. Intern splicing
   4. Covalent changes

Inhibitors of Protein Synthesis

The favorite target for antibiotics is translation only. In general antibiotics are the compounds produced by bacteria or fungi which inhibit the growth of other organisms. Most of the antibiotics are harmless to the higher organism and it only interferes with the protein synthesis of bacteria because eukaryotes and prokaryotes are sufficiently different in their translation process. The following are the various inhibitors of protein synthesis.

1. **Streptomycin:** It inhibits the initiation of protein synthesis by causing misreading of mRNA and interfering with the normal pairing between codons and anticodons.
2. **Tetracycline:** Binding of aminoacyl tRNA to ribosomal complex is inhibited by tetracycline. Eukaryotic protein synthesis can also be blocked by tetracycline but eukaryotic cell membrane is not permeable to tetracycline; hence it does not happen.
3. **Puromycin:** It is structurally related to aminoacyl tRNA. Into the growing polypeptide chain puromycin is incorporated by entering into the A-site. In both eukaryotes and prokaryotes, protein synthesis is prevented by puromycin.
4. **Chloramphenicol:** It is a competitive inhibitor of *peptidyl transferase*. Hence, it interferes with peptide chain elongation.
5. **Erythromycin:** It binds with 50S subunit of bacterial ribosome and inhibits translocation.
6. **Diphtheria toxin:** It inactivates the elongation factor eEF_2. Hence, eukaryotes prevent translocation in protein synthesis.

PROBABLE QUESTIONS

PART – A: Multiple Choice Questions

1. Nucleotide contains which of the following?
   (a) Nitrogen base (b) Sugar
   (c) Phosphate group (d) All of them
2. Numbering of purine follows which pattern?
   (a) Anti-clockwise (b) Clockwise
   (c) Either (a) or (b) (d) Both (a) and (b)
3. Which of the following is not a pyrimidine base?
   (a) Uracil (b) Guanine
   (c) Orotate (d) Thymine
4. Which of the following is not a purine base?
   (a) Orotate (b) Guanine
   (c) Xanthine (d) Uric acid

5. Which of the following compound is not involved in the synthesis of pyrimidine?
   (a) Glutamine (b) Aspartate
   (c) N^{10}-formyl THF (d) CO_2
6. Numbering of pyrimidine follows which pattern?
   (a) Anti-clockwise (b) Clockwise
   (c) Either (a) or (b) (d) Both (a) and (b)
7. Which is the rate limiting enzyme of purine biosynthesis?
   (a) *PRPP glutamyl ketotransferase* (b) *PRPP glutamyl methyltransferase*
   (c) *RPP glutamyl aminotransferase* (d) *PRPP glutamyl sulphotranaferase*
8. What is the end product of purine metabolism?
   (a) Xanthine (b) Uric acid
   (c) Hypoxanthine (d) IMP
9. What is the end product of pyrimidine metabolism?
   (a) Acetyl CoA (b) Uric acid
   (c) Ammonia (d) Xanthine
10. Reye's syndrome is a metabolic disorder of ______________.
    (a) Purine (b) Cholesterol
    (c) Bile acids (d) Pyrimidine
11. Which of the following is not a pyrimidine base?
    (a) Uracil (b) Guanine
    (c) Orotate (d) Thymine
12. Which of the following is not a purine base?
    (a) Orotate (b) Guanine
    (c) Xanthine (d) Uric acid
13. Synthesis of protein from RNA is known as______________?
    (a) Replication (b) Transcription
    (c) Translation (d) All of them
14. DNA synthesis is continuous in which strand?
    (a) Lagging (b) Leading
    (c) Either (a) or (b) (d) Both (a) and (b)
15. Which performs proof reading activity?
    (a) *DNA polymerase-I* (b) *DNA polymerase-II*
    (c) *DNA polymerase-III* (d) *DNA polymerase-IV*
16. Which enzyme separates the strands of DNA?
    (a) *DNA ligase* (b) *DNA polymerase*
    (c) *DNA gyrase* (d) *DNA helicase*
17. The metabolic disorder of DNA replication is ____________.
    (a) Ataxia telangiectasia (b) Fanconis anemia
    (c) Cockaynes syndrome (d) All of them
18. Which is the promoter region of transcription?
    (a) TATA box (b) CAAT box
    (c) Either (a) or (b) (d) Both (a) and (b)

19. Which is the initiating codon?
    (a) AUG (b) UAA
    (c) UAG (d) UGA
20. An amino group donated by glutamine is attached at C-1 of PRPP, this results in ___________
    (a) 5-Phosphoribosylamine (b) 4-Phosphoribosylamine
    (c) 3-Phosphoribosylamine (d) 2-Phosphoribosylamine
21. The first intermediate with a complete purine ring is ___________
    (a) Inosinate (b) Formate
    (c) Aspartate (d) Glycine
22. Which of the following is an important precursor in the purine pathway?
    (a) Glycine (b) Aspartate
    (c) Glutamine (d) Leucine
23. Which of the following is an important precursor in pyrimidine pathway?
    (a) Glycine (b) Aspartate
    (c) Glutamine (d) Leucine
24. In the first committed step of pyrimidine biosynthesis, the reaction is catalyzed by ___________.
    (a) *Adenylate kinase* (b) *Aspartate transcarbamoylase*
    (c) *Dihyhroorotase* (d) *Cytidylate synthase*
25. Phosphorylation of AMP to ADP is promoted by ___________.
    (a) *Adenylate kinase* (b) *Aspartate transcarbamoylase*
    (c) *Dihyhroorotase* (d) *Cytidylate synthase*
26. CTP is formed from UTP by the action of ___________
    (a) *Adenylate kinase* (b) *Aspartate transcarbamoylase*
    (c) *Dihyhroorotase* (d) *Cytidylate synthase*
27. Conversion of dUMP to dTMP is catalyzed by ___________
    (a) *Thymidylate synthase* (b) *Dihydrofolate reductase*
    (c) *Dihyhroorotase* (d) *Cytidylate synthase*
28. *Adenosine deaminase* deaminates adenosine to ___________
    (a) Hypoxanthine (b) Inosine
    (c) Xanthine (d) Guanosine
29. Which of the following is degraded to methylmalonyl semialdehyde?
    (a) Glutamine (b) Tyrosine
    (c) Thymine (d) Leucine
30. The phenomenon of twisting around itself by a molecule to relieve helical stress is ___________
    (a) Supercoiling (b) Coiling
    (c) Elongation (d) Compression
31. When there is no net bending of the DNA axis upon itself, the DNA is said to be in a ___________
    (a) Elongated state (b) Compressed state
    (c) Relaxed state (d) Denatured state
32. Over-twisting of a molecule results in ___________
    (a) Negative supercoiling (b) Positive supercoiling
    (c) Elongation (d) Compression

33. Changing twist from the relaxed state requires adding energy and increases the ___________
    (a) Forces in molecule
    (b) Stress along molecule
    (c) Strain over molecule
    (d) None of the above
34. The enzyme responsible for the removal of supercoiling in replicating DNA ahead of the replication fork is ___________
    (a) *Topoisomerase*
    (b) *Primase*
    (c) *DNA polymerase*
    (d) *Helicase*
35. Which type of *topoisomerases* generally relaxes DNA by removing negative supercoiling?
    (a) Type-I
    (b) Type-II
    (c) Type-III
    (d) Type-IV
36. The type of *topoisomerases* that can introduce negative supercoils is ___________
    (a) Type-I
    (b) Type-II
    (c) Type-III
    (d) Type-IV
37. The type-I enzyme(s) is/are ___________
    (a) *Topoisomerases-I and III*
    (b) *Topoisomerases-II*
    (c) *Topoisomerase-IV*
    (d) *Topoisomerases-I and IV*
38. Under-winding is measured in terms of ___________
    (a) Supercoiling
    (b) Linking difference
    (c) Positive supercoiling
    (d) Negative supercoiling
39. Which type of supercoiling takes the form of extended right-handed coils?
    (a) Plectonemic supercoiling
    (b) Solenoidal supercoiling
    (c) Negative supercoiling
    (d) Positive supercoiling
40. The DNA threads which appear inside the nucleus at the time of cell division?
    (a) Spindle fiber
    (b) Centrioles
    (c) Asters
    (d) Chromosomes
41. Chromatin is composed of ___________
    (a) DNA
    (b) DNA and proteins
    (c) DNA, RNA and proteins
    (d) None of the above
42. What is DNA replication?
    (a) Conservative
    (b) Non-conservative
    (c) Semi-conservative
    (d) None of the above
43. Eukaryotes differ from prokaryote in mechanism of DNA replication due to ___________
    (a) Use of DNA primer rather than RNA primer
    (b) Different enzyme for synthesis of lagging and leading strand
    (c) Discontinuous rather than semi-discontinuous replication
    (d) Unidirectional rather than semi-discontinuous replication
44. Which of the following is true about *DNA polymerase*?
    (a) It can synthesize DNA in the 5′ to 3′ direction
    (b) It can synthesize DNA in the 3′ to 5′ direction
    (c) It can synthesize mRNA in the 3′ to 5′ direction
    (d) It can synthesize mRNA in the 5′ to 3′ direction

45. What is the reaction in DNA replication catalyzed by *DNA ligase*?
   (a) Addition of new nucleotides to the leading strand
   (b) Addition of new nucleotide to the lagging strand
   (c) Formation of a phosphodiester bond between the 3′-OH of one Okazaki fragment and the 5′-phosphate of the next on the lagging strand
   (d) Base pairing of the template and the newly formed DNA strand
46. Which of the following reactions is required for proof reading during DNA replication by *DNA polymerase-III*?
   (a) 5′ to 3′ *exonuclease* activity (b) 3′ to 5′ *exonuclease* activity
   (c) 3′ to 5′ *endonuclease* activity (d) 5′ to 3′ *endonuclease* activity
47. Which of the following enzyme remove supercoiling in replicating DNA ahead of the replication fork?
   (a) *DNA polymerase* (b) *Helicase*
   (c) *Primase* (d) *Topoisomerase*
48. DNA unwinding is done by ____________
   (a) *Ligase* (b) *Helicase*
   (c) *Topoisomerase* (d) *Hexonuclease*
49. Which of the following enzymes is the principal replication enzyme in *E. coli*?
   (a) *DNA polymerase-I* (b) *DNA polymerase-II*
   (c) *DNA polymerase-III* (d) None of the above
50. Which enzyme is used to join bits of DNA?
   (a) *DNA polymerase* (b) *DNA ligase*
   (c) *Endonuclease* (d) *Primase*
51. Which of the following has the self-repairing mechanisms?
   (a) DNA and RNA (b) DNA, RNA and protein
   (c) Only DNA (d) DNA and protein
52. Which of the following involves remarkable capacity of a short segment of DNA to move from one place to another?
   (a) DNA transposition (b) DNA replication
   (c) Translation (d) Transcription
53. Which of the following process occurs between DNA molecules of very similar sequences?
   (a) Homologous genetic recombination (b) Site specific recombination
   (c) Non-homologous recombination (d) Replicative recombination
54. Transcription is catalyzed by ____________
   (a) DNA-dependent *RNA polymerase* (b) RNA-dependent *DNA polymerase*
   (c) *Reverse transcriptase* (d) *DNA ligase*
55. Where does *RNA polymerase* bind DNA?
   (a) Promoter (b) Operator
   (c) Enhancer (d) None of the above
56. Which of the following is true about RNA synthesis?
   (a) Synthesis of RNA is always in the 5′ to 3′ direction
   (b) *RNA polymerase* requires a primer for initiating transcription
   (c) "U" is inserted opposite "T" in transcription
   (d) New nucleotides are added on the 2′-OH of the ribose sugar

57. What is the role of sigma factor in bacterial *RNA polymerase*?
    (a) Catalyzing RNA synthesis
    (b) Positioning *RNA polymerase* correctly on the DNA template
    (c) Terminating RNA synthesis
    (d) Unwinding DNA template

58. TBP stands for?
    (a) *TATA box polymerase* (b) TATA box binding protein
    (c) Transcription associated factor (d) Transcription factor binding protein

59. Actinomycin-D is an inhibitor of ___________
    (a) Transcription (b) Translation
    (c) Replication (d) None of the above

60. Number of hydrogen bonds that form between "U" and "A" in a Watson-Crick base pair interactions?
    (a) 0 (b) 1
    (c) 2 (d) 3

61. Repressors bind to ___________
    (a) Promoter (b) Enhancer
    (c) Operator (d) Hormone response element

62. RNA primer is removed from the Okazaki fragment by ___________
    (a) *DNA polymerase-I* (b) *DNA polymerase-II*
    (c) *DNA polymerase-III* (d) *RNA polymerase*

63. Binding of the prokaryotic DNA dependent *RNA polymerase* to promoter site is inhibited by ___________
    (a) Rifampicin (b) Tetracycline
    (c) Puromycin (d) Streptomycin

64. Which of the following is an incorrect statement about m-RNA?
    (a) Cap is added to the 5′ end
    (b) Introns are removed and exons are spliced together
    (c) Histone mRNAs lack 5′ cap
    (d) Poly-A tail is added to the 3′ end

Key for Multiple Choice Questions

1. (d)	2. (a)	3. (b)	4. (a)	5. (c)
6. (b)	7. (c)	8. (b)	9. (a)	10. (d)
11. (b)	12. (a)	13. (c)	14. (b)	15. (c)
16. (d)	17. (d)	18. (c)	19. (a)	20. (a)
21. (a)	22. (a)	23. (b)	24. (b)	25. (a)
26. (d)	27. (a)	28. (b)	29. (c)	30. (a)
31. (c)	32. (b)	33. (b)	34. (a)	35. (a)
36. (b)	37. (a)	38. (b)	39. (a)	40. (d)

41. (c)	42. (c)	43. (c)	44. (a)	45. (c)
46. (b)	47. (d)	48. (b)	49. (c)	50. (b)
51. (c)	52. (a)	53. (a)	54. (a)	55. (a)
56. (a)	57. (b)	58. (b)	59. (a)	60. (c)
61. (c)	62. (a)	63. (a)	64. (b)	

PART – B: Short Answers

1. List out nitrogen bases present in nucleic acid and draw the chemical structure of any one nitrogen base.
2. Write a note on nomenclature of nucleotides.
3. What is the importance of DNA & RNA?
4. How AMP & GMP is synthesized from IMP?
5. Note on Salvage pathway for purine nucleotide synthesis.
6. How deoxyribonucleotides are synthesized from ribonucleotides?
7. What is genetic code? Write characteristic features of genetic code.
8. What are frame shift mutations? Write the consequences of the same.
9. Explain the role of various *DNA polymerases* in prokaryotic replication process.
10. Write the mechanism of inhibition of protein synthesis by chloramphenicol.
11. Name the enzymes involved in DNA replication.
12. What is nucleotide?
13. Define mutagen. Explain various types of mutagens.
14. Write a note on inhibitors of protein synthesis.
15. What is semi-conservative DNA replication?
16. What is meant by mutation?
17. Outline the role of ribosomes in protein synthesis.
18. What are nucleosides?
19. What is hyperuricemia & uricosuria?
20. Write a note on gout?
21. Explain Chargaff's rule.
22. Write a note on denaturation of DNA strands.
23. What is central dogma of life?
24. Explain Okazaki fragments.
25. Write a note on Wobble hypothesis.

PART – C: Long Answers

1. How purine nucleotides are degraded?
2. Enumerate the biosynthesis and degradation of uric acid?
3. Explain the composition of nucleic acid.
4. Explain the structure of DNA.
5. Write a detailed note on structure of RNA?
6. Explain various metabolic disorders of purine metabolism.
7. Write a detailed note on organization of mammalian genome.
8. Write in detail prokaryotic translation process.
9. Explain in detail DNA replication process in prokaryotes.
10. Explain DNA repair mechanisms.

11. Outline various steps involved in eukaryotic protein synthesis.
12. Write about various steps involved in protein synthesis.
13. Write about the different types of enzymes involved in DNA replication process. Discuss the following DNA repair mechanism: a) Base excision repair; b) SOS repair
14. Write about metabolic diseases associated with defective nucleic acid metabolism.
15. Write about DNA replication mechanism. Discuss about the different types of DNA replication and repair mechanisms.
16. Describe various types of mutations.
17. Explain the mechanism and function of DNA replication.
18. Write about catabolism of purine nucleotides.
19. Write a note on transcription & translation.
20. Explain replication in detail.
21. Explain the biosynthesis of purines.
22. Sketch the biosynthesis of pyrimidines.
23. Enumerate the salient features of DNA replication & its regulation.
24. Explain the transcription taking place in eukaryotes
25. Write about catabolism of pyrimidine nucleotides.

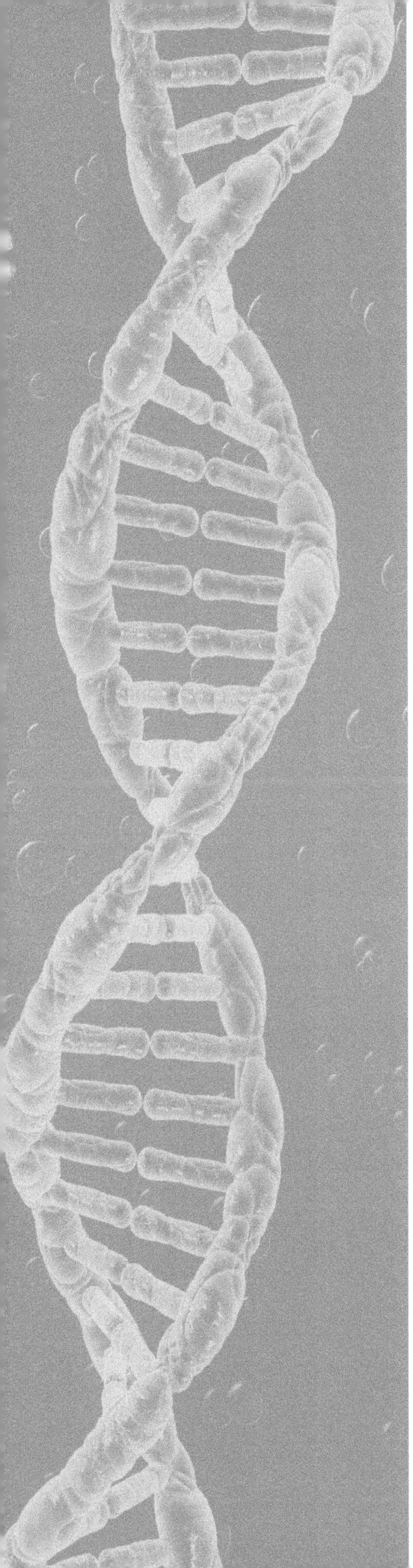

PART - III
Clinical Biochemistry

7

Introduction to Clinical Chemistry

Clinical chemistry is also known as medical biochemistry or clinical biochemistry or chemical pathology. Clinical chemistry is the branch of chemistry that is generally concerned with the analysis of body fluids for diagnostic and therapeutic purposes. In other words, clinical chemistry is an applied form of biochemistry whereas medicinal chemistry involves basic research for drug development.

Simple chemical reactions were used in the late 19th century for testing various components of blood and urine. From this only clinical chemistry, discipline originated. Since then several other advanced techniques have been applied which includes the use and measurement of enzyme activities by spectrophotometry, electrophoresis, and immunoassay techniques. Currently, many clinical urine tests and blood tests are performed extensively for diagnostic purposes. Nowadays to compensate high workload most of the clinical laboratories are highly automated with typical of a hospital laboratory. In addition, tests performed in the clinical laboratories are closely monitored and quality controlled.

Under chemical pathology, all biochemical tests are performed. Any kind of body fluid can be used in the biochemical tests but mostly biochemical tests are performed on serum or plasma. After removal of all blood cells, the yellow watery part of blood left after blood has been allowed to clot is commonly known as serum. Centrifugation is generally used for this purpose which easily packs the denser blood cells and platelets to the bottom of the centrifuge tube and leaving the liquid serum fraction resting above the packed cells. This initial step before analysis has recently been included in instruments that operate on the "integrated system" principle. When centrifuging the blood *without* clotting the essence obtained the same as the serum is known as plasma. Before clotting occurs, plasma is obtained by centrifugation. Depending upon the type of test required, sample is decided.

700 different kind of tests are performed in a large medical laboratory.

Classification of Clinical Chemistry Laboratory

Clinical chemistry laboratory is broadly classified into following types.

1. General or routine clinical chemistry laboratory (usual urine and blood tests are performed in this laboratory. **Example:** Liver and kidney function tests).
2. Advanced clinical chemistry laboratory (advanced tests are performed using elaborate techniques such as electrophoresis methods).
3. Clinical endocrinology laboratory (hormone tests are performed for the diagnosis of endocrine disorders).
4. Toxicology laboratory (toxicity tests are performed for the study of drugs of abuse and other chemicals).
5. Therapeutic drug monitoring (tests are performed to monitor therapeutic activity of drugs to adjust the doses).
6. Urine analysis laboratory (chemical analysis of urine for a wide array of diseases, along with other fluids such as CSF and effusions)
7. Fecal analysis laboratory (test are performed for analysis of feces mostly for detection of gastrointestinal disorders).

Common Clinical Chemistry Tests

The followings are the common clinical chemistry tests performed in clinical chemistry laboratory.

1. Electrolytes (sodium, potassium, chloride and bicarbonate)
2. Renal or kidney function tests (creatinine and blood urea nitrogen)
3. Liver function tests (total protein (serum), albumin, globulin, A/G ratio (albumin-globulin), protein electrophoresis, urine protein, bilirubin (direct; indirect; total), *aspartate transaminase* (*AST*), *alanine transaminase* (*ALT*), *gamma-glutamyl transpeptidase* (*GGT*) and *alkaline phosphatase* (*ALP*)).
4. Cardiac markers (H-FABP, troponin, myoglobin, CK-MB and B-type natriuretic peptide (BNP)).
5. Minerals (calcium, magnesium, phosphate, and potassium).
6. Blood disorders (iron, transferrin, TIBC, vitamin B_{12}, vitamin-D and folic acid)
7. Miscellaneous (glucose, C-reactive protein, glycated hemoglobin (HbA1c), uric acid, arterial blood gases ([H^+], P_{CO_2}, P_{O_2}), adrenocorticotropic hormone (ACTH), toxicological screening and forensic toxicology (drugs and toxins), neuron-specific *enolase* (NSE) and fecal occult blood test (FOBT)).

The followings are the set of commonly ordered tests which are combined into a panel as follows.

1. **Basic metabolic panel (BMP) tests:** It comprises eight test such as sodium, potassium, chloride, bicarbonate, blood urea nitrogen (BUN), creatinine, glucose, and calcium.
2. **Comprehensive metabolic panel (CMP) tests:** It comprises fourteen tests along with the above eight BMP, it includes total protein, albumin, *alkaline phosphatase* (*ALP*), *alanine amino transferase* (*ALT*), *aspartate amino transferase* (*AST*) and bilirubin.

Role of the Clinical Chemist in Clinical Chemistry Laboratory

Clinical chemist or lab technicians of the clinical chemistry laboratory are skilled workers that work with complex systems or perform highly technical, mechanical or diagnostic tests in medical or scientific laboratories. The followings are the role of clinical chemist in clinical chemistry laboratory.

1. Working closely with patients. Hence, responsiveness is necessary because the patients might be in pain or under emotional pressure.
2. Providing information for patient diagnosis and treatment by performing laboratory tests.
3. Receiving and labeling samples (blood, toxic, tissue etc.).
4. Performing routine and non-routine tests and analyses using the appropriate technical equipment and instruments.
5. Designing and executing laboratory test according to standard procedures.
6. Making observations and interpret findings.
7. Conducting experiments using refined scientific methods under defined conditions to verify/reject various types of hypotheses.
8. Optimizing lab procedures and succeed in producing reliable and important results that can be used to make a difference.
9. Performing quality control and calibrate equipment if necessary.
10. Maintaining equipment in proper working order and maintaining a clean work area.
11. Organizing and store all chemical substances, fluids and compressed gases according to safety instructions.
12. Recording all data and results in specified forms (paper and electronic) with accuracy and responsibility.
13. Ensuring that all safety guidelines are followed strictly at all times.
14. Using computers and perform mathematical calculations for the preparation of graphs.
15. Serving as technical resource by participating in staff training, answering questions of other

professionals, participating in educational opportunities, reading professional publications, maintaining personal networks and participating in professional organizations.
16. Excellent physical condition and endurance.
17. Keeping up to date with relevant scientific and technical developments.
18. Ability to work autonomously and under pressure.
19. Identifying and communicating abnormal patient conditions by alerting supervisory personnel, the pathologist, the patient physician, or nurse; reporting mandated information to the public health department or other designated officials.
20. Maintaining patient confidence by keeping laboratory information confidential.
21. Serving and protecting the hospital community by adhering to professional standards, hospital policies and procedures, federal, state, and local requirements.
22. Toxicology clinical chemist identifies the presence or quantity of drugs of abuse, therapeutic drugs, and toxic substances by operating toxicology instrumentation and performing manual methods for the performance of drug screens, blood alcohol levels, and carbon monoxide levels.
23. General clinical chemist provides test results for patient diagnosis and treatment by conducting experiments either manually or through instrumentation, operating chemistry equipment; performing hand chemistries.
24. Hematology clinical chemist provides test results for patient diagnosis and treatment by operating hematology, urinalysis, and coagulation equipment; performing manual methods of differentials.
25. Immunology clinical chemist provides test results for patient diagnosis and treatment by operating equipment such as the gamma counter, spectrophotometer, densitometer, and through methods such as radioimmunoassay, enzyme immunoassay, and serological testing.
26. Microbiology clinical chemist provides physician with information for treatment of patient infection by performing technical procedures for the identification or susceptibility of bacteria, parasites, fungi, and mycobacteria.
27. Blood bank clinical chemist ensures the patient of receiving compatible blood/blood components by completing blood typing, antibody screening, compatibility testing, and antibody identification procedures.
28. Blood bank clinical chemist assures future retrieval of patient transfusion information by preparing patient packets and maintaining blood bank database.

Organelle Malfunction

The functions and malfunctions result of various cellular organelles are listed in Table 7.1.

Table 7.1 Functions & malfunctions of various cellular organelles.

S. No.	Name of organelle	Functions	Malfunction results
1	Nucleolus	It is the most conspicuous domain in the eukaryotic cell which is involved in the synthesis of rRNA (ribosomal RNA) and biogenesis of ribosome.	Ribosomes are not produced.
2	Lysosomes	Cell organelle filled with enzymes needed to break down certain materials in the cell, such as large food particles or old parts of the cell. May be found only in animal cells.	Increased waste product which leads to decreased stability of the cell. Plant cell don't have lysosomes.
3	Cell membrane	The thin, flexible barrier around a cell which controls what enters and leaves the cell.	Harmful things enter into the cell due to breakage of cell membrane.
4	Ribosomes	A small particle in the cell involved in the synthesis of proteins.	Protein synthesis becomes difficult.

Table 7.1 Contd...

S. No.	Name of organelle	Functions	Malfunction results
5	Cytoplasm	Fluid present between the cell membrane and the nucleus which helps to protect organelles.	No support for the organelles in the cell leads to unable to move around in the cell.
6	Mitochondria	An organelle containing enzymes responsible for producing energy by metabolism or respiration.	No energy leads to lethargic feeling.
7	Endoplasmic reticulum	A cell structure that forms a maze of passage ways in which proteins and other materials are carried from one part of the cell to another.	Some proteins would no longer have a home and proteins would no longer have a way to get around the cell.
8	Nuclear membrane	The nuclear membrane is also known as nuclear envelope which is a double membrane layer that separates the contents of the nucleus from the rest of the cell.	No protection for the main control center of the cell.
9	Golgi body	A cell structure that helps to make and pack materials to be transported out of the cell or for storage inside the cell.	Difficulty in distributing materials by cells.
10	Chloroplast	An organelle found in the cells of plants and some other organisms that captures the energy from sunlight and converts it into chemical energy (photosynthesis).	Plant cell will be unable to produce food for itself.
11	Cell Wall	The structure outside of the cell membrane that is used to provide support and protection. Present in plants, algae, fungi, and many prokaryotes.	Some bacteria damage plants by releasing enzymes that break down this protective, strong outer barrier.
12	Vacuole	Sac like storage structure in the cell used to store water, nutrients, and even toxic substances.	No storage for the cells and shape is loosed by plant cells.
13	Nucleus	A part of the cell containing hereditary information and is responsible for growth and reproduction. Nucleus is the "command center" of the cell.	The cell would be out of control.
14	Cytoskeleton	Cellular structures that helps the cell to maintain shape and/or move.	Affect synaptic signals and organelle or vesicle trafficking.
15	Cilia	Hair-like projections on the cell surface use structures motion or the movement of fluid over a cell.	Defective and dysfunctional functioning in motile and non-motile cilia affects multiple systems, causing blindness, deafness, chronic respiratory infections, kidney disease, heart disease, infertility, obesity and diabetes.
16	Flagellum	Most often a single whip-like projection on the cell surface that allows a cell to move.	Movement of cell is blocked.
17	Centriole	A cellular structure in an animal cell that helps to organize cell division.	Impairment in cell division organization.

Cell Malfunction

A failure of cell to operate or function in the normal or correct manner is called cell malfunction. Malfunctioning of cells happened when they lack what they need or exposed to something harmful. No disease unless cells malfunction. Today we experience thousands of different diseases. All these diseases are merely the effects of thousands of combinations of deficiencies and toxicities acting through a combination of the environment, inherited genes, and our thoughts, beliefs, and emotions. Preventing and reversing cellular malfunction leads to preventing or reversing of disease. There are number of reasons for cell malfunction but here cell malfunction due to diet is explained.

Cellular sodium/potassium ratio: Minerals such as sodium and potassium are critical to normal functioning of cell but they must be in balance. For normal cell functions, low sodium and high, potassium is necessary with sodium/potassium ratio of 1:4. Eating plenty of fresh fruits and vegetables made this as possible leads to normal cell function. When there is imbalance in the sodium/potassium ratio due to modern dietary practices such as too much salt especially in processed foods, less consumption of fresh fruits and vegetables may lead to cellular malfunction. Cells function like little batteries. Due to the difference in the amount of sodium outside the cell and the amount of potassium inside the cell electrical charge is created in the cell. Change in sodium/potassium ratio inside each cell damages the 'battery of life', which interfere seriously with the body's self-regulation and repair functions. For example, cancer metastasis is accelerated when there is increase in the dietary sodium of laboratory animals. This cellular malfunction may be prevented and reversed by consuming less salt and eat more fresh fruits and vegetables.

Cellular pH: Abnormal cellular pH is another common reason for cellular malfunction. 7.4 is the normal cellular pH and it is critical to maintain it. Certain functions of cells are inhibited and others functions of the cells are enhanced when the cellular pH is too acidic or too alkaline which leads to cellular malfunction and disease. Too much cellular acidity commonly may cause cancer. Acidity of the cell is increased from a diet rich in acid-forming foods such as white flour, sugar, cola drinks and milk products. A powerful acidic effect is produced when colas combine sugar with phosphoric acid. Diet rich in alkaline foods are fresh fruits and vegetables. Hence malfunction of the cell due to cellular pH can be prevented and reversed by avoiding acid forming foods and consuming alkaline foods with mineral supplements by balance the cellular pH to normal.

Cellular membranes: Another common cause of disease is improperly constructed cell membranes. Each cell has a wall called the cell membrane. Through the membrane only everything is going in or out of the cell. Cell membrane acts like a 'gatekeeper' making sure only the right things go in and out. Cellular malfunction and disease occur due to improperly constructed cell membranes. Construction of cell membrane with proper building materials is essential to prevent and reverse disease. The 1:1 ratio of omega-6 to omega-3 oils is essential in order to construct cell membrane with proper building materials. The ratio of omega-6 to omega-3 oils in the vegetable and hydrogenated oils common to our diet is 20:1 leads to wrong building materials. The preferred building materials can be obtained by using fish and flaxseed oils.

Inflammatory process: Inflammation is a common process to almost all disease. Free radicals are generated by inflammation which damages DNA, cell membranes, and cellular machinery leads to ageing and disease. It is necessary to prevent or reverse inflammation to prevent or reverse aging and disease. Pro-inflammatory products are milk products, white flour, sugar, meat, farmed fish and processed oils. Consumption of low in anti-inflammatory chemicals and high pro-inflammatory chemicals leads to chronic inflammation and disease. Avoiding inflammatory foods and eating a diet rich in antioxidant supplements, fresh fruits, and vegetables prevents and reverses inflammation.

Proper nutrition in the womb: A growing fetus must be supplied with all the raw materials it needs to maximize lifelong health. In addition, it must be protected from toxins that could disrupt its delicate construction process. Early on-set of major chronic diseases are due to poor nutrition in utero and during infancy. For detoxification also good nutrition is required. Detoxification pathways and toxins persist without nutrients to support leads to more damage.

Toxicity: Mercury is one of the toxins among the many toxins passed from mother to child causing disease. From vaccinations, dental fillings and fish, mercury interferes with enzymes that control arranging fetal brain in organized way. Brain functions including learning, behavior and higher-level thinking are affected even minor changes in brain structure. It also affects control of the immune, hormonal, and digestive systems.

Another toxic problem is fluoride. Enormous health risk to the unborn such as lowering their IQs and dumbing down our population due to fluoridated water, toothpaste, and fluoride-contaminated foods. In artificial sweetener the compound aspartame is present which breaks down into a number of highly toxic chemicals that can damage fetal DNA, alter brain function, and contribute to cancer.

Cell Cycle

In all living organisms cell division is a very important process. DNA replication and cell growth take place during the division of a cell. In a coordinated way all these processes such as cell division, DNA replication, and cell growth, have to take place to ensure correct division and formation of progeny cells containing intact genomes. Cell cycle is defined as the sequence of events by which a cell duplicates its genome, synthesizes the other constituents of the cell and eventually divides into two daughter cells.

Phases of cell cycle

A typical eukaryotic cell cycle is illustrated by human cells in culture (Figure 7.1). From organism to organism and also from cell type to cell type duration of cell cycle can vary but usually cells divide once in approximately every 24 hours. There are two basic phases in the cell cycle as follows.

1. Interphase or Resting phase
2. Mitosis phase or M-phase

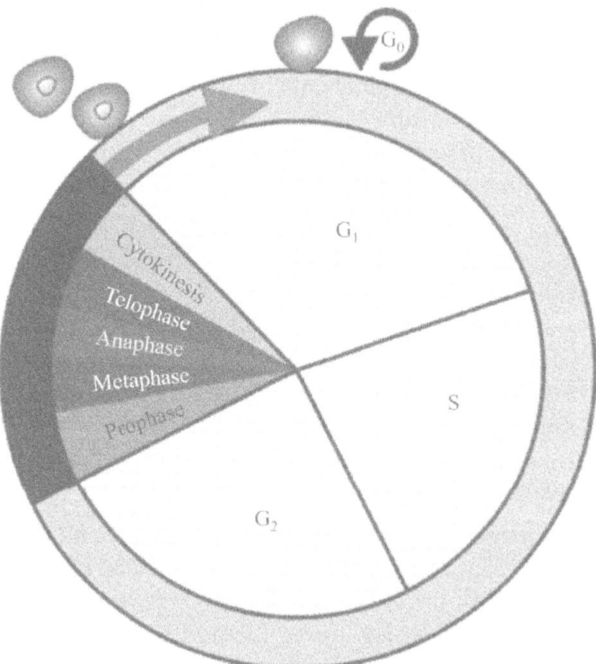

Figure 7.1 Phases of cell cycle.

The actual cell division or mitosis occurs is represented in the M-phase and the phase between two successive M-phases are represented by the interphase. 95% of the duration of cell cycle is occupied by interphase only and the remaining 5 % by M-phase. Corresponding to the karyokinesis i.e. nuclear division the M-phase starts, and with cytokinesis (division of cytoplasm) it usually ends.

Interphase or resting phase: In an orderly manner both cell growth and DNA replication take place for division and the time required for the process is known as interphase. The followings are three sub-phases of interphase. They are,

1. G_1-phase (Gap 1)
2. S-phase (Synthesis)
3. G_2-phase (Gap 2)

The interval between mitosis and initiation of DNA replication is known as G_1 phase. In this phase the cell does not replicate its DNA but it continuously grows and is metabolically active. The period of replication or DNA synthesis takes place is called as synthesis or S-phase. The amount of DNA per cell is doubled during this time but there is no increase in the chromosome number. During the S-phase, in animal cell nucleus DNA replication begins, and in the cytoplasm the centriole duplicates. In preparation for mitosis, proteins are synthesized while cell growth continues during the G_2-phase.

Quiescent stage (G_0) is the inactive stage of the cell cycle in which cells do not divide further and exit G_1-phase. Depending on the requirement no longer proliferation takes place in the cell and the cells remain metabolically active in this stage. In the diploid somatic cells, only mitotic cell division is seen in animals but not in haploid cells (Male honey bee's exception). Whereas in plants mitotic divisions is seen in both haploid and diploid cells.

M-phase or mitosis phase: All components of the cell are mainly reorganized in this phase. Hence this phase is the most dramatic period of the cell cycle. This phase is also called as equational division because the number of chromosomes in both the parent and progeny cells are same. Karyokinesis (nuclear division) involves four different stages as following,

1. Prophase
2. Metaphase
3. Anaphase
4. Telophase

Prophase: The very first stage of karyokinesis of mitosis is prophase followed by S- and G_2- phases of interphase. Chromosomal material condensation is initiated in the prophase and during the chromatin condensation process the chromosomal material becomes untangled. The new DNA molecules formed are not distinguished in the S- and G_2- phases but intertwined. During S-phase of interphase the centrosome undergone duplication, begins to move towards opposite poles of the cell in prophase. The following characteristic indicates the completion of prophase.

1. Compact mitotic chromosomes are formed by condensation of chromosomal material. At the centromere two chromatids attached together composed chromosomes are seen.
2. During interphase centrosome undergone duplication, begins to move towards opposite poles of the cell. Each centrosome radiates out microtubules called asters. Mitotic apparatus is formed by the spindle fibers together with two asters.

When the cells are viewed under the microscope, the end of prophase do not show Golgi complexes, endoplasmic reticulum, nucleolus and the nuclear envelope.

Metaphase: Second phase of mitosis is started by complete disintegration of the nuclear envelope marks leads to spread of the chromosomes through the cytoplasm of the cell. Condensation of chromosomes is completed at metaphase and can be viewed clearly under the microscope. At this stage it is most easy to study the morphology of chromosomes. Two sister chromatids made metaphase chromosome and centromere hold two sister chromatids together. At the surface of the centromeres the small disc-shaped structures present is called as kinetochores. These kinetochores serve as the sites of attachment of spindle fibers to the chromosomes that are moved into position at the centre of the cell. All the chromosomes coming to lie at the equator with one chromatid of each chromosome connected by its kinetochore to spindle fibers from one pole and its sister chromatid connected by its kinetochore to spindle fibers from the opposite pole are the characterization of the metaphase. Metaphase plate is the plane of alignment of the chromosomes at metaphase. The following features are the two key features of metaphase.

1. To the kinetochores of chromosomes, spindle fibers are attached.
2. Chromosomes are moved to spindle equator and get aligned along metaphase plate through spindle fibers to both poles.

Anaphase: Simultaneously each chromosome arranged at the metaphase plate splits and the two daughter chromatids (daughter chromosomes of the future daughter nuclei) begin their migration towards the two opposite poles at the onset of anaphase. The centromere of each chromosome remains directed towards the pole as each chromosome moves away from the equatorial plate. Hence the arms of the chromosome trails behind at the leading edge. The followings are the characterization of anaphase stage.

1. Centromeres split and chromatids separate.
2. Chromatids move to opposite poles.

Telophase: The chromosomes reach their respective poles decondense and lose their individuality at this telophase stage of karyokinesis. At each of the two poles each set of chromatin material tends to collect and the individual chromosomes can no longer be seen. The following are the key events of this stage,

1. At opposite spindle poles chromosomes cluster and their identity is lost as discrete elements.
2. At each pole around the chromosome clusters nuclear envelope develops forming two daughter nuclei.
3. Reformation of nucleolus, Golgi complex and endoplasmic reticulum.

Cytokinesis: Cell division gets completed at the end of cytokinesis which is the process of division of cell itself into two daughter cells by the separation of cytoplasm. In the plasma membrane appearance of a furrow indicates the achievement of cytokinesis in an animal cell. Gradually the furrow deepens and joins in the centre ultimately divides the cell cytoplasm into two.

Mutations

Base composition and sequence of genetic macromolecule DNA is highly stable. (Even though, from gradual change in DNA is not totally exempted). A change in the DNA structure of a gene is referred as mutation and the chemicals or substances inducing mutations are collectively known as mutagens. The change that takes place in DNA on mutation is reflected in various processes such as replication, transcription and translation. Mutations are broadly classified into two major types as follows.

1. Point mutation
2. Frame shift mutation

Point mutation:

It occurs by replacement of one base pair by another base pair and it is schematically represented in Figure 7.2. Point mutation is further sub-classified into two types as a) Transition and b) Transversion.

Transition: In this mutation, a purine (or pyrimidine) base is replaced by another purine (or pyrimidine) base. **Example:** Adenine is replaced by guanine or vice versa and thymine is replaced by cytosine or vice versa.

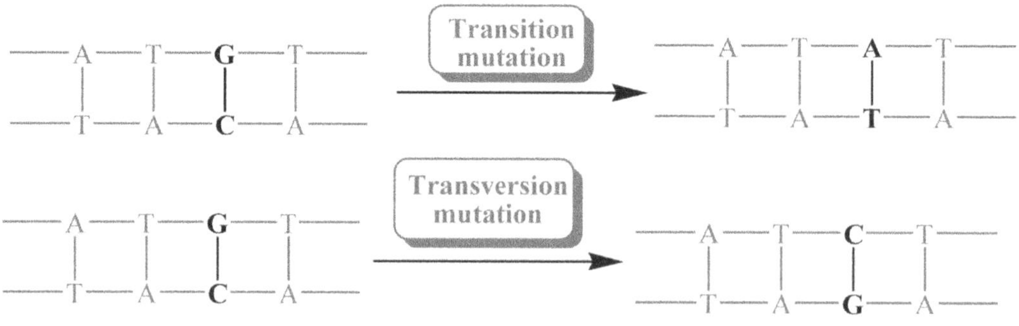

Figure 7.2 Point mutation.

Transversion: In this type of mutation, a purine base is replaced by a pyrimidine base or a pyrimidine base is replaced by a purine base. **Example:** Adenine is replaced by thymine or vice versa and guanine is replaced by cytosine or vice versa.

Consequences: The following are the consequences of point mutations and are presented in Figure 7.3.

1. **Silent mutation:** In this case no detectable effects are seen because the changed base in the codon of mRNA may code for same amino acid. **Example:** Serine is coded by UCA and the change in third base results in UCU (third base altered) which also codes for serine only.
2. **Missense mutation:** In this case the changed base in the codon of mRNA may code for different amino acid. **Example:** UCA codes for serine; whereas ACA (first base altered) codes for threonine.

With regards to the functions of a protein molecule the missense or mistaken amino acid may be unacceptable or partially acceptable or acceptable. For missense mutation the classical example is Sickle-cell anemia.

3. **Nonsense mutation:** In few cases the changed codon may be nonsense or termination codon. In this case at that point the altered codon terminates protein synthesis by stopping signal. **Example:** UCA codes for serine; whereas UAA (second base altered) is the termination codon.

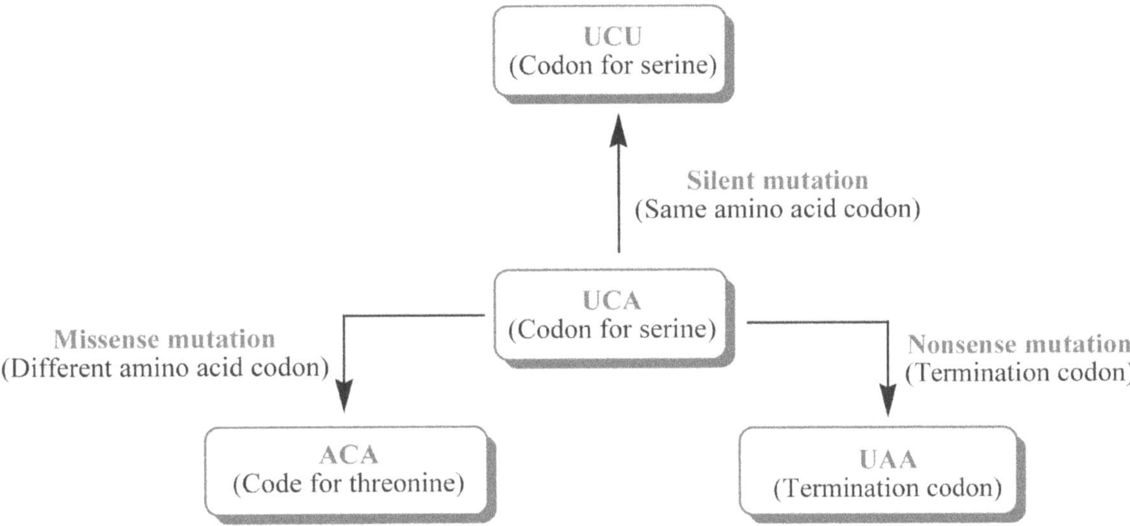

Figure 7.3 Consequences of point mutation.

Frame shift mutation:

Insertion or deletion of one or more base pairs in DNA leads to occurrence of frame shift mutation. Frame shift mutation is further classified into two types as, a) Insertion mutation (Due to insertion of one or more base pairs) and b) Deletion mutation (Due to deletion of one or more base pairs). Two types of frame shift mutations are presented schematically in Figure 7.4.

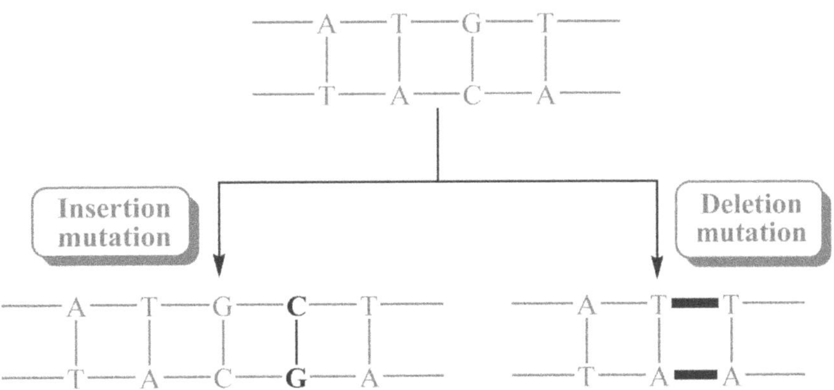

Figure 7.4 Frameshift mutation.

Consequences: The reading frame of the mRNA is altered (Hence, known as frame shift) due to insertion or deletion of base in a gene. The missing base or added base was not recognized by the machinery of mRNA which contains codons. The process of translation continues as there is no punctuation in the reading of codons. Ultimately several altered amino acids are present in synthesized protein and / or results in prematurely terminated protein.

Mutation and cancer:

DNA mutation produces permanent alteration in the structure which has been implicated in the etiopathogenesis of cancer.

PROBABLE QUESTIONS

PART – A: Multiple Choice Questions

1. Which of the following test comes under basic metabolic panel test?
   (a) Total protein test (b) Albumin test
   (c) Blood urea nitrogen (BUN) test (d) Bilirubin test
2. Which of the following test comes under comprehensive metabolic panel test?
   (a) Sodium test (b) *Aspartate amino transferase (AST)* test
   (c) Creatinine test (d) Glucose test
3. Which of the following test not comes under basic metabolic panel test?
   (a) Bicarbonate test (b) Calcium test
   (c) Creatinine test (d) *Alkaline phosphatase (ALP)* test
4. Which of the following test not comes under comprehensive metabolic panel test?
   (a) Chloride test (b) *Alanine amino transferase (ALT)* test
   (c) Total protein test (d) Albumin test
5. Which of the followings are role of the clinical chemist in clinical chemistry laboratory?
   (a) Responsiveness is necessary because the patients might be in pain or under emotional pressure
   (b) Receiving and labeling samples
   (c) Making observations and interpret findings
   (d) All the above
6. ______________________ is involved in the synthesis of rRNA (ribosomal RNA) and biogenesis of ribosome.
   (a) Cell membrane (b) Nucleolus
   (c) Lysosome (d) Mitochondria
7. Which cell organelle is filled with enzymes needed to break down certain materials in the cell, such as large food particles or old parts of the cell and it may be found only in animal cells?
   (a) Lysosome (b) Nucleolus
   (c) Cell membrane (d) Cytoplasm
8. Malfunctions of which organelle results in increased waste product which leads to decreased stability of the cell.
   (a) Mitochondria (b) Endoplasmic reticulum
   (c) Nuclear membrane (d) Lysosome
9. The thin, flexible barrier around a cell which controls what enters and leaves the cell is known as ______________________.
   (a) Cell membrane (b) Mitochondria
   (c) Ribosomes (d) Nucleolus
10. Which of the following one occurs due to malfunction of cell membrane?
    (a) Ribosomes are not produced (b) Harmful things enter into the cell
    (c) Protein synthesis becomes difficult (d) No energy leads to lethargic feeling

11. ______________ is a small particle in the cell involved in the synthesis of proteins.
    (a) Endoplasmic reticulum (b) Ribosome
    (c) Cytoplasm (d) Nucleolus
12. ____________ is fluid present between the cell membrane and the nucleus which helps to protect organelles.
    (a) Cytoplasm (b) Nucleolus
    (c) Mitochondria (d) Ribosome
13. Which is an organelle containing enzymes responsible for producing energy by metabolism or respiration?
    (a) Golgi body (b) Endoplasmic reticulum
    (c) Nucleolus (d) Mitochondria
14. Malfunctions of which cellular organelle leads to lethargic feeling.
    (a) Mitochondria (b) Nucleus
    (c) Golgi body (d) Cytoskeleton
15. Which is a cell structure that forms a maze of passageways in which proteins and other materials are carried from one part of the cell to another?
    (a) Golgi body (b) Lysosome
    (c) Ribosome (d) Endoplasmic reticulum
16. Some proteins would no longer have a home and proteins would no longer have a way to get around the cell is due to malfunction of which cellular organelle.
    (a) Endoplasmic reticulum (b) Golgi body
    (c) Nucleolus (d) Nuclear membrane
17. Which is a double membrane layer that separates the contents of the nucleus from the rest of the cell?
    (a) Lysosome (b) Cytoskeleton
    (c) Nuclear membrane (d) Mitochondria
18. A cell structure that helps to make and pack materials to be transported out of the cell or for storage inside the cell.
    (a) Mitochondria (b) Golgi body
    (c) Endoplasmic reticulum (d) Lysosome
19. An organelle found in the cells of plants and some other organisms that captures the energy from sunlight and converts it into chemical energy (photosynthesis).
    (a) Cell Wall (b) Vacuole
    (c) Cilia (d) Chloroplast
20. The structure outside of the cell membrane that is used to provide support and protection is known as ________________.
    (a) Endoplasmic reticulum (b) Cell Wall
    (c) Lysosome (d) Vacuole
21. ______________________ is saclike storage structure in the cell used to store water, nutrients, and even toxic substances.
    (a) Vacuole (b) Nucleus
    (c) Cell Wall (d) Ribosome

22. Which is a part of the cell containing hereditary information and is responsible for growth and reproduction?
    (a) Lysosome (b) Golgi body
    (c) Cilia (d) Nucleus
23. ____________ is the "command center" of the cell.
    (a) Cell Wall (b) Nucleus
    (c) Endoplasmic reticulum (d) Cytoskeleton
24. The cell would be out of control due to malfunction of ____________.
    (a) Lysosome (b) Cytoskeleton
    (c) Cell Wall (d) Nucleus
25. ______________ are the cellular structures that helps the cell to maintain shape and/or move.
    (a) Cytoskeleton (b) Ribosome
    (c) Nucleus (d) Vacuole
26. Malfunctions of ___________________ affect synaptic signals and organelle or vesicle trafficking?
    (a) Nucleolus (b) Cilia
    (c) Cell membrane (d) Cytoskeleton
27. ____________________ is a hair-like projections on the cell surface use structures motion or the movement of fluid over a cell.
    (a) Centriole (b) Cilia
    (c) Flagellum (d) Nuclear membrane
28. Defective and dysfunctional functioning in motile and non-motile ______________ affects multiple systems, causing blindness, deafness, chronic respiratory infections, kidney disease, heart disease, infertility, obesity and diabetes.
    (a) Cilia (b) Golgi body
    (c) Endoplasmic reticulum (d) Lysosome
29. ____________________ is most often a single whip-like projection on the cell surface of microorganism that allows a cell to move.
    (a) Flagellum (b) Centriole
    (c) Cilia (d) Vacuole
30. Movement of cell is blocked in microorganism due to malfunction of ____________.
    (a) Cell wall (b) Lysosome
    (c) Flagellum (d) Ribosome
31. ____________________ is a cellular structure in an animal cell that helps to organize cell division.
    (a) Endoplasmic reticulum (b) Mitochondria
    (c) Ribosome (d) Centriole
32. Malfunction of centriole causes which of the following?
    (a) Impairment in cell division organization
    (b) Movement of cell is blocked
    (c) Affect synaptic signals and organelle or vesicle trafficking
    (d) No storage for the cells and shape is loosed by plant cells
33. For normal cell functions, which of the following is necessary?
    (a) High sodium and high potassium (b) High sodium and low potassium
    (c) Low sodium and high potassium (d) Low sodium and low potassium

34. For normal cell functions, the ratio between sodium and potassium should be__________.
    (a) 1:1 (b) 1:4
    (c) 4:1 (d) 1:2
35. __________ ratio of omega-6 to omega-3 oils is essential in order to construct cell membrane with proper building materials
    (a) 1:1 (b) 1:4
    (c) 4:1 (d) 1:2
36. Interphase of cell cycle is otherwise known as ______________.
    (a) Prophase (b) Metaphase
    (c) Anaphase (d) Resting phase
37. The phase between two successive M-phases are represented by the __________.
    (a) Metaphase (b) Telophase
    (c) Interphase (d) Prophase
38. In M-phase of cell cycle "M" indicates ______________.
    (a) Minor (b) Metaphase
    (c) Major (d) Mitosis
39. In an orderly manner both cell growth and DNA replication take place for division and the time required for the process is known as _____________.
    (a) M-phase (b) Interphase
    (c) Metaphase (d) Anaphase
40. Which of the following phase is not a sub-phase of interphase?
    (a) G_1-phase (b) G_2-phase
    (c) S-phase (d) Prophase
41. The interval between mitosis and initiation of DNA replication is known as __________ and in this phase the cell does not replicate its DNA but it continuously grows and is metabolically active.
    (a) G_1-phase (b) G_2-phase
    (c) S-phase (d) M-phase
42. The period of replication or DNA synthesis takes place is called as _________.
    (a) G_1-phase (b) G_2-phase
    (c) S-phase (d) M-phase
43. In preparation for mitosis, proteins are synthesized while cell growth continues during the ___________.
    (a) G_1-phase (b) G_2-phase
    (c) S-phase (d) M-phase
44. All components of the cell are mainly reorganized in which phase of cell cycle?
    (a) Resting phase (b) Mitosis phase
    (c) G_1-phase (d) S-phase
45. Which of the following one is not an stage of karyokinesis.
    (a) Prophase (b) Telophase
    (c) Interphase (d) Anaphase
46. Which of the following is types of point mutation?
    (a) Transition & Transversion (b) Insertion & Deletion
    (c) Transition & Deletion (d) Insertion & Transversion

47. Which of the following is types of frameshift mutation?
    (a) Transition & Transversion
    (b) Insertion & Deletion
    (c) Transition & Deletion
    (d) Insertion & Transversion
48. In which mutation no detectable effects are seen because the changed base in the codon of mRNA may code for same amino acid.
    (a) Silent mutation
    (b) Missense mutation
    (c) Nonsense mutation
    (d) Insertion mutation
49. In which mutation the changed base in the codon of mRNA may code for different amino acid.
    (a) Nonsense mutation
    (b) Silent mutation
    (c) Deletion mutation
    (d) Missense mutation
50. In which mutation altered codon terminates protein synthesis by stopping signal?
    (a) Insertion mutation
    (b) Silent mutation
    (c) Nonsense mutation
    (d) Missense mutation

Key for Multiple Choice Questions

1. (c)	2. (b)	3. (d)	4. (a)	5. (d)
6. (b)	7. (a)	8. (d)	9. (a)	10. (b)
11. (b)	12. (a)	13. (d)	14. (a)	15. (d)
16. (a)	17. (c)	18. (b)	19. (d)	20. (b)
21. (a)	22. (d)	23. (b)	24. (d)	25. (a)
26. (d)	27. (b)	28. (a)	29. (a)	30. (c)
31. (d)	32. (a)	33. (c)	34. (b)	35. (a)
36. (d)	37. (c)	38. (d)	39. (b)	40. (d)
41. (a)	42. (c)	43. (b)	44. (b)	45. (c)
46. (a)	47. (b)	48. (a)	49. (d)	50. (c)

PART – B: Short Answers

1. List out various types of clinical chemistry laboratory.
2. List out various common clinical chemistry test.
3. What is basic metabolic panel (BMP) tests?
4. What is comprehensive metabolic panel (CMP) tests?
5. Write the functions and malfunction results of nucleolus.
6. Write a note on functions and malfunction results of lysosome.
7. Explain the functions and malfunction results of cell membrane.
8. Write a short note on ribosome.
9. Write a note on functions and malfunction results of mitochondria.
10. Explain the functions and malfunction results of endoplasmic reticulum.
11. Write a short note on Golgi body.
12. Write a note on cellular sodium/ potassium ratio.

13. How pH changes affect cellular functions?
14. What are the different phases of cell cycle?
15. What is interphase of cell cycle?
16. Explain the three sub-phases of interphase.
17. What is quiescent stage?
18. What is mitosis phase of cell cycle?
19. Explain karyokinesis.
20. Write a note on prophase.
21. Define cytokinesis.
22. Write a short note on mutation.
23. Explain the term point mutation.
24. What is frame shift mutation?
25. Explain the different consequences of point mutations.

PART – C: Long Answers

1. Write a detailed note on clinical chemistry laboratory.
2. Explain various common clinical chemistry tests performed in clinical chemistry laboratory.
3. List out various role of clinical chemist in clinical chemistry laboratory.
4. Explain the functions and malfunctions result of various cellular organelles in detail.
5. Explain cell malfunction specifically due to diet.
6. What is cell cycle? Explain the various stages of cell cycle with suitable diagram.
7. Define and classify mutation. Explain any one type of mutation in detail.

8

Kidney Function Tests or Renal Function Tests

Urinary System

The urinary system is otherwise known as the renal system or urinary tract. The major excretory system of the body is the urinary system and it is the body's drainage system for the eventual removal of urine. The major functions of the urinary system are,

1. Removal of waste products from the body
2. Storage of urea and uric acid (particularly) before excretion
3. Regulation of blood volume and blood pressure
4. Regulation of electrolytes and metabolites
5. Regulation of homeostasis of blood pH
6. Production of red blood cells (kidney contributes) and
7. Helps to synthesize the active form of vitamin-D i.e., ca**lcitriol.**

The urinary system refers to the structures that produce and transport urine to the point of excretion. The urinary system consists of

1. Two kidneys (to secrete urine)
2. Two ureters (to transport urine from the kidney to the bladder)
3. One bladder (to collects urine from kidney *via* ureter and store it temporarily) and
4. One urethra (to pass urine from the bladder to the exterior).

The renal arteries extensively supply blood to the kidneys and via the renal vein, it leaves the kidney. Generally, after filtration of blood and further processing *via* the ureters wastes in the form of urine exit the kidney. Ureters are the tubes made of smooth muscle fibers that propel urine towards the urinary bladder. Urine is stored and subsequently expelled from the body from the urinary bladder by urination (voiding) *via* urethra. The urethra is a tube that connects the urinary bladder to the urinary meatus for the removal of urine from the body. Only in the length of the urethra the male and female urinary systems differ. Through a filtration of blood, urine is formed in the kidneys. Then the urine is passed to the bladder through the ureters and stored in the bladder. Finally, the urine is passed to the outside of the body from the bladder through the urethra during urination. In a healthy human, every day about 800 to 2,000 ml of urine are excreted. Depending upon the kidney function and fluid intake this amount may vary. The urinary system is diagrammatically presented in Figure 8.1.

Kidney:

The kidneys are reddish-brown bean-shaped organs found in the vertebrates. They receive blood from the paired renal arteries; blood exits into the paired renal veins. Each kidney is attached to a ureter, a tube that carries excreted urine to the bladder. In the retroperitoneal space, two kidneys are located on the left and right. Just below the waist between the peritoneum and posterior wall of the abdomen, kidneys are exactly located. The position is posterior to the peritoneum of the abdominal cavity; hence, it is commonly known as retroperitoneal space. Position of the liver causes asymmetry within the abdominal cavity; hence, the right kidney being slightly lower and smaller than the left kidney. The left kidney is approximately at the vertebral level T_{12} to L_3 and the right is slightly lower. Just below the diaphragm and posterior to the liver the right kidney sits; whereas, below the diaphragm and posterior to the spleen the left kidney sits. An adrenal gland is present on top of each kidney. An 11th and 12th rib partially protect the upper parts of the kidneys. Two layers of fat namely the perirenal fat (present between renal fascia and renal capsule) and pararenal fat (superior to the renal fascia) surrounds each kidney with its adrenal gland. Structure of kidney is presented in Figure 8.2.

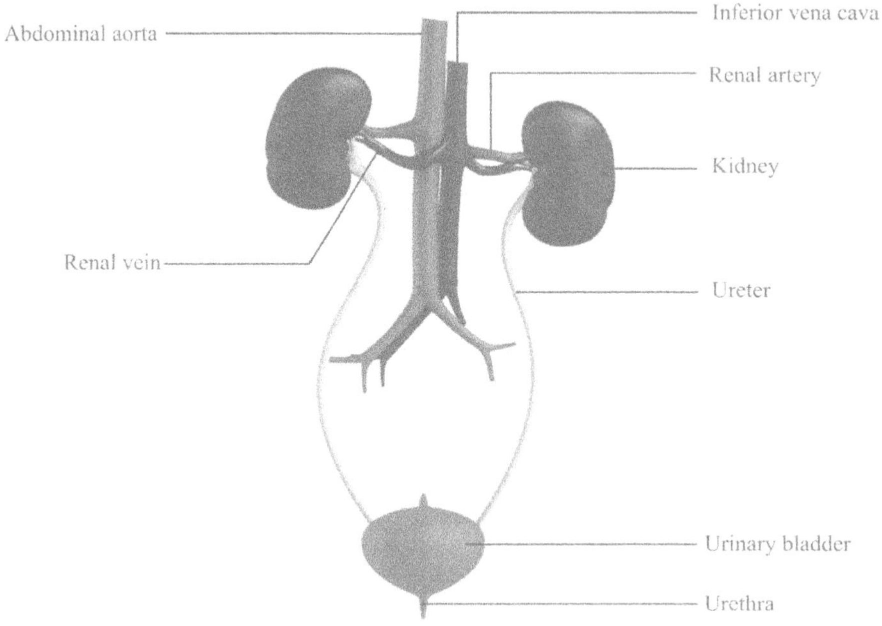

Figure 8.1 Urinary system.

External anatomy: The length of the kidney is 10 to 12 cm; width of the kidney is 5 to 7 cm and thickness of the kidney is 3 cm. A convex and a concave border are present in kidney. Renal hilum or renal hilus is the recessed area on the concave border. The renal artery enters the kidney and the renal vein and ureter leaves the kidney in renal hilum only. Three layers of tissues surround the kidney. They are,

1. **Deep inner layer (Renal capsule):** It is made up of a smooth transparent sheet of dense irregular connective tissue. It serves as barrier against trauma and used to maintain shape.
2. **Middle layer (Adipose capsule):** It is a mass of fatty tissues surrounding the renal capsule. It protects the kidney from trauma and holds the kidney within abdominal cavity.
3. **Superficial inner layer (Renal fascia):** It is a thin layer of dense irregular connective tissue surrounds adipose capsule. It anchors the kidney to the surrounding structures and the abdominal wall.

Internal anatomy: The functional substance, or parenchyma, of the kidney is divided into two major structures namely a) the outer renal cortex (superficial light red area) and b) the inner renal medulla (deep darker reddish-brown inner area). Grossly, these structures take the shape of 8 to 18 cone-shaped renal lobes, each containing renal cortex surrounding a portion of medulla called a renal pyramid. Renal columns are the projections of the cortex is present between the renal pyramids. The urine producing functional structures of the kidney i.e., nephrons separates the renal cortex and renal medulla. The renal corpuscle is the initial filtering portion of a nephron and is located in the renal cortex. A renal tubule follows this and that passes from the adrenal cortex deep into the medullary pyramids. A medullary ray is a part of the renal cortex which is a collection of renal tubules that drain into a single collecting duct. Urine is emptied into a minor calyx by the tip or papilla of each pyramid. Latter, minor calyces empty urine into major calyces and major calyces empty urine into the renal pelvis. This becomes the ureter. The renal artery enters at the hilum, and the ureter and renal vein exit the kidney at the hilum. These structures are surrounded by hilar fat and lymphatic tissue with lymph nodes. Renal sinus is a fat-filled cavity present adjacent to the hilar fat. The renal pelvis and calyces are collectively present in the renal sinus and from the renal medullary tissue it separates these structures.

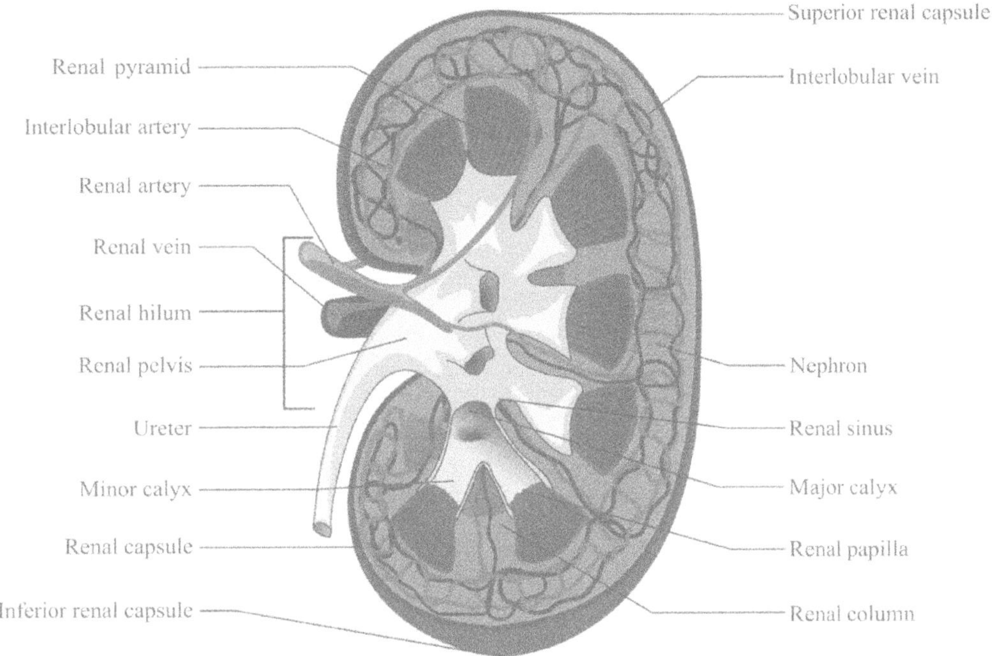

Figure 8.2 Structure of the kidney.

Nephron: The microscopic structural and functional unit of the kidney is known as nephron and is composed of a renal corpuscle and a renal tubule. Glomerulus (a tuft of capillaries) and an encompassing Bowman's capsule or glomerular capsules are present in the renal corpuscle. From the Bowman's capsule, the renal tubule extends. Both renal tubule and Bowman's capsule are composed of epithelial cells with a lumen and are connected. In each kidney, about 1 to 1.5 million nephrons are present in a healthy adult. Blood is filtered as it passes through three layers: the endothelial cells of the capillary wall, its basement membrane, and between the foot processes of the podocytes of the lining of the capsule. Diagram of a long *juxtamedullary nephron* and of a short *cortical nephron* is presented in Figure 8.3.

Blood is converted into urine by four mechanisms in the nephron. They are a) filtration, b) reabsorption, c) secretion and d) excretion. The followings are the major parts of the nephron.

1. **Proximal convoluted tubule:** It reabsorbs more than half of the filtered salt and water and all filtered organic solutes primarily glucose and amino acids into the peritubular capillaries.
2. **Loop of Henle:** It enables the organism to produce concentrated urine by rendering the interstitial fluid hypertonic and not by increasing the tubular concentration. The descending limb is permeable to water; hence water flows freely out of the descending limb by osmosis until the tonicity of the filtrate and interstitium equilibrate. The ascending limb is impermeable to water and actively pumps sodium out of the filtrate and made filtrate hypotonic.
3. **Distal convoluted tubule:** It reabsorbs more calcium and secretes more phosphate in presence of parathyroid hormone. It reabsorbs more sodium and secretes more potassium in the presence of aldosterone. More sodium is secreted in the presence of atrial natriuretic peptide.
4. **Collection duct:** Normally it is impermeable to water and it becomes permeable in the presence of antidiuretic hormone (ADH).

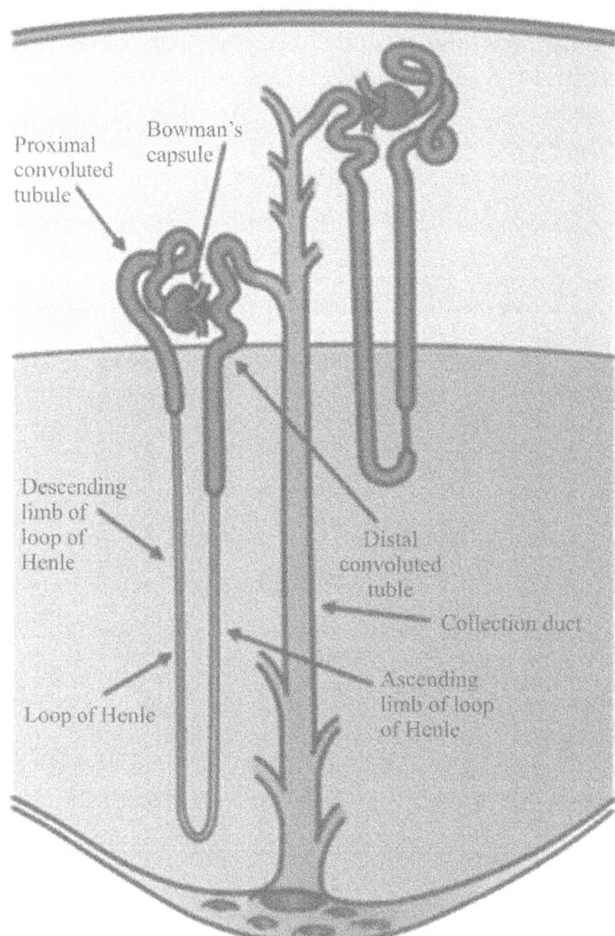

Figure 8.3 Diagram (left) of a long *juxtamedullary nephron* and (right) of a short *cortical nephron*.

Juxtaglomerular apparatus (JGA): It is a specialized region associated with the nephron, but separate from nephron. It produces and secretes the enzyme *renin* or *angiotensinogenase* into the circulation which cleaves angiotensinogen into angiotensin.

Urine Analysis

Urine is an excretory product formed by the kidneys. The composition of urine is not only a mirror of renal function. It is also a mirror of many physiological and metabolic processes occurring in the body. Hence, a quick and convenient method for obtaining considerable diagnostic value is the analysis of urine. In general, depends on several factors the composition of urine greatly varies. The followings are the chief constituents of urine.

1. Water
2. Inorganic constituents
3. Organic constituents

Urine collection:

The composition of urine may considerably vary within a day; hence 24 hours of urine is preferred for examination. This 24-hour urine is collected by asking the person to void in the morning for example 6 AM. Discard this urine and collect all the urine passed during the day and night till next day 6 AM and collect the urine of 6 AM on next day morning also. Mix well all the urine sample collected throughout the day. Soon after the collection of the sample it is better to examine it. A preservative like thymol crystal, few drops of formaldehyde or toluene is added to the urine sample to prevent the growth of bacteria and molds if the delay is unavoidable.

Physical examination:

1. **Urine volume or urine output:** The volume of urine output for 24 hours is collected and measured. The normal daily output of urine is 800 ml to 2000 ml and it may vary from 600 ml to 2500 ml under certain physiological conditions. If the increased output of urine is observed it may know as polyuria and it occurs in diabetes mellitus, diabetes insipidus, chronic renal failure and after use of drugs like diuretics, salicylate and digitalis. If the decreased output of urine is observed it may know as oliguria and it occurs in nephritis, fever, diarrhoea and vomiting, bilateral obstruction of the uterus, renal stone and Addison's disease. If urine formation is suppressed then the condition is known as anuria and it mainly occurs during shock, acute nephritis and incompatible blood transfusion, mercury poisoning and bilateral stone formation.
2. **Appearance:** The clarity of urine is observed. In general, normal urine is clear and transparent when freshly collected. On standing it may become turbid due to precipitation of mucoproteins and nucleoproteins. In alkaline and acid urine ammonium urate and other urates are precipitated, respectively. Fresh urine itself looks milky or turbid due to presence of pus or bacterial cells (occurs in urinary tract infection) or presence of chyle (occurs in filariasis) or casts or crystals. On adding chyle will dissolve but microscopic examination is needed in other cases.
3. **Color:** The color of the urine is observed. Amber yellow is the color of normal urine due to the presence of pigments such as urochrome, uroerythrin, uroporphyrin and coproporphyrin. Based on the urinary output the color may deepen or lighten. Abnormal color of urine may due to the presence of other pigments or drugs or dyes, etc.
   (a) In hepatic and obstructive jaundice, the urine may be deep yellow or greenish-yellow due to the presence of bile pigments.
   (b) The urine becomes pink to red color due to presence of a) hemoglobin in various conditions, b) porphyrins in porphyria and c) pyridium - a drug.
   (c) Brown or black color urine due to presence of melanin in malignant melanoma.
   (d) Brownish-yellow color urine due to laxatives such as rhubarb and senna.
   (e) When freshly voided the urine is normal in color. But on standing, darkens due to presence of homogentisic acid in alkaptonuria.
4. **Odor:** The odor of urine is observed. The aromatic odor is the characteristic odor of normal urine due to presence of some volatile organic acids. In ketoacidosis, the fruity odor is observed due to presence of acetone. In phenylketonuria, the mousy odor is observed due to the presence of phenylacetyl glutamine. In certain urinary tract infection (UTI), an ammoniacal odor is observed due to microorganism. Abnormal urine odor is also produced by certain foods and drugs.
5. **pH:** The pH of urine is tested mostly using litmus paper. Normal urine is usually slightly acidic. Sometimes it may be slightly alkaline also. The pH of urine may vary depends on nature of the diet. Protein-rich diet produces acidic urine and fruits and vegetables produce alkaline urine. The urine is acidic in clinical conditions like fever, diabetes mellitus, starvation and diarrhea. The urine is acidic basic in clinical conditions like severe vomiting and urinary tract infections (UTI). Ingestion of alkalis like sodium bicarbonate may also produce alkaline urine.
6. **Specific gravity:** The specific gravity of urine is determined by urinometer. The specific gravity of normal urine is 1.012 to 1.024. Specific gravity is increased in conditions that are accompanied with low urine volume like acute glomerulonephritis, diabetes mellitus, fever and dehydration. Specific gravity is decreased in conditions that are accompanied by increased urine volume like diabetes insipidus and chronic glomerulonephritis.

Chemical examination for inorganic constituents:

1. **Test for chloride:** To 2 ml of urine sample in a test tube add few drops of concentrated nitric acid and 2 ml 10 % silver nitrate solution. Formation of a curdy white precipitate indicates the presence of

chloride in urine sample. In this test, chloride present in the urine sample reacts with silver nitrate in the presence of concentrated nitric acid and precipitated as white color silver chloride.

Take **2 ml of urine sample** in a test tube

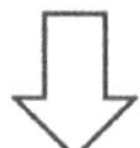

Add **few drops of concentrated nitric acid and 2 ml 10 % silver nitrate** solution

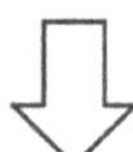

Formation of a **curdy white precipitate**

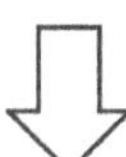

Indicates the **presence of chloride** in urine sample

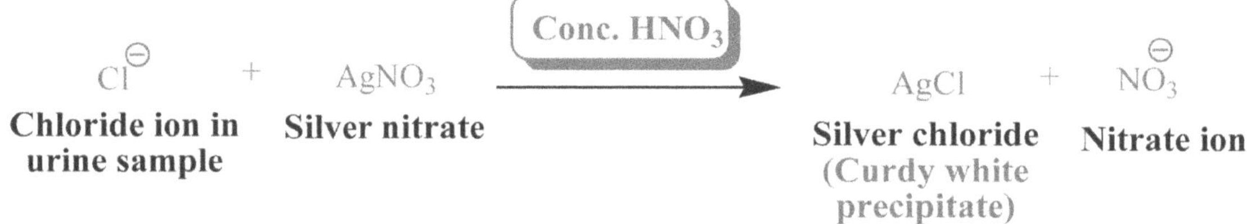

2. **Test for sulphate:** To 2 ml of urine sample in a test tube, add two drops of concentrated hydrochloric acid and 2 ml 10 % barium chloride solution. Formation of thick white precipitate which is insoluble in concentrated hydrochloric acid indicates the presence of sulphate in urine sample. In this test, sulphate present in the urine sample reacts with barium chloride in the presence of concentrated hydrochloric acid and precipitated as white color barium sulphate.

Take **2 ml of urine sample** in a test tube

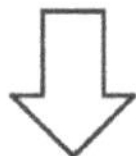

Add **two drops of concentrated hydrochloric acid and 2 ml 10 % barium chloride solution**

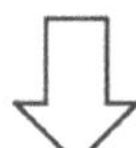

Formation of a **thick white precipitate**
(Insoluble in concentrated hydrochloric acid)

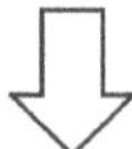

Indicates the **presence of sulphate** in urine sample

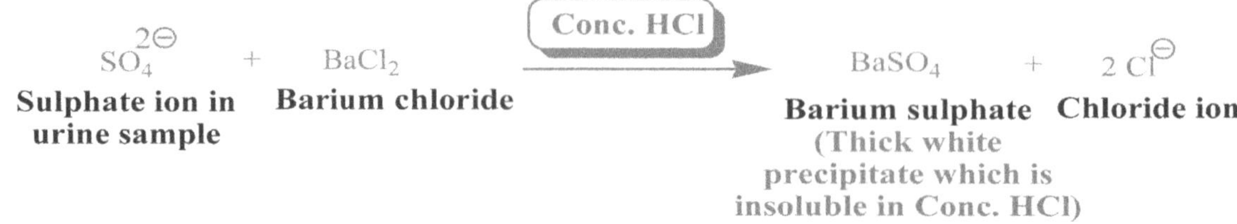

3. **Test for calcium:** To 5 ml of urine sample in a test tube, add five drops of 1 % acetic acid and 5 ml 2 % potassium oxalate solution. Formation of white precipitate indicates the presence of calcium in the urine sample. In this test, calcium present in urine sample reacts with potassium oxalate in the presence of 1 % acetic acid and precipitated as white color calcium oxalate.

Take **5 ml of urine sample** in a test tube

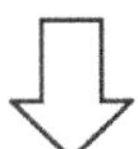

Add **five drops of 1 % acetic acid and 5 ml 2 % potassium oxalate solution**

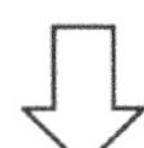

Formation of a **white precipitate**

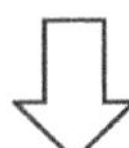

Indicates the **presence of calcium** in urine sample

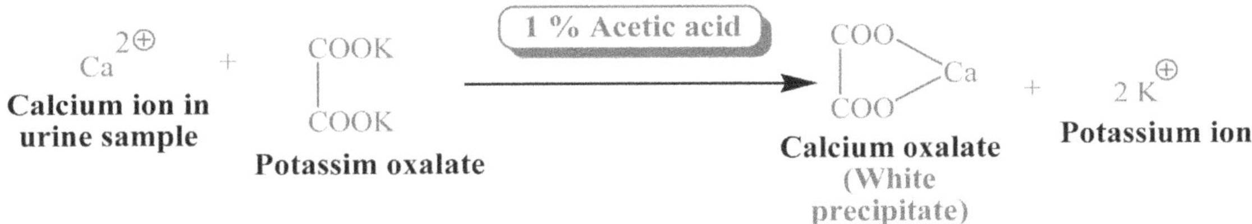

4. **Test for phosphate:** To 3 ml of urine sample in a test tube, add 3 ml of concentrated nitric acid and 3 ml of ammonium molybdate solution. Heat the mixture to boil in the water-bath. Formation of canary-yellow precipitate indicates the presence of phosphate in urine sample. In this test, phosphate present in urine sample reacts with ammonium molybdate in the presence of concentrated nitric acid and precipitated as canary-yellow color ammonium phosphomolybdate.

Take **3 ml of urine sample** in a test tube

Add **3 ml of concentrated nitric acid and 3 ml of ammonium molybdate solution**

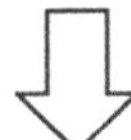

Heat the mixture to boil in the water-bath

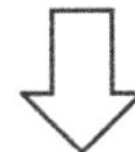

Formation of a **canary-yellow precipitate**

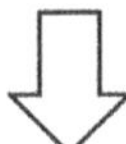

Indicates the **presence of phosphate** in urine sample

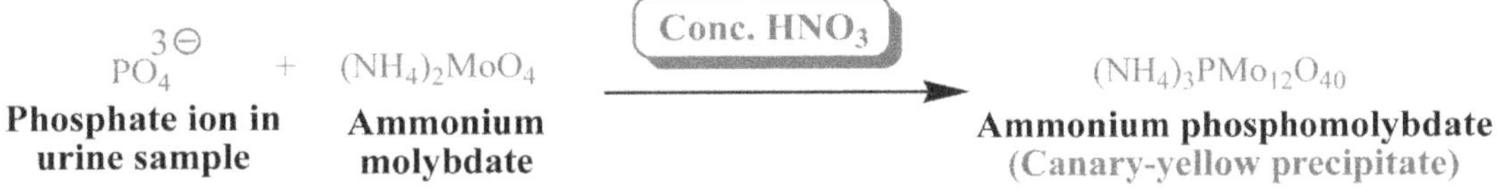

5. **Test for ammonia:** Heat 5 ml of urine sample in a test tube to boil and hold the piece of moist red litmus paper over the mouth of test tube. Turning of red litmus into blue indicates the presence of ammonia in urine sample. In this test, ammonia present in the urine sample is evolved as gas when heated and it changes red litmus into blue color.

Heat **5 ml of urine sample** in a test tube

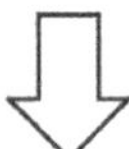

Hold the piece of **moist red litmus paper over the mouth of test tube**

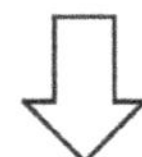

Turning of red litmus into blue

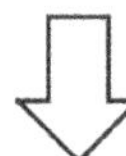

Indicates the **presence of ammonia** in urine sample

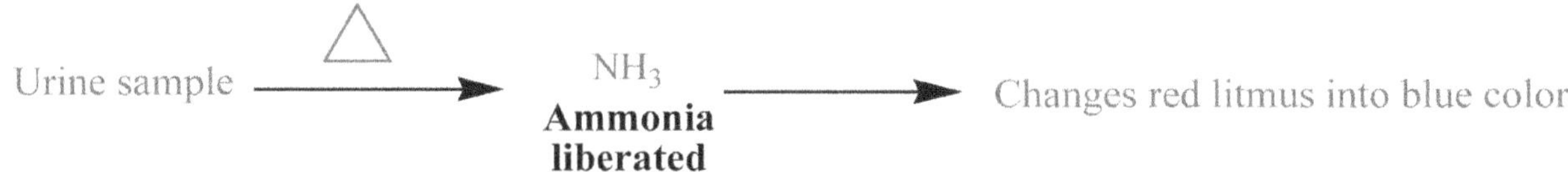

6. **Test for bicarbonate:** To 5 ml of urine sample in a test tube, add few ml of dilute hydrochloric acid and lime water. Turning of lime water into milky white indicates the presence of bicarbonate in the urine sample. In this test, bicarbonate present in urine sample reacts with dilute hydrochloric acid and liberates carbondioxide which turns lime water into milky white.

Take **5 ml of urine sample** in a test tube

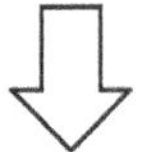

Add **few ml of dilute hydrochloric acid and lime water**

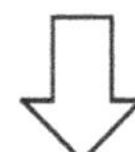

Turning of lime water into milky white

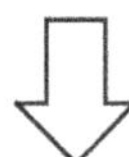

Indicates the **presence of bicarbonate** in urine sample

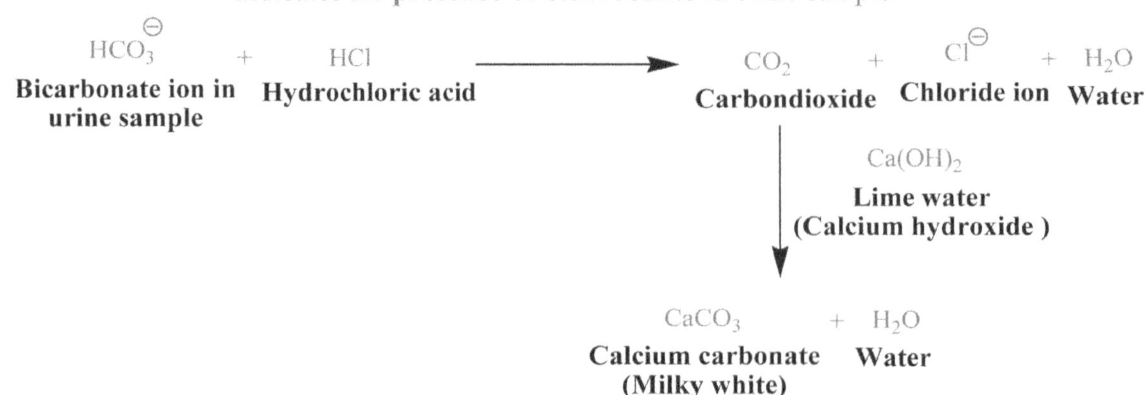

Chemical examination for organic constituents:

1. **Test for urea:**

   (a) **Sodium hypobromite test:** To 5 ml of urine sample in a test tube, add 1 ml of freshly prepared alkaline sodium hypobromite solution. Formation of a brisk effervescence of nitrogen gas indicates the presence of urea in urine sample. In this test, urea present in urine sample decomposed when reacting with sodium hypobromite and liberates nitrogen and carbondioxide gas. The carbondioxide gas formed is absorbed by sodium hydroxide and produced sodium carbonate. Hence the evolved nitrogen gas gives brisk effervescence.

Take **5 ml of urine sample** in a test tube

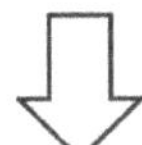

Add **1 ml of freshly prepared alkaline sodium hypobromite solution**

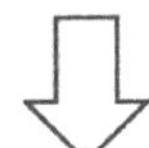

Formation of a **brisk effervescence of nitrogen gas**

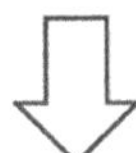

Indicates the **presence of urea** in urine sample

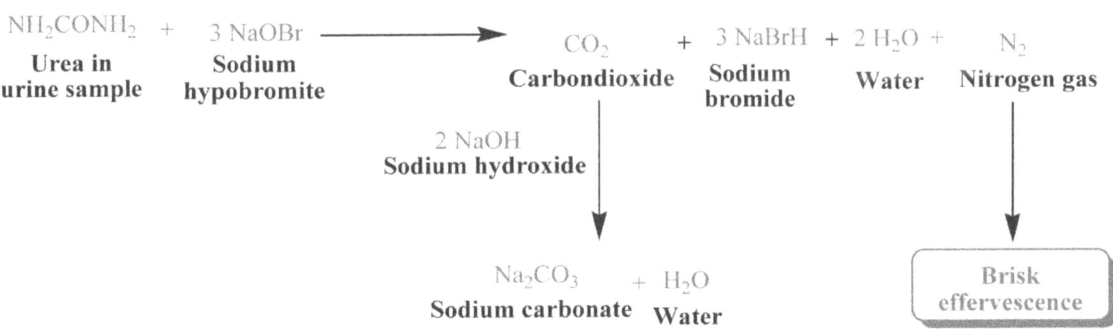

   (b) ***Urease* test:** To 5 ml of urine sample in a test tube, add a small amount of soya bean meal or jack bean meal and one to two drops of phenol red indicator. Mix well the mixture and allow to stand for 10 to 15 minutes. The change of yellow color of solution into red color indicates the presence of urea in the urine sample. In this test, *urease* enzyme present in soya bean meal or jack bean meal hydrolyzes urea present in urine sample and liberates ammonia and carbondioxide. The evolved ammonia changes the yellow color of phenol red indicator into red color (pH: 6.7 to 8.3).

   (c) **Test for peptide linkages and proteins (Biuret test or Piotrowski's test):** Perform this test with solid urea. Heat gently about 1 g of solid urea in porcelain dish over a small flame. The urea melts and continues to heat until it solidifies again. Cool and dissolve the residue in 3 ml of 10 % sodium hydroxide. Add one or two drops of 0.5 % copper sulphate solution to this and mix well. The appearance of purplish-violet color indicates the presence of urea in the sample. In this test, melted and resolidified urea reacts with copper sulphate in the presence of sodium hydroxide and produced purplish-violet color biuret.

Take **5 ml of urine sample** in a test tube

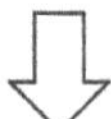

Add a **small amount of soya bean meal or jack bean meal and one to two drops of phenol red indicator**

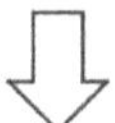

Mix well the mixture and allow to stand for 10 to 15 minutes

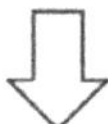

Change of yellow color of solution into red color

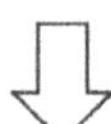

Indicates the **presence of urea** in urine sample

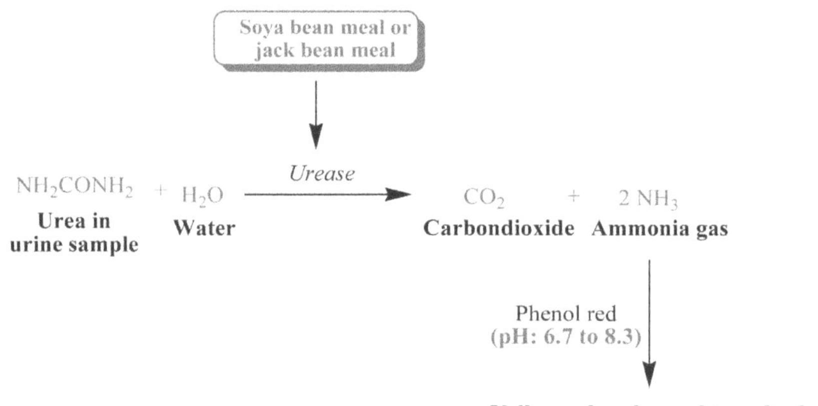

Heat 1g solid urea in porcelain dish over a small flame

Urea melts

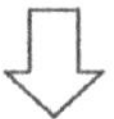

Continues to heat untill it solidifies again

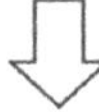

Cool & dissolve the residue in 3 ml of 10% sodium hydroxide

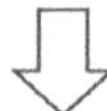

Add 1 or 2 drops of 0.5% copper sulphate solution & mix well

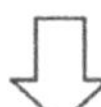

Appearance of purplish-violet color

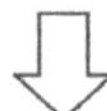

Indicates presence of urea in urine sample

$NH_2-C(=O)-NH_2$ **Urea in urine sample (Excess)** $\xrightarrow{180\ °C}$ $NH_2-C(=O)-NH-C(=O)-NH_2$ **Biuret (Carbamylurea)** $\xrightarrow[\text{NaOH Sodium hydroxide}]{\text{CuSO}_4 \text{ Copper sulphate}}$ **Biuret complex (Purplish-violet color)** ($Cu^{2\oplus}$ coordinated by the N–H of two biuret molecules)

2. **Test for uric acid:**

   (a) **Phosphotungstic reduction test or Benedict's test for uric acid:** To 5 ml of urine sample in a test tube, add a pinch of sodium carbonate and mix well. Add five drops of Benedict's uric acid reagent (a mixture of sodium tungstate, arsenic pentoxide, phosphoric acid and concentrated hydrochloric acid) to the above solutions and mix well. Formation of blue color indicates the presence of uric acid in the urine sample. In this test, uric acid present in urine sample reduces colorless arsenophosphotungstate of Benedict's uric acid reagent to blue colored arsenophosphotungstite in the presence of alkaline sodium carbonate.

Take **5 ml of urine sample** in a test tube

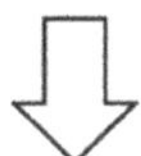

Add **five drops of Benedict's uric acid reagent** and mix well.

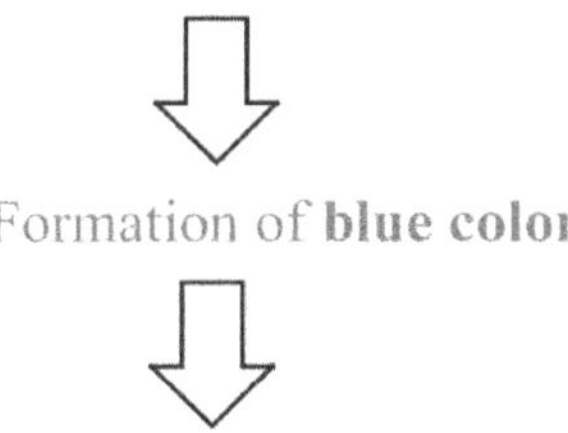

Indicates the **presence of uric acid** in urine sample

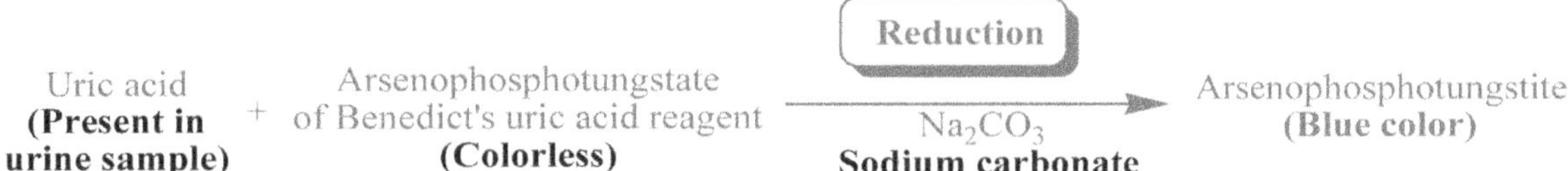

   (b) **Schiff's test:** Wet a piece of filter paper with few drops of ammoniacal silver nitrate solution and add 2 drops of urine sample. Formation of black color on the paper indicate the presence of uric acid in urine sample. In this test, uric acid present in urine sample reduces colorless ammoniacal silver nitrate to black metallic silver.

Wet a piece of filter paper with few drops of ammoniacal silver nitrate solution

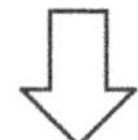

Add 2 drops of urine sample

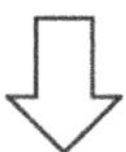

Formation of **black color on the paper**

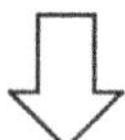

Indicates the **presence of uric acid** in urine sample

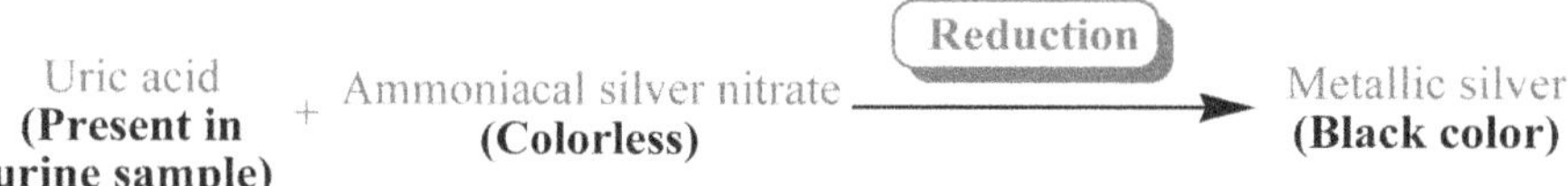

(c) **Murexide test for solid uric acid:** To a 100 ml of urine sample in a beaker, add 5 ml of concentrated hydrochloric acid, mix and allow to stand for 24 hours. Filter the separated uric acid crystals and use for this test. To a small pinch of solid uric acid separated from urine sample in a clean and dry porcelain dish, add two to three drops of concentrated nitric acid and heat gently over a small flame until dry. Cool and add a drop of dilute ammonia. Formation of purplish-red color indicates the presence of uric acid. In this test, uric acid is initially oxidized to dialuric acid and alloxan by concentrated nitric acid. Later, obtained dialuric acid and alloxan are condensed to form alloxantin. When dilute ammonia is added, it reacts with alloxantin and forms purplish-red color ammonium purpurate i.e., murexide.

Take a **100 ml of urine sample** in a beaker

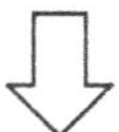

Add **5 ml of concentrated hydrochloric acid**, mix and allow to stand for 24 hours

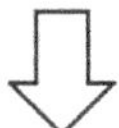

Filter the separated uric acid crystals

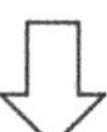

Take a **small pinch of solid uric acid** separated from urine sample in a clean and dry porcelain dish

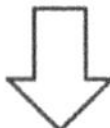

Add **two to three drops of concentrated nitric acid and** heat gently over a small flame until dry

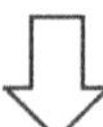

Cool and add a **drop of dilute ammonia**

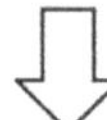

Formation of **purplish-red color**

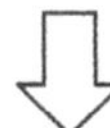

Indicates the **presence of uric acid** in urine sample

Oxidation
Conc. HNO_3

Uric acid (Present in urine sample)

Dialuric acid + Alloxan

Rewritten

Condensation

Alloxantin

$- 2 H_2O$ Water
$2 NH_3$ Dilute ammonia

Murexide or Ammonium purpurate (Purplish-red color)

3. **Test for creatinine:**
   (a) **Jaffe's test:** To 5 ml of urine sample in a test tube, add 2 ml of the saturated picric acid solution and 0.5 ml of 10 % sodium hydroxide solution. Mix well the solution and keep aside for 5 minutes. Formation of deep orange color indicates the presence of creatinine in the urine sample. In this test, the creatinine present in urine sample is reacted with picric acid in the presence of alkaline sodium hydroxide to produce deep orange color creatinine picrate.

Creatinine + Picric acid **(Present in urine sample)** —NaOH / Sodium hydroxide→ Creatinine picrate **(Deep orange colour)**

   (b) **Weyl's test:** To 5 ml of urine sample in a test tube, 5 drops of sodium nitroprusside solution and 2 ml of sodium hydroxide solution were added. Formation of red color and soon it changes to yellow color indicates the presence of creatinine in the urine sample. In this test, creatinine present in urine sample is reacted with sodium nitroprusside in presence of alkaline sodium hydroxide to produce red color and soon it changes to yellow color.

Take **5 ml of urine sample** in a test tube

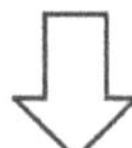

Add 2 ml of the saturated picric acid solution and 0.5 ml of 10 % sodium hydroxide solution

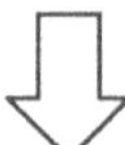

Mix well the solution and keep aside for 5 minutes

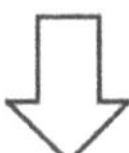

Formation of **deep orange** color

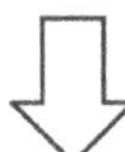

Indicates the **presence of uric acid** in urine sample

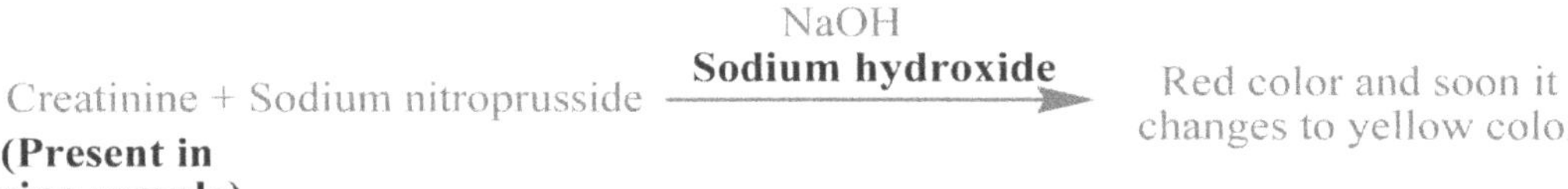

Chemical examination for abnormal constituents:

1. **Test for proteins:**

   (a) **Sulphosalicylic acid test:** To 3 ml of clear urine (Filter if turbid) in a test tube, add 1 ml of 20 % sulphosalicylic acid. Formation of white precipitate indicates the presence of protein in urine sample. This test is employed for preliminary screening of urine for proteins and is not specific for albumin and globulin.

Take **3 ml of clear urine** (Filter if turbid) in a test tube

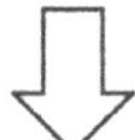

Add 1 ml of 20 % sulphosalicylic acid

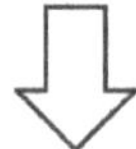

Indicates the **presence of protein** in urine sample

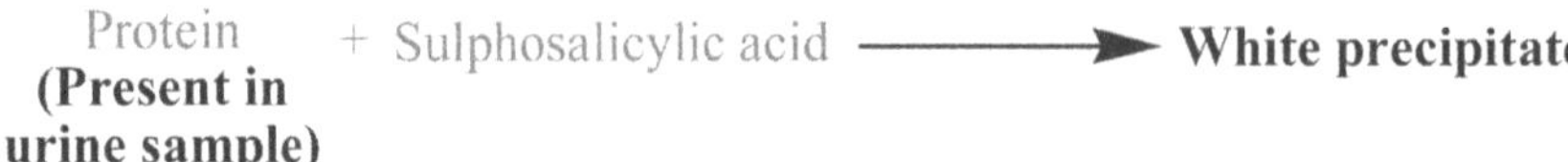

   (b) **Heller's test:** To 3 ml of concentrated nitric acid in a test tube, add 2 ml of urine along the sides of test tube. Formation of a white ring at the junction of two layers indicates the presence of protein in the urine sample. This test is more specific than sulphosalicylic acid test.

Take **3 ml of concentrated nitric acid** in a test tube

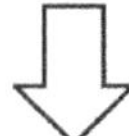

Add **2 ml of urine** along the sides of test tube

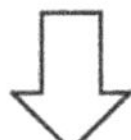

Formation of white ring at the junction of two layers

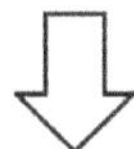

Indicates the **presence of protein** in urine sample

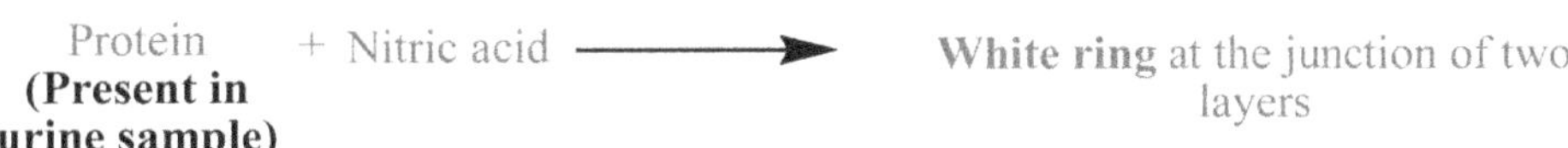

Protein **(Present in urine sample)** + Nitric acid ⟶ **White ring** at the junction of two layers

(c) **Heat coagulation test:** In a test tube take 2 ml of urine and heat it. Formation of coagulation indicates the presence of albumin and globulin in the urine sample.

Take **2 ml of urine** in a test tube

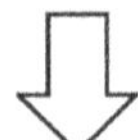

Heat the sample solution

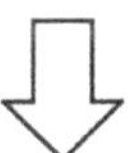

Formation of coagulation

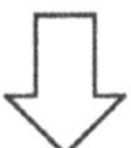

Indicates the **presence of protein** such as albumin and globulin in urine sample

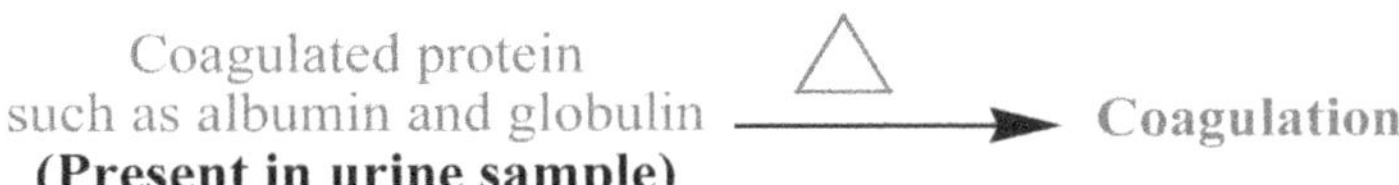

Coagulated protein such as albumin and globulin **(Present in urine sample)** $\xrightarrow{\triangle}$ **Coagulation**

(d) **Heat & acetic acid test:** Heat the upper half of 5 ml urine sample (Lower half act as control) in a test tube and add few drops of 1 % acetic acid. The appearance of cloudy white precipitate in the heated portion indicates the presence of albumin and globulin in the urine sample.

Heat the upper half of 5 ml urine sample (Lower half act as control) in a test tube

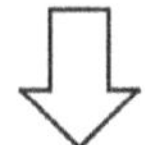

Add few drops of 1 % acetic acid

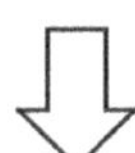

Appearance of cloudy white precipitate

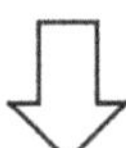

Indicates the **presence of protein** such as albumin and globulin in urine sample

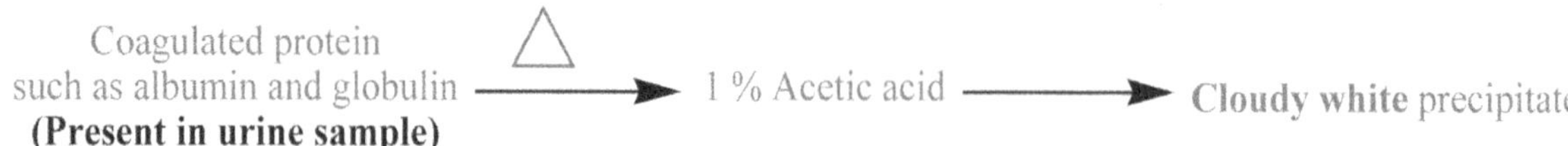

Coagulated protein such as albumin and globulin **(Present in urine sample)** —△→ 1 % Acetic acid ——→ **Cloudy white** precipitate

2. **Test for carbohydrates (reducing sugars):**
   To a 5 ml of Benedict's reagent in a test tube, add 8 drops of urine and boil for 2 minutes and cool. Formation of green / greenish-yellow / yellow / orange / brick-red precipitate indicates the presence of reducing sugars particularly glucose in urine sample. The appearance of green color indicates presence of trace amount of glucose in urine sample; greenish-yellow color indicates presence of 0.5 % glucose in urine sample; yellow color indicates presence of 1 % glucose in urine sample; orange color indicates presence of 1.5 % glucose in urine sample; and brick-red color indicates the presence of 2 % & above glucose in urine sample.

Take **5 ml of Benedict's reagent** in a test tube

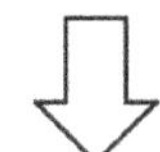

Add 8 drops of urine

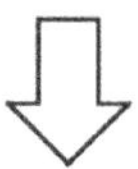

Boil for 2 minutes & cool it

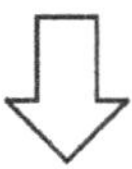

Formation of **green / greenish-yellow / yellow / orange / brick-red precipitate**

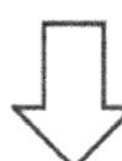

Indicates the **presence of reducing sugar**s particularly glucose in urine sample

Carbohydrates particularly reducing sugars **(Present in urine sample)** + Benedict's reagent ——→ **Green / greenish-yellow / yellow / orange / brick red** precipitate

3. **Test for ketone bodies:**
   (a) **Rothera's test:** To a 5 ml of urine sample in a test tube, add ammonium sulphate until saturation. To this mixture add 2-3 drops of freshly prepared 5 % sodium nitroprusside solution, mix well and add 1 ml of concentrated ammonium hydroxide along the sides of test tube without mixing. Formation of a purple ring at the junction of two layers indicates the presence of ketone bodies such as acetone and acetoacetic acid in urine sample. This test does not respond to ketone bodies like β-hydroxybutyric acid.
   (b) **Gerhard's test:** To a 5 ml of urine sample in a test tube, add 10 % ferric chloride solution drop by drop until maximum precipitate appears and filter it. To the filtrate, add a few drops of 10 % ferric chloride solution. The appearance of wine-red color indicates the presence of ketone bodies such as acetoacetic acid in the urine sample.

Take **5 ml of** urine sample in a test tube

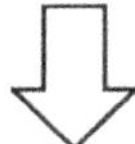

Add **ammonium sulphate** until saturation

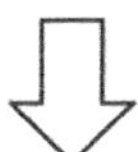

Add **2-3 drops of freshly prepared 5 % sodium nitroprusside solution and mix well**

Add **1 ml of concentrated ammonium hydroxide** along the sides of test tube without mixing

Formation of a **purple ring at the junction** of two layers

Indicates the **presence of ketone bodies such as acetone and acetoacetic acid** in urine sample

Ketone bodies particularly acetone and acetoacetic acid **(Present in urine sample)** + Ammonium sulphate + Sodium nitroprusside

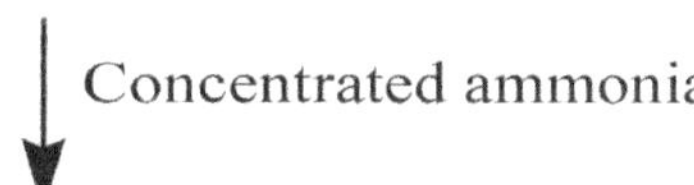

Purple ring at the junction of two layers

Take **5 ml of urine sample** in a test tube

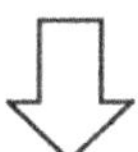

Add 10 % ferric chloride solution drop by drop until maximum precipitate appears and filter it

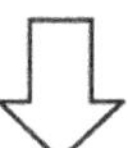

To the filtrate, add a **few drops of 10 % ferric chloride** solution

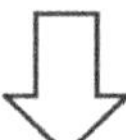

Appearance of **wine-red color**

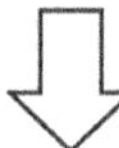

Indicates the **presence of ketone bodies such as acetoacetic acid** in urine sample

Ketone bodies particularly acetoacetic acid **(Present in urine sample)** + Ferric chloride ⟶ **Wine-red** color

4. **Test for bile salts (Hay's test):**
   To a 5 ml of urine sample in a test tube, sprinkle sulphur powder over the surface of urine. If sulphur sinks to the bottom of the test tube it indicates the presence of bile salts.

Take **5 ml of urine sample** in a test tube

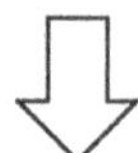

Sprinkle sulphur powder over the surface of urine

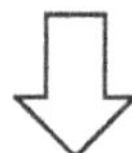

Sulphur sinks to the bottom of the test tube

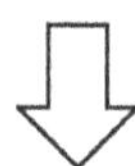

Indicates the **presence of bile salts in** urine sample

Bile salts **(Present in urine sample)** + Sulphur powder ⟶ Sulphur sinks to the bottom of test tube

5. **Test for bile pigments:**
   (a) **Fouchet's test:** To a 5 ml of urine sample in a test tube, add 5 ml of 10 % barium chloride, and 1 mg magnesium sulphate. Mix well and filter after 5 minutes. Dry the obtained precipitate and treat with Fouchet's reagent (Ferric chloride + trichloro acetic acid). The appearance of green or blue color indicates the presence of bile pigments in urine sample.

Take **5 ml of urine sample** in a test tube

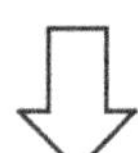

Add **5 ml of 10 % barium chloride, and 1 mg magnesium sulphate**

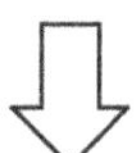

Mix well and filter after 5 minutes

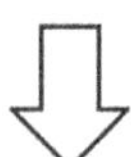

Dry the obtained precipitate and treat with **Fouchet's reagent**

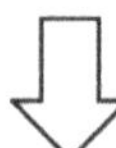

Appearance of green or blue color

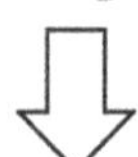

Indicates the **presence of bile pigments** in urine sample

Bile pigments **(Present in urine sample)** + Barium chloride + Magnesium sulphate + Fouchet's reagent

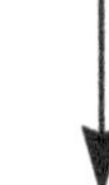

Green or blue color

6. **Test for blood:**

Pus present in the urine sample may also respond to this test. However, if urine is acidified with acetic acid and boiled, blood will still give the tests whereas pus will not.

(a) **Benzidine test:** To a 2 ml of urine sample in a test tube, add a mixture of 2-3 drops of benzidine solution and 2 drops of hydrogen peroxide. Appearance of green color immediately and disappearance in a few seconds indicates the presence of blood in urine sample.

Take **2 ml of urine sample** in a test tube

⇩

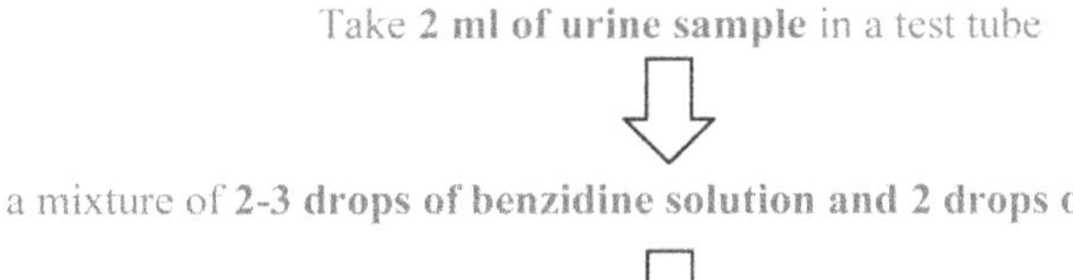

Add a mixture of **2-3 drops of benzidine solution and 2 drops of hydrogen peroxide**

⇩

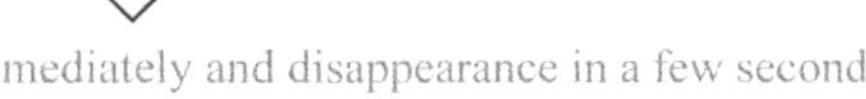

Appearance of green color immediately and disappearance in a few seconds

⇩

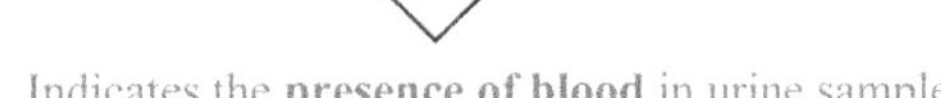

Indicates the **presence of blood** in urine sample

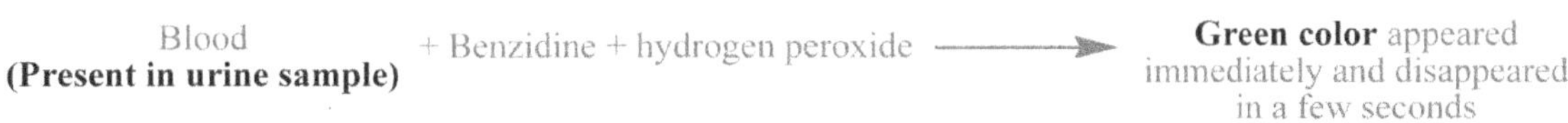

Blood **(Present in urine sample)** + Benzidine + hydrogen peroxide ⟶ **Green color** appeared immediately and disappeared in a few seconds

(b) ***o*-Toluidine test:** To five drops of urine sample in a test tube, add about 5 mg of solid *o*-toluidine and mix well. Place a drop of this mixture on a small piece of Whatman filter paper No. 1 on a white porcelain tile. To this add one drop of acid peroxide reagent. Appearance of blue-green color indicates the presence of blood in urine sample.

Take **five drops of urine sample** in a test tube

Add about **5 mg of solid *o*-toluidine** and mix well

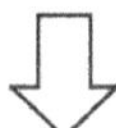

Place a drop of this mixture on a **small piece of Whatman filter paper No. 1** on a white porcelain tile

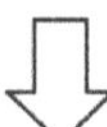

Add **one drop of acid peroxide reagent**

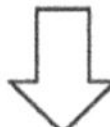

Appearance of **blue-green color**

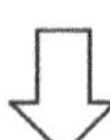

Indicates the **presence of blood** in urine sample

Blood **(Present in urine sample)** + *o*-Toluidine + Acid-peroxide reagent ⟶ Blue-green color

Recently, abnormal constituents present in the urine sample are detected using some dip-strip or read-strips. In this plastic strip, for different abnormal constituent separate reagent areas are present. When the strip is dipped in urine, the color developed on the different reagent area is compared with a standard color chart after specific time intervals. These strips are expensive but convenient and time-saving one.

Organ Function Test

Proper functioning of various vital organs of biological systems or body is determined by using organ function test. **Example:** Kidney function test, liver function test, gastric function test, pancreatic function test, thyroid function test, etc.

Functions of Kidney

Kidney is the vital organ of the body because it performs several important biochemical functions as follows:

1. **Maintenance of homeostasis:** Kidney plays an important role in the maintenance of water, electrolyte and acid-base balance in the biological systems.
2. **Waste products excretion:** Kidney excretes metabolic waste products produced in the body. Kidney excretes the end products of protein & nucleic acid metabolism including urea, creatinine, creatine, uric acid, phosphate and sulphate.
3. **Retention of vital substances:** Kidney reabsorbs and retains some important constituents which are biologically important for body. **Example:** Electrolytes, glucose, amino acids, etc.
4. **Hormonal function:** Kidney can act as endocrine organs through secretion of following substances.
   (a) **Erythropoietin:** It is a peptide hormone stimulates the synthesis & formation of hemoglobin and erythrocytes.
   (b) **Calcitriol:** It is chemically 1, 25-dihydroxy cholecalciferol. It is the active form of vitamin-D which regulates calcium absorption from the gut.
   (c) **Renin:** It is a proteolytic enzyme liberated by kidney. It stimulates the formation of angiotensin–II which leads to the production of aldosterone. Angiotensin–II & aldosterone are the hormones involved in the regulation of electrolyte balance.

Types of Kidney Function Test

Kidney function test is defined as the tests which are used to assess the functions of kidney. As the kidney plays a vital role in biological system the disturbed function of kidneys may leads to severe complications. Hence, it is necessary to determine the improper functioning or deficient functioning of kidney as early as possible. There are several tests which are useful to assess the functioning of kidney but these entire test gives positive report only after $2/3^{rd}$ of the kidney cells are damaged. Kidney function tests are broadly classified into four major types.

1. **Glomerular function test or clearance test:** These tests are used to assess the functions of glomerular filtration or clearance ability of the kidney. **Example:** Inulin clearance test, urea clearance test and creatinine clearance test.
2. **Tubular function test:** These tests assess the functions of kidney based on tubular re-absorption. **Example:** Urine concentration test, urine dilution test and urine acidification test.
3. **Analysis of serum / blood:** These tests are based on the estimation of certain substance present in serum or blood. **Example:** Blood urea estimation, serum creatinine estimation, serum protein estimation, and serum electrolyte estimation.
4. **Urine analysis test:** These tests are based on analysis of urine sample for the presence of some abnormal constituents. **Example:** Volume of urine, pH of urine, specific gravity of urine, presence of abnormal constituents like proteins, reducing sugars, bile salts, bile pigments, etc.

Glomerular Function Test

It is the most important renal function test used to find out the abnormalities of the kidney. **It is also known as "clearance test"**. These tests are based on glomerular function and measuring the glomerular filtration rate (GFR). Compare to other tests, these tests will provide accurate results.

Clearance tests: Clearance is defined as the volume of plasma that would be completely cleared of particular substances per minute or ml of plasma which contains the amount of that particular substances excreted by kidney per minute. The unit of clearance is ml/min and can be calculated by using the following formula.

$$C = \frac{U \times V}{P}$$

Where, C = Clearance of substance (in ml/min)
U = Concentration of substance in urine (in mmol/l or mg/dl)
V = Volume of urine excreted per minute (in ml)
P = Concentration of substance in plasma (in mmol/l or mg/dl)

The clearance of a given substance is determined by its mode of excretion. The maximum rate at which the plasma cleared of any substances is equal to GFR. This can be easily calculated by measuring the clearance of a plasma compound which is freely filtered by the glomerulus and is neither absorbed nor secreted in the tubule. The substance which is used to determine the GFR is inulin and (chromium) ^{51}Cr-EDTA. Inulin is hetero polysaccharides which are composed of fructose units and is administered through *i.v.* route to measure GFR.

In normal practice, the substances which are already present in the biological system is used to determine the clearance. **Example:** Creatinine and urea. Creatinine is secreted by the tubules; hence, creatinine clearance (-145 ml/min) is marginally higher than the GFR. Whereas urea is partially re-absorbed by the tubules, hence urea clearance (-75 ml/min) is less than the GFR.

The substance called "Diodrast" (Diiodopyridone acetic acid) is generally used as a contrast medium to take urinary tract X-rays. Diodrast and para-amino hippuric acid (PAH) are the peculiar substances as they are entirely excreted by a single passage of blood through kidneys. It is partly filtered by the glomerulus and mostly excreted by the tubules. The clearance of PAH is around 700 ml/min (1200 ml if expressed as blood). Hence, clearance of PAH represents the renal plasma flow.

Creatinine Clearance Test

Creatinine is an excretory substance obtained from creatinine phosphate which is largely present in the muscle. The concentration of creatinine excretion in the biological system is rather constant and is not altered by body metabolism or dietary factors. Creatinine is filtered by the glomeruli and only marginally secreted by the tubules. The creatinine clearance value is closer to GFR. Hence it is a very sensitive test and gives accurate results to assess the renal glomerular function.

Creatinine clearance is defined as the volume (ml) of plasma that would be completely cleared of creatinine per minute. The normal value of creatinine clearance is 120 to 145 ml/min. In women, these values are slightly lower. Recently, body surface area is used to express creatinine clearance.

Procedure: Creatinine clearance is determined by two different methods with slight modification. They are 1) Older or conventional or traditional method; 2) Latest or new method.

Older or conventional or traditional method: According to conventional method, collect 24 hours of urine and determine the creatinine content. Measure the plasma concentration of creatinine also. From this, calculate the creatinine clearance by using the following formula.

$$C = \frac{U \times V}{P}$$

Where, C = Clearance of creatinine (in ml/min)
U = Concentration of creatinine in urine (in mmol/l or mg/dl)
V = Volume of urine excreted per minute (in ml) [Volume of urine excreted/min (in ml) = volume of urine collected in 24 hours / 24 × 60]
P = Concentration of creatinine in plasma (in mmol/l or mg/dl)

Collect 24 hours of urine

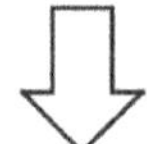

Measure the volumes of urine

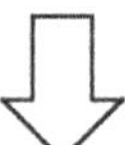

Determine the creatinine content

Measure the plasma concentration of creatinine also

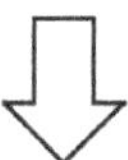

Calculate the creatinine clearance

Latest or new method: The procedure is slightly modified in new method. Accordingly, collect one hour urine sample after giving water instead of 24 hours urine collection. Measure the volumes of urine. Estimate the content of creatinine in plasma and urine. From this, calculate creatinine clearance by using the same formula mentioned in the traditional method.

Collect one hour urine

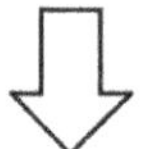

Measure the volumes of urine

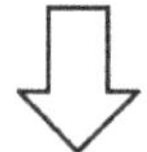

Determine the creatinine content

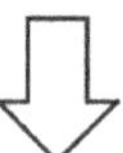

Measure the plasma concentration of creatinine also

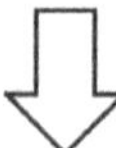

Calculate the creatinine clearance

Significance: Creatinine clearance of less than 75 % of the standard value indicates the decreased GFR due to renal damage. It is one of the sensitive tests used to detect early damage of the kidney function, often before the clinical manifestations are seen.

Urea Clearance Test

Urea is the end product of protein metabolism; hence, urea clearance test is influenced by protein content of the diet. Consequently, this test is not as sensitive as creatinine clearance test for assessing functions of the kidney. Urea is filtered from glomeruli and partially reabsorbed by the renal tubules. Therefore, compare to GFR, urea clearance is less. Even though in several laboratories urea clearance test is traditionally used to assess kidney functions. Urea clearance is defined as the volume (in ml) of plasma that would be completely cleared of urea per minute.

Procedure:

1. **Maximum urea clearance:** Measure the concentration of urea in urine and plasma and volume of urine excreted per minute. From this calculate urea clearance by using the following formula.

$$C_m = \frac{U \times V}{P}$$

Where, C_m = Maximum urea clearance (in ml/min)
U = Concentration of urea in urine (in mg/ml)
V = Volume of urine excreted per minute (in ml)
P = Concentration of urea in plasma (in mg/ml)

Measure the concentration of urea in urine

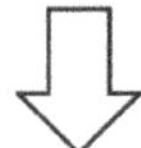

Measure the concentration of urea in plasma

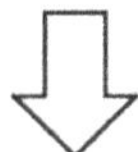

Measure the volume of urine excreted per minute

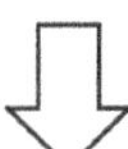

Calculate the urea clearance

The above formula is valid only when volume of urine excreted per minute is more than 2 ml. This urea clearance is known as maximum urea clearance (C_m). The normal value of maximum urea clearance is 75 ml per minute.

2. **Standard urea clearance:** When the volume of urine excreted per minute is less than 2 ml it was observed that urea clearance is changing drastically. This is known as standard urea clearance (C_s). It is calculated by using the following formula which is obtained by modifying the above formula.

$$C_s = \frac{U \times \sqrt{V}}{P}$$

Where, C_s = Standard urea clearance (in ml/min)
U = Concentration of urea in urine (in mg/ml)
V = Volume of urine excreted per minute (in ml)
P = Concentration of urea in plasma (in mg/ml)

The normal value of standard urea clearance is 54 ml per minute.

Significance: Urea clearance test is used to find out the proper functioning of kidneys. If a urea clearance value is less than 75 % of the standard value it indicates the renal damage. When the urea clearance is decreased below 50 % normal then blood urea level as such increase.

Estimation of Creatinine in Blood

Principle:

Creatinine is a substance obtained from creatinine phosphate. Creatinine in blood is estimated by Folin modified method using a photoelectric calorimeter. In this Folin Wu i.e., protein-free blood is used. In this method, creatinine (unknown) contained in the filtrate is treated with picric acid in alkaline medium to obtain red colored creatinine picrate. Optical density of this red colored creatinine picrate thus obtained is compared with that of standard solution, similarly converted by picric acid to creatinine picrate. By using colorimetric principle, concentration of creatinine in blood can be calculated.

$$\text{Creatinine + Picric acid} \xrightarrow{\text{NaOH}} \text{Creatinine picrate (Red in color)}$$

Preparation of reagents:

1. **Folin Wu filtrate:** Take 1 ml of blood, 1 ml of 10 % sodium tungstate solution, 1 ml of 2/3 N sulphuric acid and 7 ml water in 10 ml volumetric flask. Mix well, allow to stand for 10 min and filter it. Color of the precipitate should be chocolate and the Folin Wu filtrate is nearly neutral.
2. **10 % Sodium tungstate solution:** Dissolve 10 g of sodium tungstate in 50 ml of water and dilute to 100 ml using distilled water.
3. **2/3 N Sulphuric acid:** Add 1.8 ml of concentrated sulphuric acid into 98.2 ml of water.
4. **Creatinine stock solution:** Dissolve 0.1 g of creatinine or 0.16106 g of creatinine zinc chloride in 10 ml 1 N hydrochloric acid and dilute the whole to 100 ml with distilled water (0.1 g or 100 mg creatinine in 100 ml. Therefore, 1 ml creatinine stock solution contains 1 mg of creatinine).
5. **Standard creatinine solution:** Dilute 1 ml of creatinine stock solution (1 mg) to 500 ml with water (1 mg creatinine in 500 ml standard creatinine solution. Therefore,1 ml standard creatinine solution contains 0.002 mg of creatinine; Hence 5 ml standard creatinine solution contains 0.01 mg of creatinine).
6. **1 % Picric acid:** Dissolve 1 g of picric acid in 25 ml of water and dilute to 100 ml using distilled water.
7. **10 % Sodium hydroxide:** Dissolve 10 g of sodium hydroxide in 50 ml of water and dilute to 100 ml using distilled water.

Procedure:

1. **Preparation of unknown sample:** Label the flask as "U" and pipette out 5 ml of Folin Wu filtrate. Add 2 ml of 1% picric acid and mix well. Add 0.5 ml of 10 % sodium hydroxide solution. Allow to stand for 15 min and obtain the optical density from photoelectric colorimeter by using green filter (530 nm).
2. **Preparation of standard sample:** Label the flask as "S" and pipette out 5 ml of standard creatinine solution. Add 2 ml of 1 % picric acid and mix well. Add 0.5 ml of 10 % sodium hydroxide solution. Allow to stand for 15 min and obtain the optical density from photoelectric colorimeter using green filter (530 nm).
3. **Preparation of blank sample:** Label the flask as "B" and pipette out 5 ml of distilled water. Add 2 ml of 1 % picric acid and mix well. Add 0.5 ml of 10 % sodium hydroxide solution. Allow to stand for 15 min and obtain the optical density from photoelectric colorimeter using green filter (530 nm).

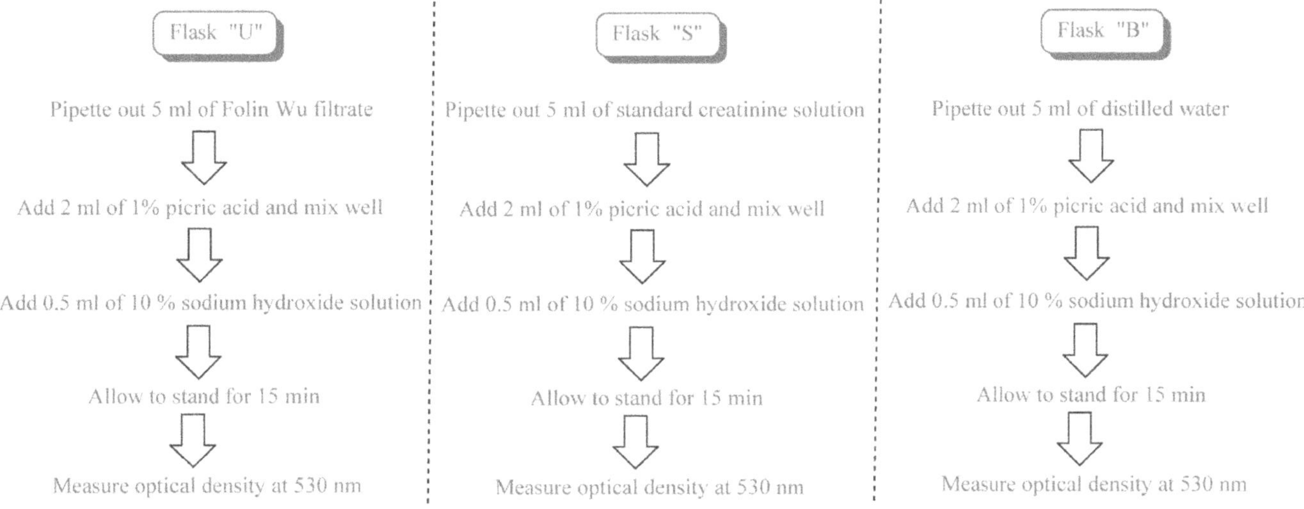

4. **Calculation:** Finally, calculate the percentage of creatinine present in blood by using the following formula.

$$\text{Concentration of creatinine in 0.5 ml blood (or) 5 ml of filtrate} = \frac{E_u}{E_s} \times C_s = \frac{E_u}{E_s} \times 0.01 \; mg \; creatinine$$

$$\text{Concentration of creatinine in 100 ml blood} = \frac{\left(\frac{E_u}{E_s} \times 0.01\right)}{0.5} \times 100 = \frac{E_u}{E_s} \times 2 \; mg$$

Where, E_u = Optical density of unknown blood sample
E_s = Optical density of standard creatinine solution
C_s = Concentration of standard creatinine solution.

Significance: Estimation of serum creatinine along with blood urea is used as a diagnostic test to assess the kidney function. Normal concentration of creatinine in 100 ml of blood is 0.7 - 2.0 mg. In whole blood the creatinine range is higher. Serum creatinine increases in all the conditions in which serum urea increases; Even though for renal dysfunction serum creatinine is a more specific and sensitive indicator as it is not influenced by exogenous factors as in case of urea. In kidney diseases the serum creatinine level generally increases. Increase of serum creatinine is indicative of severity of kidney diseases as it is the last substance increase in serum followed by urea and uric acid.

Estimation of Creatinine in Urine

Principle:

Creatinine is a substance obtained from creatinine phosphate. Creatinine in urine is estimated by Folin Wu modified method using photoelectric calorimeter. In this method urine sample containing creatinine is treated with picric acid in an alkaline medium to obtain red-colored creatinine picrate. The optical density of this red color solution is compared with that of standard solution similarly converted by picric acid to creatinine picrate. By using colorimetric principle concentration of creatinine in urine is calculated.

$$\text{Creatinine} + \text{Picric acid} \xrightarrow{\text{NaOH}} \text{Creatinine picrate}$$

(Red in color)

Preparation of reagents:

1. **Standard creatinine solution:** Dissolve 0.1 g of creatinine or 0.16106 g of creatinine zinc chloride in 10 ml 1 N hydrochloric acid and dilute the whole to 100 ml with distilled water (0.1 g or 100 mg creatinine in 100 ml. Therefore, 0.5 ml creatinine stock solution contains 0.5 mg of creatinine).

2. **1 % Picric acid:** Dissolve 1 g of picric acid in 25 ml of water and dilute to 100 ml using distilled water.
3. **10 % Sodium hydroxide:** Dissolve 10 g of sodium hydroxide in 50 ml of water and dilute to 100 ml using distilled water.

Procedure:

Take two 50 ml standard flask and label as 'S' for standard and 'U' for an unknown sample. In standard flask 'S', add 0.5 ml standard creatinine solution, 1 ml of 10 % sodium hydroxide and 10 ml of 1 % picric acid. Then, dilute to 50 ml with distilled water. Mix and allow to stand for 15 minutes. In the standard flask 'U' add 0.5 ml of urine sample instead of 0.5 ml standard creatinine solution in the above procedure and repeat it. Measure the colors obtained on both standard and unknown using photoelectric colorimeter, at 530 nm (green filter). Finally, calculate the percentage of creatinine present in urine by using the following formula.

$$\text{Concentration of creatinine in 0.5 ml urine} = \frac{E_u}{E_s} \times C_s = \frac{E_u}{E_s} \times 0.5 \text{ mg creatinine}$$

$$\text{Concentration of creatinine in 100 ml urine} = \frac{\left(\frac{E_u}{E_s} \times 0.5\right)}{0.5} \times 100 = \frac{E_u}{E_s} \times 100 \text{ mg}$$

Where,
E_u = Optical density of unknown urine sample
E_s = Optical density of standard creatinine solution
Cs = Concentration of standard creatinine solution.

Flask "S"	Flask "U"
Pipette out 0.5 ml of standard creatinine solution	Pipette out 0.5 ml of urine sample (Dilute if necessary)
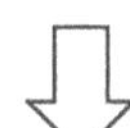	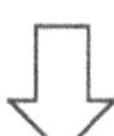
Add 1 ml of 10 % sodium hydroxide solution	Add 1 ml of 10 % sodium hydroxide solution
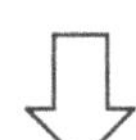	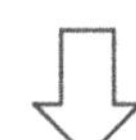
Add 10 ml of 1 % picric acid and mix well	Add 10 ml of 1 % picric acid and mix well
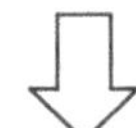	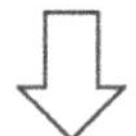
Dilute to 50 ml with distilled water	Dilute to 50 ml with distilled water
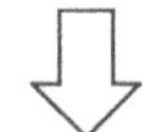	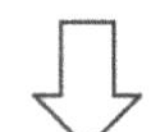
Mix and allow to stand for 15 minutes	Mix and allow to stand for 15 minutes
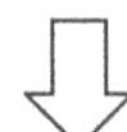	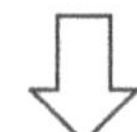
Measure optical density at 530 nm	Measure optical density at 530 nm

Significance: The normal daily excretion of creatinine in male is 1.04 to 2.35 g and in female it is 0.7 to 1.5 g. Creatinine synthesis in the body is related to the total muscle mass and its excretion is constant unless the muscle mass changes. Creatinine excretion is not influenced by dietary factors. Urine creatinine estimation is used to calculate creatinine clearance and GFR measurement. Creatinine clearance is decreased in advanced renal failure, all kind of renal diseases and in post renal conditions. In general, urine creatinine is more in muscle disorders like myasthenia gravis, muscular atrophy and myositis.

Estimation of Urea in Blood and Urine

Urea is the end product of protein metabolism. Urea is generally catabolized by an enzyme called *urease* and produces ammonia and carbondioxide.

$$\underset{\textbf{Urea}}{NH_2CONH_2 + H_2O} \xrightarrow[\textit{Urease}]{} \underset{\textbf{Ammonia}}{2\,NH_3 + CO_2}$$

The liberated ammonia can be estimated by different methods. They are,

1. Direct Nesslerization method (Reaction with Nessler's reagent)
2. Berthelot reaction (Reaction with phenol in presence of hypochlorite)
3. Diacetylmonoxime method (Direct reaction of urea with diacetyl monoxime)

All these three methods are used for the estimation of urea in plasma or blood. In general, the Nesslerization method is used to estimate the urea present in urine.

1. **Nesslerization or Nessler's method:**

   Principle: In this method, a protein free filtrate (Folin Wu filtrate) is initially prepared using sodium tungstate and sulphuric acid. Later, the protein free filtrate is treated with *urease* enzyme by which ammonium carbonate is liberated. This reaction takes place in the presence of acetate buffer. Finally, the liberated ammonium carbonate is treated with Nessler's reagent in the presence of gum ghatti that produces colored substances. The intensity of the color complex formed is measured at 540 nm.

$$\underset{\textbf{Urea}}{NH_2CONH_2 + 2\,H_2O} \xrightarrow[\textit{Urease}]{\text{Acetate buffer}} \underset{\textbf{Ammonium carbonate}}{(NH_4)_2CO_3}$$

$$\text{Ammonium carbonate} + \text{Nessler's reagent} \xrightarrow{\text{Gum ghatti}} \underset{(\lambda_{max} = 540\text{ nm})}{\textbf{Colored complex}}$$

Preparation of reagents:

1. **Folin Wu filtrate:** Take 1 ml of blood, 1 ml of 10 % sodium tungstate solution, 1 ml of 2/3 N sulphuric acid, and 7 ml water in a 10 ml volumetric flask. Mix well; allow to stand for 10 min and then filter. The color of the precipitate should be chocolate and the Folin Wu filtrate is nearly neutral.
2. **10 % Sodium tungstate solution:** Dissolve 10 g of sodium tungstate in 50 ml of water and dilute to 100 ml using distilled water.
3. **2/3 N Sulphuric acid:** Add 1.8 ml of concentrated sulphuric acid into 98.2 ml of water.
4. ***Urease* solution:** Shake 0.5 g of jack bean meal and 20 ml of 30 % ethanol vigorously for 10 min. Later, centrifuge the obtained solution for 10 min at 1500 rpm. Collect and use the supernatant liquid. This solution must be prepared fresh every day.
5. **Acetate buffer:** Dissolve 20 g of sodium acetate in 50 ml of water and add 2.1 ml of 10 % acetic acid. Finally, dilute the solution to 100 ml using distilled water.
6. **Gum ghatti solution:** Wrap 2 g of gum ghatti in a muslin cloth and immerse in 100 ml of water for 24 hours. Later, filter the liquid through the filter paper.
7. **Nessler's reagent:** Dissolve 30 g of potassium iodide in 20 ml of water. Add 22.5 g of iodine to the solution and dissolve it by stirring. To the above solution, add 30 g of mercury and mix well until the yellow color of iodine is lost in the supernatant liquid. Then, cool the solution in running tap water and test the supernatant liquid for the presence of iodine using starch. If no blue color is obtained, add the iodine little by little until the supernatant liquid gives positive results for the presence of iodine. Then, made the volume up to 200 ml using water. Add the above mixture to 975 ml 10 % NaOH and stirr well. If the precipitate is obtained, then allow the solution to settle down and separate the clear supernatant liquid for use.
8. **Urea stock solution:** Dissolve 300 mg of urea in 100 ml of water and dilute to 1000 ml using distilled water (300 mg urea in 1000 ml. Therefore, 1 ml urea stock solution contains 0.3 mg of urea).

9. **Standard urea solution:** Dilute 15 ml of urea stock solution to 100 ml with water ($15 \times 0.3 = 4.5$ mg urea in 100 ml standard urea solution. Therefore, 1 ml standard urea solution contains 0.045 mg of urea. Hence, 5 ml standard urea solution contains 0.225 mg of urea).

Procedure:

Take three 25 ml standard volumetric flasks and label as standard, blank and unknown. In the unknown flask, take 5 ml of Folin Wu filtrate; and in the standard flask, take 5 ml of standard urea solution; in the blank flask, take 5 ml of water. To all these standard volumetric flasks, add 5 drops of *urease* solution, and 0.5 ml of acetate buffer and stir well. Incubate all standard volumetric flask for 15 minutes at 50 °C. Finally, made the volume up to 25 ml using distilled water. Take 10 ml of the above solution into the corresponding labeled test tubes containing 2 drops of gum ghatti. To this, add 1 ml of Nessler's reagent, stir well, and allow to stand for 10 min. Measure the intensity of the color obtained in the standard and unknown tubes against the blank at 540 nm. Calculate the concentration of urea present in the unknown sample using the following formula.

$$\textit{Concentration of urea in 0.5 ml blood (or) 5 ml of filtrate} = \frac{E_u}{E_s} \times C_s = \frac{E_u}{E_s} \times 0.225\ mg\ urea$$

$$\textit{Concentration of urea in 100 ml blood} = \frac{\left(\frac{E_u}{E_s} \times 0.225\right)}{0.5} \times 100 = \frac{E_u}{E_s} \times 45\ mg$$

Where, E_u = Optical density of unknown blood sample

E_s = Optical density of standard urea solution

C_s = Concentration of standard urea solution.

Take three 25 ml standard volumetric flasks and label as standard, blank and unknown

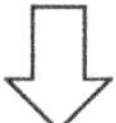

In the unknown flask, take 5 ml of Folin Wu filtrate; and in the standard flask, take 5 ml of standard urea solution; in the blank flask, take 5 ml of water

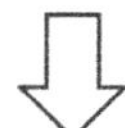

Add 5 drops of *urease* solution, and 0.5 ml of acetate buffer

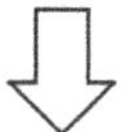

Stir well and incubate for 15 minutes at 50 °C

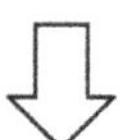

Made the volume up to 25 ml using distilled water

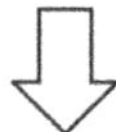

Take 10 ml of the above solution into the corresponding labeled test tubes containing 2 drops of gum ghatti

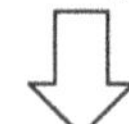

Add 1 ml of Nessler's reagent

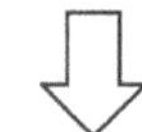

Stir well, and allow to stand for 10 min

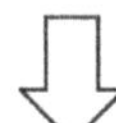

Measure the intensity of the color obtained in the standard and unknown tubes against the blank at 540 nm

2. **Berthelot method:**

Principle: Urea is generally catabolized by an enzyme called *urease* and produces ammonia and carbondioxide. In this method, the ammonia liberated from urea by *urease* is reacting with phenol in the presence of hypochlorite and produces indophenols. Later, indophenol reacts with sodium hydroxide and produces a blue color complex. In this reaction, sodium nitroprusside acts as a catalyst. The absorbance is measured at 630 nm.

$$\underset{\textbf{Urea}}{NH_2CONH_2} + H_2O \xrightarrow[\textit{Urease}]{\text{Buffer}} \underset{\textbf{Ammonia}}{2\,NH_3 + CO_2}$$

$$\text{Ammonia} + \text{Phenol} \xrightarrow{\text{Hypochlorite}} \text{Indophenol}$$

Indophenol → (Sodium nitroprusside | NaOH) → **Blue color** complex
(λ_{max} = 630 nm)

Preparation of reagents:

1. **Folin Wu filtrate:** Take 1 ml of blood, 1 ml of 10 % sodium tungstate solution, 1 ml of 2/3 N sulphuric acid, and 7 ml water in 10 ml volumetric flask. Mix well; allow to stand for 10 min and then filter. The color of the precipitate should be chocolate and the Folin Wu filtrate is nearly neutral.
2. **10 % Sodium tungstate solution:** Dissolve 10 g of sodium tungstate in 50 ml of water and dilute to 100 ml using distilled water.
3. **2/3 N Sulphuric acid:** Add 1.8 ml of concentrated sulphuric acid into 98.2 ml of water.
4. **Buffered *urease* solution:** Prepare 1% w/v EDTA in water & adjust the pH to 6.5. Use the above solution to prepare 0.15 % w/v of *urease* solution. Store the prepared urease solution at 4 °C.
5. **Phenol nitroprusside solution:** Dissolve 50 g of phenol and 250 mg of sodium nitroprusside in 250 ml of water and dilute it to 1000 ml using distilled water. Later, dilute 20 ml of the above solution to 100 ml with distilled water.
6. **Hypochlorite solution:** Dissolve 25 g of sodium hydroxide and 2.1 g of sodium hypochlorite in 250 ml of water and dilute to 1000 ml using distilled water. Later, dilute 20 ml of the above solution to 100 ml with distilled water.
7. **Standard urea solution:** Dissolve 100 mg of urea in 50 ml of water and dilute to 100 ml using distilled water. (100 mg urea in 100 ml standard urea solution. Therefore, 1 ml standard urea solution contains 1 mg of urea. Hence, 0.02 ml standard urea solution contains 0.02 mg of urea).

Procedure:

Take three test tubes and label as standard, blank, and unknown. To all test tubes, add 0.2 ml of buffered *urease* solution. In the unknown test tube, add 0.02 ml of Folin Wu filtrate; in the standard test tube, add 0.02 ml of standard urea solution and in the blank test tube, add 0.02 ml of water. Incubate all three tubes for 15 minutes at 37 °C. To all test tubes, add 5 ml of phenol nitroprusside solution and mix well. Then, add 5 ml hypochlorite solution to all three test tubes. Finally, incubate all three tubes for 15 minutes at 37 °C. Measure the intensity of the color obtained in the standard and unknown against the blank at 630 nm. Calculate the concentration of urea present in the unknown sample using the following formula.

$$\textit{Concentration of urea in 0.002 ml blood (or) 0.02 ml of filtrate} = \frac{E_u}{E_s} \times C_s = \frac{E_u}{E_s} \times 0.02\ \textit{mg urea}$$

$$\text{Concentration of urea in 100 ml blood} = \frac{\left(\frac{E_u}{E_s} \times 0.02\right)}{0.002} \times 100 = \frac{E_u}{E_s} \times 1000\ mg$$

Where, E_u = Optical density of unknown blood sample
E_s = Optical density of standard urea solution
C_s = Concentration of standard urea solution.

Take three test tubes and label as standard, blank, and unknown

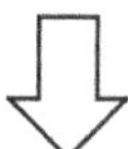

In the unknown test tube, add 0.02 ml of Folin Wu filtrate; in the standard test tube, add 0.02 ml of standard urea solution and in the blank test tube, add 0.02 ml of water

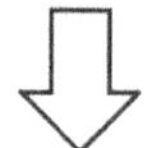

Add 0.2 ml of buffered *urease* solution

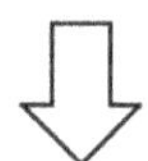

Incubate for 15 minutes at 37 °C

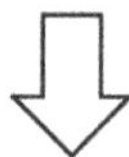

Add 5 ml of phenol nitroprusside solution and mix well

Add 5 ml hypochlorite solution

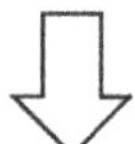

Incubate for 15 minutes at 37 °C

Measure the intensity of the color obtained in the standard and unknown against the blank at 630 nm

3. **Diacetyl monoxime method:**

Principle: In this method, urea is directly reacted with diacetylmonoxime under the acidic condition in the presence of thiosemicarbazide and cadmium ion to produce rose-purple color diazine derivative. The intensity of the color complex formed is measured at 540 nm. In this method, serum is directly analyzed without removal of protein.

$$\text{Urea + Diacetylmonoxime} \xrightarrow[\text{Acid}]{\text{Thiosemicarbazide, Cadmium ion}} \text{Diazide derivative } \textbf{(Rose-purple color)}\ (\lambda_{max} = 540\ nm)$$

Preparation of reagents:

1. **Diacetylmonoxime solution:** Dissolve 2 g of diacetylmonoxime in 50 ml of water and dilute to 100 ml using distilled water. Store it in a brown color bottle in refrigerator.

2. **Urea solution:** Dissolve 2.6 mg of urea in 50 ml of water and dilute to 100 ml using distilled water.
3. **Urea nitrogen reagent:** Add 44 ml concentrated sulphuric acid and 66 ml 85 % ortho phosphoric acid slowly to 100 ml of water present in 1 liter volumetric flask. After cooling to the room temperature, add 50 mg of thiosemicarbazide and 2 g cadmium sulphate and 10 ml urea solution to the above mixture. Finally, dilute the above solution to 1000 ml with distilled water. Store it in a brown color bottle in the refrigerator.
4. **Standard urea solution (High):** Dissolve 100 mg of urea in 50 ml of water and dilute to 100 ml using distilled water. Add few drops of chloroform as preservatives. Store it in a brown color bottle in the refrigerator. (100 mg urea in 100 ml standard urea solution. Therefore, 1 ml standard urea solution contains 1 mg of urea; hence, 0.02 ml standard urea solution contains 0.02 mg of urea).
5. **Standard urea solution (Low):** Dissolve 50 mg of urea in 50 ml of water and dilute to 100 ml using distilled water. Add few drops of chloroform as preservative. Store it in brown color bottle in the refrigerator. (50 mg urea in 100 ml standard urea solution. Therefore, 1 ml standard urea solution contains 0.5 mg of urea. Hence, 0.02 ml standard urea solution contains 0.01 mg of urea).

Procedure:

Take four test tubes and label as standard high, standard low, blank and unknown. To the all test tubes, add 5 ml of urea nitrogen reagent. In the unknown tube, take 0.02 ml of serum and in the standard high tube, take 0.02 ml of standard urea solution (high). In the standard low tube, take 0.02 ml of standard urea solution (low) and in the blank tube, take 0.02 ml of water. Mix well all four test tubes and to each tube, add 0.5 ml of diacetylmonoxime solution. Heat the test tubes in a boiling water bath for 12 min, followed by immerse in cool water for 5 min. Measure the intensity of the color obtained in standard (high), standard (low), and unknown against the blank at 540 nm. Calculate the concentration of urea present in the unknown sample using the following formula.

Using standard urea high

$$\text{Concentration of urea in 0.02 ml of serum} = \frac{E_u}{E_{sh}} \times C_s = \frac{E_u}{E_{sh}} \times 0.02\ mg\ urea$$

$$\text{Concentration of urea in 100 ml blood} = \frac{\left(\frac{E_u}{E_{sh}} \times 0.02\right)}{0.02} \times 100 = \frac{E_u}{E_{sh}} \times 100\ mg$$

or

Using standard urea low

$$\text{Concentration of urea in 0.02 ml of serum} = \frac{E_u}{E_{sl}} \times C_s = \frac{E_u}{E_{sl}} \times 0.01\ mg\ urea$$

$$\text{Concentration of urea in 100 ml blood} = \frac{\left(\frac{E_u}{E_{sl}} \times 0.01\right)}{0.02} \times 100 = \frac{E_u}{E_{sl}} \times 50\ mg$$

Where, E_u = Optical density of unknown blood sample
E_{sh} = Optical density of standard urea solution (high)
E_{sl} = Optical density of standard urea solution (low)
C_s = Concentration of standard urea solution.

Take four test tubes and label as standard high, standard low, blank and unknown

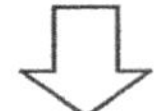

Add 5 ml of urea nitrogen reagent to all test tubes

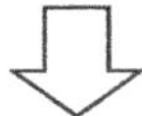

In the unknown tube, take 0.02 ml of serum and in the standard high tube, take 0.02 ml of standard urea solution (high). In the standard low tube, take 0.02 ml of standard urea solution (low) and in the blank tube, take 0.02 ml of water

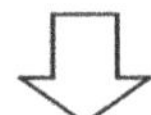

Mix well all four test tubes and to each tube, add 0.5 ml of diacetyl monoxime solution

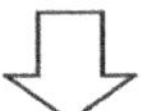

Heat the test tubes in a boiling water bath for 12 minutes, followed by immerse in cool water for 5 min

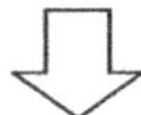

Measure the intensity of the color obtained in standard (high), standard (low), and unknown against the blank at 540 nm

Non-protein nitrogen (NPN): Other than protein, all nitrogen containing substances are termed as non-protein nitrogen (NPN). It includes urea, creatinine, creatine, uric acid, peptides, amino acids, etc. NPN concentration in the blood is 20 to 40 mg/dl for normal healthy people. 60 is the molecular weight of urea and half of it, i.e. 28 is contributed by the two nitrogen atoms. The blood urea concentration is 60 mg and half of it i.e. 28 mg is blood urea nitrogen (BUN). Hence, BUN is equal to 1/2 NPN or NPN is equal to 2 BUNs. The estimation of BUN or NPN is used in some countries rather than the estimation of urea for the kidney function assessment. The normal ratio of BUN and serum creatinine is 10:1 to 15:1.

Significance: The normal serum urea ranges from 20 to 45 mg/100 ml. The serum urea level is highly influenced by dietary protein. High protein diet increases the serum urea level, whereas low protein diet decreases the serum urea level. In general, serum urea level is increased in various renal diseases like glomerulonephritis, pyelonephritis, renal tuberculosis, renal carcinoma, polycystic kidneys, etc. In addition, urinary tract obstruction, dehydration, shock, hematemesis and increased tissue breakdown may also increase serum urea levels. The serum urea is decreased in acute hepatic insufficiency. During the first and second trimester of pregnancy, a slight decrease in the serum urea occurs.

Estimation of Uric Acid in Blood

Principle:

In general, uric acid is estimated by its reducing property. It reduces phosphotungstic acid to phosphotungstus acid. Phosphotungstic acid is colorless and the formed phosphotungstus acid is blue in color. This reaction takes place in the presence of alkaline conditions. In older methods, sodium cyanide (NaCN) is used, whereas in newer methods, sodium cyanide is replaced by sodium carbonate (Na_2CO_3). This newer method is also known as the **Caraway method of uric acid estimation.** The intensity of the developed blue color was measured photometrically at 700 nm or using red filters.

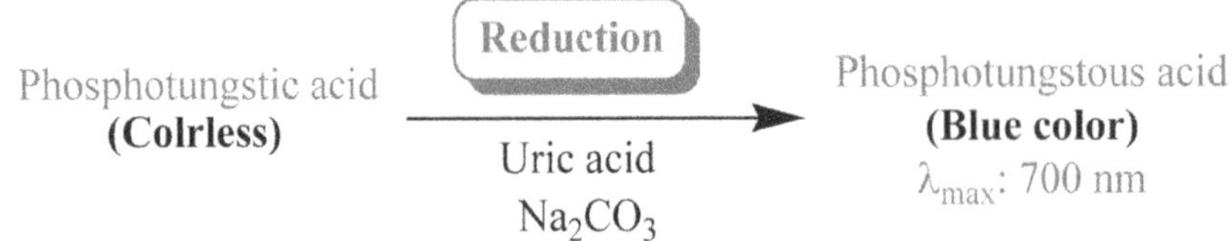

Preparation of reagents:

1. **Folin Wu filtrate:** Take 1 ml of blood, 1 ml of 10 % sodium tungstate solution, 1 ml of 2/3 N sulphuric acid and 7 ml water in a 10 ml volumetric flask. Mix well; allow to stand for 10 min and then filter it. The color of the precipitate should be chocolate and the Folin Wu filtrate is nearly neutral.
2. **10 % Sodium tungstate solution:** Dissolve 10 g of sodium tungstate in 50 ml of water and dilute to 100 ml using distilled water.
3. **2/3 N Sulphuric acid:** Add 1.8 ml of concentrated sulphuric acid into 98.2 ml of water.
4. **10 % Sodium carbonate solution:** Dissolve 10 g of sodium carbonate in 50 ml of water and dilute to 100 ml using distilled water.
5. **Phosphotungstic acid solution:** Dissolve 50 g of sodium tungstate in 400 ml water and add 40 ml of 85 % phosphoric acid to the above solution. Then, reflux the mixture in a water bath for 2 hours and dilute the whole to 500 ml with distilled water. 10 ml of the above solution is further diluted to 100 ml using distilled water.
6. **Standard uric acid solution:** Dissolve 60 mg of lithium carbonate in 20 ml water and heat it to 60 °C. Then add 100 mg of uric acid to the solution and stirr well until uric acid dissolves. To this mixture, add 2 ml 40 % formalin and 1 ml of 50 % acetic acid with stirring. Dilute the obtained solution to 100 ml using distilled water. Further dilute 0.5 ml of the above solution to 100 ml using distilled water. (100 mg uric acid in 100 ml solution. Therefore, 1 ml solution contains 1 mg of uric acid; 0.5 ml solution contains 0.5 mg of uric acid. Hence, 0.5 mg uric acid is present in 100 ml standard uric acid solution; Therefore, 5 ml standard uric acid solution contains 0.025 mg of uric acid).

Procedure:

Take three test tubes and label as standard, blank and unknown. In the unknown test tube, take 5 ml of Folin Wu filtrate; in the standard test tube, take 5 ml of standard uric acid solution and in the blank test tube, take 5 ml of water. To all test tubes, add 1 ml of 10 % sodium carbonate solution and 1 ml of phosphotungstic acid solution and mix well. Finally, heat all three tubes in a water bath for 35 min at 25 °C. Measure the intensity of the color obtained in the standard and unknown against blank at 700 nm or using red filter. Calculate the concentration of the uric acid present in the unknown sample using the following formula.

$$\textit{Concentration of uric acid in } 0.5 \textit{ ml of blood (or) } 5 \textit{ ml of filtrate} = \frac{E_u}{E_s} \times C_s = \frac{E_u}{E_s} \times 0.025\, mg \textit{ uric acid}$$

$$\textit{Concentration of uric acid in } 100 \textit{ ml blood} = \frac{\left(\frac{E_u}{E_s} \times 0.025\right)}{0.5} \times 100 = \frac{E_u}{E_s} \times 5\, mg$$

Where, E_u = Optical density of unknown blood sample

E_s = Optical density of standard uric acid solution

C_s = Concentration of standard uric acid solution.

Significance: The normal serum uric acid ranges from 2 to 6.5 mg/100 ml in men and post-menopausal women; and 2 to 5.5 mg/100 ml in pre-menopausal women. The serum uric acid level estimation is mainly useful for the diagnosis of gout in which serum uric acid level is characteristically increased. In general, the serum uric acid level is markedly increased in various renal diseases like renal failure and leukemia. In addition, other diseases like lobar pneumonia, megaloblastic anemia, polycythemia, multiple myeloma, myocardial infarction, eclampsia and psoriasis may also increase the serum uric acid levels. In healthy people, the serum uric acid is increased during high intake of organ meats rich in nucleic acid. Less commonly decreased serum uric acid is seen and may occur in Wilson's disease, familial periodic paralysis, and Fanconi syndrome.

Take three test tubes and label as standard, blank and unknown

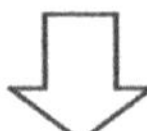

In the unknown test tube, take 5 ml of Folin Wu filtrate;
in the standard test tube, take 5 ml of standard uric acid solution
and in the blank test tube, take 5 ml of water

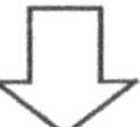

Add 1 ml of 10 % sodium carbonate solution and 1 ml of
phosphotungstic acid solution to all three test tubes and mix well

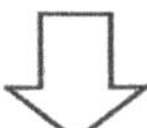

Heat all three tubes in a water bath for 35 minutes at 25 °C

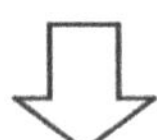

Measure the intensity of the color obtained in the standard
and unknown against blank at 700 nm or using red filter

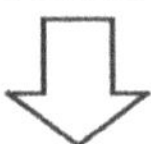

Calculate the concentration of the uric
acid present in the unknown sample

Estimation of Uric Acid in Urine

For estimating uric acid in urine, the same method i.e, estimation of uric acid in plasma is used. Instead of Folin Wu filtrate, urine (1 in 10 diluted with water) was used in an unknown test tube. The obtained results are multiplied by dilution factor 10. If protein is not present, then it may be diluted 1 in 100 with water.

Urine Concentration / Dilution Test

Kidneys play an important role in the maintenance of fluid balance in the biological system. Renal tubular functions of the kidney are easily estimated by the urine concentration or dilution test. Renal tubular plays an important role in the re-absorption of fluids. Hence, any defect in renal or renal tubular ultimately alters the specific gravity of the urine. The urine concentration or dilution test is based on simple measurement of specific gravity of urine. The specific gravity of the urine depends on the concentration of solutes present in the urine. The specific gravity of urine can be determined by the following two methods namely 1) Urine concentration test, 2) Urine dilution test.

1. **Urine concentration test:**

   This test is performed by the following ways. After taking a normal dinner, restrict the patients to take water overnight. Later in the morning, collect urine samples three times with a 1 hour intervals. Measure the specific gravity of the collected three urine samples. The normal specific gravity of a urine concentrated sample is 1.025. If the renal tubule is functioning properly, then the specific gravity of any one urine sample collected must be greater than 1.025. In case none of the urine samples specific gravity is more than 1.025, it indicates abnormalities in the kidney function, particularly renal tubular function. In another method instead of water deprivation, anti-diuretic hormone is administered and measured the specific gravity of collected urine.

After taking a normal dinner, restrict the patients to take water overnight

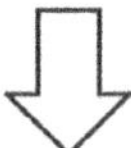

Later in the morning, collect urine samples three times with a 1 hour intervals

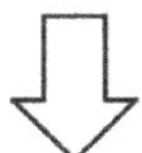

Measure the specific gravity of the collected three urine samples

2. **Urine dilution test:**
   In this method, the urine is diluted by consuming more water and the specific gravity of the urine is determined. After fasting overnight, empty the stomach in the morning. Later, consume 1200 ml of water within 30 min. After that, collect a urine sample every hour for the next four hours and estimate its specific gravity. The normal urine dilution specific gravity value is 1.003. If no abnormalities are present, then anyone one of these urine samples specific gravity must be less than 1.003. In case all urine samples specific gravity is more than 1.003, it indicates the abnormalities of kidney function, specifically the renal tubular function.

After fasting overnight, empty the stomach in the morning

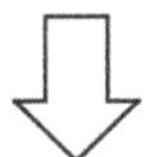

Consume 1200 ml of water within 30 min

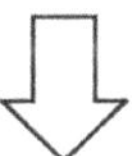

Collect a urine sample every hour for the next four hours

Estimate the specific gravity of urine sample

Osmolality:

It is the other parameter used in urine concentration or dilution test which indirectly estimates the specific gravity of urine. Hence, urine osmolality measurements are also helpful for assessing tubular function of the kidney. Osmolality is related to specific gravity and the osmolality of the urine is variable. The osmolality of normal urine varies from 500 to 1200 mosm/kg. (mosm means milliosmole). The normal osmolality of plasma is 300 mosm/kg. The ratio of the urine and plasma osmolality is between 2 to 4. The protein or high molecular weight substances free urine with 800 mosm/kg has a specific gravity of 1.020. Hence, based on the deviation of above mentioned osmolality, we can easily determine the specific gravity of the urine indirectly.

Urinary Tract Calculi (Kidney Stones)

Kidney stones, or renal calculi, are solid masses made of crystals. Kidney stones usually originate in kidneys. Nevertheless, it can develop anywhere along the urinary tract, which consists of kidneys, ureters, bladder and urethra.

Types:

Not all kidney stones are made up of the same type of crystals. The different types of kidney stones are 1) Calcium kidney stone, 2) Uric acid kidney stone, 3) Struvite kidney stone, 4) Cystine stone.

Calcium stones are the most common type of urinary tract calculi. These stones are mainly made up of calcium oxalate and they also contain calcium phosphate or maleate. The risk of developing this type of stone is reduced by consuming a low oxalate diet and avoiding high oxalate foods like potato chips, peanuts, chocolate, beets, spinach, etc. Even though some kidney stones are made of calcium, getting enough calcium in the diet can prevent stones formation.

Compared to women, uric acid kidney stone is more common in men. It mainly occurs in gout or chemotherapy patients. When the urine is too acidic, this type of stone develops. The acidity of the urine is increased due to a purine rich diet. Purine is a colorless substance mainly present in animal proteins like fish, shellfish, and meats.

Struvite kidney stone is more common in women with urinary tract infections (UTIs). It may cause urinary obstruction due to its large size. Kidney infection is the most common reason for this type of stone. It can be prevented by treating an underlying infection.

Cystine kidney stones are rare and occur in cystinuria patients. Cystine is leaked from the kidney into the urine.

Risk factors:

Less urine formation (Less than 1 liter/day) is the most important reason for kidney stones. It is most common in premature infants with kidney problems. However, it mostly occurs in people between the ages of 20 and 50. Many factors increase the chance of kidney stone formation. They are 1) Obesity, 2) Dehydration, 3) Hyperparathyroidism, 4) Protein, salt or glucose rich diet, 5) Inflammatory bowel disease (IBD) causing increased absorption of calcium, 6) Gastric bypass surgery, 7) Drugs like triamterene, diuretic, antiseizure drugs, calcium-based antacid, etc.

Symptoms:

The major symptom is severe pain known as renal colic. Until the stone begins to move down the ureters the symptoms of kidney stones may not occur. The pain of renal colic comes and goes. One side back or abdomen pain is the other symptoms. Various other symptoms of kidney stones can include 1) blood in the urine (red, pink, or brown urine), 2) vomiting, 3) nausea, 4) discolored or foul-smelling urine, 5) chills, 6) fever, 7) frequent need to urinate, 7) urinating small amounts of urine. In case if the kidney stone is small no pain or symptoms appear because the stone easily passes through the urinary tract.

Diagnostic tests:

1. Blood tests for calcium, phosphorus, uric acid, and electrolytes.
2. Blood urea nitrogen (BUN) and creatinine to assess kidney functioning.
3. Urinalysis to check for crystals, bacteria, blood, and white cells.
4. Examination of passed stones to determine their type.
5. Obstruction can be rule out by the following tests like abdominal X-rays, intravenous pyelogram (IVP), retrograde pyelogram, ultrasound of the kidney (the preferred test), MRI scan of the abdomen and kidneys and abdominal CT scan.

Treatment:

1. Analgesics are used to relieve pain.
2. Antibiotics are used to treat infections.
3. Allopurinol is used for uric acid stones.
4. Thiazide diuretics are used for prevention of calcium stones.
5. Sodium bicarbonate or sodium citrate is used to decrease the acidity of urine.
6. Phosphorus solutions are used for prevention of calcium stones.
7. Removal of urinary tract calculi by surgery like ureteroscopy, shock wave lithotripsy, percutaneous nephrolithotomy, etc.

PROBABLE QUESTIONS

PART – A: Multiple Choice Questions

1. What is the major excretory system of the body?
   (a) Respiratory system (b) Urinary system
   (c) Digestive system (d) Nervous system
2. What are the major functions of urinary system?
   (a) Removal of waste products from the body
   (b) Used for digestion of food
   (c) System helps to absorb oxygen
   (d) Used to maintain blood flow to all parts of the body
3. Urinary system helps to synthesize the active form of which vitamin?
   (a) Vitamin-A (b) Vitamin-C
   (c) Vitamin-D (d) Vitamin-K
4. Which organ secretes urine?
   (a) Liver (b) Kidney
   (c) Lung (d) Heart
5. What is function of ureters?
   (a) To transport urine from the bladder
   (b) To transport urine from the bladder to the kidney
   (c) To transport urine from the kidney to the bladder
   (d) To pass urine from the bladder to the exterior.
6. What is function of urethra?
   (a) To pass urine from the bladder to the exterior
   (b) To transport urine from the bladder
   (c) To transport urine from the bladder to the kidney
   (d) To transport urine from the kidney to the bladder.
7. In a healthy human, how much urine to be excreted per day?
   (a) 500 to 1,000 ml (b) 800 to 2,000 ml
   (c) 1,000 to 2,500 ml (d) 1,500 to 3,000 ml
8. What is the shape of the kidney?
   (a) Oval (b) Round
   (c) Bean (d) Square
9. Where the kidney is exactly located?
   (a) Between the peritoneum and posterior wall of the abdomen
   (b) Between the peritoneum and posterior wall of the back-bone
   (c) Between the peritoneum and posterior wall of the chest
   (d) Between the peritoneum and anterior wall of the abdomen.
10. Why the right kidney being slightly lower and smaller than the left kidney?
    (a) Position of the liver causes asymmetry within the abdominal cavity
    (b) Position of the heart causes symmetry within the abdominal cavity

(c) Position of the lungs causes asymmetry within the abdominal cavity
(d) Position of the intestine causes asymmetry within the abdominal cavity

11. Which of the following ribs are partially protecting the upper parts of the kidneys?
 (a) 09th and 10th (b) 11th and 12th
 (c) 13th and 14th (d) 15th and 16th
12. What is the length of the kidney?
 (a) 8 to 9 cm (b) 9 to 14 cm
 (c) 10 to 12 cm (d) 15 to 18 cm
13. What is the width of the kidney?
 (a) 3 to 4 cm (b) 4 to 9 cm
 (c) 5 to 7 cm (d) 7 to 14 cm
14. What is the thickness of the kidney?
 (a) 2 cm (b) 3 cm
 (c) 4 cm (d) 5 cm
15. Which of the following is not a layer of tissues surrounds the kidney?
 (a) Renal capsule (b) Adipose capsule
 (c) Renal fasicia (d) Renal hilum
16. Parenchyma, grossly take the shape of ___________ cone shaped renal lobes?
 (a) 8 to 18 (b) 8 to 14
 (c) 8 to 18 (d) 19 to 28
17. Each renal cortex surrounded by a portion of medulla is known as _______________.
 (a) Renal pyramid (b) Renal capsule
 (c) Renal fasicia (d) Renal hilum
18. Which of the following one is microscopic structural and functional unit of the kidney?
 (a) Neuron (b) Nerve
 (c) Nephron (d) Renal hilum
19. In each kidney, about ____________ million nephrons are present in a healthy adult.
 (a) 1 (b) 1 to 1.5
 (c) 2 to 2.5 (d) 3 to 3.5
20. Which of the following is not a mechanism in converting blood into urine in the nephron?
 (a) Filtration (b) Reabsorption
 (c) Inhalation (d) Excretion
21. Which of the following is not the chief constituents of urine?
 (a) Water (b) Blood
 (c) Inorganic constituents (d) Organic constituents
22. Which preservative is added to the urine sample to prevent the growth of bacteria and molds?
 (a) Thymol crystal, few drops of formaldehyde
 (b) Thymol blue, few drops of benzaldehyde
 (c) Thymol crystal, few drops of chloroform
 (d) Thymol crystal, few drops of benzene

23. If increased output of urine is observed it may know as ____________ and it occurs in which condition?
    (a) Hyper urea, diabetes insipidus
    (b) Hypo urea, diabetes insipidus
    (c) Polyuria, diabetes mellitus
    (d) None of the above
24. Turbidity of the urine is due to presence of ____________.
    (a) Mucoproteins and nucleoproteins
    (b) Haptoglobin
    (c) Prealbumin
    (d) Fibrinogen
25. How the specific gravity of urine is determined?
    (a) Thermometer
    (b) Urinometer
    (c) Spigmomanometer
    (d) Colorimeter
26. What is the specific gravity of normal urine?
    (a) 1.012 to 1.024
    (b) 1.535 to 1.538
    (c) 2.012 to 2.024
    (d) 3.093 to 3.095
27. In chemical examination of chlorides, in presence of concentrated nitric acid ____________ reacts with chloride and produce white precipitate.
    (a) $MgSO_4$
    (b) $NaNO_2$
    (c) $AgNO_3$
    (d) $BaCl_2$
28. In test for sulphate, in presence of concentrated hydrochloric acid ____________ reacts with sulphate and produce white precipitate
    (a) $MgSO_4$
    (b) $NaNO_2$
    (c) $AgNO_3$
    (d) $BaCl_2$
29. In chemical examination of calcium, in presence of acetic acid ____________ reacts with calcium and produce white precipitate.
    (a) $K_2C_2O_4$
    (b) $MgSO_4$
    (c) $NaNO_2$
    (d) $BaCl_2$.
30. What changes will happen when moist litmus paper is exposed to ammonia?
    (a) Blue to red
    (b) Red to blue
    (c) Red to black
    (d) Red to colorless.
31. Which color will form when uric acid is reacted with Benedict's uric acid reagent?
    (a) White
    (b) Brick-red
    (c) Black
    (d) Blue
32. Which color will form when creatinine is reacts with picric acid in presence of strong alkali?
    (a) Black
    (b) Purple
    (c) Deep orange
    (d) Blue
33. Which of the following test is used for identification of creatinine?
    (a) Jaffe's test
    (b) Benedict's test
    (c) Weyl's test
    (d) Barford's test
34. What is the name of test which is used for determination of proteins in urine?
    (a) Jaffe's test
    (b) Sulpho salicylic acid test
    (c) Weyl's test
    (d) Benedict's test
35. Gerhard's test is used to identify which components present in urine?
    (a) Bile salts
    (b) Proteins
    (c) Carbohydrates
    (d) Ketone bodies

36. Which of the following test is used for determination of bile salts in urine?
    (a) Jaffe's test (b) Hay's test
    (c) Weyl's test (d) Fouchet's test.
37. Bile pigments present in urine is identified by using which test?
    (a) Weyl's test (b) Jaffe's test
    (c) Fouchet's test (d) Benedict's test.
38. Which of the following is not a function of kidney?
    (a) Maintenance of homeostasis (b) Hormonal function
    (c) Waste products excretion (d) Blood circulation
39. Which of the following is not a kidney function test?
    (a) Glomerular function test or clearance test (b) Estimation of creatinine
    (c) Estimation of uric acid (d) Estimation of bilirubin
40. Which formula is used in clearance test?
    (a) $C= U \times P/V$ (b) $C=V \times P/U$
    (c) $C= U \times V/P$ (d) $C= U \times P$
41. Which of the following are risk factors for urinary tract calculi?
    (a) Obesity (b) Dehydration
    (c) Hyperparathyroidism (d) All the above
42. Which of the following is not a urinary tract calculi?
    (a) Calcium kidney stone (b) Uric acid kidney stone
    (c) Sodium kidney stone (d) Struvite kidney stone
43. Which of the following is not a treatment for urinary tract calculi?
    (a) Ureteroscopy (b) Analgesics & antibiotics
    (c) Kidney transplantation (d) Decrease the acidity of urine
44. Renal capsule is the_______________ layer of tissues surrounds the kidney?
    (a) Deep inner layer (b) Superficial inner layer
    (c) Middle layer (d) Superficial middle layer
45. Which layer of tissues surrounds the kidney which protects the kidney from trauma and holds the kidney within abdominal cavity?
    (a) Renal fascia (b) Middle layer
    (c) Deep inner layer (d) Superficial inner layer
46. Which layer of tissues surrounds the kidney which anchors the kidney to the surrounding structures and the abdominal wall?
    (a) Renal capsule (b) Adipose capsule
    (c) Superficial inner layer (d) Deep inner layer
47. Which layer of tissues surrounds the kidney which serves as barrier against trauma and used to maintain shape?
    (a) Adipose capsule (b) Middle layer
    (c) Renal fascia (d) Renal capsule
48. Which is the microscopic structural and functional unit of the kidney?
    (a) Nephron (b) Ureter
    (c) Renal capsule (d) Major calyx

49. Which part of the nephron reabsorbs more calcium and secretes more phosphate in presence of parathyroid hormone?
    (a) Loop of Henle (b) Distal convoluted tubule
    (c) Proximal convoluted tubule (d) Collection duct
50. Which part of the nephron is impermeable to water and it becomes permeable in the presence of antidiuretic hormone (ADH)?
    (a) Distal convoluted tubule (b) Proximal convoluted tubule
    (c) Collection duct (d) Loop of Henle

Key for Multiple Choice Questions

1 (b)	2 (a)	3 (c)	4 (b)	5 (c)
6 (a)	7 (b)	8 (c)	9 (a)	10 (a)
11 (b)	12 (c)	13 (c)	14 (b)	15 (d)
16 (a)	17 (a)	18 (c)	19 (b)	20 (c)
21 (b)	22 (a)	23 (c)	24 (a)	25 (b)
26 (a)	27 (c)	28 (d)	29 (a)	30 (b)
31 (d)	32 (c)	33 (a)	34 (b)	35 (d)
36 (b)	37 (c)	38 (d)	39 (d)	40 (a)
41 (d)	42 (c)	43 (c)	44 (a)	45 (b)
46 (c)	47 (d)	48 (a)	49 (b)	50 (c)

PART – B: Short Answers

1. List out the major functions of the urinary system.
2. Write a short note on external anatomy of kidney.
3. What is nephron?
4. What is juxtaglomerular apparatus?
5. List out various physical examination tests used in urine analysis and explain any one test.
6. Write a note on chemical examination for inorganic constituents in urine analysis.
7. How presence of chlorine in urine is identified?
8. Write the test used for identification of sulphate present in urine.
9. Write a note on chemical test used for identification of calcium present in urine.
10. Write the test used for identification of phosphate present in urine.
11. Write a note on chemical test used for identification of ammonia present in urine.
12. How presence of bicarbonate in urine is identified?
13. What is sodium hypobromite test?
14. Write a note on *urease* test.
15. Explain Biuret test or Piotrowski's test.
16. How uric acid presence in urine is identified?
17. Write a short note on Murexide test for solid uric acid.
18. What is Jaffe's test?
19. Write about Weyl's test.
20. What is urine concentration test? Write the diagnostic significance.

21. Write about metabolic acidosis and compensatory mechanism for its correction.
22. What is cystinuria? Write its clinical consequence.
23. What is creatinine clearance? Write its diagnostic significance.
24. Explain urinary tract calculi.
25. Write short notes on phenyl ketonuria.

PART – C: Long Answers

1. Write a note on Heller's test, sulphosalicylic acid test and heat & acetic acid test.
2. Write a detailed note on tests used for identification of carbohydrates and ketone bodies in urine.
3. How presence of bile salts, bile pigments and blood in urine is identified?
4. What is organ function test? List out major functions of kidney and add a note on types of kidney function test.
5. Write a detailed note on glomerular function test.
6. Explain clearance test in detail with any one example.
7. How creatinine is quantitatively estimated? Explain with procedure.
8. Write the basic principle and procedure involved in the estimation of urea in blood and urine.
9. Explain Nessler's method and Berthelot method of urea estimation.
10. Write a detailed note on estimation of uric acid in serum and urine.
11. What is the importance of specific gravity of urine? Explain urine concentration and urine dilution test.
12. What is kidney stone? Explain the types of kidney stones along with symptoms, diagnostic tests and treatment of kidney stones.
13. List out various renal function test and explain the tests based on glomerular function of kidneys.
14. List out various abnormal constituents present in urine sample. Explain the tests used to detect glucose, proteins and ketone bodies in urine.
15. Write notes on urinary calculi.
16. Classify kidney function tests? Describe any two tests.
17. Describe abnormal constituents of urine.
18. Explain urinary system with a neat labeled diagram.
19. Write a detailed note on kidney.
20. Draw a neat labeled diagram of nephron and explain its biological functions.
21. Explain urine analysis with suitable test.
22. Explain various physical examination tests used in urine analysis.
23. Write a note on various chemical tests used for identification of inorganic constituents in urine.
24. Write a note on chemical examination of urine for presence of organic constituents.
25. Explain organ function test with suitable example.

9

Liver Function Test

In the human body, liver is the largest solid organ and the largest gland. This vital organ carries out more than 500 roles in the human body and it is the only organ that can regenerate. It is classified as a part of the digestive system and the roles of the liver include detoxification, protein synthesis, and the production of chemicals that help in the digestion of food. In the industrialized world alcohol abuse is one of the major causes of liver problems.

Structure of Liver

The liver is a reddish-brown with a rubbery texture weighs approximately 1.5 kg (for men ranging from 0.97 to 1.86 kg and for women ranging from 0.6 to 1.77 kg) and has a width of about 15 cm or 6 inches. It is located in the right upper quadrant of the abdominal cavity; rests just below the diaphragm, to the right of the stomach and overlies the gallbladder or simply it is situated above and to the left of the stomach and below the lungs. The only organ heavier and larger than the liver is the skin.

The liver is wedge-shaped organ (roughly triangular in shape) and consists of two lobes such as a larger right lobe and a smaller left lobe. The liver is connected to two large blood vessels such as portal vein and hepatic artery and common hepatic duct unlike most organs. From the entire digestive system (GIT, spleen and pancreas) digested nutrient-rich blood is carried by the portal vein and from the heart (aorta) oxygenated blood is carried via the celia plexus by the hepatic artery. The blood vessels are sub divided into small capillaries known as liver sinusoids, with each ending in a lobule. The functional unit of the liver is lobules and it consists of millions of hepatic cells called hepatocytes which are the basic metabolic cells. The lobules are held together by a fine, dense, irregular, fibroelastic connective tissue layer extending from the fibrous capsule covering the entire liver known as Glisson's capsule. This extends into the structure of the liver, by accompanying the blood vessels (veins and arteries), ducts, and nerves at the hepatic hilum. The whole surface of the liver except for the bare area is covered in a serous coat derived from the peritoneum, and this firmly adheres to the inner Glisson's capsule. This protects the liver from physical damage and helps to hold it in place. Blood is removed from the liver through three hepatic veins. Structure of liver is presented in Figure 9.1.

Lobes: When viewed from above the liver is grossly divided into two parts such as right lobe and left lobe; whereas when viewed from below the liver is divided into four parts namely left lobe, right lobe, caudate lobe and quadrate lobe. Falciform ligament is a band of tissue that keeps it anchored to the diaphragm which separates the left and right lobes. Between the right and left lobes, the two additional lobes are located from below one in front of the other. Cantlie's line is an imaginary line running from the left of the vena cava and all the way forward to divide the liver and gallbladder into two halves. The left side of the liver is further divided in to two sections by ligamentum venosum and round ligament of the liver (ligamentum teres). This left portion is divided into four segments by porta hepatis which can be numbered in an anticlockwise manner starting at the caudate lobe as I. Seven segments can be seen from this parietal view and in the visceral view only eighth segment is visible.

Surfaces: On the diaphragmatic surface, the liver is covered by a thin, double-layered membrane, the peritoneum (helps to reduce friction against other organs) apart from a triangular bare area where it connects to the diaphragm. The shape of the diaphragm is accommodated in this surface covers the convex shape of the two lobes. Falciform ligament and the right and left triangular ligaments are formed from the peritoneum folds back on itself. These peritoneal ligaments are not related to the anatomic ligaments in joints. Though they serve as surface landmarks the right and left triangular ligaments have no known functional importance. Liver is attached to the posterior portion of the anterior body wall by the falciform ligament. The inferior surface or visceral surface is uneven and concave. It is covered in peritoneum apart from where it attaches the gallbladder and the porta hepatis. The fossa of gall bladder lies to the right of the quadrate lobe, occupied by the gallbladder with its cystic duct close to the right end of porta hepatis.

Impressions: The various adjacent structures and organs are accommodated on the surface of the liver produces several impressions. The two impressions one behind the other and separated by a ridge is underneath the right lobe and to the right of the gallbladder fossa. Hepatic flexure forms a shallow colic impression in front and part of the right kidney and part of the suprarenal gland accommodating the deeper renal impression one behind. A small, triangular, depressed area on the liver is the suprarenal impression. It is located immediately above the renal impression and close to the right of the fossa between the bare area and the caudate lobe. Devoid of peritoneum is the greater part of the suprarenal impression and it lodges the right suprarenal gland. The third is medial to the renal impression and slightly marked impression lying between it and the neck of the gall bladder due to descending portion of the duodenum is known as the duodenal impression. Gastric impression is present behind and to the left of the inferior surface of the left lobe of the liver. Over the upper front surface of the stomach this is molded, and to the right of this is a rounded eminence, the tuber omentale, which fits into the concavity of the lesser curvature of the stomach and lies in front of the anterior layer of the lesser omentum.

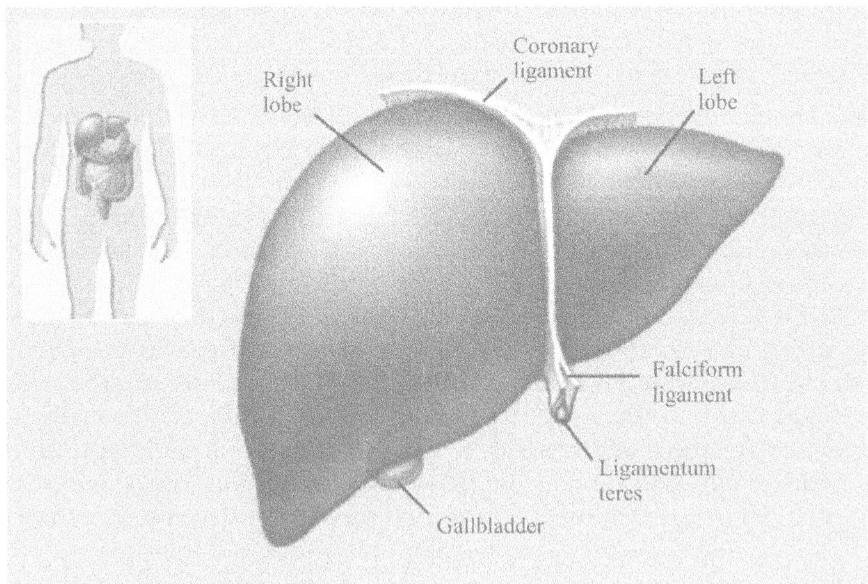

Figure 9.1 Structure of liver.

Biological Functions of Liver

Liver is the major organ of biological system and it is the central organs of body's metabolism. Liver performs several diversified biological functions. The major biological functions of liver are, 1) Metabolic function, 2) Excretory function, 3) Protective function, 4) Detoxification function, 5) Hematological function, and 6) Storage function.

1. **Metabolic functions of liver:** Liver is the enzyme factory of biological systems; hence, almost all metabolism of biomolecules takes place in liver. It actively participates in the metabolism of biomolecules such as carbohydrates, proteins, lipids, minerals and vitamins. Because of this metabolic function of liver many compounds are biosynthesized and degraded in liver.
2. **Excretory function of liver:** Liver is also involved in excretions of some compounds from biological systems. Liver excretes bile pigments, bile salts and cholesterol into intestine .
3. **Protective function of liver:** Biological system is protected by liver also. In liver Kupffer cells are present. These cells are responsible for phagocytosis (engulfment of microorganism) and protect biological system from microorganisms. Hence, liver is involved in elimination of foreign compounds and protecting the biological system from foreign compounds.
4. **Detoxification function of liver:** In biological system, liver plays a major role in conversion of several toxic compounds into non-toxic compound. For example, ammonia is toxic to biological system and liver detoxifies ammonia into urea which is excreted in urine. Xenobiotic metabolism is defined as a series of biochemical reactions taking place in biological systems to convert the foreign substances such as drugs, cosmetics, pollutants, food additives, waste product produced in normal metabolism, etc, which is often toxic into non-toxic or less toxic and more easily excretable form.
5. **Hematological functions of liver:** Liver is involved in the synthesis of blood mainly in the embryo. It is also involved in formation of plasma proteins including blood clotting factors. Moreover, it also involved in destruction of erythrocytes.
6. **Storage function of liver:** Many substances are stored in the liver and utilized when it is needed by the biological system. The following substances like glycogen, vitamin-A, vitamin-D, vitamin-B_{12}, trace elements iron is stored in liver.

Causes of Liver Damage

The liver can be damaged by the following substances (or) processes. They are 1) Viruses (Hepatitis A and hepatitis B virus), 2) Toxic chemical substances like aflatoxins, carbon tetrachloride, etc. 3) Alcohol, 4) Hepatocellular carcinoma, 5) Autoimmune hepatitis, etc.

Liver Function Test (LFT)

Liver function test (LFT) is defined as the biochemical investigations used to assess the capability of liver to carry out any of its biological function. Hence LFT is used to detect the abnormalities of liver and also the extent of liver damages. Liver is the major organ of biological system and it is the central organs of body's metabolism. Liver performs several diversified biological functions. Hence the following facts must be considered while performing LFT.

1. Liver is the biggest biochemical factory performs several biological functions. Hence, liver damage may not affect all biological functions of liver and it performs many of its functions almost normally.
2. It is very important to select the particular right liver function test otherwise the results may not be significant since liver performs several diversified functions, the function that is assessed in LFT may not be the one that is adversely affected.

Classification:

Liver function tests are broadly classified into many types as follows,

1. Liver function test based on metabolic capacity of liver: **Example:** Galactose tolerance test, and antipyrine clearance test.
2. Liver function test based on excretory functions of liver. **Example:** Estimation of bile pigments, estimation of bile salts, and estimation of bromosulphthalein.
3. Liver function test based on detoxification function of liver. **Example:** Hippuric acid synthesis.
4. Liver function test based on hematological functions of liver or synthetic functions of liver. **Example:** Estimation of serum albumin, and estimation of prothrombin time.

5. Liver function test based on serum enzymes derived from liver. **Example:** Estimation of *alkaline phosphatase*, estimation of *transaminase*, estimation of *γ-glutamoyl transpeptidase*, and estimation of *5-nucleotidase*.

   The various liver functions and the common serum or plasma markers for the impaired functions of liver are listed in Table 9.1.

Table 9.1 List of hepatic functions with its common markers for impaired functions.

S. No.	Functions of liver	Common serum or plasma markers for the impaired functions
1	Drug metabolism	Increased half life of drugs
2	Protein synthesis	Decreased albumin and increased prothrombin time
3	Protein catabolism	Increased urea and increased ammonia
4	Lipid metabolism	Increased cholesterol and increased triglycerides
5	Heme metabolism	Increased bilirubin
6	Bile acid metabolism	Increased bile acids
7	Enzymes	Increased *alanine transaminase*, increased *aspartate transaminase*, and increased *γ-glutamyltranspeptidase*

Metabolism of Bile Pigments

The life span of erythrocytes is only 120 days. After 120 days the erythrocytes are removed from the circulation and taken up by the macrophages of the reticuloendothelial (RE) system in the spleen and liver. In macrophages erythrocytes are degraded into non-protein heme and the protein part globin by cleaving. This protein part globin may be degraded into individual amino acids or as such it is reutilized for the formation of hemoglobin. The formed amino acids may undergo its own metabolism including participation in fresh globin synthesis. About 80 % of the heme subjected for degradations is obtained from erythrocytes only. The remaining 20 % are obtained from immature RBC, cytochromes and myoglobin.

Later, heme is converted into biliverdin (Green pigment) in presence of enzyme *heme oxygenase* (The substrate is "heme" and the type of reaction involved is "oxidation") which utilizes NADPH + H^+ and oxygen and breaks the methenyl bridges present in between two pyrrole rings (A and B ring). In the mean time, ferrous (Fe^{2+}) is oxidized into ferric (Fe^{3+}) ion. Carbon monoxide is also released during this reaction. In amphibian and birds, the biliverdin is excreted as such, whereas in mammals it further undergoes degradations.

In the next step, the methenyl bridge present between pyrrole ring C and D of biliverdin is reduced to methylene group and forms bilirubin (Yellow pigment). *Biliverdin reductase* (The substrate is "biliverdin" and the type of reaction involved is "reduction") catalyzes this reaction which is a NADPH + H^+ dependent soluble enzyme. The term bile pigments are used to collectively represent bilirubin and its derivatives like biliverdin.

Bilirubin is insoluble in aqueous solution because it is lipophilic in nature. Hence, it is transported into plasma in a non-covalently bound form to albumin as bilirubin-albumin complex. Albumin has two binding sites namely high affinity site (about 25 mg of bilirubin per 100 ml of plasma tightly binds at this site) and low affinity sites (Rest of bilirubin binds loosely at this site). The latter one easily detaches from the albumin and enters into the tissues. Some times bilirubin may enter into the CNS and cause damage to the neurons because certain drugs like sulfonamides and salicylates can displace the bilirubin from albumin.

Once albumin-bilirubin complex enters into the liver, the dissociated bilirubin was taken up by the sinusoidal surface of the hepatocytes through a carrier mediated active transport system. In liver, bilirubin binds with a specific intracellular protein namely ligandin. More over bilirubin in liver undergoes glucuronic acid conjugation by reacting with two moles of UDP glucuronate and produces bilirubin diglucuronide which is water soluble and liberates free UDP. This reaction is catalyzed by the enzyme called *bilirubin glucuronyl transferase* (The substrate is "bilirubin" and the group transferred is "glucuronide") of smooth endoplasmic reticulum. This enzyme can be induced by number of drugs such as phenobarbital. When excess bilirubin is there bilirubin monoglucuronide may also accumulate in the body.

Later, conjugated bilirubin is excreted into the bile canaliculi against a concentration gradient which then enters into the bile. This transport of bilirubin diglucuronide is energy dependent, active and rate limiting process. Almost all the bilirubin (> 98 %) enters into the bile are conjugated form only.

The specific bacterial enzymes present in the intestine namely *β-glucuronidase* (The substrate is "bilirubin glucuronide" and the type of reaction involved is "hydrolysis") hydrolyzes the bilirubin glucuronide into bilirubin. Later bilirubin is converted into urobilinogen which is a colorless compound and a small part of it may get reabsorbed into the circulation. In the kidney, urobilinogen can be converted into yellow color compound urobilin and excreted in urine. The characteristic yellow color of the urine is due to urobilin only. A major part of the urobilinogen is converted into stercobilin by the intestinal bacteria. This formed stercobilin is excreted along with feces. The characteristic brown color of the feces is due to stercobilin only.

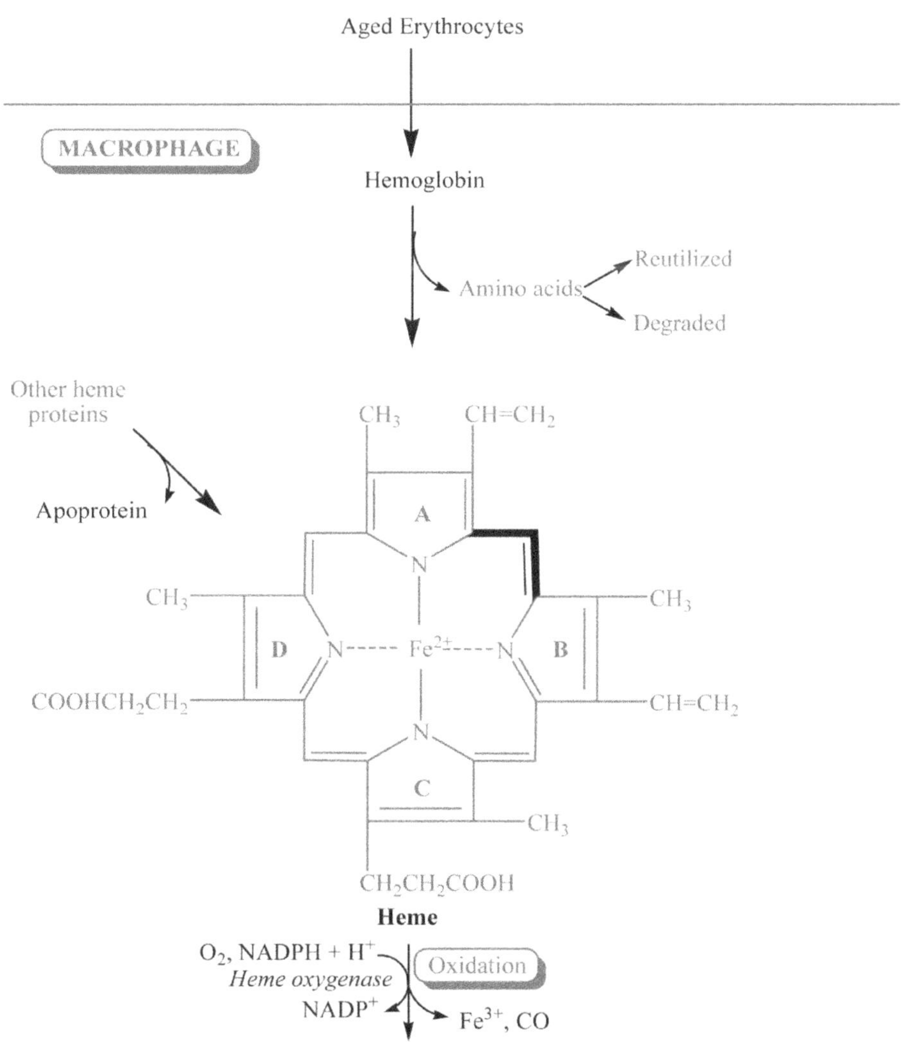

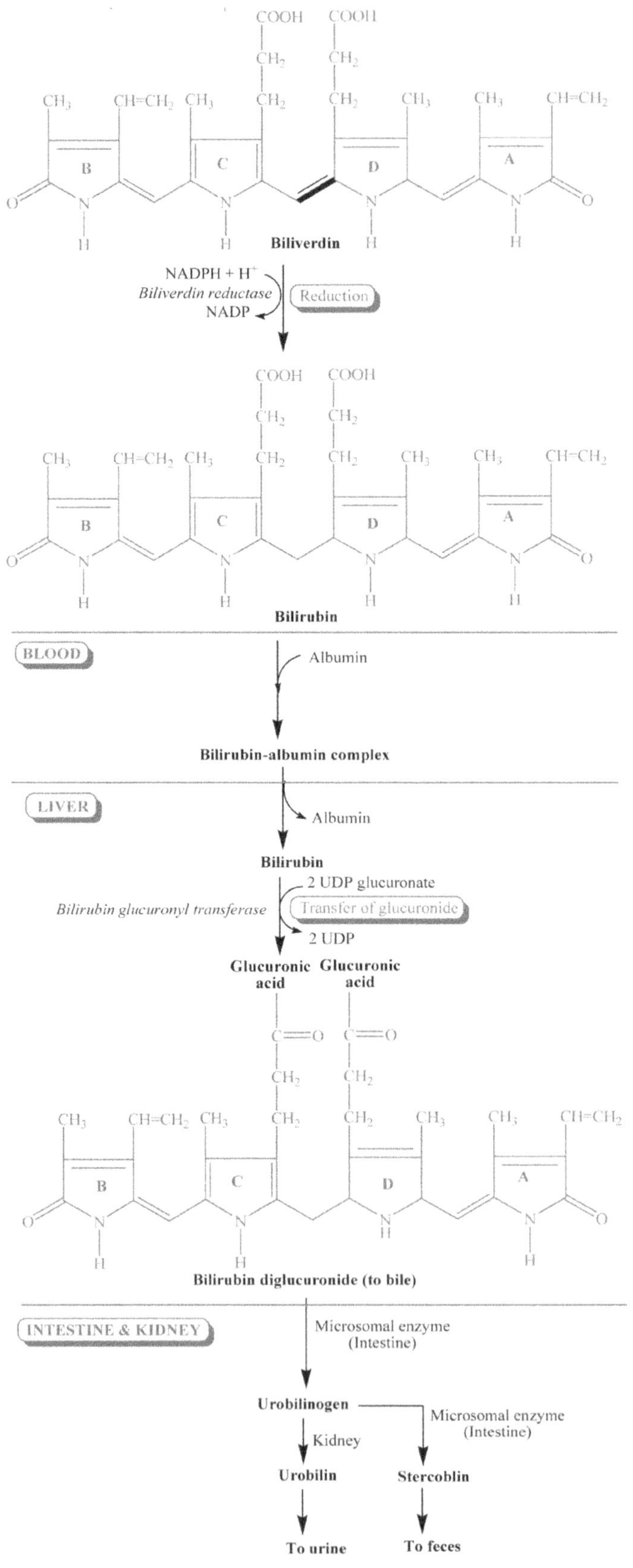

COOH COOH
CH_2 CH_2
CH_3 $CH{=}CH_2$ CH_3 CH_2 CH_2 CH_3 CH_3 $CH{=}CH_2$
B C D A
O N N N N O
H H H H
Biliverdin

NADPH + H^+
Biliverdin reductase (Reduction)
NADP

COOH COOH
CH_2 CH_2
CH_3 $CH{=}CH_2$ CH_3 CH_2 CH_2 CH_3 CH_3 $CH{=}CH_2$
B C D A
O N N N N O
H H H H
Bilirubin

BLOOD

Albumin

Bilirubin-albumin complex

LIVER

Albumin

Bilirubin

2 UDP glucuronate
Bilirubin glucuronyl transferase (Transfer of glucuronide)
2 UDP

Glucuronic acid **Glucuronic acid**
C=O C=O
CH_2 CH_2
CH_3 $CH{=}CH_2$ CH_3 CH_2 CH_2 CH_3 CH_3 $CH{=}CH_2$
B C D A
O N N N N O
H H H H
Bilirubin diglucuronide (to bile)

INTESTINE & KIDNEY

Microsomal enzyme (Intestine)

Urobilinogen

Kidney → **Urobilin** → **To urine**

Microsomal enzyme (Intestine) → **Stercoblin** → **To feces**

Liver Function Test Based on Excretory Functions of Liver

The excretory function of liver can be assessed by estimating the following compounds like bile salts, bile pigments and bromosulphthalein present in serum.

Estimation of Bilirubin

Bilirubin is the excretory end product of heme metabolism and it is a yellow color bile pigment. In liver bilirubin undergoes conjugation and produces bilirubin diglucuronide. Later, it enters in intestine where it is converted to urobilinogen further to urobilin and stercobilin (urobilin is the substances which is responsible for yellow color of urine and stercobilin is the substance which is responsible for brown color of feces).

The normal serum bilirubin levels are 0.2 to 1 mg/dl. Bilirubin is present in both conjugated and unconjugated form in liver. The normal conjugated bilirubin serum level is 0.2 to 0.4 mg/dl. In the conjugated form 75 % are diglucuronide and 25 % are monoglucuronide. The normal unconjugated bilirubin level in serum is 0.2 to 0.6 mg/dl.

Following are the various tests used to determine the bilirubin levels. They are 1) Icterus test, 2) Van den Bergh reaction, 3) Fouchet's test and Gmelin's test.

Estimation of Bilirubin in Serum

1. **Icterus Test**
   This is very simple but outdated test used to determine serum bilirubin. This test is based on yellow color of serum due to bilirubin. It is useful for the immediate diagnosis of neonatal jaundice.
2. **Van Den Bergh Reaction**
   This test is a very sensitive test used to estimate the level of bilirubin in serum. Generally, normal serum gives negative test to Van den Bergh reaction.

Mechanism of reaction:

This test is based on Ehrlich's diazo reaction. Van den Bergh reagent is composed of equal volumes of sulphanilic acid in dilute hydrochloric acid and sodium nitrite ($NaNO_2$). The basic principle behind the Van den Bergh reaction is diazotized sulphanilic acid forms purple colored azobilirubin on reaction with bilirubin.

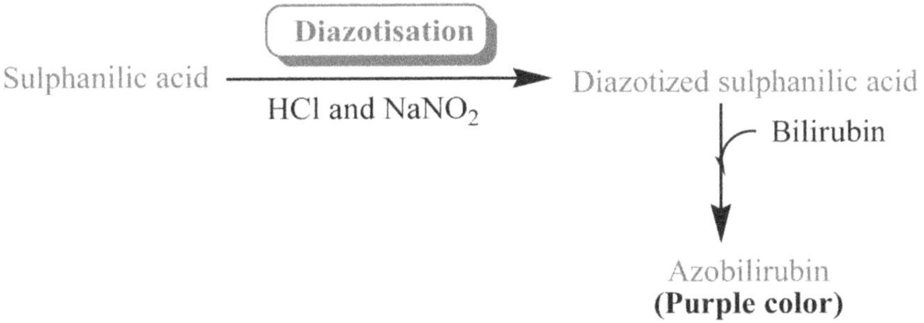

Procedure (Direct and indirect reactions):

As such bilirubin is insoluble in water whereas conjugated bilirubin is soluble in water. In case of direct positive Van den Bergh reaction, conjugated bilirubin reacts immediately with Van den Bergh reagent and produces purple color within 30 seconds.

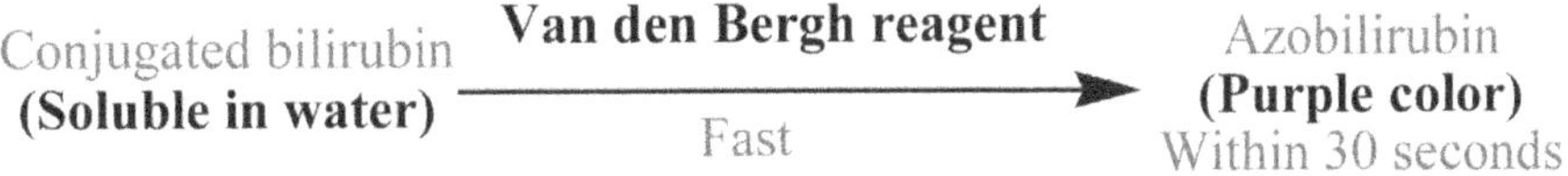

In case of indirect positive Van den Bergh reaction, methanol or alcohol is added to dissolve the unconjugated bilirubin which later reacts with Van den Bergh reagent and produces purple color within 30 minutes.

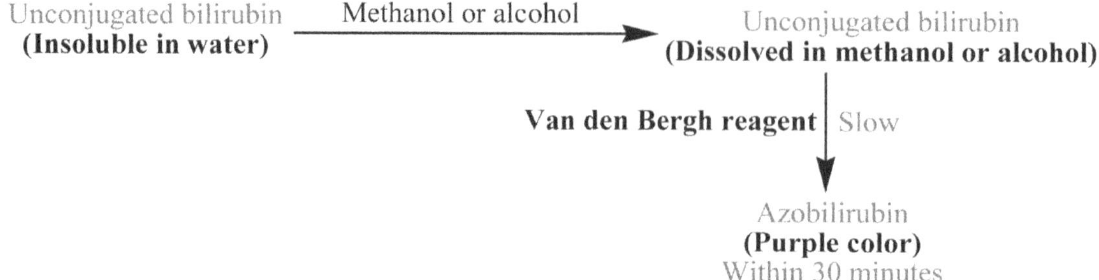

If both unconjugated and conjugated bilirubins are present in high concentrations in serum then the purple color is developed immediately. Later the violet color intensity is increased when methanol or alcohol is added. This type of reaction is known as biphasic reaction.

Significance:

Nature of the jaundice is easily identified using Van den Bergh reaction because type of jaundice is characterized by increased serum unconjugated bilirubin (hemolytic jaundice) or serum conjugated bilirubin (obstructive jaundice) or both (hepatic jaundice). In Van den Bergh reaction, the types of jaundice are differentiated as follows, a) Hemolytic jaundice gives indirect positive in Van den Bergh reaction, b) Obstructive jaundice gives direct positive in Van den Bergh reaction, and c) Hepatic jaundice gives biphasic in Van den Bergh reaction.

Tests based on Van Den Bergh Reaction

There are two different methods for estimation of serum bilirubin based on Van den Bergh reaction. They are 1) Malloy-Evelyn method (Simple method), 2) Jendrassik-Grof method (Accurate method). Hemolyzed samples should be avoided because hemoglobin interferes in both methods and light exposure of sample should also be avoided because bilirubin is destroyed by light.

1. MALLOY-EVELYN METHOD

Principle:

Azobilirubin is formed by reaction of bilirubin with Ehrlich's diazo reagent. The obtained red purple color is estimated using colorimeter. Later methanol (concentration that does not precipitate proteins) is added to measure the unconjugated bilirubin.

Bilirubin + Ehrlich's diazo reagent ⟶ Azobilirubin **(Red purple color)**

Reagents:

1. **Diazo reagent:**
   - (a) **Solution A:** Dissolve 1 g of sulphanilic acid in 15 ml of concentrated hydrochloric acid and dilute to 1000 ml with distilled water.
   - (b) **Solution B:** Dissolve 0.5 g of sodium nitrite in 25 ml of water and dilute to 100 ml with distilled water.
   - (c) **Diazo reagent:** Just before use, mix 10 ml of solution A and 0.3 ml of solution B and use within 30 minutes.
2. **Blank diazo reagent:** Add 15 ml of concentrated hydrochloric acid to 900 ml of water slowly and dilute to 1000 ml with distilled water.
3. **Standard bilirubin solution:** Dissolve 10 mg of bilirubin in 50 ml of chloroform (Heat gently to dissolve bilirubin) and dilute to 100 ml using chloroform. 10 ml of the above solution is further diluted to 100 ml using chloroform. (10 mg bilirubin in 100 ml solution. Therefore 1 ml solution contains 0.1 mg of bilirubin; 10 ml solution contains 1 mg of bilirubin. Hence, 1 mg bilirubin is

present in 100 ml standard bilirubin solution; Therefore, 2 ml standard bilirubin solution contains 0.02 mg of bilirubin).

4. **Standard methyl red solution:** Dissolve 290 mg of methyl red in 50 ml of glacial acetic acid and dilute to 100 ml with glacial acetic acid. Add 1 ml of the above solution to 5 ml glacial acetic acid and add the solution of 14.4 g sodium acetate trihydrate in 50 ml water and made the volume to 1000 ml using distilled water. (Measure the absorbance of standard methyl red solution at 540 nm against water. This absorbance is generally equal to the absorbance of bilirubin whose concentration is 10 mg/100 ml. Standard methyl red solution is used to standardize standard bilirubin solution because bilirubin solutions are unstable).

Procedure:

Take three test tubes and label as standard, blank and unknown. In unknown test tube take 0.2 ml serum and 1.8 ml water; in standard test tube take 2 ml of standard bilirubin solution and in blank test tube take 2 ml of water. Add 0.5 ml of diazo reagent to standard and unknown test tubes and mix well. Add 0.5 ml of blank diazo reagent to blank test tube and mix well. Finally, add 2.5 ml of methanol to all three tubes and mix well. Measure the intensity of the color obtained in standard and unknown against blank at 540 nm or using green filter after 30 minutes. Calculate the concentration of bilirubin present in unknown sample using the following formula.

$$\text{Concentration of total bilirubin in 0.2 ml serum} = \frac{E_u}{E_s} \times C_s = \frac{E_u}{E_s} \times 0.02\ mg\ bilirubin$$

$$\text{Concentration of total bilirubin in 100 ml serum} = \frac{\left(\frac{E_u}{E_s} \times 0.02\right)}{0.2} \times 100 = \frac{E_u}{E_s} \times 10\ mg$$

Where, E_u = Optical density of unknown serum sample

E_s = Optical density of standard bilirubin solution

C_s = Concentration of standard bilirubin solution

Take three test tubes and label as standard, blank and unknown

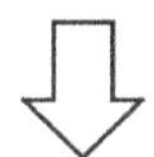

Add 5 ml of Biuret reagent to all three test tubes

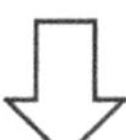

Add 0.1 ml of serum in unknown test tube, 0.1 ml of standard protein solution in standard test tube and 0.1 ml of water in blank test tube

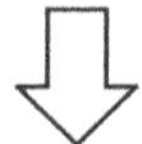

Mix well all three tubes individually

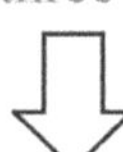

Finally, measure the intensity of the violet color obtained in standard and unknown against blank at 540 nm or using green filter after 30 minutes

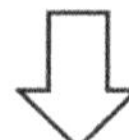

Calculate the concentration of total protein present in unknown sample

Concentration of conjugated bilirubin in 100 ml serum is measured by substituting methanol with water and the concentration of unconjugated bilirubin in 100 ml serum is calculated by difference i.e., Concentration of unconjugated bilirubin = Concentration of total bilirubin - Concentration of conjugated bilirubin.

2. JENDRASSIK-GROF METHOD

Principle:

Azobilirubin is formed by reacting bilirubin with diazo reagent in the presence of sodium acetate and caffeine benzoate. In this method, sodium acetate acts as a buffer and caffeine benzoate accelerates the reaction. Excess diazo reagent is destroyed and the reaction was stopped by adding ascorbic acid. Later, the purple color azobilirubin formed is converted to blue azobilirubin by treating with strong alkaline tartrate solution. The intensity of the blue color is estimated using colorimeter. Caffeine benzoate is omitted to measure the conjugated bilirubin.

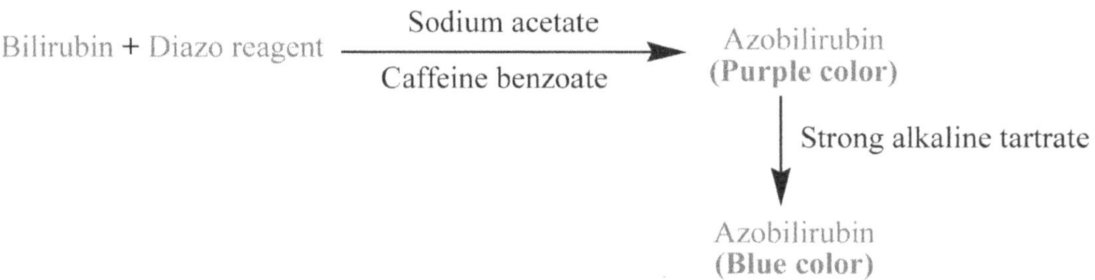

Reagents:

1. **0.05 N Hydrochloric acid:** Dilute 4.2 ml of concentrated hydrochloric acid to 1000 ml with distilled water.
2. **Caffeine benzoate reagent:** Dissolve 50 g of caffeine, 75 g of sodium benzoate and 125 g of sodium acetate in 500 ml of warm water. Cool the solution, add 1 g of disodium EDTA and mix well. Dilute the solution to 1000 ml using distilled water.
3. **Diazo reagent:**
   (a) **Solution A:** Dissolve 1 g of sulphanilic acid in 15 ml of concentrated hydrochloric acid and dilute to 1000 ml with distilled water.
   (b) **Solution B:** Dissolve 0.5 g of sodium nitrite in 25 ml of water and dilute to 100 ml with distilled water.
   (c) **Diazo reagent:** Just before use, mix 10 ml of solution A and 0.3 ml of solution B and use within 30 minutes.
4. **Blank diazo reagent:** Add 15 ml of concentrated hydrochloric acid to 900 ml of water slowly and dilute to 1000 ml with distilled water.
5. **4 % Ascorbic acid solution:** Dissolve 4 g of ascorbic acid in 25 ml of water and dilute to 100 ml with distilled water.
6. **Alkaline tartrate solution:** Dissolve 100 g of sodium hydroxide and 350 g of sodium tartrate in 500 ml of water. After cooling, dilute the solution to 1000 ml with distilled water.
7. **Stock bilirubin solution:** Dissolve 10 mg of bilirubin in 50 ml of chloroform (Heat gently to dissolve bilirubin) and dilute to 100 ml with chloroform. Further, dilute the stock bilirubin solution as follows.
8. **Standard bilirubin solution:** Prepare this solution from the stock bilirubin solution as follows.

Solution name	S_1	S_2	S_3	S_4	S_5
Stock bilirubin solution (in ml)	0.2	0.4	0.6	0.8	1.0
Chloroform (in ml)	0.8	0.6	0.4	0.2	0.0
Concentration of bilirubin (mg/100 ml)	2	4	6	8	10

Procedure:

Total and direct bilirubin is measured separately and indirect bilirubin is calculated by difference.

Total bilirubin: Take two test tubes and label as total and total blank. In both the test tube add 0.3 ml water and 0.2 ml serum. Add 2 ml of caffeine benzoate reagent to both the test tubes and mix well. Add 0.5 ml of diazo A solution and 0.5 ml of diazo reagent to total blank and total test tube, respectively. Mix well the two test tubes separately and keep aside for 10 minutes. Add 1 ml of alkaline tartrate solution to both the test tubes and mix well. Measure the absorbance of total test tube at 600 nm against total blank test tube.

Take two test tubes and label as total and total blank

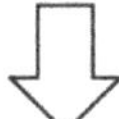

In both the test tube add 0.3 ml water and 0.2 ml serum

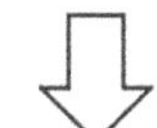

Add 2 ml of caffeine benzoate reagent to both the test tubes and mix well

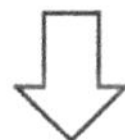

Add 0.5 ml of diazo A solution and 0.5 ml of diazo reagent to total blank and total test tube, respectively

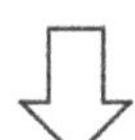

Mix well the two test tubes separately and keep aside for 10 minutes

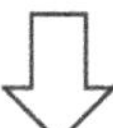

Add 1 ml of alkaline tartrate solution to both the test tubes and mix well

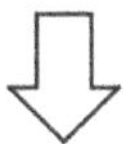

Measure the absorbance of total test tube at 600 nm against total blank test tube

Direct bilirubin: Take two test tubes and label as direct and direct blank. In both the test tube, add 0.3 ml water and 0.2 ml serum. Add 2 ml of caffeine benzoate reagent to direct blank test tube and 2 ml of 0.05 N hydrochloric acid to direct test tube. Mix well the two test tubes individually. Add 0.5 ml of diazo A solution to direct blank test tube and 0.5 ml of diazo reagent to direct test tube. Mix well the two test tubes separately and add 0.1 ml of ascorbic acid solution to both the test tube one minute latter and mix well. Measure the absorbance of direct test tube at 600 nm against direct blank test tube.

Analyze the different concentration containing standard bilirubin solutions in the same way as serum. Draw a calibration curve by taking concentration of bilirubin on "X" axis and absorbance on "Y" axis. Measure the concentration of bilirubin present in serum from the calibration curve.

Take two test tubes and label as direct and direct blank

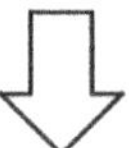

In both the test tube add 0.3 ml water and 0.2 ml serum

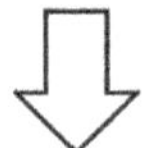

Add 2 ml of caffeine benzoate reagent to direct blank test tube and 2 ml of 0.05 N hydrochloric acid to direct test tube

Mix well the two test tubes separately and add 0.1 ml of ascorbic acid solution to both the test tube one minute latter and mix well

Measure the absorbance of direct test tube at 600 nm against direct blank test tube

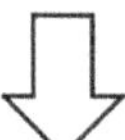

Analyze the different concentration containing standard bilirubin solutions in the same way as serum

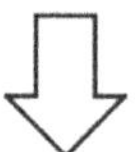

Draw a calibration curve by taking concentration of bilirubin on "X" axis and absorbance on "Y" axis

Measure the concentration of bilirubin present in serum from the calibration curve

Estimation of Bilirubin in Urine

Conjugated bilirubin is soluble in water, hence it is excreted in urine, whereas unconjugated bilirubin is insoluble in water, hence it is not excreted in urine. Presence of bilirubin in urine can be detected by using the following tests like a) Fouchet's test, and 2) Gmelin 's test.

1. **Fouchet's test**

   Principle:

   This test is based on oxidation of bilirubin into biliverdin. In this test, initially barium chloride reacts with urinary sulphates and forms a barium sulphate precipitate. In this formed barium sulphate precipitate bilirubin is adsorbed. Ferric chloride oxidizes the adsorbed bilirubin in presence of trichloroacetic acid to biliverdin.

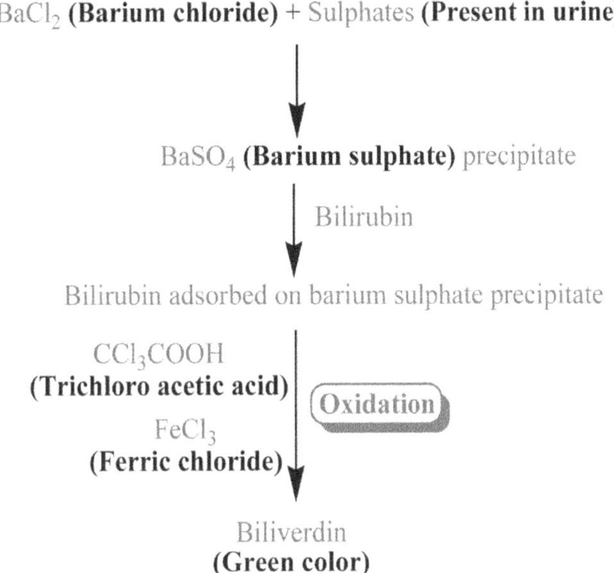

Reagents:

1. **10 % Barium chloride solution:** Dissolve 10 g of barium chloride in 25 ml of water and dilute to 100 ml with distilled water.
2. **10 % Ferric chloride solution:** Dissolve 10 g of ferric chloride in 25 ml of water and dilute to 100 ml with distilled water.
3. **25 % Trichloro acetic acid solution:** Dissolve 25 g of trichloro acetic acid in 25 ml of water and dilute to 100 ml with distilled water.
4. **Fouchet's reagent:** Mix 10 ml of 10 % ferric chloride solution with 90 ml of 25 % trichloroacetic acid solution.

Procedure:

To 10 ml of urine solution, add 5 ml of barium sulphate solution and mix well. Filter the solution using filter paper and dry the filter paper. Add few drops of Fouchet's reagent on the filter paper and dry it. Appearance of green color on the filter paper indicates the presence of bilirubin.

To 10 ml of urine solution, add 5 ml of barium sulphate solution and mix well

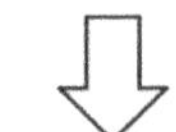

Filter the solution using filter paper and dry the filter paper

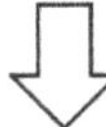

Add few drops of Fouchet's reagent on the filter paper and dry it

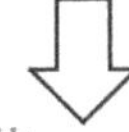

Appearance of green color on the filter paper indicates the presence of bilirubin

2. **Gmelin's test**

Principle:

It is a simple qualitative method used for identifying bilirubin in urine. Urine is layered over nitric acid and if bilirubin is present, various colored rings are seen at the junctions. This test is based on oxidation of bilirubin into biliverdin. In this test, nitric acid is used as an oxidizing agent which oxidizes bilirubin into various oxidized products like biliverdin, etc.

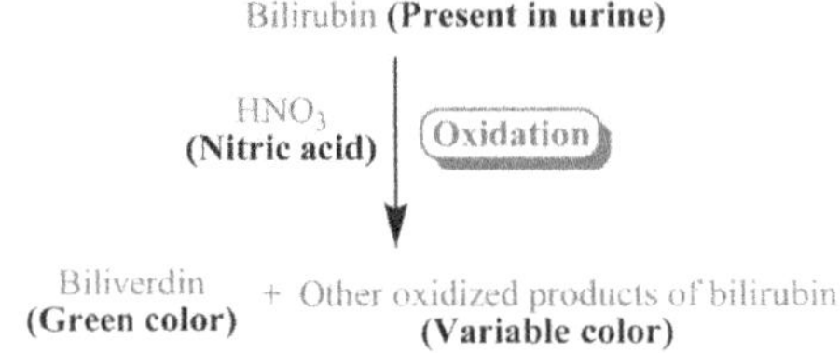

Procedure:

In a test tube, take 5 ml of the urine sample. Add 5 ml of concentrated nitric acid. If bile pigments are present different colored rings are appear between the two layers due to oxidation of bilirubin into various chemical products. If bilirubin is present blue, green and violet rings appear. Gmelin's test is not sensitive, hence a positive result always indicates the presence of bile pigments but a negative result does not exclude the presence of small quantities of bile pigments.

In a test tube, take 5 ml of the urine sample

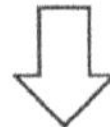

Add 5 ml of concentrated nitric acid

⇩

If bile pigments are present different colored rings are appear between the two layers due to oxidation of bilirubin into various chemical products

Estimation of Urobilinogen in Urine

Hemoglobin breaks into bilirubin and enters the intestine where it is transformed into urobilinogen by the action of bacteria and excreted as urobilin which gives yellow color to urine. In addition, urobilinogen in the intestine is reduced to brown color stercobilin which gives color to feces by the action of intestinal bacteria. Some part of urobilinogen is absorbed into the portal circulation and reaches the liver, metabolized and excreted into the bile. Traces of urobilinogen escaped from the liver is carried to kidney and excreted in the urine. Urobilinogen is colorless but the urobilin which is the oxidized form of urobilinogen is a brown pigment. Absence of urobilinogen indicates obstructive jaundice.

Principle:

Urobilinogen in urine is estimated by using Ehrlichs aldehyde reagent. Urobilinogen is one of the bile pigments found in urine in case of liver defects, (epidemic icterus, and cirrhosis) or as a result of excessive formation of bilirubin (hemolytic jaundice). The normal concentrations of urobilinogen in urine are up to 1.0 mg/dl in random sample or 0.5 to 4 mg/dl in 24 hours sample or 0.5 to 4.0 Ehrlich units/day or 0.1 to 1.0 Ehrlich units/2 hours (One Ehrlich unit is approximately equal to 1 mg of urobilinogen). The normal concentrations of urobilinogen in feces are 75 to 400 Ehrlich units/day. In an acidic medium, the colorless urobilinogen reacts with Ehrlich's aldehyde reagent and forms pink-red condensing products. Medications may cause false positive results. False negative reactions can be caused by high nitrite concentrations. Pigmented urine can interfere with detection of urobilinogen.

Urobilinogen + Ehrlich's aldehyde reagent —Acid medium→ Condensing products **(Pink-red color)**

Reagents:

1. **Ehrlich's aldehyde reagent:** Dissolve 4 g of *p*-dimethylamino benzaldehyde in 100 ml of concentrated hydrochloric acid and add 100 ml of distilled water.

Procedure:

To 10 ml of urine sample add 1.0 ml Ehrlich's aldehyde reagent. Mix well and allow to stand for about 10 minutes. Observe the color developed by looking down into the tube held over a white surface.

Appearance of pink-red color indicates the presence of urobilinogen. The same method can be used for estimation of urobilinogen in feces also. Exception is treating stool aqueous extract with the alkaline ferrous hydroxide to reduce urobilin to urobilinogen. The rest of the procedure is same.

To 10 ml of urine sample add 1.0 ml Ehrlich's aldehyde reagent

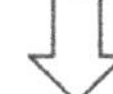

Mix well and allow to stand for about 10 minutes

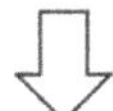

Observe the color developed by looking down into the tube held over a white surface

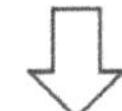

Appearance of pink-red color indicates the presence of urobilinogen

Significance:

Urobilinogen estimation is used to assess liver function. This is the earliest sign of liver disease. This test is positive in hemolytic anemia. In obstructive jaundice, there is no urobilinogen in urine; in hemolytic jaundice urine urobilinogen is increased and in hepatocellular jaundice urobilinogen level in urine becomes normal. Increased urobilinogen is seen in clinical conditions like cirrhosis due to alcohol or viral diseases or chemicals, biliary obstruction, biliary tract infection, cholangitis, hepatotoxic drugs (amino salicylic acid, phenothiazine and penicillin), due to increased RBCs destruction in hemolytic anemia, pernicious anemia and malaria, acute hepatitis, pulmonary infarction, hematoma and excessive ecchymosis. Decreased urobilinogen is seen in conditions like gallstones, biliary obstruction, biliary tract infection (severe), pancreatic cancer (head of the pancreas) and use of drugs such as aspirin, chloramphenicol, insulin, phenytoin, streptomycin, tetracycline, methyldopa, and sulphonamide.

Bromsulphthalein Test or BSP Test or Dye Test

Principle:

Bromsulphthalein (BSP) is a non-toxic dye used to estimate the excretory functions of liver. It is entirely excreted by the liver through bile. If excretory function of liver is normal, the bromsulphthalein (BSP) dye administered must be cleared from serum (almost 95 %) within 45 minutes of administration. If the dye is retained for a longer time in the serum then it is an indication of the abnormalities in liver function particularly in excretory function.

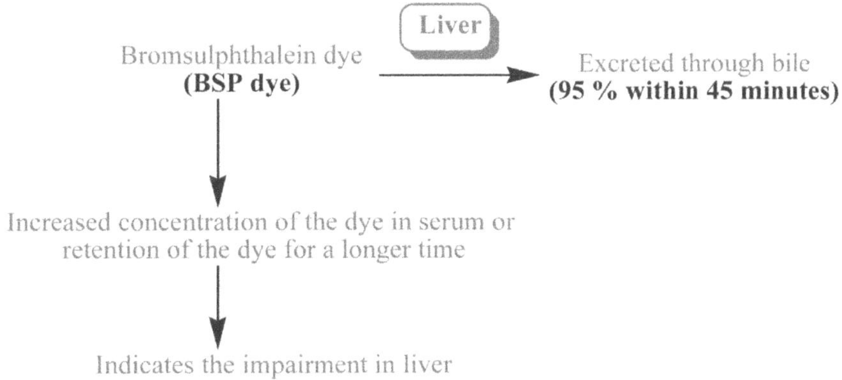

Procedure:

Administer bromsulphthalein (BSP) dye at a dose of 5 mg/kg body weight intravenously. Measure the serum concentration of bromsulphthalein (BSP) at 45 minutes and 2 hours after administration of BSP dye. In normal conditions only less than 5 % of the dye is retained at the end of 45 minutes. Increased concentration of the dye in serum or retention of the dye for a longer time indicates the impairment in liver.

Administer bromsulphthalein (BSP) dye at a dose of 5 mg/kg body weight intravenously

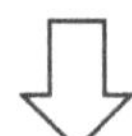

Measure the serum concentration of bromsulphthalein (BSP) at 45 minutes and 2 hours after administration of BSP dye

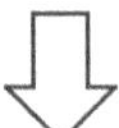

In normal conditions only less than 5 % of the dye is retained at the end of 45 minutes

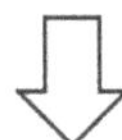

Increased concentration of the dye in serum or retention of the dye for a longer time indicates the impairment in liver

Significance:

Bromsulphthalein (BSP) dye test is a quite sensitive test used to assess the abnormalities of liver with specific reference to excretory function.

Liver Function Tests based on Serum Proteins

The following are the important liver function estimation tests which are based on serum proteins. They are,

1. Estimation of serum total proteins.
2. Estimation of serum albumin and globulin.
3. Estimation of prothrombin time.

1. Estimation of Serum Total Protein (Biuret Method)

Serum contains many different varieties of protein. Out of these, the two proteins which constitute the bulk of the total amount of protein in serum is albumin and globulin. Generally, Biuret method is used for the estimation of total proteins in serum.

Principle:

The basic principle involved in the Biuret method is chelation of cupric ion with peptide bonds of protein in alkaline medium. In this method, alkaline medium is provided by sodium potassium tartrate which helps to keep cupric ions in solution. The formed chelates are violet in color and the intensity of the color is proportional to the number of peptide bonds which in turns depends upon the amount of proteins present in the sample. The intensity of the violet color chelates are measured colorimetrically at 540 nm or using a green filter.

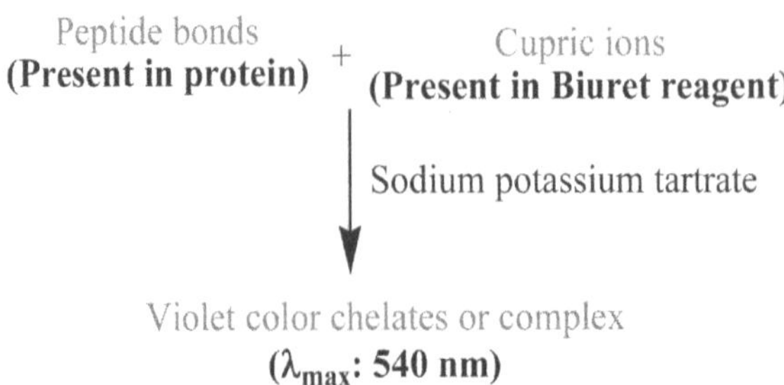

Reagents:

1. **Biuret reagent:** Dissolve 3 g of copper sulphate in 50 ml of water. To this solution, add 9 g of sodium potassium tartrate, 5 g of potassium iodide and sodium hydroxide solution (Dissolve 24 g sodium hydroxide in 100 ml of water). Finally, made the volume up to 1000 ml with distilled water. Store the reagent in a well stoppered polythene bottle.
2. **Biuret blank:** Prepare the solution in the same way like Biuret reagent without copper sulphate.
3. **Standard protein solution:** Dissolve 6 g of bovine albumin in 25 ml of water and dilute to 100 ml with distilled water (6 g bovine albumin in 100 ml solution. Therefore 1 ml solution contains 0.06 g of bovine albumin; Hence 0.1 ml standard protein solution contains 0.006 g of bovine albumin).

Procedure:

Take three test tubes and label as standard, blank and unknown. Add 5 ml of Biuret reagent to all three test tubes. Add 0.1 ml of serum in unknown test tube, 0.1 ml of standard protein solution in standard test tube and 0.1 ml of water in blank test tube. Mix well all three tubes individually. Finally, measure the intensity of the violet color obtained in standard and unknown against blank at 540 nm or using green filter after 30 minutes. Calculate the concentration of total protein present in unknown sample using the following formula.

$$\text{Concentration of total protein in 0.1 ml serum} = \frac{E_u}{E_s} \times C_s = \frac{E_u}{E_s} \times 0.006 \text{ g total protein}$$

$$\text{Concentration of total protein in 100 ml serum} = \frac{\left(\frac{E_u}{E_s} \times 0.006\right)}{0.1} \times 100 = \frac{E_u}{E_s} \times 6 \text{ g}$$

Where, E_u = Optical density of unknown serum sample
E_s = Optical density of standard protein solution
C_s = Concentration of standard protein solution

Take three test tubes and label as standard, blank and unknown

Add 5 ml of Biuret reagent to all three test tubes

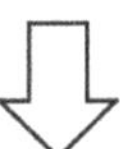

Add 0.1 ml of serum in unknown test tube, 0.1 ml of standard protein solution in standard test tube and 0.1 ml of water in blank test tube

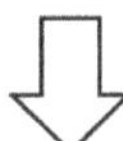

Mix well all three tubes individually

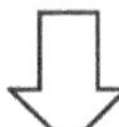

Finally, measure the intensity of the violet color obtained in standard and unknown against blank at 540 nm or using green filter after 30 minutes

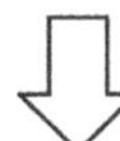

Calculate the concentration of total protein present in unknown sample

The above procedure is applicable for clear and non-hemolyzed samples. If the serum is icteric, lipemic or hemolyzed, an additional test tube should be prepared as serum blank. In this test tube mix 5 ml of Biuret blank with 0.1 ml of serum and measure the absorbance after 30 minutes against blank. Subtract the absorbance of the serum blank from the unknown sample before calculation.

Significance:

The normal serum total proteins is 6 to 8 g/100 ml in adults. In neonates the values are lower, rise gradually in infancy and reaches the adults level in childhood. During pregnancy the level will decrease. Serum total proteins will increase in clinical conditions like dehydration due to hemoconcentration, multiple myeloma, macroglobulinemia, chronic infections, chronic liver diseases and auto immune diseases. Serum total proteins will decrease in clinical conditions like nephrotic syndrome, untreated diabetes mellitus, hyperthyroidism, wasting disease, protein under nutrition, intestinal malabsorption and protein losing enteropathy. Also decreased serum total proteins occur in shock, burns, crush injuries, hemorrhage, etc. due to hemodilution.

2. **Estimation of Serum Albumin and Globulin**

Albumin and globulins are the two major proteins present in the serum. There are several sub-classes in globulins. Various techniques like salt fractionation, alcohol fractionation and electrophoresis are used to separate different types of proteins. But clinically useful formations are obtained from serum albumin, serum globulin and the ratio of albumin and globulin (A:G) without measuring the sub-classes of globulins. The colorimetric estimation of albumin is simple than globulin. Hence, total proteins and albumin are estimated in serum and concentration of globulin is obtained by difference. Recently bromocresol green (BCG) method is used for the estimation of albumin in serum.

Principle:

The basic principle involved in the bromocresol green (BCG) method is protein error of indicators. The color of indicator is changed when protein binds to an indicator. Only albumin binds to bromocresol green (BCG) among various serum proteins. This binding of albumin changes the color of bromocresol green (BCG) which is estimated colorimetrically. The intensity of the color change is measured colorimetrically at 630 nm or using a red filter. Buffer is used to maintain the pH of the reaction constant.

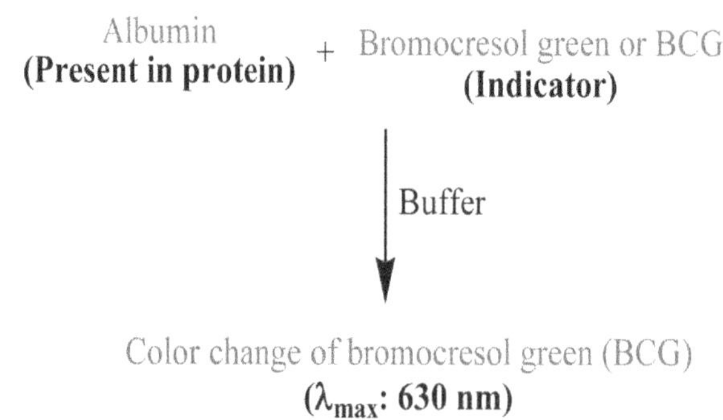

Reagents:

1. **0.1 N Sodium hydroxide:** Dissolve 0.42 g of sodium hydroxide in 25 ml of water and dilute to 100 ml with distilled water.
2. **Succinate buffer:** Dissolve 11.8 g of succinic acid in 800 ml of water. Adjust the pH of the solution to 4.0 using 0.1 N sodium hydroxide. Finally, make up the volume to 1000 ml with distilled water. Store this solution in a refrigerator.
3. **BCG solution:** Dissolve 419 mg of bromocresol green in 10 ml of 0.1 N sodium hydroxide and dilute to 1000 ml with distilled water. Store this solution in a refrigerator.
4. **Buffered BCG solution:** Mix 250 ml of above prepared buffer with 750 ml of succinate buffer. Adjust the pH of the mixture to 4.2 using 0.1 N sodium hydroxide solution. To this add 4 ml of 30 % Brij-35 solution and mix well.

5. **Standard albumin solution:** Dissolve 4 g of bovine albumin in 25 ml of water and dilute to 100 ml with distilled water. Add 50 mg of sodium azide to the above solution as preservative. (4 g bovine albumin in 100 ml solution. Therefore, 1 ml solution contains 0.04 g of bovine albumin; Hence, 0.02 ml standard albumin solution contains 0.0008 g of bovine albumin).

Procedure:

Take three test tubes and label as standard, blank and unknown. To all three tubes, add 4 ml of buffered BCG solution. In unknown test tube add 0.02 ml serum; in standard test tube add 0.02 ml of standard albumin solution and in blank test tube add 0.02 ml of water. Mix well all three tubes individually. Measure the intensity of the color obtained in standard and unknown against blank at 630 nm or using red filter after 5 minutes. Calculate the concentration of albumin present in unknown sample using the following formula.

$$\text{Concentration of albumin in 0.02 ml serum} = \frac{E_u}{E_s} \times C_s = \frac{E_u}{E_s} \times 0.0008 \text{ g albumin}$$

$$\text{Concentration of albumin in 100 ml serum} = \frac{\left(\frac{E_u}{E_s} \times 0.0008\right)}{0.02} \times 100 = \frac{E_u}{E_s} \times 4 \text{ g}$$

Where, E_u = Optical density of unknown serum sample
E_s = Optical density of standard albumin solution
C_s = Concentration of standard albumin solution

Take three test tubes and label as standard, blank and unknown

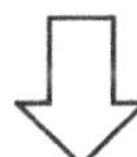

To all three tubes, add 4 ml of buffered BCG solution

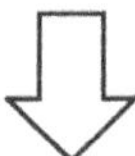

In unknown test tube add 0.02 ml serum; in standard test tube add 0.02 ml of standard albumin solution and in blank test tube add 0.02 ml of water

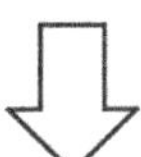

Mix well all three tubes individually

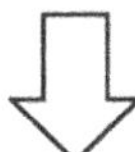

Measure the intensity of the color obtained in standard and unknown against blank at 630 nm or using red filter after 5 minutes

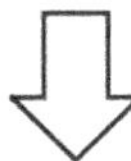

Calculate the concentration of albumin present in unknown sample

Significance:

The normal serum albumins are 3.7 to 5.3 g/100 ml, serum globulin is 1.8 to 3.6 g/100 ml and the ratio of albumin and globulin (A:G) is 2:1 (Ranges from 1.2:1 to 2.5:1).

Serum albumin will decrease in clinical conditions like protein under nutrition, intestinal malabsorption, protein losing enteropathy, wasting disease, liver disease, nephrotic syndrome and hemodilution. A severe decrease or near absence of albumin is seen in analbuminaemia which is a genetic disease with autosomal recessive inheritance. Serum albumin will increase in clinical conditions like dehydration due to hemoconcentration.

Decreased serum globulin levels occur in shock, burns, hemorrhage, etc due to hemodilution. Serum globulin will increase in clinical conditions like multiple myeloma, macroglobulinemia, chronic infections, chronic liver diseases and auto immune diseases. The A:G ratio may be decreased or reversed in these conditions.

3. **Estimation of Prothrombin Time (PT)**

The *extrinsic* pathway and common pathway of coagulation are evaluated by assays like the prothrombin time (PT) and its derived measures like prothrombin ratio (PR) and international normalized ratio (INR). This also known as *protime INR* and *PT/INR*. Independent of the testing methods, results of prothrombin time tests are standardized by using INR (international normalized ratio). Hence, PT test is also known as INR test. Most of the blood clotting factors is protein in nature. All blood clotting factors are synthesized in liver. Hence, liver impairment may lead to decreased concentration of plasma clotting factor. In laboratory this can be easily estimated by measuring the prothrombin time. Compared to normal people the prothrombin time is prolonged in liver damage patients. The clotting factors half-life is very short, hence changes in prothrombin time occurs quickly. Prothrombin time is used to estimate acute and chronic liver damages. It also helps in prognosis. Synthesis of many clotting factors like factors-II, VII, IX and X depends on vitamin-K. Hence, prolonged prothrombin time occurs in vitamin K deficiency also. Before drawing conclusion, the above one must be ruled out by estimating prothrombin time before and after administration of vitamin-K.

Principle:

The prothrombin time is the time plasma takes to clot after addition of tissue factor which is obtained from animals such as rabbits, or recombinant tissue factor, or from brains of autopsy patients. This measures the quality of the *extrinsic pathway* as well as the *common pathway* of coagulation. The speed of the *extrinsic pathway* is greatly affected by the levels of functional factor-VII in the body. Factor-VII has a short half-life and the carboxylation of its glutamate residues requires vitamin-K. The PT can be prolonged as a result of deficiencies in vitamin-K, warfarin therapy, malabsorption, or lack of intestinal colonization by bacteria (such as in newborns). In addition, poor factor-VII synthesis (due to liver disease) or increased consumption (in disseminated intravascular coagulation) may also prolong the prothrombin time.

Procedure

The prothrombin time is estimated in an automated instrument at normal human body temperature i.e., 37 °C. In a test tube containing liquid sodium citrate (anticoagulant), add unknown blood sample and mix well. Later, separate the blood cells from blood plasma by centrifugation. In case of newborns, use a capillary of whole blood sample. Extract a sample of the plasma from the test tube and place into a measuring test tube. For an accurate measurement, fix the ratio of blood to citrate. To reverse the effects of citrate and enabling the blood to clot again, add an excess of calcium suspended in a phospholipid. Finally, add tissue factor commonly known as factor-III in order to activate the extrinsic/tissue factor clotting cascade pathway. Optically measure the time taken by the sample to clot. Mechanical measurements are used in some laboratories to avoid interferences from lipemic and icteric samples.

In a test tube containing liquid sodium citrate (anticoagulant), add unknown blood sample and mix well

Later, separate the blood cells from blood plasma by centrifugation (In case of newborns, use a capillary of whole blood sample)

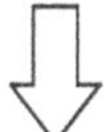

Extract a sample of the plasma from the test tube and place into a measuring test tube

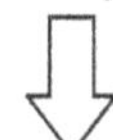

To reverse the effects of citrate and enabling the blood to clot again, add an excess of calcium suspended in a phospholipid

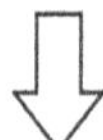

Finally, add tissue factor commonly known as factor III in order to activate the extrinsic/tissue factor clotting cascade pathway

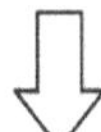

Optically measure the time taken by the sample to clot (Mechanical measurements are used in some laboratories to avoid interferences from lipemic and icteric samples)

The ISI value indicates how a particular batch of tissue factor is compared to an international reference tissue factor. The ISI is usually between 0.94 and 1.40 for more sensitive and 2.0–3.0 for less sensitive thromboplastins. The INR is the ratio of a patient's prothrombin time to a normal (control) sample, raised to the power of the ISI value for the analytical system being used. Calculate the INR from the below mentioned formula.

$$INR = \left(\frac{PT_{test}}{PT_{normal}} \right)^{ISI}$$

Significance:

Prothrombin time (PT) is a blood test used to measure how long it takes the blood to clot. Bleeding problems are checked by using prothrombin time. PT is also used to check the activity of coagulating agents and also for determining clotting tendency of blood in the conditions like warfarin dosage, liver damage, and vitamin-K status. In general, PT is used for the measurement of the coagulation factors like I (fibrinogen), II (prothrombin), V (proaccelerin), VII (proconvertin), and X (Stuart–Prowar factor). Activated partial thromboplastin time (aPTT) is used for measurement of the *intrinsic* pathway and common pathway of coagulation. Hence, PT is often used in combination with aPTT.

The normal prothrombin time is usually around 12 to 13 seconds; INR in absence of anticoagulant is 0.8 to 1.2 and INR in presence of anticoagulant like warfarin is 2 to 3. Depending on the indication for anticoagulation in some cases, the target range of INR may be as high as 2.5 to 3.5 if more intense anticoagulation is required. In general, a high INR indicates a higher risk of bleeding, while a low INR suggests a higher risk of developing a clot.

Selected Serum Enzyme Tests

Several enzymes present in the liver cells are released into the circulation when the liver cell is damaged. Hence, liver function is estimated by measuring these selected enzymes level in serum. But specific to liver no single enzymes are present even though for liver function test valuable information is obtained from serum enzymes. The followings are some selected serum enzymes used for estimation of LFT.

1. *Transaminases* or *aminotransferases (SGOT* and *SGPT)*
2. *Alkaline phosphatase*
3. *Acid phosphatase*
4. *Lactate dehydrogenase*

Estimation of Serum Glutamate Oxaloacetate Transaminase (SGOT) and Serum glutamete pyruvate transaminase (SGPT)

Serum glutamate oxaloacetate transaminase (*SGOT*) is otherwise known as *aspartate transaminase* (*AST*) or *aspartate aminotransferase* (*ASAT*). This enzyme catalyzes the conversion of aspartate and α-ketoglutarate into oxaloacetate and glutamate, respectively. This reaction is reversible in nature.

Aspartate + α- Keto glutarate ⇌ (Transamination; *Serum glutamate oxaloacetate transaminase (SGOT)*, PLP) Oxaloacetate + Glutamate

Serum glutamate pyruvate transaminase (*SGPT*) is otherwise known as *alanine transaminase* (*ALT*) or *alanine aminotransferase* (*ALAT*). This enzyme catalyzes the conversion of alanine and α-ketoglutarate into pyruvate and glutamate, respectively. This reaction is reversible in nature.

Alanine + α- Keto glutarate ⇌ (Transamination; *Serum glutamate pyruvate transaminase (SGPT)*, PLP) Pyruvate + Glutamate

Principle:

At 37 °C, serum is incubated with substrate (In case of *SGOT*, aspartate and α-ketoglutarate and in case of *SGPT* alanine and α-ketoglutarate). Using phosphate buffer, the pH is maintained at 7.5 throughout the procedure. Aniline citrate reagent is added after a fixed interval to terminate the reaction. Later, pyruvate is treated with 2,4-dinitro phenyl hydrazine and converted into a corresponding colored phenylhydrazone for its measurement (In case of *SGPT*, aniline citrate reagent converts oxaloacetate present into pyruvate). By running a blank experiment initial concentration of pyruvate is measured. During the incubation period, pyruvate concentration is increased due to presence of *SGOT* and *SGPT*. Hence, the velocity of reaction is measured indirectly from the concentration of pyruvate which is directly proportional to concentration of *SGOT* and *SGPT* because pH, temperature and substrate concentration are kept constant.

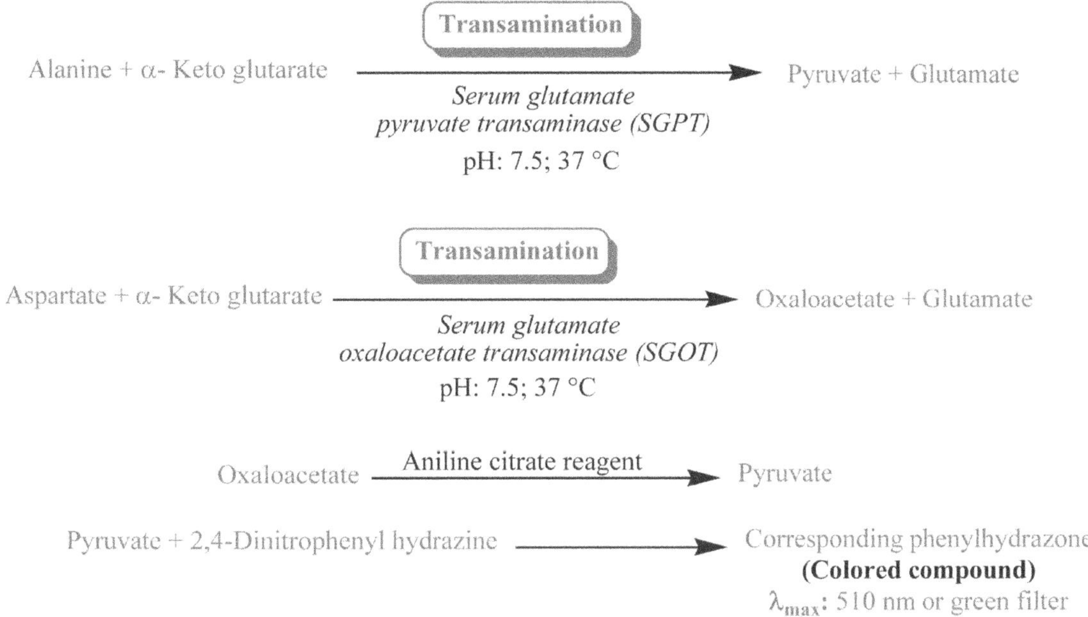

Reagents:

1. **Phosphate buffer:** Dissolve 9.976 g of disodium hydrogen phosphate ($Na_2HPO_4 . 2H_2O$) and 1.452 g of potassium hydrogen phosphate (KH_2PO_4) in 500 ml of water and dilute to 1000 ml with distilled water.
2. **10 % Sodium hydroxide:** Dissolve 10 g of sodium hydroxide in 25 ml of water and dilute to 100 ml with distilled water.
3. **Buffered substrate:**
   (a) ***SGOT* substrate:** Dissolve 300 mg of L-aspartic acid and 50 mg of α-ketoglutaric acid in 30 ml of phosphate buffer. Using 10 % sodium hydroxide adjust the pH to 7.5. Finally, dilute the solution to 100 ml using phosphate buffer. Store this solution in a refrigerator.
   (b) ***SGPT* substrate:** Dissolve 5 g of DL-alanine and 20 mg of α-ketoglutaric acid in 30 ml of phosphate buffer. Using 10 % sodium hydroxide adjust the pH to 7.5. Finally, dilute the solution to 100 ml using phosphate buffer. Store this his solution in a refrigerator.
4. **Aniline citrate reagent:** Dissolve 50 g of citric acid in 50 ml of water and add 50 ml of aniline solution.
5. **2,4-Dinitrophenyl hydrazine (DNPH) reagent:** Dissolve 200 mg of 2,4-dinitro phenyl hydrazine in 85 ml of concentrated hydrochloric acid and 100 ml of water. Mix well and dilute to 1000 ml with distilled water.
6. **0.4 N Sodium hydroxide:** Dissolve 1.6 g of sodium hydroxide in 25 ml of water and dilute to 100 ml with distilled water.
7. **Standard pyruvic acid solution:** Dilute 0.8 ml (equivalent to 1 g or 1000 mg) of pure pyruvic acid to 100 ml with distilled water. Further, one ml of this solution is diluted to 100 ml using distilled water. (1000 mg pyruvic acid in 100 ml solution. Therefore, 1 ml solution contains 10 mg of pyruvic acid; 10 mg pyruvic acid in 100 ml solution. Hence, 1 ml standard pyruvic acid solution contains 0.1 mg or 100 µg of pyruvic acid).

Procedure:

Take two test tubes and label as blank and unknown. To both two tubes, add 1 ml of buffered substrate (*SGOT* substrate for *SGOT* and *SGPT* substrate for *SGPT*). Keep test tubes at 37 °C in incubator for few minutes in order to get temperature equilibrium. In unknown test tube add 0.2 ml serum, mix and place in incubator. Note down the time. To each tube, add 0.1 ml of aniline citrate reagent after 60 minutes in case of *SGOT* and after 30 minutes in case of *SGPT*, respectively. Add 0.2 ml of serum to the blank test tube and mix well. Keep the tubes at room temperature for 20 minutes. To each test tube add 1 ml of DNPH reagent, mix and keep aside for 20 minutes. Add 10 ml of 0.4 N sodium hydroxide to each test tube, mix and allow to stand for 30 minutes. Finally, measure the intensity of the color obtained in unknown and blank against water at 510 nm or using green filter.

Take two test tubes and label as blank and unknown

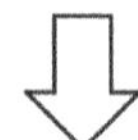

To both two tubes, add 1 ml of buffered substrate (*SGOT* substrate for *SGOT* and *SGPT* substrate for *SGPT*)

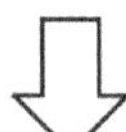

Keep test tubes at 37 °C in incubator for few minutes in order to get temperature equilibrium

In unknown test tube add 0.2 ml serum, mix and place in incubator (Note down the time)

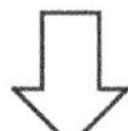

To each tube, add 0.1 ml of aniline citrate reagent after 60 minutes in case of *SGOT* and after 30 minutes in case of *SGPT*, respectively

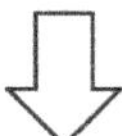

Add 0.2 ml of serum to the blank test tube and mix well. Keep the tubes at room temperature for 20 minutes

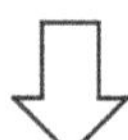

To each test tube add 1 ml of DNPH reagent, mix and keep aside for 20 minutes

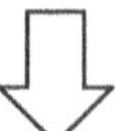

Add 10 ml of 0.4 N sodium hydroxide to each test tube, mix and allow to stand for 30 minutes

Finally, measure the intensity of the color obtained in unknown and blank against water at 510 nm or using green filter

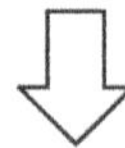

Calculate the concentration of *SGOT* and *SGPT* from the standard calibration curve

Calculate the concentration of *SGOT* and *SGPT* from the standard calibration curve. Plot the standard calibration curve using a series of standards which are prepared as mentioned in Table 9.2.

Table 9.2 Preparation of standard solution for calibration curve.

S. No.	Standard	Standard pyruvic acid solution (in ml)	Water (in ml)	*SGOT* (in IU/l)	*SGPT* (in IU/l)
1	S_1	3.5	6.5	0.0	0.0
2	S_2	4.0	6.0	4.1	6.5
3	S_3	4.5	5.5	9.6	15.2
4	S_4	5.5	4.5	21.0	28.5
5	S_5	6.5	3.5	38.0	46.0
6	S_6	7.5	2.5	65.0	62.0
7	S_7	9.5	0.5	-	101.0

Take 1 ml of each standard solution and add 1 ml of DNPH reagent, mix and keep aside for 20 minutes. Add 10 ml of 0.4 N sodium hydroxide to each standard, mix and stand for 30 minutes. Finally, measure the intensity of the color obtained in all standards against water at 510 nm or using green filter. Plot the calibration curve by taking *SGOT* or *SGPT* concentration on "X" axis and its absorbance on "Y" axis. Measure the concentration of *SGOT* or *SGPT* of unknown sample from the calibration curve after subtracting the absorbance of blank from that of unknown. RBC is rich in *SGOT* and *SGPT*, hence avoid hemolysis.

Take 1 ml of each standard solution and add 1 ml of DNPH reagent, mix and keep aside for 20 minutes

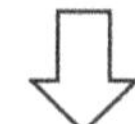

Add 10 ml of 0.4 N sodium hydroxide to each standard, mix and stand for 30 minutes

Finally, measure the intensity of the color obtained in all standards against water at 510 nm or using green filter

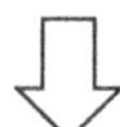

Plot the calibration curve by taking *SGOT* or *SGPT* concentration on "X" axis and its absorbance on "Y" axis

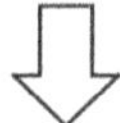

Measure the concentration of *SGOT* or *SGPT* of unknown sample from the calibration curve after subtracting the absorbance of blank from that of unknown

Significance:

The normal *SGOT* is 4 to 17 IU/l and the normal *SGPT* is 3 to 15 IU/l. It is useful for the diagnosis of myocardial infarction, viral hepatitis, muscle trauma and myopathies. The increase in *SGOT* is far greater than *SGPT* in myocardial infarction. In case of viral hepatitis and toxic liver damage the reverse take place. Mostly, *SGOT* level only increase in muscle trauma and myopathies. *SGOT* level begins to increase in 10 to 12 hours, reaches peak at 48 hours and return to normal in 5 to 7 days in myocardial infarction.

Estimation of Serum *Phosphatases*

In a variety of tissues serum *phosphatases* are present. These are group of enzymes which produces phosphoric acid from monophosphoric acid esters by hydrolysis. They are broadly classified into two categories based on its optimum pH as, 1) *Alkaline phosphatase* (Active at pH above 10), 2) *Acid phosphatase* (Active at pH 5 to 6). Each class is a mixture of many enzymes.

Estimation of Serum *Alkaline Phosphatase*

Principle:

The activity of serum *alkaline phosphatase* is measured from the velocity of reaction catalyzed by the enzyme present in unknown sample under ideal conditions. In such conditions the velocity of reaction is directly proportional to concentration of enzyme. This method of estimation of serum *alkaline phosphatase* is called as **Kind and King method**. In this method phenyl phosphate is converted to phenol by *alkaline phosphatase*. 4-Aminophenazone was reacted with the liberated phenol and produce red purple color compound in the presence of alkaline oxidizing agents. The intensity of the red purple color obtained is measured at 520 nm or using green filter. Sodium carbonate-sodium bicarbonate buffer is used to maintain the pH at 10.

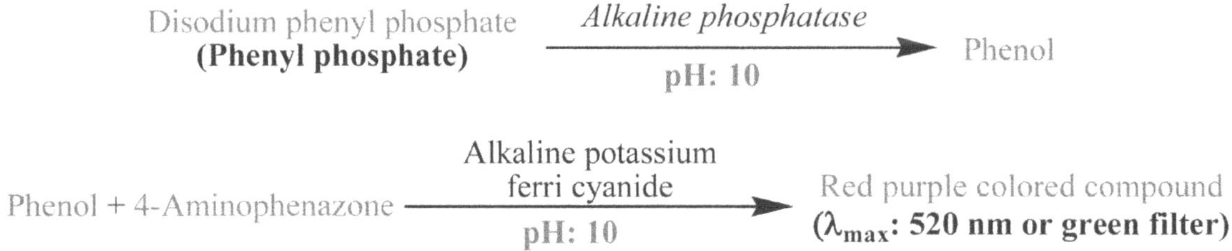

Reagents:

1. **Phenyl phosphate solution:** Dissolve 2.18 g of disodium phenyl phosphate in 500 ml of water and dilute to 1000 ml with distilled water. Heat the solution to boil and cool. Add 1 to 2 drops of chloroform as a preservative. Store this solution in a refrigerator.
2. **Buffer solution:** Dissolve 6.36 g of anhydrous sodium carbonate and 3.36 g of sodium bicarbonate in 500 ml of water and dilute to 1000 ml with distilled water.
3. **Buffered substrate:** Mix 500 ml of phenyl phosphate solution and 500 ml of buffer solution. Store this solution in a refrigerator.
4. **0.5 M Sodium hydroxide:** Dissolve 20 g of sodium hydroxide in 500 ml of water and dilute to 1000 ml with distilled water.
5. **0.5 M Sodium bicarbonate:** Dissolve 42 g of sodium bicarbonate in 500 ml of water and dilute to 1000 ml with distilled water.
6. **4-Aminophenazone reagent:** Dissolve 6 g of 4-aminophenazone in 500 ml of water and dilute to 1000 ml with distilled water.
7. **Potassium ferricyanide solution:** Dissolve 24 g of potassium ferricyanide in 500 ml of water and dilute to 1000 ml with distilled water.
8. **0.1 N Hydrochloric acid:** Dilute 8.4 ml of concetrated hydrochloric acid to 1000 ml with distilled water.
9. **Standard phenol solution:** Dissolve 1 g of pure crystalline phenol in 500 ml 0.1 N hydrochloric acid and dilute to 1000 ml with 0.1 N hydrochloric acid. Further dilute one ml of this solution to 100 ml with distilled water. (1 g or 1000 mg phenol in 1000 ml solution. Therefore, 1 ml solution contains 1 mg of phenol; 1 mg phenol in 100 ml solution. Hence, 1 ml standard phenol solution contains 0.01 mg of phenol).

Procedure:

Take four test tubes and label as standard, blank, control and unknown. Take 2 ml of buffered substrate in unknown and control test tubes and keep in incubator at 37 °C for few minutes. Take 1.1 ml of buffer in standard and blank test tubes. Add 1 ml of standard phenol solution to standard test tube and 1 ml water in blank test tube. Keep these two test tubes in room temperature. Add 0.1 ml of serum to unknown test tube and incubate for exactly 15 minutes at 37 °C. Remove unknown and control test tubes from the incubator. To all four tubes add 0.8 ml of sodium hydroxide and 1.2 ml of sodium bicarbonate and mix well. Add 0.1 ml of serum to control test tube. Add 1 ml of 4-aminophenazone reagent to all test tubes and mix well. Later, add 1 ml of potassium ferricyanide solution to all test tubes and mix well. Finally, measure the intensity of the red-purple color obtained in standard, control and unknown against blank at 520 nm or using green filter. Calculate the concentration of serum *alkaline phosphatase* present in unknown sample using the following formula.

$$\textit{Concentration of alkaline phosphatase in } 0.1 \textit{ ml serum} = \frac{E_u - E_c}{E_s} \times C_s$$

$$= \frac{E_u - E_c}{E_s} \times 0.01 \textit{ KA alkaline phosphatase}$$

Take four test tubes and label as standard, blank, control and unknown

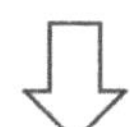

Take 2 ml of buffered substrate in unknown and control test tubes and keep in incubator at 37 °C for few minutes

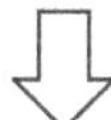

Take 1.1 ml of buffer in standard and blank test tubes

Add 1 ml of standard phenol solution to standard test tube and 1 ml water in blank test tube (Keep these two test tubes in room temperature)

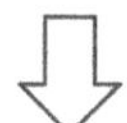

Add 0.1 ml of serum to unknown test tube and incubate for exactly 15 minutes at 37 °C

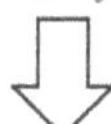

Remove unknown and control test tubes from the incubator

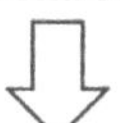

To all four tubes add 0.8 ml of sodium hydroxide and 1.2 ml of sodium bicarbonate and mix well

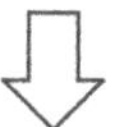

Add 0.1 ml of serum to control test tube

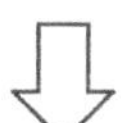

Add 1 ml of 4-aminophenazone reagent to all test tubes and mix well

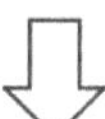

Add 1 ml of potassium ferricyanide solution to all test tubes and mix well

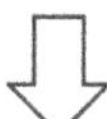

Measure the intensity of the red-purple color obtained in standard, control and unknown against blank at 520 nm or using green filter

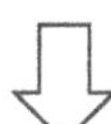

Calculate the concentration of serum *alkaline phosphatase* present in unknown sample

$$\textit{Concentration of alkaline phosphatase in 100 ml serum} = \frac{\left(\frac{E_u - E_c}{E_s} \times 0.01\right)}{0.1} \times 100$$

$$= \frac{E_u - E_c}{E_s} \times 10\,KA$$

Where, E_u = Optical density of unknown serum sample

E_c = Optical density of control

E_s = Optical density of standard phenol solution

C_s = Concentration of standard phenol solution

King-Armstrong (KA) units are used to express the results. 1 KA unit correspond to liberation of 1 mg of phenol by 100 ml of serum under test conditions. Phenol liberated by the enzyme is represented from the difference between unknown and control.

Significance:

The normal serum *alkaline phosphatase* level is 4 to 17 KA units/100 ml in adults and 17 to 33 KA units/100 ml in children. The activity of serum *alkaline phosphatase* is increased in clinical conditions like hepatitis, obstructive jaundice, liver cancer, bone cancer, rickets, osteomalacia, hyperparathyroidism, Paget's disease and last trimester of pregnancy. The activity of serum *alkaline phosphatase* is decreased in clinical conditions like achondroplasia, cretinism, severe anemia, hypophosphatasia and kwashiorkor.

Estimation of Serum Acid Phosphatase

Like serum *alkaline phosphatase* estimation serum *acid phosphatase* is also estimated with the following changes.

1. Citric acid-sodium citrate buffer (pH 4.9) is used instead of sodium carbonate–sodium bicarbonate buffer (pH 10.0). [**Preparation of citric acid-sodium citrate buffer solution:** Dissolve 21 g of crystalline citric acid in 100 ml distilled water. Add 188 ml of 1 M sodium hydroxide (Dissolve 40 g of sodium hydroxide in 500 ml of water and dilute to 1000 ml with distilled water) and dilute to 500 ml with distilled water. Adjust the pH of the solution to 4.9 using sodium hydroxide or hydrochloric acid].
2. For serum *acid phosphatase* estimation, the incubation period is 60 minutes instead of 15 minutes in serum *alkaline phosphatase* estimation.

Significance:

The normal serum *acid phosphatase* level is 1 to 5 KA units/100 ml. It is mainly used for the diagnosis of prostate cancer. The serum *acid phosphatase* level is normal until the tumor is confined within the capsule of prostate and it considerably increases when tumor breaks through the capsule. Small increase is common after rectal palpation of prostate, passage of catheter and in acute retention of urine.

Estimation of Serum *Lactate Dehydrogenase*

Serum *lactate dehydrogenase* (NAD^+ involved reaction the enzymes are "*dehydrogenase*" and the substrate is "lactate") is otherwise known as *LDH*. The systemic name of *LDH* is *L-lactate-NAD⁺ oxidoreductase* and it catalyses the interconversion of lactate and pyruvate. This reaction is reversible in nature.

$$CH_3-\underset{OH}{\overset{H}{C}}-COOH \xrightleftharpoons[\textit{Lactate dehydrogenase (LDH)}]{NAD^+ \rightarrow NADH + H^+} CH_3-\underset{\|}{C}(=O)-COOH$$

Lactate — Redox reaction — Pyruvate

Principle:

The basic principle involved in the estimation of serum *lactate dehydrogenase* is colorimetric estimation of decreased pyruvate concentration. Pyruvate and NADH are incubated with serum at 37 °C and the pH is maintained using buffer. Initial and final concentration of pyruvate in the system is measured from the color reaction of pyruvate with 2,4-dinitrophenylhydrazine. Pyruvate is reacted with 2,4-dinitrophenylhydrazine and forms corresponding colored phenylhydrazone derivatives. The intensity of the color obtained is measured at 510 nm or using green filters. From the decreased concentration of pyruvate serum *lactate dehydrogenase* is estimated.

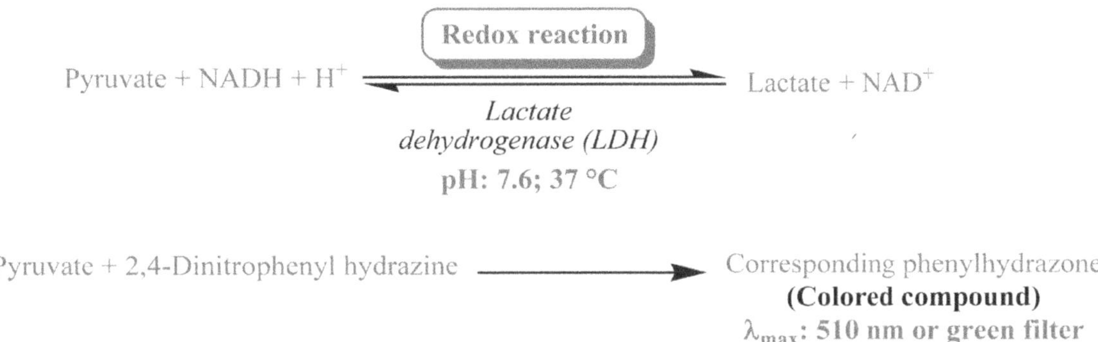

Reagents:

1. **Buffer solution:** Dissolve 10 g of dipotassium hydrogen phosphate trihydrate ($K_2HPO_4 \cdot 3H_2O$) or 7.7 g of dipotassium hydrogen phosphate (K_2HPO_4) in 250 ml water. Add 200 mg of pyruvic acid or 259 mg of sodium pyruvate to the above solution. Mix well and add 8 ml of 0.3 M phosphoric acid. Adjust the pH to 7.6. Finally, dilute the solution to 1000 ml with distilled water. Add a drop of chloroform as preservative. Store this solution in a refrigerator.
2. **Buffered substrate:** Immediately before testing dissolve 10 mg of NADH in 10 ml of buffer solution.
3. **2,4-Dinitrophenyl hydrazine (DNPH) reagent:** Dissolve 200 mg of 2,4-dinitrophenyl hydrazine in 85 ml of concentrated hydrochloric acid and 100 ml of water. Mix well and dilute to 1000 ml with distilled water.
4. **0.4 N Sodium hydroxide:** Dissolve 16 g of sodium hydroxide in 500 ml of water and dilute to 1000 ml with distilled water.
5. **0.3 M Phosphoric acid:** Dilute 2 ml of 85 % phosphoric acid to 100 ml with distilled water.

Procedure:

Take two test tubes and label as blank and unknown. Take 1 ml of buffered substrate in both the test tubes. Add 0.02 ml of serum in unknown test tube and 0.02 ml water in blank test tube. Incubate both tubes for 45 minutes at 37 °C. Add 1 ml of 2,4-dinitrophenyl hydrazine (DNPH) reagent to both test tubes, mix well and allow to stand for 30 minutes at room temperature. Finally, measure the intensity of the color obtained in blank and unknown against water at 510 nm or using green filter.

Calculate the concentration of serum *LDH* present in unknown sample from the standard calibration curve. Prepare a series of standards and plot standard curve as follows.

S. No.	Standard	Buffered substrate (in ml)	Water (in ml)	*LDH* (in units/ml)
1	S_1	1.0	0.0	0
2	S_2	0.8	0.2	300
3	S_3	0.6	0.4	700
4	S_4	0.4	0.6	1000
5	S_5	0.2	0.8	1500
6	S_6	0.1	0.9	2000

Take two test tubes and label as blank and unknown

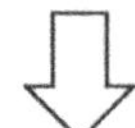

Take 1 ml of buffered substrate in both the test tubes

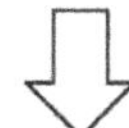

Add 0.02 ml of serum in unknown test tube and 0.02 ml water in blank test tube (Incubate both tubes for 45 minutes at 37 °C)

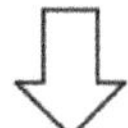

Measure the intensity of the color obtained in blank and unknown against water at 510 nm or using green filter

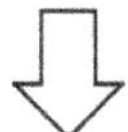

Calculate the concentration of serum *LDH* present in unknown sample from the standard calibration curve

Add 1 ml of DNPH reagent to each buffered standard, mix well and keep aside for 20 minutes. Add 10 ml of 0.4 N sodium hydroxide to each standard, mix and stand for 30 minutes. Measure the intensity of the color obtained in all standards against water at 510 nm or using green filter. Plot the calibration curve by taking *LDH* concentration on "X" axis and its absorbance on "Y" axis. Measure the concentration of *LDH* present in unknown sample from the calibration curve after subtracting the absorbance of blank from that of unknown. RBC is rich in *LDH*, hence avoid hemolysis. Don't use oxalate as an anticoagulant if the assay is performed on plasma.

Add 1 ml of DNPH reagent to each buffered standard, mix well and keep aside for 20 minutes

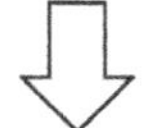

Add 10 ml of 0.4 N sodium hydroxide to each standard, mix and stand for 30 minutes

Measure the intensity of the color obtained in all standards against water at 510 nm or using green filter

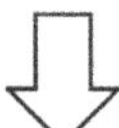

Plot the calibration curve by taking *LDH* concentration on "X" axis and its absorbance on "Y" axis

Measure the concentration of *LDH* present in unknown sample from the calibration curve after subtracting the absorbance of blank from that of unknown

Significance:

The normal serum *LDH* level is 200 to 450 KA units/100 ml. The activity of serum *LDH* is increased in clinical conditions like myocardial infarction, pulmonary infarction, viral hepatitis, muscle injuries, acute lymphoblastic leukemia, pernicious anemia and generalized carcinomatosis. *LDH* level begins to increase in 12 to 14 hours after infarction, reaches peak at 48 to 72 hours and return to normal in 7 to 10 days in myocardial infarction.

PROBABLE QUESTIONS

PART – A: Multiple Choice Questions

1. Which of the following function is not performed by liver?
   (a) Metabolic function (b) Excretory function
   (c) Protective function (d) Reproductive function
2. Which of these tests are not an example of liver function tests based on metabolic capacity of liver?
   (a) Galactose tolerance test (b) Antipyrine clearance test
   (c) Estimation of bile pigments (d) Both a & b
3. Which of the following are functions of liver?
   (a) Drug metabolism (b) Protein synthesis
   (c) Protein catabolism (d) All of the above
4. What is the normal serum bilirubin levels?
   (a) 0.1 to 0.5 mg/dl (b) 0.2 to 1.0 mg/dl
   (c) 0.3 to 1.5 mg/dl (d) 0.4 to 2.0 mg/dl
5. Which of the following test is used to determine the bilirubin levels?
   (a) Fouchet's test (b) Sackett's test
   (c) Liebermann–Burchard's test (d) Benedict's test.
6. In case of direct positive Van den Bergh reaction, conjugated bilirubin reacts immediately with Van den Bergh reagent and produces ____________________.
   (a) Red color (b) Purple color
   (c) Pink color (d) Blue color
7. In Sackett's method, at which wavelength the intensity of the green colored complexes is measured spectrophotometrically?
   (a) 680 nm (b) 580 nm
   (c) 620 nm (d) 520 nm
8. Kim and Goldberg method are a direct method of the estimation of ____________.
   (a) Bilirubin (b) Cholesterol
   (c) Creatinine (d) Urobilinogen
9. What is the composition of lipoproteins?
   (a) Only lipid (b) Only protein
   (c) Lipid and protein (d) Lipid and carbohydrate
10. The method which utilizes a highly specific affinity of an antibody for its antigen is known as ________.
    (a) Immunochemical methods (b) Immunoelectrophoresis
    (c) Immunofixation (d) Immunoprecipitation
11. The functional unit of the liver is lobules and it consists of millions of hepatic cells known as ____________.
    (a) Hepatocytes (b) Haematocytes
    (c) Heparocytes (d) Osteocytes
12. What is the normal prothrombin time?
    (a) 2 to 3 seconds (b) 5 to 10 seconds
    (c) 12 to 13 seconds (d) 22 to 23 seconds

13. Liver function test (LFT) is used to detect the
    (a) Anatomy of liver
    (b) Abnormalities and damages of liver
    (c) Anatomy of kidney
    (d) Abnormalities and damages of kidney
14. Which of the following are the causes for liver damage?
    (a) Viruses (Hepatitis-A and hepatitis-B virus)
    (b) Toxic chemical substances
    (c) Alcohol
    (d) All of the above
15. What is the life span of erythrocytes?
    (a) 120 days
    (b) 160 days
    (c) 200 days
    (d) 240 days
16. The liver undergoes glucuronic acid conjugation in the presence of which of the following enzyme?
    (a) *Heme oxygenase*
    (b) *Biliverdin reductase*
    (c) *Bilirubin glucuronyl transferase*
    (d) *Peroxidase*
17. What is the color obtained in Malloy-Evelyn method used for estimation of bilirubin?
    (a) Red-green color
    (b) Red-purple color
    (c) Blue-green color
    (d) Blue-purple color
18. Which of the following binding sites are present in albumin?
    (a) Two high affinity sites and two low affinity sites
    (b) One high affinity site and one low affinity site
    (c) Two high affinity sites and one low affinity site
    (d) One high affinity site and two low affinity sites
19. Which of the following one is responsible for the characteristic yellow color of the urine?
    (a) Bilirubin
    (b) Urobilin
    (c) Biliverdin
    (d) Stercobilin
20. Which of the following one is responsible for the characteristic brown color of the feces?
    (a) Urobilin
    (b) Bilirubin
    (c) Stercobilin
    (d) Biliverdin
21. Van den Bergh reaction test is a very sensitive test used to estimate ________________ in the body fluid.
    (a) Cholesterol
    (b) Bilirubin
    (c) Triglycerides
    (d) Creatinine
22. What is the basic principle involved in the Biuret method of serum total protein estimation?
    (a) Chelation of cuprous ion with peptide bonds of protein in alkaline medium
    (b) Chelation of cupric ion with peptide bonds of protein in alkaline medium
    (c) Chelation of cuprous ion with peptide bonds of protein in acidic medium
    (d) Chelation of cupric ion with peptide bonds of protein in acidic medium
23. Which of the following enzymes are not used for estimation of liver function test?
    (a) *Transaminase*
    (b) *Alkaline phosphatase*
    (c) *Gluco kinase*
    (d) *Acid phosphatase*
24. What is the indicator used in estimation of serum albumin and globulin?
    (a) Methylene blue
    (b) Phenol red
    (c) Bromocresol green
    (d) Methyl orange

25. Which enzyme catalyzes the conversion of aspartate and α-ketoglutarate into oxaloacetate and glutamate?
   (a) *Serum glutamate oxaloacetate transaminase* (b) *Serum glutamate pyruvate transaminase*
   (c) *Acid phosphatase* (d) *Alkaline phosphatase*
26. What is the rough shape of liver?
   (a) Oval (b) Square
   (c) Rectangle (d) Triangle
27. Cantlie's line is an imaginary line running from the left of the vena cava and all the way forward to divide the ___________ and _____________ into two halves?
   (a) Liver & gallbladder (b) Kidney & intestine
   (c) Gallbladder & intestine (d) Liver & kidney
28. Which test is not a liver function test based on excretory functions of liver?
   (a) Estimation of bile pigments (b) Estimation of albumin
   (c) Estimation of bile salts (d) Estimation of bromsulphthalein
29. Which test is a liver function test based on detoxification functions of liver?
   (a) Hippuric acid synthesis (b) Galactose tolerance test
   (c) Estimation of bile pigments (d) Estimation of prothrombin time
30. Which of the following test is a liver function test based on hematological functions of liver?
   (a) Estimation of bromsulphthalein (b) Antipyrine clearance test
   (c) Estimation of *transaminase* (d) Estimation of serum albumin
31. Which test is not a liver function test based on serum enzymes derived from liver?
   (a) Estimation of *alkaline phosphatase* (b) Estimation of *esterase*
   (c) Estimation of *transaminase* (d) Estimation of *γ-glutamoyl transpeptidase*
32. Antipyrine clearance test is a liver function test which is based on ________________.
   (a) Excretory functions of liver (b) Detoxification function of liver
   (c) Hematological functions of liver (d) Metabolic capacity of liver
33. What is the color of biliverdin?
   (a) Blue (b) Red
   (c) Green (d) Yellow
34. What is the color of bilirubin?
   (a) Green (b) Yellow
   (c) Red (d) Blue
35. Which enzyme is responsible for synthesis of biliverdin from heme?
   (a) *Heme oxygenase* (b) *Heme reductase*
   (c) *Biliverdin reductase* (d) *Biliverdin oxygenase*
36. Which enzyme is responsible for synthesis of bilirubin from biliverdin?
   (a) *Biliverdin oxygenase* (b) *Biliverdin reductase*
   (c) *Heme oxygenase* (d) *Heme reductase*
37. Which enzyme is responsible for synthesis of urobilinogen from bilirubin diglucuronide?
   (a) *Heme reductase* (b) *Biliverdin oxygenase*
   (c) *Heme oxygenase* (d) *Microsomal enzyme*

38. What is the end product of heme metabolism?
    (a) Urea (b) Bilirubin
    (c) Hippuric acid (d) Glucose
39. Which test is not used to determine the bilirubin levels?
    (a) Icterus test (b) Van den Bergh reaction
    (c) Fouchet's test (d) Biuret test
40. Which of the following bilirubin test is based on Ehrlich's diazo reaction?
    (a) Gmelin's test (b) Fouchet's test
    (c) Icterus test (d) Van den Bergh reaction
41. Which chemical is not present in Van den Bergh reagent?
    (a) Hydrochloric acid (b) Acetic acid
    (c) Sulphanilic acid (d) Sodium nitrite
42. Which results are obtained for hemolytic jaundice in Van den Bergh reaction?
    (a) Indirect positive (b) Direct positive
    (c) Indirect negative (d) Direct positive & indirect positive
43. Which results are obtained for obstructive jaundice in Van den Bergh reaction?
    (a) Direct negative (b) Direct positive & indirect positive
    (c) Direct positive (d) Indirect positive
44. Which results are obtained for hepatic jaundice in Van den Bergh reaction?
    (a) Direct positive (b) Indirect positive
    (c) Direct negative (d) Direct positive & indirect positive
45. Which of the following statement is wrong?
    (a) Conjugated bilirubin is soluble in water
    (b) Conjugated bilirubin is insoluble in water
    (c) Unconjugated bilirubin is insoluble in water
    (d) Conjugated bilirubin is excreted in urine
46. Which test is based on oxidation of bilirubin into biliverdin?
    (a) Van den Bergh reaction (b) Icterus test
    (c) Biuret test (d) Gmelin's test & Fouchet's test
47. What is the role of nitric acid in Gmelin's test?
    (a) Oxidizing agent (b) Reducing agent
    (c) Dehydrating agent (d) Complexing agent
48. Which compound is estimated using Ehrlich's aldehyde reagent?
    (a) Bilirubin (b) Biliverdin
    (c) Urobilinogen (d) Creatinine
49. What is the composition of Ehrlich's aldehyde reagent?
    (a) *p*-Dimethylamino benzaldehyde in acetic acid
    (b) *p*-Dimethylamino benzaldehyde in hydrochloric acid
    (c) *p*-Dimethylamino benzoic acid in acetic acid
    (d) *p*-Dimethylamino benzoic acid in hydrochloric acid

50. Serum total proteins will increase in which clinical condition?
   (a) Dehydration (b) Nephrotic syndrome
   (c) Untreated diabetes mellitus (d) Hyperthyroidism

Key for Multiple Choice Questions

1 (d)	2 (c)	3 (d)	4 (b)	5 (a)
6 (b)	7 (a)	8 (b)	9 (c)	10 (a)
11 (a)	12 (c)	13 (b)	14 (d)	15 (a)
16 (c)	17 (b)	18 (b)	19 (b)	20 (c)
21 (b)	22 (b)	23 (c)	24 (c)	25 (a)
26 (d)	27 (a)	28 (b)	29 (a)	30 (d)
31 (b)	32 (d)	33 (c)	34 (b)	35 (a)
36 (b)	37 (d)	38 (b)	39 (d)	40 (d)
41 (b)	42 (a)	43 (c)	44 (d)	45 (b)
46 (d)	47 (a)	48 (c)	49 (b)	50 (a)

PART – B: Short Answers

1. What are all the different causes of liver damage?
2. Write a short note on metabolic functions of liver.
3. Write a note on detoxification function of liver.
4. What is liver function test?
5. What facts must be considered while performing liver function test?
6. Classify liver function test with suitable example.
7. How biliverdin is biosynthesized in macrophage?
8. Write the reaction involved in the conversion bilirubin from biliverdin.
9. What is urobilin and stercobilin?
10. What is icterus test? and add a note on its significance.
11. Write the mechanism involved in the Van den Bergh reaction.
12. List out the significance of Van den Bergh reaction.
13. Write the basic principle involved in the Malloy-Evelyn method of serum bilirubin estimation.
14. Write the basic principle involved in the Jendrassik-Grof method of serum bilirubin estimation.
15. How presence of bilirubin in urine can be detected?
16. What is Gmelin's test?
17. What is Ehrlich's aldehyde reagent? Write the composition and uses of Ehrlich's aldehyde reagent.
18. Write a short note on dye test.
19. What is the basic principle involved in the Biuret method of serum total protein estimation?
20. What is BCG method?
21. List out the significance of prothrombin time.
22. Write a note on *SGOT*.
23. Explain the liver enzyme tests.
24. Write a short note on bile pigments.
25. How the activity of serum *alkaline phosphatase* is measured?

PART – C: Long Answers

1. With a neat labeled diagram explain the structure of liver.
2. List out various biological functions of liver and explain each and every function in detail.
3. Define and classify liver function test with suitable example. Explain any one liver function test in detail.
4. How bile pigments are metabolized? Explain with suitable chemical reaction.
5. Explain various liver function tests and explain the tests based on excretory functions of liver.
6. What is liver function tests? and explain the tests based on metabolic capacity of liver.
7. Define and classify liver function test. Explain the tests based on detoxification function of liver.
8. Explain various liver function tests and explain the tests based on hematological functions of liver.
9. What is liver function tests? and explain the tests based on serum enzymes derived from liver.
10. How serum bilirubin is estimated?
11. Write the principle, procedure and significance of Van den Bergh reaction.
12. Write a detailed note on Malloy-Evelyn method.
13. Explain Jendrassik-Grof method.
14. Write the principle and procedure involved in Fouchet's test and Gmelin's test.
15. How urobilinogen in urine is estimated? Explain with procedure.
16. Explain dye test for excretory function of liver.
17. Explain various liver function tests and explain the tests based on synthetic function of liver.
18. How serum total proteins are estimated by Biuret method?
19. Write the principle and procedure involved in the estimation of serum albumin and globulin.
20. Explain prothrombin time estimation with its significance.
21. Write a detailed note on estimation of *serum glutamate oxaloacetate transaminase.*
22. Write the principle, and procedure involved in *serum glutamate pyruvate transaminase* estimation.
23. How serum *alkaline phosphatase* are estimated?
24. Write the principle and procedure involved in the estimation of serum *acid phosphatase.* Add a note on significance of serum *acid phosphatase.*
25. Explain estimation of serum *lactate dehydrogenase* along with significance of *lactate dehydrogenase.*

10

Lipid Profile Tests

Lipoproteins

Lipoproteins are molecular complexes composed of lipids and proteins. It is a type of conjugated lipid in which protein is the prosthetic group attached to lipid. In blood, lipoproteins are used as transport vehicles for lipids. In addition, lipoproteins also deliver lipid components such as triacyl glycerol, cholesterol, etc., to various tissues for utilization.

Lipoprotein **(Conjugated lipid)** ⟶ Lipid **(Fatty acid + Alcohol)** + Protein **(Prosthetic group or Conjugating group)**

Structure:

Basically, lipoproteins are composed of neutral lipid core (with triacyl glycerol and/or cholesteryl ester) surrounded by coat shell of cholesterol, apoproteins, and phospholipids. Lipoproteins are soluble in aqueous solution because the polar portions (amphiphilic) of cholesterol and phospholipids are oriented outwards toward the surrounding water and the non-polar portions orients inwards toward the lipid molecules within the particles. Hence, the complex serves to emulsify the fats in the extracellular fluids. Special kinds of proteins, called apolipoproteins are embedded in the outer shell, both stabilizing the complex and giving it a functional identity that determines its fate. General structure of lipoprotein complex is depicted in Figure 10.1.

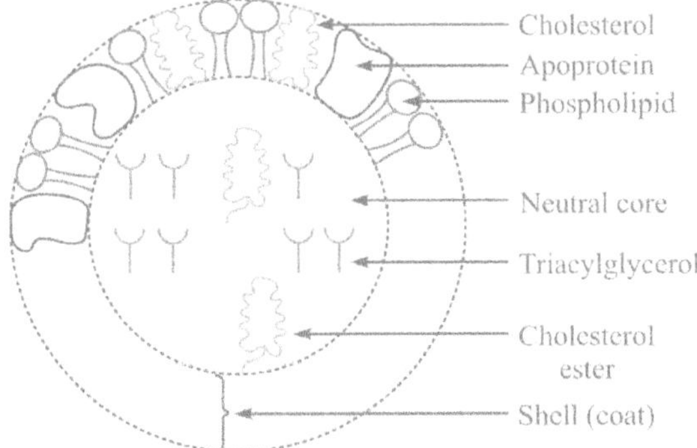

Figure 10.1 General structure of lipoprotein complex.

Apoprotein is also known as apolipoprotein. Apoprotein is defined as the protein components present in the lipoproteins. Apoproteins act as the structural components of lipoproteins. It acts as ligands for lipoprotein receptors. It also guides the formation of lipoproteins. It serves as an activator or inhibitor of enzymes involved in the metabolism of lipoproteins.

Composition:

Lipoproteins are composed of lipids and proteins and their composition may vary depending on the type of lipoprotein. In general, the amount of lipid present in lipoprotein may vary from 60 to 98 % and the amount of protein present in lipoprotein may vary from 2 to 40 %. The various lipid components present in the lipoproteins are 1) Triacylglycerol, 2) Cholesterol in both free form and esterified form, 3) Phospho lipids and 4) Free fatty acid. Based on the type of lipoproteins, the composition of the lipid components may also vary. Normally in various lipoproteins the amount of triacyl glycerol, cholesterol (Free and ester), phospholipids and free fatty acids present may vary from 12 to 88 %, 4 to 59 %, 8 to 47 % and 0 to 1 %, respectively. The approximate percentage compositions of various lipoproteins are summarized in the Table 10.1.

Table 10.1 Percentage compositions of various lipoproteins.

S. No.	Components	Chylomicrons	VLDL	LDL	HDL
Lipoprotein composition (in %)					
1	Protein	2	10	20	40
2	Total lipid	98	90	80	60
Total lipid composition (in %)					
3	Triacyl glycerol	88	55	12	12
4	Cholesterol (Free & ester)	4	24	59	40
5	Phospholipid	8	20	28	47
6	Free fatty acid	0	1	1	1

Classification:

Lipoproteins present in human plasma are broadly classified into five different types according to their separation by electrophoresis. They are 1) Chylomicrons, 2) Very low-density lipoproteins (VLDL), 3) Low-density lipoproteins (LDL), 4) High-density lipoproteins (HDL), and 5) Free fatty acids. The various characteristic (such as electrophoretic mobility, density, diameter and apoproteins type) of different lipoproteins are summarized in the Table 10.2. The electrophoretic mobility of plasma (serum) lipoproteins are presented in Figure 10.2.

Table 10.2 Characteristic of human plasma lipoproteins.

S. No.	Characteristic	Chylomicrons	VLDL	LDL	HDL
1	Electrophoretic mobility	Origin	Pre-β	β	α
2	Density	< 0.96	0.96 – 1.006	1.006 – 1.063	1.063 – 1.21
3	Diameter (in mm)	100 – 1000	30 – 90	20 – 25	10 – 20
4	Apoproteins type	AI, AII, B_{48}	B_{100}, CI, CII, CHI, E	B_{100}	AI, AII, CI, CII, CIII, D, E

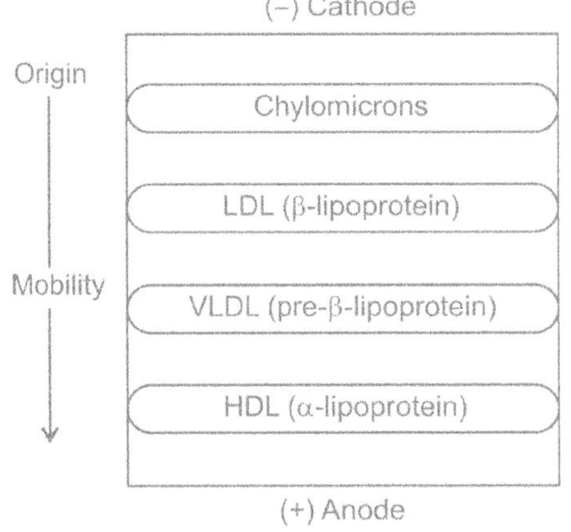

Figure 10.2 Electrophoretic mobility of plasma (serum) lipoproteins.

1. **Chylomicrons:** Chylomicrons are synthesized in the intestine. They contain high quantities (98 %) of lipids and low quantities (2 %) of proteins. Among all lipoproteins the density of chylomicrons (less than 0.96) is the least and the size of chylomicrons is large. They are useful for transporting exogenous (dietary) triacyl glycerol to various tissues. During the electrophoresis separation, the chylomicrons are present in the negative end of the electrodes (cathode) i.e., present near to the origin itself.
2. **Very low-density lipoproteins (VLDL):** VLDL is synthesized in the liver and the intestine. It is composed of lipids (90 %) and proteins (10 %). The density of VLDL (0.96 - 1.006) lies in between that of chylomicrons and LDL. They are useful for the transport of endogenously synthesized triacyl glycerol to various tissues. During the electrophoresis separation, VLDL is present in between chylomicrons and LDL.
3. **Low-density lipoproteins (LDL):** LDL is formed from VLDL in the blood circulation. It is commonly known as **bad cholesterol**. It is composed of lipids (80 %) and proteins (20 %). The density of LDL (1.006 - 1.063) lies in between VLDL and HDL density. They are useful for transporting cholesterol from liver to other tissues. During the electrophoresis separation, LDL is present in between VLDL and HDL.
4. **High-density lipoproteins (HDL):** Mostly, HDL is synthesized in the liver. It is commonly known as **good cholesterol**. It is composed of lipids (60 %) and proteins (40 %) . Among all lipoproteins, the density of HDL (1.063 - 1.210) is higher. They are useful for the transport of cholesterol from peripheral tissues to the liver. During the electrophoresis separation, HDL is present near the positive end of the electrodes (anode). Through ultracentrifugation, three fractions of HDL are identified. They are HDL-1, HDL-2, and HDL-3.
5. **Free fatty acid–albumin complex:** During circulation, free fatty acids are usually present in bound form with the albumin. 20 to 30 molecules of free fatty acids can be holed by one molecule of albumin. They cannot be separated by the electrophoresis technique.

Functions:

1. Chylomicrons are useful for transporting exogenous (dietary) triacyl glycerol to various tissues.
2. VLDLs are useful for transporting the endogenously synthesized triacyl glycerol to various tissues.
3. LDLs are useful for transporting cholesterol from liver to other tissues.
4. HDLs are useful for transporting cholesterol from peripheral tissues to the liver.
5. Lipoproteins, specifically HDL, plays important role in the inflammatory process.
6. Apoproteins act as structural components of lipoproteins.
7. Apoproteins act as ligands for lipoprotein receptors.
8. Apoproteins also guide the formation of lipoproteins.
9. Apoproteins serves as the activators or inhibitors of enzymes involved in the metabolism of lipoproteins.

Estimation of Serum Total Cholesterol

Serum cholesterol can be determined by two different methods. They are 1) Chemical method (Liebermann-Burchard reaction-based method i.e., Sackett's method and Kim and Goldberg method), 2) Enzymatic method (*Cholesterol oxidase* method).

Estimation of Serum Total Cholesterol by Sackett's Method

Principle:

In this method, cholesterol is extracted from a protein-free filtrate using a mixture of alcohol and ether. The extracted cholesterol is evaporated leaving a residue. The obtained residue is dissolved in chloroform. Finally, the extracted cholesterol is treated with Liebermann–Burchard's reagent that results in the formation of a green colored complex. The intensity of the green colored complexes is measured spectrophotometrically or colorimetrically at 680 nm or using a red filter.

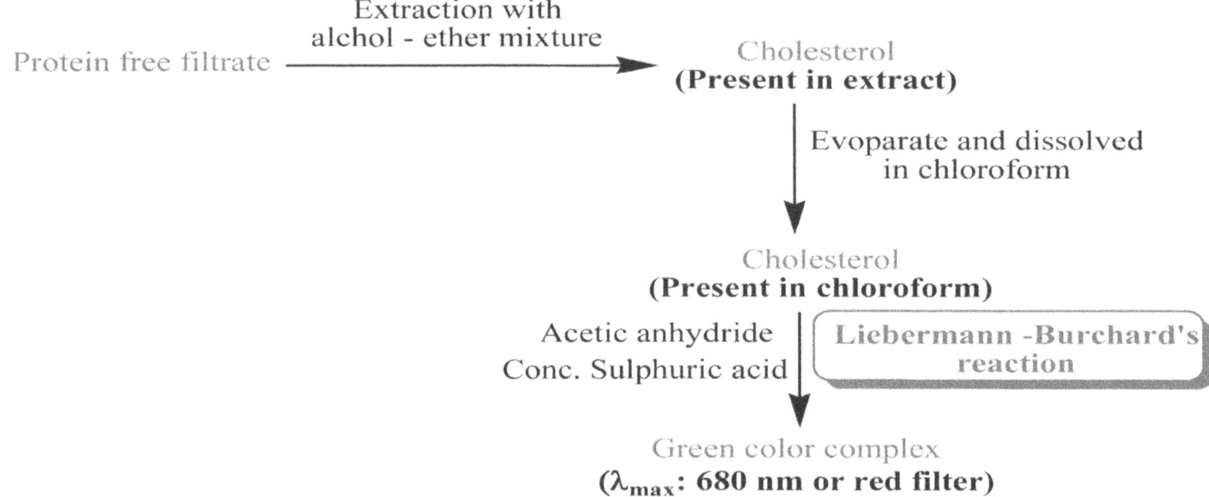

Reagents:

1. **Alcohol-ether mixture:** Mix ethanol and ether in the ratio of 3:1 i.e., mix 75 ml of alcohol with 25 ml of ether to get 100 ml alcohol-ether mixture.
2. **Acetic anhydride-sulphuric acid mixture (Liebermann-Burchard's reagent):** Mix acetic anhydride and concentrated sulphuric acid in the ratio of 20:1 i.e., mix 95.2 ml of acetic anhydride with 4.8 ml of concentrated sulphuric acid to get a 100 ml acetic anhydride-sulphuric acid mixture.
3. **Standard cholesterol solution:** Dissolve 200 mg of cholesterol in 25 ml of chloroform and dilute to 100 ml with chloroform. Dilute 4 ml of the above solution to 100 ml using chloroform (200 mg cholesterol in 100 ml solution. Therefore, a 1 ml solution contains 2 mg of cholesterol; A 4 ml solution contains 8 mg cholesterol; Hence, there will be 8 mg cholesterol in 100 ml standard cholesterol solution. Therefore, 5 ml of standard cholesterol solution contain 0.4 mg of cholesterol).

Procedure:

To 12 ml of alcohol-ether mixture, add 0.2 ml of serum slowly in dry centrifuge tube. Shake the mixture vigorously for 1 minute after corking the tube and keep aside for 30 minutes. Centrifuge the tubes for 5 minutes at 1500 rpm. Separate the supernatant liquid in small beaker and evaporate it on a hot plate or steam bath. Extract the cholesterol using 2 ml chloroform twice in a dry tube and make up the volume to 5 ml with chloroform. Label the tube as unknown.

To 12 ml of alcohol-ether mixture, add 0.2 ml of serum slowly in dry centrifuge tube

⇩

Shake the mixture vigorously for 1 minute after corking the tube and keep aside for 30 minutes

⇩

Centrifuge the tubes for 5 minutes at 1500 rpm

⇩

Separate the supernatant liquid in small beaker and evaporate it on a hot plate or steam bath

⇩

Extract the cholesterol using 2 ml chloroform twice in a dry tube and make up the volume to 5 ml with chloroform (Label the tube as unknown)

Take two test tubes and label as standard and blank, respectively. In the standard test tube take 5 ml of standard cholesterol solution and in blank test tube take 5 ml of chloroform. To all three tubes, add 2 ml of acetic anhydride–sulphuric acid mixture (Liebermann–Burchard's reagent), mix well, and keep in the dark for 15 minutes. Finally, measure the intensity of the green color obtained in the standard and unknown against blank at 680 nm or using a red filter. Calculate the concentration of total cholesterol present in the unknown sample using the following formula.

$$\textit{Concentration of total cholesterol in 0.2 ml serum} = \frac{E_u}{E_s} \times C_s = \frac{E_u}{E_s} \times 0.4 \textit{ mg total cholesterol}$$

$$\textit{Concentration of total cholesterol in 100 ml serum} = \frac{\left(\frac{E_u}{E_s} \times 0.4\right)}{0.2} \times 100 = \frac{E_u}{E_s} \times 200 \textit{ g}$$

Where, E_u = Optical density of unknown serum sample

E_s = Optical density of standard cholesterol solution

C_s = Concentration of standard cholesterol solution

Take two test tubes and label as standard and blank, respectively

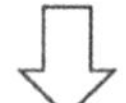

In the standard test tube take 5 ml of standard cholesterol solution and in blank test tube take 5 ml of chloroform

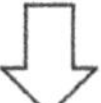

To all three tubes, add 2 ml of acetic anhydride-sulphuric acid mixture (Liebermann-Burchard's reagent), mix well, and keep in the dark for 15 minutes

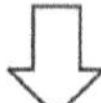

Measure the intensity of the green color obtained in the standard and unknown against blank at 680 nm or using a red filter

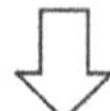

Calculate the concentration of total cholesterol present in the unknown sample

Estimation of Serum Total Cholesterol by Kim and Goldberg Method

Principle:

Kim and Goldberg method is a direct method of the estimation of cholesterol using Liebermann-Burchard's reagent containing acetic acid, acetic anhydride and sulphuric acid. In this method, the serum is directly treated with Liebermann-Burchard's reagent. Acetic acid is used to dissolve cholesterol. Latter the dissolved cholesterol undergoes Liebermann-Burchard's reaction with acetic anhydride and sulphuric acid resulting in a green-colored complex formation. The intensity of the green-color complexes is measured spectrophotometrically or colorimetrically at 625 nm or using a red filter.

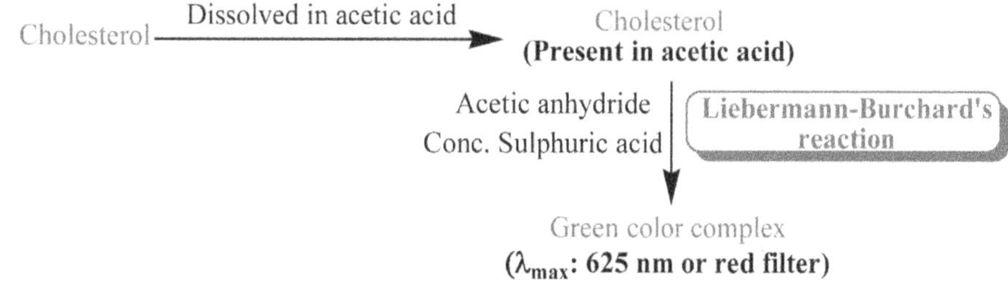

Reagents:

1. **Stable Liebermann–Burchard's reagent:** Cool acetic anhydride and concentrated sulphuric acid in ice-water or freezer. Mix 220 ml of cold acetic anhydride and 200 ml of glacial acetic acid. Add 30 ml of cold concentrated sulphuric acid and mix well. Store in a brown-colored bottle at 4 °C. This reagent is stable for 6 months.
2. **Standard cholesterol solution:** Dissolve 200 mg of cholesterol in 25 ml of glacial acetic acid and dilute to 100 ml with glacial acetic acid. Store in a brown-colored bottle at room temperature. (200 mg cholesterol in a 100 ml solution. Therefore, 1 ml solution contains 2 mg of cholesterol; hence, 0.1 ml standard cholesterol solutions contain 0.2 mg of cholesterol).

Procedure:

Take three test tubes and label as unknown, standard, and blank. Take 6 ml of stable Liebermann–Burchard's reagent in all three test tubes. Add 0.1 ml of serum, 0.1 ml of standard cholesterol solution, and 0.1 ml of water in unknown, standard and blank test tubes, respectively. Shake the mixtures vigorously and incubate all test tubes for 18 minutes at 37 °C. Measure the intensity of the green color obtained in the standard and unknown tubes against the blank one at 625 nm or using a red filter. Calculate the concentration of total cholesterol present in the unknown sample using the following formula:

$$\textit{Concentration of total cholesterol in 0.1 ml serum} = \frac{E_u}{E_s} \times C_s = \frac{E_u}{E_s} \times 0.2 \; \textit{mg total cholesterol}$$

$$\textit{Concentration of total cholesterol in 100 ml serum} = \frac{\left(\frac{E_u}{E_s} \times 0.2\right)}{0.1} \times 100 = \frac{E_u}{E_s} \times 200 \; g$$

Where, E_u = Optical density of unknown serum sample

E_s = Optical density of standard cholesterol solution

C_s = Concentration of standard cholesterol solution

Dry and hemolyze all test tubes and don't use icteric sera.

Take three test tubes and label as unknown, standard, and blank

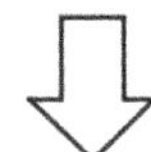

Take 1 ml of reagent in all three test tubes

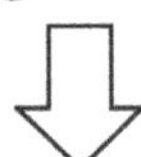

Add 20 µl of serum, 20 µl of standard cholesterol solution and 20 µl of water in the unknown, standard, and blank test tubes, respectively

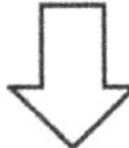

Shake the test tubes well and incubate all test tubes for 5 minutes at 37 °C

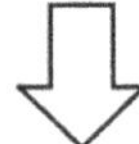

Measure the intensity of the red color obtained in the standard and unknown ones against blank at 505 nm or using a green filter

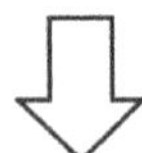

Calculate the concentration of total cholesterol present in the unknown sample

Estimation of Serum Total Cholesterol by Enzymatic Method

Principle:

Cholesterol esterase hydrolyzes cholesterol esters. Bacterial *cholesterol oxidase* oxidizes cholesterol into cholest-4-en-3-one and hydrogen peroxide. The liberated hydrogen peroxide forms a red-colored complex by reacting with phenol and amino-4-antipyrin in the presence of *peroxidase* enzyme. The intensity of the red-colored complex is measured spectrophotometrically or colorimetrically at 505 nm or using a green filter.

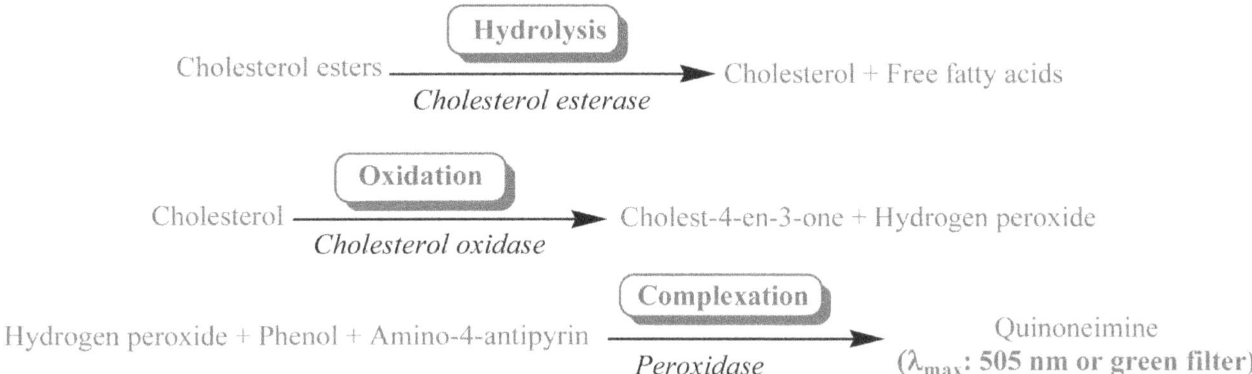

Reagents:

1. **Buffer solution:** Mix 50 mmol/l PIPES buffer (pH: 6.9) and 24 mmol/l phenol.
2. **Reagent:** Dissolve 250 U/l *cholesterol esterase*, 250 U/l *cholesterol oxidase*, 1000 U/l *peroxidase*, 0.5 mmol/l amino-4-antipyrin and 2.5 mmol/l sodium chloride in 10 ml of buffer solution.
3. **Standard cholesterol solution:** Prepare standard solutions in a concentration of 5.17 mmol/l which is equal to 200 mg of cholesterol in 100 ml solutions or 2 g of (2000 mg) cholesterol in 1 l (1000 ml) solution.

Procedure:

Take three test tubes and label as unknown, standard, and blank. Take 1 ml of reagent in all three test tubes. Add 20 µl of serum, 20 µl of standard cholesterol solution and 20 µl of water in the unknown, standard, and blank test tubes, respectively. Shake the test tubes well and incubate all test tubes for 5 minutes at 37 °C. Measure the intensity of the red color obtained in the standard and unknown ones against blank at 505 nm or using a green filter. Calculate the concentration of total cholesterol present in the unknown sample using the following formula:

$$\textit{Concentration of total cholesterol in serum} = \frac{E_u}{E_s} \times C_s$$

Where, E_u = Optical density of unknown serum sample

E_s = Optical density of standard cholesterol solution

C_s = Concentration of standard cholesterol solution (If C_s = 5.17 then the unit is mmol/l; If C_s = 200 then the unit is mg/100 ml; If C_s = 2 then the unit is g/l)

Significance:

The normal serum cholesterol is 150-240 mg/100 ml in a healthy person and the level is increased with age and may go up to 300 mg/100 ml. The desirable serum cholesterol level is 200 mg/100 ml. If the serum cholesterol level is > 240 mg/100 ml then it indicates a high risk of developing coronary artery disease. The borderline serum cholesterol level is 201 to 239 mg/100 ml. The serum cholesterol level is increased (hypercholesterolemia) in the clinical conditions like hypothyroidism, uncontrolled diabetes mellitus, obstructive jaundice, nephrotic syndrome, during ether anesthesia and xanthomatosis. Serum cholesterol level is decreased (hypocholesterolemia) in the clinical conditions like hyperthyroidism, anemia (except hemorrhagic), wasting disease, hepatocellular damage, acute infections, intestinal obstruction and terminal states of a variety of diseases.

Take three test tubes and label as unknown, standard, and blank

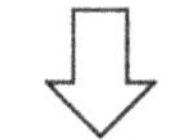

Take 1 ml of reagent in all three test tubes

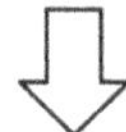

Add 20 µl of serum, 20 µl of standard cholesterol solution and 20 µl of water in the unknown, standard, and blank test tubes, respectively

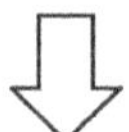

Shake the test tubes well and incubate all test tubes for 5 minutes at 37 °C

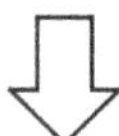

Measure the intensity of the red color obtained in the standard and unknown ones against blank at 505 nm or using a green filter

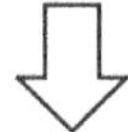

Calculate the concentration of total cholesterol present in the unknown sample

Estimation of Serum HDL Cholesterol

Principle:

A mixture of phosphotungstic acid and magnesium chloride precipitates LDL fraction. Hence, after the centrifugation, the supernatant liquid contains only HDL cholesterol. This HDL cholesterol is hydrolyzed by *cholesterol esterase*. Bacterial *cholesterol oxidase* oxidizes HDL cholesterol into HDL cholest-4-en-3-one and hydrogen peroxide. The liberated hydrogen peroxide forms a red-colored complex by reacting with phenol and amino-4-antipyrin in the presence of *peroxidase* enzyme. The intensity of the red-colored complexes is measured spectrophotometrically or colorimetrically at 505 nm or using a green filter.

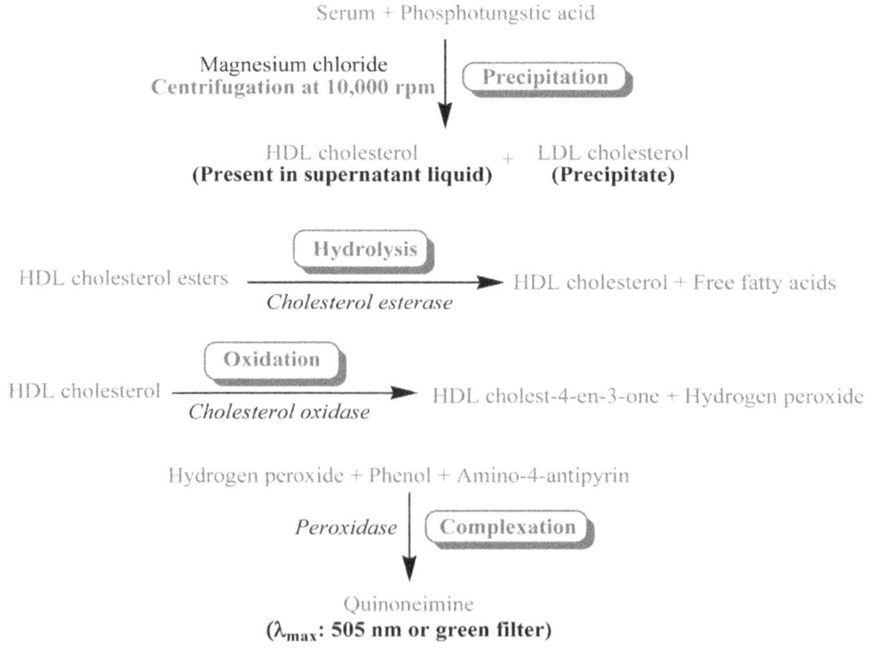

Reagents:

1. **Precipitating reagent:** Mix 32 g/l phosphotungstic acid and 0.4 mmol/l magnesium chloride.
2. **Buffer solution:** Mix 50 mmol/l PIPES buffer (pH: 6.9) and 24 mmol/l phenol.

3. **Reagent:** Dissolve 250 U/l *cholesterol esterase*, 250 U/l *cholesterol oxidase*, 1000 U/l *peroxidase*, 0.5 mmol/l amino-4-antipyrin and 2.5 mmol/l sodium chloride in 10 ml of buffer solution.
4. **Standard HDL cholesterol solution:** Prepare standard HDL cholesterol solutions in a concentration of 1.3 mmol/l which is equal to 50 mg HDL cholesterol in 1 dl solution.

Procedure:

Add 50 µl of precipitating reagent to 500 µl plasma into the marked Eppendorf tubes. Mix the solution thoroughly and centrifuge at 10,000 rpm for 15 minutes. Separate the clear supernatant liquid (Only contain HDL cholesterol) and use it for the estimation of HDL cholesterol.

Add 50 µl of precipitating reagent to 500 µl plasma into the marked Eppendorf tubes

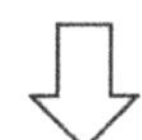

Mix the solution thoroughly and centrifuge at 10,000 rpm for 15 minutes

Separate the clear supernatant liquid (Only contain HDL cholesterol)

Take three test tubes and label as unknown, standard and blank. Take 1 ml of reagent in all three test tubes. Add 20 µl of supernatant liquid prepared as above, 20 µl of standard HDL cholesterol solution, and 20 µl of water in the unknown, standard and blank test tube, respectively. Shake well the mixtures and incubate all test tubes for 5 minutes at 37 °C. Measure the intensity of the red color obtained in the standard and unknown tubes against the blank at 505 nm or using a green filter. Calculate the concentration of the HDL cholesterol present in unknown sample using the following formula.

$$\textit{Concentration of HDL cholesterol in serum} = \frac{E_u}{E_s} \times C_s$$

Where, E_u = Optical density of unknown serum sample

E_s = Optical density of standard HDL cholesterol solution

C_s = Concentration of standard HDL cholesterol solution (If C_s = 1.3 then the unit is mmol/l; If C_s = 50 then the unit is mg/dl)

Take three test tubes and label as unknown, standard and blank

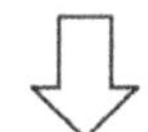

Take 1 ml of reagent in all three test tubes

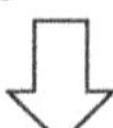

Add 20 µl of supernatant liquid prepared as above, 20 µl of standard HDL cholesterol solution, and 20 µl of water in the unknown, standard and blank test tube, respectively

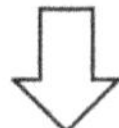

Shake well the mixtures and incubate all test tubes for 5 minutes at 37 °C

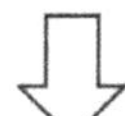

Measure the intensity of the red color obtained in the standard and unknown tubes against the blank at 505 nm or using a green filter

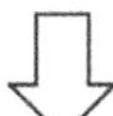

Calculate the concentration of the HDL cholesterol present in unknown sample

Significance:

The normal serum HDL cholesterol is greater than 55 and 65 mg/100 ml for males and females, respectively The atherosclerotic risk is slightly increased when serum HDL cholesterol is between 35 to 55 and 45 to 65 mg/100 ml for males and females, respectively. Additionally, the risk is greatly increased when serum HDL cholesterol is less than 35 and 45 mg/100 ml for males and females, respectively. The prognosis of myocardial infarction also needs the evaluation of both HDL and LDL cholesterol levels. The lower the HDL cholesterol level the higher is the risk of myocardial infarction. The determination of HDL cholesterol is important for patients who have hypercholesterolemia, as well as hypertriglyceridemia. Simultaneously elevated levels of serum triglycerides and decreased levels of HDL cholesterol indicate high coronary risk.

Estimation of Serum Triglycerides

Principle:

Triglycerides undergo hydrolysis in the presence of *lipoprotein lipase* and produce glycerol and free fatty acids. Then, glycerol undergoes phosphorylation reaction by reacting with ATP in the presence of *glycerol kinase* and produce glycerol-3-phosphate with the liberation of one mole of ADP. Later, glycerol-3-phosphate is oxidized by reacting with oxygen in the presence of *glycerol-3-phosphate oxidase* resulting in the formation of dihydroxy acetone phosphate with the liberation of hydrogen peroxide. Finally, the liberated hydrogen peroxide forms a red-colored complex by reacting with amino-4-antipyrin and ESPAS reagent in the presence of *peroxidase*. The intensity of the red-coloured complexes is measured spectrophotometrically or colorimetrically at 505 nm or using a green filter.

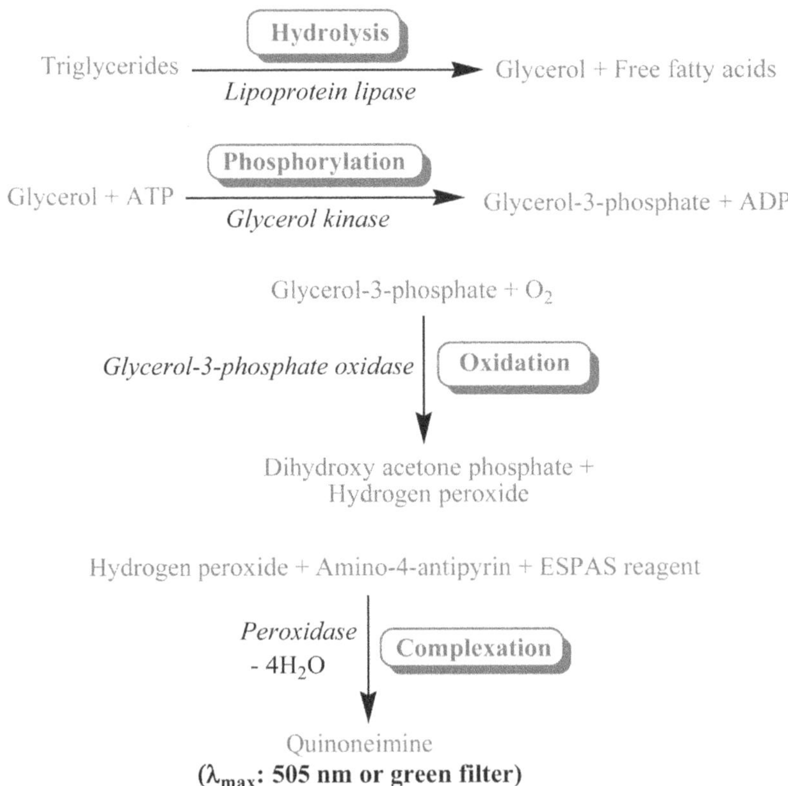

Reagents:

1. **Buffer solution:** Mix 50 mmol/l PIPES buffer (pH: 7.5) and 1 mmol/l N-ethyl-N-sulfopropyl-m-anizidine (ESPAS).

2. **Reagent:** Dissolve 1100 U/l *lipoprotein lipase,* 800 U/l *glycerol kinase,* 3000 U/l *glycerol phosphate oxidase,* 350 U/l *peroxidase,* 0.7 mmol/l 4-amino-antipyrine and 0.3 mmol/l ATP in 10 ml of buffer solution.
3. **Standard triglyceride solution:** Prepare standard glycerol solution in a concentration of 2.28 mmol/l which is equal to 200 mg glycerol in 100 ml solution or 2 g (2000 mg) glycerol in 1 l (1000 ml) solution.

Procedure:

Take three test tubes and label as unknown, standard and blank. Take 1 ml of reagent in all three test tubes. Add 20 µl of serum, 20 µl of standard triglyceride solution, 20 µl of water in the unknown, standard, and blank test tubes, respectively, and shake well. Incubate all test tubes for 5 minutes at 37 °C. Finally, measure the intensity of the red color obtained in the standard and unknown tubes against the blank tube at 505 nm or using a green filter. Calculate the concentration of the triglycerides present in the unknown sample using the following formula.

$$\text{Concentration of triglycerides in serum} = \frac{E_u}{E_s} \times C_s$$

Where, E_u = Optical density of unknown serum sample

E_s = Optical density of standard triglyceride solution

C_s = Concentration of standard triglyceride solution (If C_s = 2.28 then the unit is mmol/l; If C_s = 200 then the unit is mg/100 ml; If C_s = 2 then the unit is g/l).

Take three test tubes and label as unknown, standard and blank

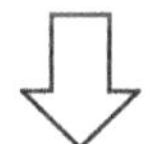

Take 1 ml of reagent in all three test tubes

Add 20 µl of serum, 20 µl of standard triglyceride solution, 20 µl of water in the unknown, standard, and blank test tubes, respectively, and shake well

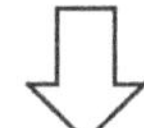

Incubate all test tubes for 5 minutes at 37 °C

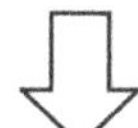

Measure the intensity of the red color obtained in the standard and unknown tubes against the blank tube at 505 nm or using a green filter

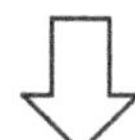

Calculate the concentration of the triglycerides present in the unknown sample

Significance:

The normal serum triglyceride is less than 150 mg/100 ml. The atherosclerotic risk is slightly increased when serum triglyceride is between 150 to 200 mg/100 ml and the risk is greatly increased when serum triglyceride is greater than 200 mg/100 ml. The determination of serum triglyceride level is important in patients (i) with decreased HDL cholesterol level, (ii) with secondary hypertriglyceridemia, and (iii) with occlusion of peripheral arteries.

Estimation of Serum LDL Cholesterol

In general serum LDL cholesterol is not estimated directly. It is usually estimated from the total cholesterol, HDL cholesterol and triglycerides indirectly. The LDL cholesterol is calculated using the below mentioned formula.

$$LDL\ cholesterol = Total\ cholesterol - \left[HDL\ cholestrol + \frac{Triglcerides}{5}\right]$$

In case of a higher concentration of triglycerides i.e., > 400 mg/ml and hyperlipoproteinemia type-I and III patients this equation will not work. In such cases LDL cholesterol is determined at pH 5.12 (isoelectric precipitation with heparin).

Significance:

The normal serum LDL cholesterol is less than 150 mg/100 ml. The atherosclerotic risk is slightly increased when the serum LDL cholesterol is between 150 to 190 mg/100 ml and the risk is greatly increased when the serum LDL cholesterol is greater than 190 mg/100 ml. The determination of LDL cholesterol is important for patients (i) of young ages with vascular diseases, (ii) with xanthomas, and (iii) secondary hypercholesterolemia. The prognosis of myocardial infarction also needs the evaluation of both HDL and LDL cholesterol levels.

Determination of lipid constituents in plasma or serum is normally done on blood drawn from patients fasting for 12 or 16 hours. The "normal" value of serum cholesterol and triglycerides varies individually and with ages. The maximal concentration of lipids can be measured in winter.

PROBABLE QUESTIONS

PART – A: Multiple Choice Questions

1. Which is prosthetic group in lipoprotein?
   (a) Protein (b) Lipid
   (c) Carbohydrate (d) Nucleic acid
2. Protein components present in the lipoproteins is known as ________________.
   (a) Apoprotein (b) Apolipoprotein
   (c) Both a & b (d) None of the above
3. The density of VLDL lies in between that of ________________ density.
   (a) Chylomicrons and HDL (b) LDL and HDL
   (c) VLDL and chylomicrons (d) Chylomicrons and LDL
4. Which among these are functions of lipoproteins?
   (a) Chylomicrons are useful for transporting exogenous triacyl glycerol to various tissues
   (b) VLDLs are useful for transporting the endogenously synthesized triacyl glycerol to various tissues
   (c) LDLs are useful for transporting cholesterol from liver to other tissues, chylomicrons and HDL
   (d) All the above
5. Which of the following methods are not useful for the estimation serum cholesterol?
   (a) Sackett's method (b) Kim and Goldberg method
   (c) Malloy-Evelyn method (d) *Cholesterol oxidase* method

6. Cholesterol reacts with Liebermann–Burchard's reagent and produce which color complex?
   (a) Red (b) Brown
   (c) Black (d) Green
7. What is the composition of Liebermann–Burchard's reagent?
   (a) Acetic anhydride–hydrochloric acid mixture
   (b) Acetone–hydrochloric acid mixture
   (c) Acetic anhydride–sulphuric acid mixture
   (d) Acetone–sulphuric acid mixture
8. In Sackett's method, the intensity of the green colored complexes formed is measured spectrophotometrically at which wavelength?
   (a) 580 nm (b) 680 nm
   (c) 780 nm (d) 880 nm
9. Which product is formed when cholesterol is oxidized by bacterial *cholesterol oxidase*?
   (a) Cholest-4-en-3-one and hydrogen peroxide (b) Cholest-4-en-2-one and hydrogen peroxide
   (c) Cholest-5-en-3-one and hydrogen peroxide (d) Cholest-5-en-2-one and hydrogen peroxide.
10. In enzymatic method, the intensity of the red colored complexes formed is measured spectrophotometrically at which wavelength?
    (a) 455 nm (b) 505 nm
    (c) 555 nm (d) 605 nm
11. Which mixture is used as the precipitating reagent in estimation of serum HDL cholesterol?
    (a) Phosphotungstic acid and potassium cyanide
    (b) Phosphoric acid and magnesium chloride
    (c) Phosphoric acid and potassium cyanide
    (d) Phosphotungstic acid and magnesium chloride
12. What is the normal serum HDL cholesterol level in male & female?
    (a) Greater than 75 and 95 mg/100 ml (b) Greater than 55 and 65 mg/100 ml
    (c) Less than 75 and 95 mg/100 ml (d) Less than 55 and 65 mg/100 ml
13. Which enzyme hydrolyses triglycerides into glycerol and free fatty acids?
    (a) *Lipoprotein lipase* (b) *Lipoprotein protease*
    (c) *Lipoprotein transferase* (d) *Lipoprotein nuclease*
14. What is the normal serum LDL cholesterol?
    (a) Less than 50 mg/100 ml (b) Less than 100 mg/100 ml
    (c) Less than 150 mg/100 ml (d) Less than 200 mg/100 ml
15. Among all lipoproteins, which lipoprotein poses higher density?
    (a) HDL (b) VLDL
    (c) Chylomicrons (d) LDL
16. Among all lipoproteins, which lipoprotein poses lower density?
    (a) VLDL (b) Chylomicrons
    (c) LDL (d) HDL
17. Where very low-density lipoproteins are synthesized?
    (a) Intestine & kidney (b) Liver & pancreas
    (c) Liver & intestine (d) Kidney & pancreas

18. What is DNPH reagent?
    (a) 1,3-Dinitrophenyl hydrazine reagent
    (b) 2,4-Dinitrophenyl hydrazine reagent
    (c) 3,5-Dinitrophenyl hydrazine reagent
    (d) 4,6-Dinitrophenyl hydrazine reagent
19. Which statement is wrong with respect to lipoproteins?
    (a) Transport vehicles for lipids
    (b) Deliver triacyl glycerol to various tissues for utilization
    (c) Deliver cholesterol to various tissues for utilization
    (d) Deliver protein to various tissues for utilization
20. In lipoproteins, neutral lipid core is surrounded by coat shell of which compound?
    (a) Carbohydrate
    (b) Cholesterol
    (c) Apoprotein
    (d) Phospholipid
21. Which statement is wrong with respect to lipoproteins?
    (a) Lipoproteins are soluble in aqueous solution
    (b) The polar portions of cholesterol and phospholipids are oriented outwards toward the surrounding water
    (c) The non-polar portions orients inwards toward the lipid molecules
    (d) The polar portions of cholesterol and phospholipids are oriented inwards toward the lipid molecules
22. Which statement is wrong with respect to apolipoproteins?
    (a) Act as the structural components of lipoproteins
    (b) Not serves as an activator or inhibitor of enzymes involved in the metabolism of lipoproteins
    (c) Acts as ligands for lipoprotein receptors
    (d) Guides the formation of lipoproteins
23. How much amount of lipid is present in lipoprotein?
    (a) 10 to 48 %
    (b) 20 to 58 %
    (c) 40 to 78 %
    (d) 60 to 98 %
24. How much amount of lipid is present in lipoprotein?
    (a) 1 to 30 %
    (b) 2 to 40 %
    (c) 3 to 50 %
    (d) 4 to 60 %
25. Which of the following are the lipid components present in the lipoproteins?
    (a) Triacylglycerol
    (b) Cholesterol in both free form and esterified form
    (c) Phospho lipids & free fatty acid
    (d) All the above
26. How much amount of triacyl glycerol is present in lipoprotein?
    (a) 2 to 58 %
    (b) 2 to 88 %
    (c) 12 to 88 %
    (d) 12 to 58 %
27. How much amount of cholesterol is present in lipoprotein?
    (a) 4 to 59 %
    (b) 14 to 59 %
    (c) 24 to 59 %
    (d) 34 to 59 %
28. How much amount of phospholipid is present in lipoprotein?
    (a) 0.8 to 47 %
    (b) 8 to 47 %
    (c) 18 to 47 %
    (d) 28 to 47 %

29. How much amount of free fatty acid is present in lipoprotein?
    (a) 0 to 1 % (b) 1 to 10 %
    (c) 10 to 20 % (d) 20 to 30 %
30. Which human plasma lipoprotein poses "α" electrophoretic mobility?
    (a) VLDL (b) Chylomicrons
    (c) LDL (d) HDL
31. What is the diameter of VLDL?
    (a) 100-1000 mm (b) 30-90 mm
    (c) 20-25 mm (d) 10-20 mm
32. Which statement is wrong with respect to chylomicrons?
    (a) Synthesized in the intestine
    (b) High density among all lipoprotein
    (c) Useful for transporting exogenous triacyl glycerol to various tissues
    (d) During the electrophoresis separation, present in the negative end of the electrodes
33. Which statement is wrong with respect to VLDL?
    (a) Synthesized in the liver and the intestine
    (b) Density lies in between that of chylomicrons and LDL
    (c) Useful for transporting exogenous triacyl glycerol to various tissues
    (d) During the electrophoresis separation, present in between chylomicrons and LDL
34. Which statement is wrong with respect to LDL?
    (a) Formed from chylomicron in the blood circulation
    (b) During the electrophoresis separation, present in between VLDL and HDL
    (c) The density lies in between VLDL and HDL
    (d) Useful for transporting cholesterol from liver to other tissues
35. Which statement is wrong with respect to HDL?
    (a) Synthesized in the liver
    (b) During the electrophoresis separation, present near the positive end of the electrodes
    (c) Useful for the transport of cholesterol from peripheral tissues to the liver
    (d) Low density among all lipoprotein
36. Which statement is wrong with respect to free fatty acid-albumin complex?
    (a) 20 to 30 molecules of free fatty acids can be holed by one molecule of albumin
    (b) They cannot be separated by the electrophoresis technique
    (c) They can be separated by the electrophoresis technique
    (d) During circulation, free fatty acids are usually present in bound form with the albumin
37. Which one is commonly known as bad cholesterol?
    (a) VLDL (b) Chylomicrons
    (c) LDL (d) HDL
38. Which one is commonly known as good cholesterol?
    (a) Chylomicrons (b) HDL
    (c) VLDL (d) LDL

39. Which one is not present in stable Liebermann–Burchard's reagent?
    (a) Hydrochloric acid (b) Acetic anhydride
    (c) Sulphuric acid (d) Glacial acetic acid
40. In enzymatic method of cholesterol estimation, liberated hydrogen peroxide reacts with which compound and produce red color complex?
    (a) Phenol (b) Amino-4-antipyrine
    (c) Both a & b (d) None of the above
41. What is the desirable serum cholesterol level?
    (a) 100 mg/100 ml (b) 200 mg/100 ml
    (c) 300 mg/100 ml (d) 400 mg/100 ml
42. Which level of serum cholesterol is known as borderline serum cholesterol level?
    (a) 1 to 39 mg/100 ml (b) 101 to 139 mg/100 ml
    (c) 201 to 239 mg/100 ml (d) 301 to 339 mg/100 ml
43. If the serum cholesterol level is ____________ then it indicates a high risk of developing coronary artery disease.
    (a) > 440 mg/100 ml (b) > 340 mg/100 ml
    (c) > 240 mg/100 ml (d) > 140 mg/100 ml
44. In which clinical condition serum cholesterol level is decreased?
    (a) Hypothyroidism (b) Uncontrolled diabetes mellitus
    (c) Obstructive jaundice (d) Wasting disease
45. In which clinical condition serum cholesterol level is increased?
    (a) Nephrotic syndrome (b) Hepatocellular damage
    (c) Anemia (except hemorrhagic) (d) Hyperthyroidism
46. The ________ the HDL cholesterol level the ____________ is the risk of myocardial infarction.
    (a) Higher & higher (b) Higher & lower
    (c) Lower & higher (d) Lower & lower
47. The determination of serum triglyceride level is important in which patients?
    (a) Patient with decreased HDL cholesterol level
    (b) Patient with secondary hypertriglyceridemia
    (c) Patient with occlusion of peripheral arteries
    (d) All the above patient
48. The atherosclerotic risk is slightly increased when the serum LDL cholesterol is between ____________________.
    (a) 50 to 90 mg/100 ml (b) 150 to 190 mg/100 ml
    (c) 250 to 290 mg/100 ml (d) 350 to 390 mg/100 ml
49. The atherosclerotic risk is greatly increased when the serum LDL cholesterol is between ____________________.
    (a) Greater than 90 mg/100 ml (b) Greater than 190 mg/100 ml
    (c) Greater than 290 mg/100 ml (d) Greater than 390 mg/100 ml
50. The determination of LDL cholesterol is important in which patients?
    (a) Patient of young age with vascular diseases
    (b) Patient with xanthomas
    (c) Patient with secondary hypercholesterolemia
    (d) All the above patients

Key for Multiple Choice Questions

1. (a)	2. (c)	3. (d)	4. (d)	5. (c)
6. (d)	7. (c)	8. (b)	9. (a)	10. (b)
11. (d)	12. (b)	13. (a)	14. (c)	15. (a)
16. (b)	17. (c)	18. (b)	19. (d)	20. (a)
21. (d)	22. (b)	23. (d)	24. (b)	25. (d)
26. (c)	27. (a)	28. (b)	29. (a)	30. (d)
31. (b)	32. (b)	33. (c)	34. (a)	35. (d)
36. (c)	37. (c)	38. (b)	39. (a)	40. (c)
41. (b)	42. (c)	43. (c)	44. (d)	45. (a)
46. (c)	47. (d)	48. (b)	49. (b)	50. (d)

PART – B: Short Answers

1. Define lipoproteins.
2. Write a note on structure of lipoproteins.
3. Explain the composition of various lipoproteins.
4. What is chylomicron?
5. What is LDL cholesterol.
6. Explain the term "VLDL".
7. Write about HDL cholesterol.
8. What is LDL and HDL ratio? Mention its clinical significance.
9. Classify lipoproteins.
10. What is free fatty acid-albumin complex?
11. List out the important functions of lipoproteins.
12. Write the basic principle involved in the estimation of serum total cholesterol by Sackett's method.
13. What is Liebermann-Burchard's reagent? Mention its use.
14. Write the basic principle involved in the estimation of serum total cholesterol by Kim and Goldberg method.
15. What is stable Liebermann-Burchard's reagent? Mention its use.
16. How serum total cholesterol is estimated by enzymatic method?
17. Write a short note on principle involved in the estimation of serum HDL cholesterol.
18. What is the principle involved in the estimation of serum triglycerides?
19. How LDL cholesterol is measured from other components of lipid profile?
20. What are apoproteins? Write their functions.
21. What are triglycerides? Explain their significance.
22. Write the significance of LDL cholesterol.
23. Write a note on significance of serum cholesterol.
24. Write the characteristic of human plasma lipoproteins.
25. Draw a neat labeled diagram of lipoprotein complex.

PART – C: Long Answers

1. Write a detailed note on lipoproteins.
2. What are lipoproteins? Explain with general structure and functions of lipoprotein.
3. Define and classify lipoprotein. Add a note on composition of various lipoprotein.
4. Classify lipoprotein and explain any one lipoprotein estimation in detail.
5. Write about the HDL and LDL cholesterols.
6. Write about lipid profile tests and their diagnostic importance.
7. How does serum total cholesterol is estimated?
8. Write a detailed note on Sackett's method.
9. How serum total cholesterol is estimated by Kim and Goldberg method.
10. Explain the enzymatic estimation of serum total cholesterol.
11. Write principle and procedure involved in the estimation of serum HDL cholesterol. Mention the significance of HDL cholesterol.
12. How serum triglyceride is estimated? Add a note on significance of triglyceride.
13. How serum LDL cholesterol is estimated? Add a note on significance of LDL cholesterol.

11

Immunochemical Techniques

Most hormones are present in the circulating blood in extremely low concentrations. The concentration of hormones present in the circulating blood may vary from picogram (pg) to nanogram (ng) level per ml (10^{-12} to 10^{-9} g/ml); whereas the concentration of other routinely determined clinical chemistry parameters may vary from microgram (µg) to milligram (mg) level per ml (10^{-6} to 10^{-3} g/ml). It is extremely difficult to measure hormone concentrations when they are this low. Hence, they need a series of sensitive analytical methods for their measurement. Serum concentrations of several hormones are lower in animals than that in humans. However, a revolutionary technique known as immunoassay was developed in the mid 20th century. This technique measured the concentrations of hormones and their end products that are present in lower concentrations. Currently, the most commonly used methods for the estimation of hormone levels are immunoassays and immunometric assays. Other useful techniques for the estimation of hormones are gas chromatography-mass spectrometry (GC-MS), high performance liquid chromatography (HPLC), and liquid chromatography-mass spectrometry (LC-MS/MS).

Immunochemistry:

Immunochemistry is an advanced area of immunology and the branch of chemistry which deals with the chemistry of the immune system. This involves the study of the properties, functions, interactions, and production of the chemical components (antibodies/immunoglobulins, toxin, epitopes of proteins like CD_4, antitoxins, cytokines/chemokines, antigens) of the immune system, immune responses along with the determination of immune materials by immunochemical assays.

Immunochemical techniques:

The method which utilizes a highly specific affinity of an antibody for its antigen is known as immunochemical methods. In tissues or cells, it detects the distribution of a given protein or antigen. Immunochemical techniques are the methods used for the immunochemical analysis. From a diagnostic and clinical point of view, these techniques are highly important because in a diseased state several proteins are altered even in a normal cell.

Terms used:

The followings are the important terms used in immunochemical techniques:

1. **Antigens:** Any foreign substances which when introduced into an animal can stimulate a specific immune response in the form of production of antibodies and specific reactive T-lymphocytes. Antigens have the ability to combine specifically with the antibodies produced or sensitized T-cells that are induced in the process. It is usually denoted by the symbol "Ag".
2. **Antibodies:** Antibodies are glycoproteins that bind specifically to the antigen that induced their formation. They are usually denoted by the symbol "Ab". Antibodies are broadly classified into two classes as, a) Monoclonal antibodies and b) Polyclonal antibodies.
   a. **Monoclonal antibodies:** They are very specific antibodies that bind only to one antigen epitope, which in turn reduces the occurrence of false positives in the immunoassay. They are the products

of a single clone of plasma cells by B-lymphocytes and are mostly prepared in a laboratory. They are directed against single epitopes – identical copies with the same structure and antigen specificity. They have an excellent specificity but poor ability to precipitate antigen. Sometimes, monoclonal is called as "monovalent" for indicating the antigen specificity.

b. **Polyclonal antibodies:** They may be produced in mammals like rabbits and sheep. Antiserum usually contains a mixture of antibodies that recognizes and binds to the same antigen, but it may attach to different epitopes. It is conventional, i.e., produced by immunization of animals with antigen. Thus, an antibody consists of a mixture of monoclonal antibodies having specificity for complex antigens. Sometimes, polyclonal is also called as "polyvalent" for indicating the antigen specificity.

3. **Epitope:** It is also known as the antigenic determinant. It is the part of an antigen that is recognized by the immune system, specifically by antibodies, B-cells, or T-cells. For example, the epitope is the specific piece of the antigen to which an antibody binds.

Characteristics:

The following are the important characteristics of the immunochemical technique:

1. It is simple, rapid, and robust.
2. This technique is highly sensitive.
3. This technique is easily automated. Hence, applicable to the regular clinical diagnostic laboratories.
4. It does not require extensive and easily destructible sample preparation.
5. It does not require expensive instrumentation.
6. Usually, the detection of this technique is based on simple photometric, fluorometric, and luminometric detection.
7. It is useful for both qualitative and quantitative measurements.

Applications:

The following are the various applications of the immunochemical technique:

1. It is used for identifying the function of the newly identified or novel proteins.
2. It is used to identify the importance of uncharacterized proteins in their natural environment.
3. It is used for the determination of species or tissues in which the protein or residues is expressed.
4. It is used to find the cell type or sub-cellular compartment in which the protein can be found.
5. During the development of an organism, it is used to detect whether there is any variation in the expression of the proteins.
6. It is useful for the diagnosis and treatment of a particular disease as this technique can offer useful information. A particular disease state may be indicated by some alteration in the normal expression pattern of a particular protein.

Principle:

A highly specific and sensitive reaction between an antigen and an antibody is the basic principle behind all the immunochemical methods. Antibodies are immunoglobins, belonging to a family of glycoproteins – IgG, IgA, IgD, IgM and IgE. Antibodies contain four polypeptide units and are often structurally visualized as the Y-shaped molecules. Out of these four, two types have two identical polypeptide units. They are known as heavy chains and light chains. A fab is the domain of antibodies site where it binds to an antigen. The epitope is the region of an antigen binding to an antibody. The antigen-antibody reaction is presented in Figure 11.1.

Quantitative precipitin curve: In general, the term affinity is used to measure the strength of the binding. At equilibrium, the concentration of an antibody-antigen complex is measured. It is often used to express affinity. In 1935, Heidelberger and Kendall proposed a quantitative precipitin curve for the measurement of the antibody-antigen complex. This method is the basis of many immunochemical techniques. In clinical laboratories, many immunochemical techniques are performed based on this precipitin curve.

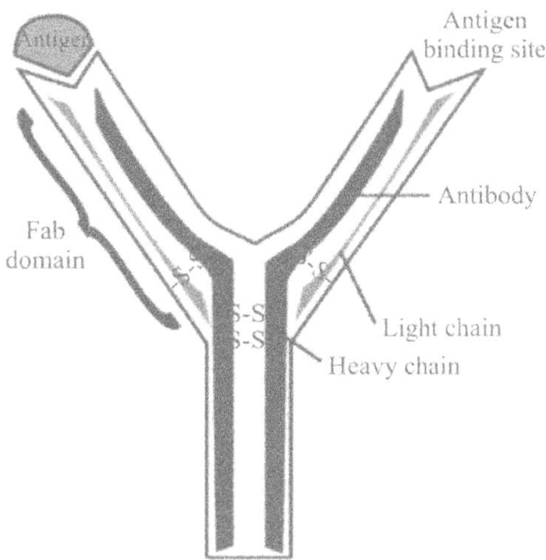

Figure 11.1 Antigen–antibody reactions.

The relationship between the antigen concentration and the amount of precipitate formed for a constant quantity of an antibody is described by the quantitative precipitin curve (Figure 11.2). From this curve three zones can be distinguished as follows:

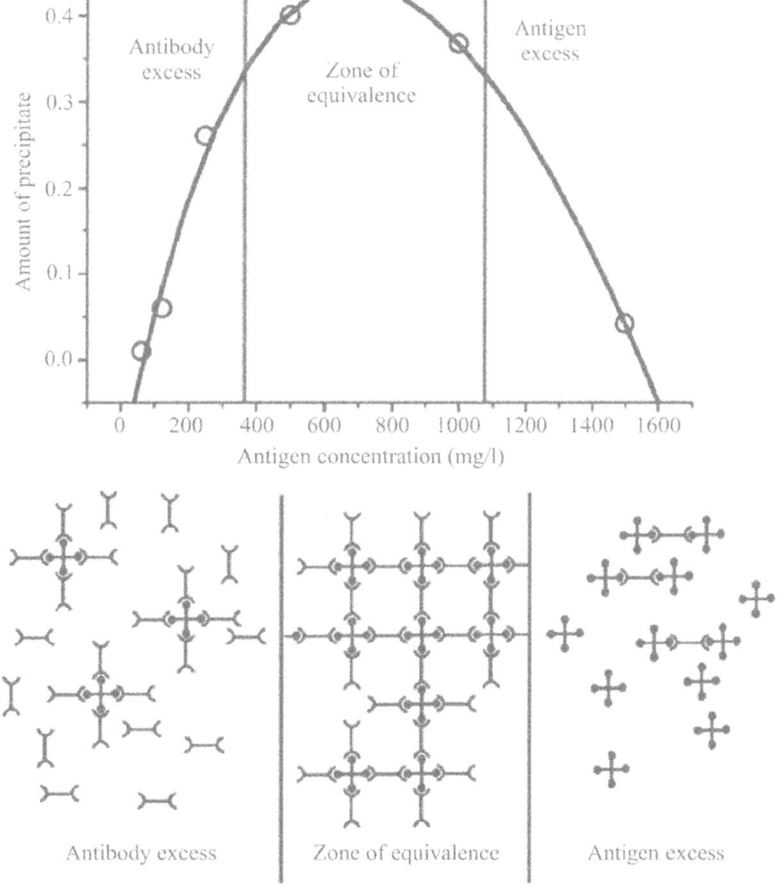

Figure 11.2 Precipitin curve.

1. **Antibody excess zone:** In this zone, fewer antigens are present in the sample and it is the first phase of the quantitative precipitin curve.
2. **Equivalence zone:** In this zone, both the antigen and antibody are cross-linked and form precipitates. Hence, no free antibody or antigen is present in this zone.
3. **Antigen excess zone:** In this zone, due to high antigen concentration, the amount of precipitate formed is reduced.

Classification: The immunochemical techniques are broadly classified into three major classes based on the type of reaction performed, reagents, and the samples used. The following are the various classes of immunochemical techniques:

1. **Particle methods:** In this method, the antigen-antibody interaction is observed. The following are the various types of particle methods:
   a. Agglutination
   b. Immunoprecipitation
   c. Immunoelectrophoresis
   d. Immunofixation
   e. Immunoturbidimetry
   f. Immunonephelometry
2. **Label methods:** In this method, either antigen or antibody is labeled and through the label concentration, the antigen-antibody reaction is observed. The following are the various types of label methods.
   a. Immunoassay
   b. Competitive binding
3. **Other methods:** The remaining methods of immunochemical techniques come under this category. The following are the various types of other methods:
   a. Immunofluorescence
   b. Immunoelectron microscopy
   c. Immunostaining
   d. Electrophoretic separation of proteins
   e. Immunoblotting
   f. Immunodetection

Particle methods:

Agglutination: In Latin, "*agglutino*" means to "glue or attach". An antibody reacts with a particulate antigen producing clumping of cells & the process is known as agglutination. The high affinity of IgM to different antigens makes it a good agglutinin among all the other antibodies. Agglutination may be either a qualitative or a quantitative test. The reaction involved in the agglutination is represented in Figure 11.3. There are different methods in agglutination which are described as follows:

1. **Direct agglutination:** Specific antibodies agglutinates antigen present on the cell surface. **Example:** Determination of the blood group (ABO typing) and the Widal test used for the diagnosis of *Salmonella typhi*.
2. **Indirect or reverse agglutination:** The antibody or antigen in a given sample is determined by using particles already coated with antigens or antibodies to be determined. **Example:** Pregnancy test using human chorionic gonadotropin (HCG) and diagnosis of rheumatoid arthritis.
3. **Agglutination inhibition:** The concentration of soluble antigen in the sample is determined by the competitive binding of an antigen.
4. **Hemagglutination:** Diseases and other viruses, blood typing, etc. are detected using red blood cells involving reactions.

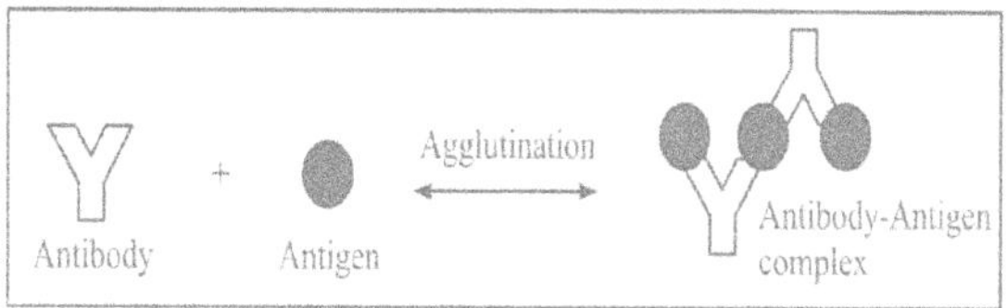

Figure 11.3 Agglutination reaction.

Immunoprecipitation: The flocculation and precipitation reactions are included in the immunoprecipitation methods. The reactants form flocculating or precipitating aggregate under suitable conditions when a solution of an antigen is mixed with its corresponding antibody. At the equivalence region, they can be assessed visually by the formation of the precipitin line. Immunoprecipitation is of two types a) Simple immunoprecipitation (reaction between one antigen and a precipitin line antibody), b) Complex immunoprecipitation (reaction of many unrelated reactants). Between the antigen and the antibody, a concentration gradient is established in simple immunoprecipitation methods. Immunoprecipitation is diagrammatically represented in Figure 11.4. **Example:** Single radial immune diffusion (SRID) (amount of antigen concentration is equal to the circular precipitin area originating from antigen well in the gel) and double immune diffusion (Precipitin line is formed by both antigen and antibody diffuse from separate wells). Based on the presence or absence of the precipitin line in complex immunoprecipitation methods, different antigens are compared with an antibody and vice versa.

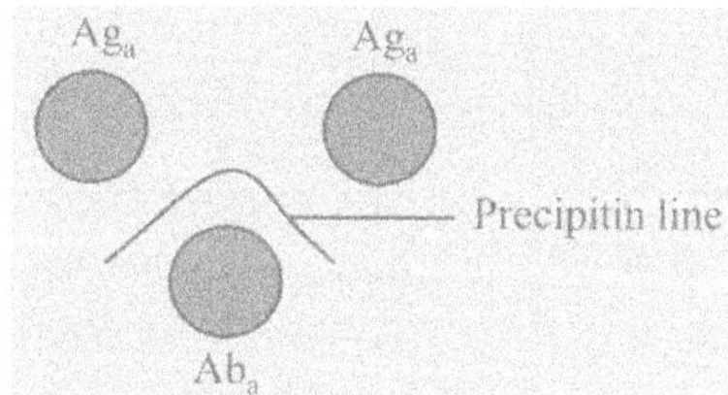

Figure 11.4 Precipitation reaction, (Ab: Antibody; Ag: Antigen)

Immunoelectrophoresis: It is a qualitative technique that is a combination of two techniques namely gel electrophoresis (components separated based on charge) and immunodiffusion (precipitin line is formed by diffusion of both antibody and antigen towards each other). Mostly, these techniques are qualitative in nature except the rocket immunoelectrophoresis which is a quantitative technique that is used to measure the antigen level in a sample. Similar to double immunodiffusion, in this method, a counter current immunoelectrophoresis is also available. The process of electrophoresis is presented in Figure 11.5 (a) and immunodiffusion is presented in Figure 11.5 (b).

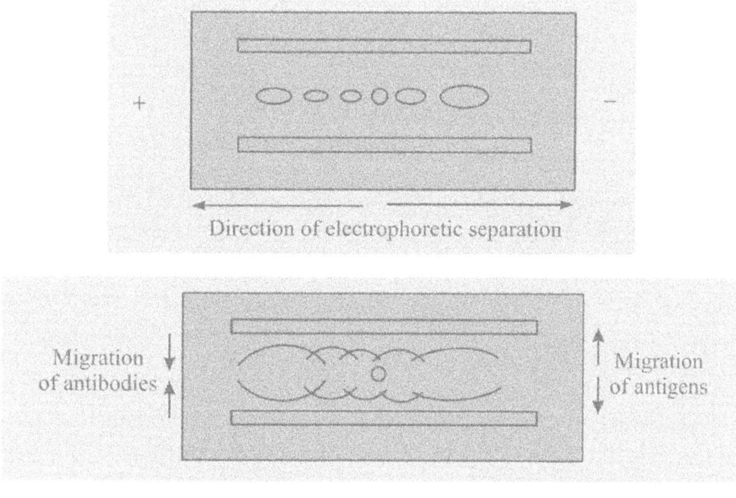

Figure 11.5 (a) Electrophoresis, (b) Immunodiffusion.

Immunofixation: Antibody present in serum, urine, and other body fluids are detected and identified by the immunofixation technique. The principle is similar to that of the immunoelectrophoresis with two stages as a) antibody protein separation by electrophoresis, b) specific antibodies with immunoprecipitation separation. It is easy to perform and evaluate. Furthermore, the technique is more sensitive. In clinical laboratories, through specific antibody, it is used for the detection of cancerous myeloma. Immunofixation is represented in Figure 11.6.

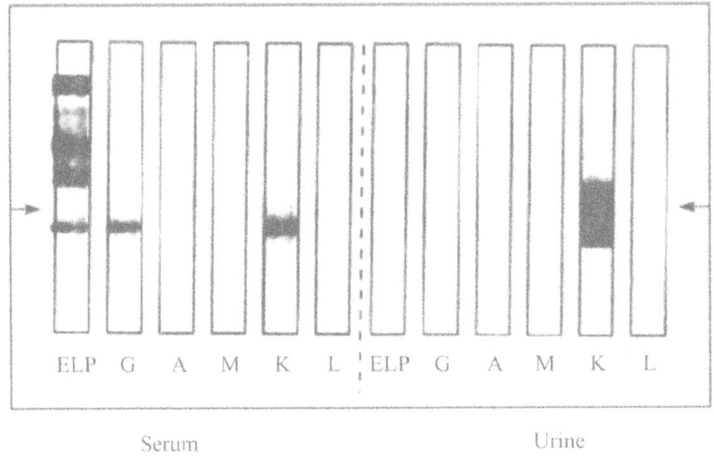

Figure 11.6 Immunofixation – serum and urine samples.

Immunoturbidimetry: Similar to a gel, the precipitin line or the curve is also formed in the solution. The cloudy appearance takes place as a result of the clumping formed when an antigen solution is combined with a specific antibody. This process is known as turbidity which is the basic principle of immunoturbidimetry. It is performed on an instrument called the spectrophotometer. In this method, the measurement is based on the intensity or the amount of light that passes through the sample. The basic principle behind turbidimetry and nephelometry is presented in Figure 11.7 (a) and 11.7 (b), respectively.

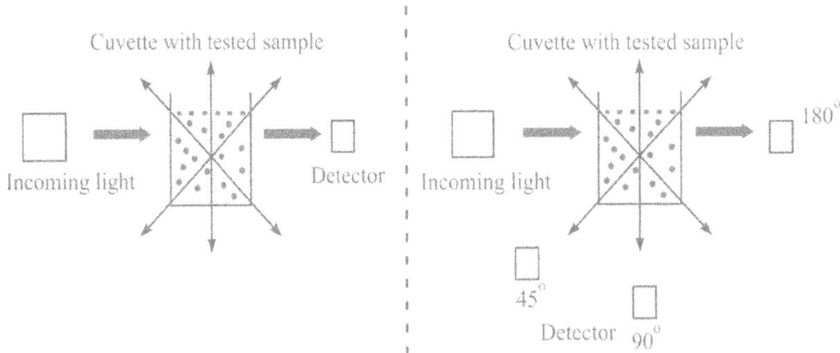

Figure 11.7 a) Turbidimetry, b) Nephelometry.

Immunonephelometry: Similar to turbidimetry, immunonephelometry also works on the same principle. However, in this method, the intensity of the scattered light from the sample is measured directly. This method is performed on an instrument called nephelometer and it uses the laser light. Both methods are more expensive but faster. The automation of these techniques increases the sensitivity of the antigen and antibody.

Label methods:

Immunoassay: Before the reaction in the immunoassay technique, either the antigen or the antibody is labeled. This increases the sensitivity of detection in the experiment over the formation of immunoprecipitate. The label can be an enzyme, radio isotope, DNA reporters, fluorogenic reporters, electroluminescent tags, etc.

Competitive binding: The basic principle involved in this technique is the competitive binding of an antigen. Firstly, an antibody is incubated to a solution having the antigen. Then, this mixture is added to the antigen-coated reaction well. If more antigens are present in the sample, fewer antibodies will bind to the coated antigen. When the labeled antibody is added to this solution, the amount of antigen present in the sample can be measured.

Other Methods

Immunofluorescence: In this technique, the presence of an antigen in a cell or a tissue is detected using an antibody labeled with a fluorescent molecule (fluorescein, rhodamine, or one of the many other fluorescent dyes). The measurement is based on the fluorescence emitted by the bound antibody.

Immunoelectron microscopy: In this method, the tissues and their components are viewed using the antibody specificity through a microscope.

Immunostaining: In this method, a specific protein in a sample is detected by using an antibody labeled with an enzyme or a dye. Western blot is the most important staining method which consists of three processes - a) electrophoretic separation of proteins in a sample, b) immunoblotting (transfer of proteins from gel to a membrane), c) immunodetection (identification using labeled antibody).

Detection:

These immunochemical techniques are used for proper detection and diagnosis of diseases and also certain body conditions. **Example:** Diagnosis of typhoid by detecting *Salmonella typhi* in blood, detection of narcotics in urine and saliva, detection of protein hormones like insulin, thyroxine, etc. and pregnancy test based on human chorionic gonadotropin (HCG) hormone level in urine.

Immunoassay

Immunoassay is a qualitative or quantitative biochemical test used to measure the presence or concentration of a macromolecule or a small molecule in a solution using usually an antibody or an antigen. "Analyte" is the term that is used to refer to the molecule detected by the immunoassay. These molecules are proteins in many cases. Other kinds of molecules, of different sizes and types, may also be detected if proper antibodies are developed with adequate properties for the immunoassay. In general, immunoassays are used for medical and research purposes to measure the presence or concentration of analytes in biological liquids such as a serum, urine, etc.

Principle:

The basic principle behind immunoassays is the ability of an antibody to recognize and bind with a specific macromolecule in a complex mixture of macromolecules. Antigen is the particular macromolecule bound by an antibody and the antibody binding site of an antigen is known as an epitope. Using immunoassay in some cases, the presence of antibodies in a solution is detected by the antigen. In other words, in some immunoassays, the analyte may be an antibody rather than an antigen.

The other important feature of all immunoassay is to produce a measurable signal in response to the binding along with the binding of an antibody to its antigen. For this purpose, chemically linking antibodies or antigens with some kind of detectable label is used in most immunoassays. In modern immunoassays, a large number of labels exist and are used for detection through different mechanisms. A lot of labels may emit radiation or produce a color change in a solution or fluoresce under the light. They can also be induced to emit light. Hence, they are easily detected.

Labels:

Immunoassay technique works on the principle of labeling either the antigen or antibody before the reaction. This increases the sensitivity of detection in the experiment along with the formation of immunoprecipitate. Immunoassays employ a variety of different labels to allow the detection of antibodies and antigens. Usually, the labels are chemically linked or conjugated to the desired antibody or antigen. The following are the various labels used in immunoassay.

1. **Enzymes:** It is the most commonly used label in immunoassays. The enzyme labeled immunoassays is known as enzyme-linked immunosorbent assay (ELISA) or enzyme immunoassay (EIA). It is a safer and efficient method. The most frequently used enzyme for labeling is *horse radish peroxidase (HRP), alkaline phosphatase (AP)* and *glucose oxidase (GO).* This is because in the presence of certain reagents these enzymes produce an observable color change. Reagents producing light or chemiluminescence are used in some cases for enzyme exposer.
2. **Radioactive isotopes:** Radioactive isotopes labeled immunoassays are known as radioimmunoassay (RIA). Using conventional methods, it is easy to measure the radioactivity emitted by bound antibody-antigen complexes. RIA is the first immunoassay developed but not used commonly because of the difficulty and potential dangers by working with radioactivity.
3. **DNA reporters:** This is a new approach in immunoassays using both real-time quantitative *polymerase* chain reaction (RT qPCR) and traditional immunoassay techniques. DNA probe is the label used in these assays and is commonly known as the real-time immuno quantitative *polymerase* chain reaction (RT iqPCR).
4. **Fluorogenic reporters:** In some modern immunoassays, fluorogenic reporters like phycoerythrin are used. **Example:** Protein microarrays.
5. **Electrochemiluminescent tags:** Electrochemiluminescence is the basis behind some labels that emit detectable light in response to electric current.
6. **Label free immunoassays:** Some immunoassays employ detection methods that don't require the modification or labeling of the components of the assay. Hence, they don't need any labels. **Example:** Surface plasmon resonance (Detect binding between an unlabeled antibody and antigens) and measuring the change in resistance on an electrode as antigens bind to it.

Classification:

Immunoassays can be broadly classified into two major classes, based on the working principles. The following are the major class of immunoassays:

1. Competitive immunoassays
   a. Competitive, homogeneous immunoassays
   b. Competitive, heterogeneous immunoassays
2. Non-competitive immunoassays
   a. One site non-competitive immunoassays
   b. Two site non-competitive immunoassays

Competitive, homogeneous immunoassays: In this method, there is a competition between the unlabeled analyte in a sample and the labeled analyte for binding with the antibody. The labeled analyte gets displaced more when more analyte is present in the sample. The amount of displaced labeled, unbound analyte is then measured. The amount of labeled, unbound analyte is proportional to the amount of analyte in the sample. Competitive, homogeneous immunoassay is represented schematically in Figure 11.8.

The amount of labeled, unbound analyte α The amount of analyte in the sample

Competitive, heterogeneous immunoassays: In this method, there is also a competition between the unlabeled analyte in a sample and labeled analyte for binding with the antibody. In the heterogeneous assays, the labeled, unbound analyte is separated or washed away, and the remaining labeled, bound analyte is measured.

One site, non-competitive immunoassays: The unknown analyte in the sample binds with the labeled antibodies. The unbound, labeled antibodies are washed away, and the bound, labeled antibodies are measured. The intensity of the signal is directly proportional to the amount of unknown analyte.

The amount of unknown analyte α The intensity of the signal

Two sites, non-competitive immunoassays: The analyte in the unknown sample is bound to the antibody site, and then the labeled antibody is bound to the analyte. The amount of labeled antibodies on the site is then measured. It will be directly proportional to the concentration of the analyte because the labeled antibody will not bind if the analyte is not present in the unknown sample. Two sites, non-competitive immunoassays is represented in Figure 11.9. This type of immunoassay is also known as a sandwich assay as the analyte is "sandwiched" between the two antibodies. **Example:** ELISA (Sandwich type ELISA method is presented in Figure 11.10).

The amount of labeled antibody α The amount of analyte in the sample

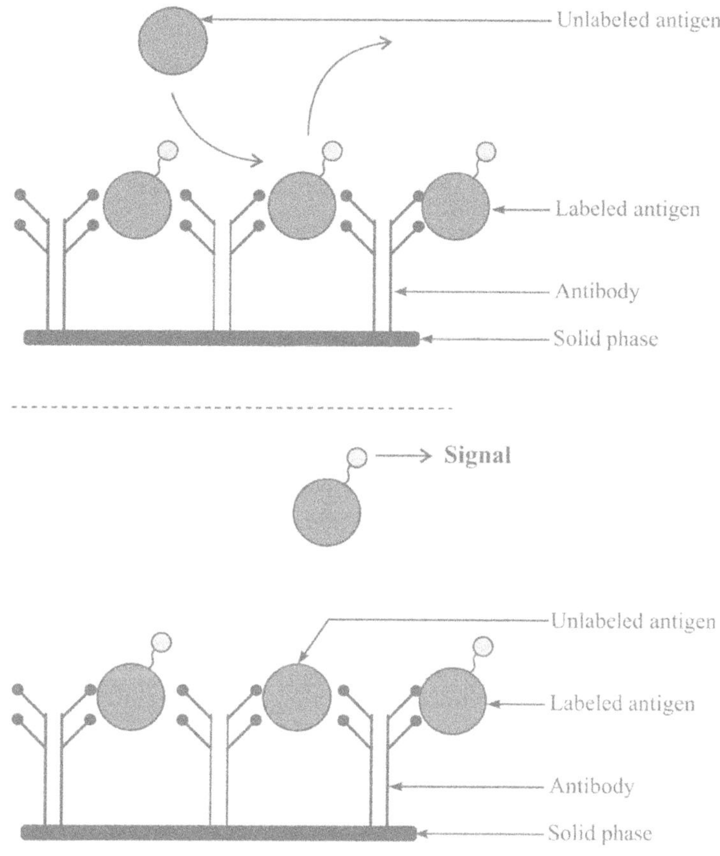

Figure 11.8 Competitive, homogeneous immunoassay.

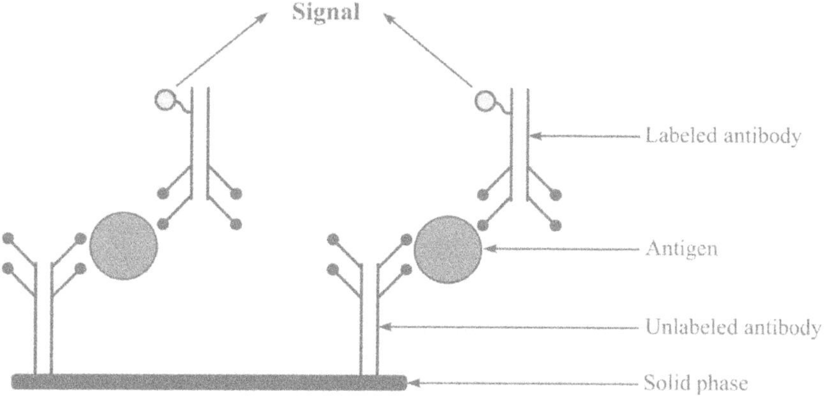

Figure 11.9 Two-site, non-competitive immunoassays.

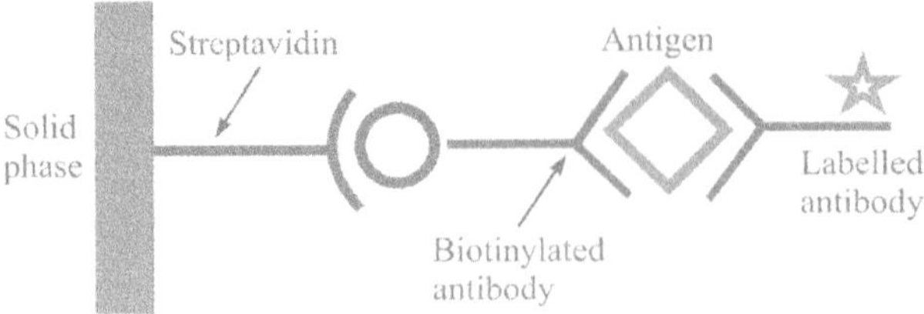

Figure 11.10 ELISA – sandwich type.

Radioimmunoassay (RIA)

This is an isotopic immune assay because it uses radioactive isotopes for labeling. In the year 1959, Solomon, Benson, and Rosalyn Yalow developed radioimmunoassay (RIA) for the estimation of insulin in human serum. In biological fluids, many compounds are present in very low concentrations (picogram i.e., 10^{-12} g or nanogram i.e., 10^{-9} g). In the estimation of these compounds, RIA made a revolution. This technique is a very specific and sensitive analytical tool for the estimation of very low concentrated compounds present in the biological fluids.

Principle:

RIA is a combination of two basic techniques like radioactivity of isotopes and the immunological reactions of antigen and antibody. Hence, this technique is called the radioimmunoassay (RIA).

The primary principle involved in RIA is the competition between labeled and unlabeled antigens to bind with antibody to form either labeled or unlabeled antigen-antibody complex. The substance to be determined is called an unlabeled antigen. When injecting this antigen to a rabbit or goat, the substance produced in the rabbit or goat is called an antibody. The substance to be determined (antigen) is specifically labeled or treated with radioactive isotopes such as ^{131}I, with known radioactivity. It is called a labeled antigen.

In RIA, the specific antibody (Ab) is subjected to react with unlabeled antigen (Ag) in the presence of known excess amount of labeled antigen (Ag^+). Hence, the labeled and unlabeled antigens (Ag^+ and Ag) compete with each other to bind with antibody (Ab) to form the corresponding antigen-antibody complex (Ag^+-Ab and Ag-Ab). Out of these two complexes, the predominant one formed is labeled antigen-antibody complex (Ag^+-Ab) due to its high concentration.

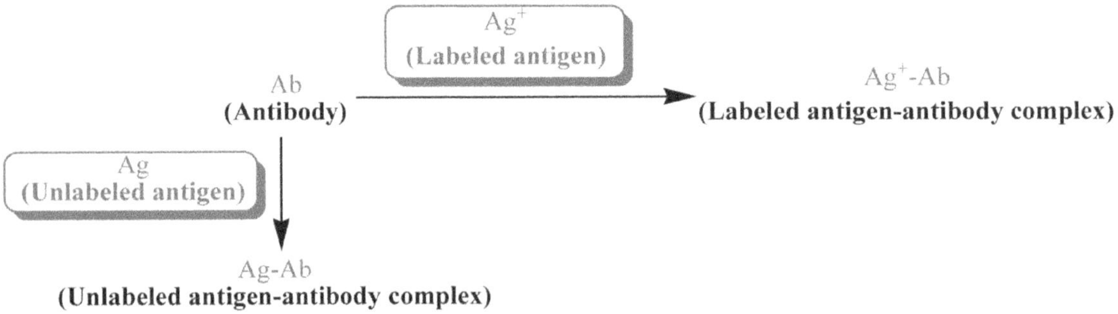

When the concentration of the unlabeled antigens (Ag) is increased, the concentration of the labeled antigen-antibody complex (Ag^+-Ab) is decreased because the unlabeled antigen (Ag) replaces labeled antigen (Ag^+) by competition.

Ag^{+}-Ab

(Labeled antigen-antibody complex)

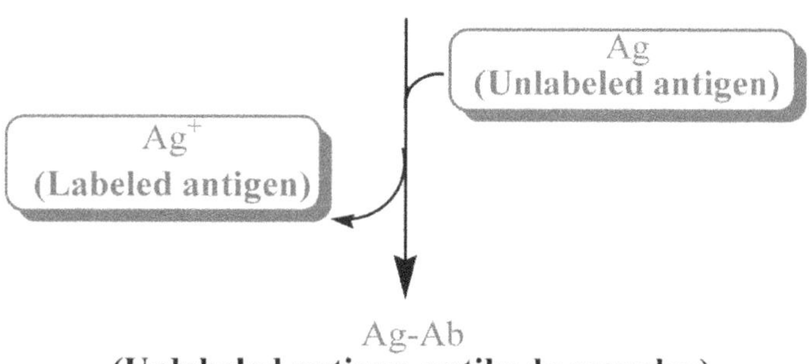

Ag-Ab

(Unlabeled antigen-antibody complex)

Hence, the concentration of labeled antigen-antibody complex (Ag^{+}-Ab) is inversely proportional to the concentration of the substance to be determined i.e., unlabeled antigens (Ag).

$$[Ag^{+} - Ab] \alpha \frac{1}{[Ag]}$$

Where, [Ag^{+}-Ab] is the concentration of labeled antigen-antibody complex and [Ag] is the concentration of substance to be determined i.e., unlabeled antigen. This relationship is almost linear. Hence, keeping the concentration of the antibody (Ab) and labeled antigen (Ag^{+}) as constant, a standard graph is obtained by changing the concentration of the unlabeled antigen (Ag). The standard graph is drawn by taking the concentration of unlabeled antigen (Ag) on the "x" axis and the concentration of labeled antigen-antibody complex (Ag^{+}-Ab) on "y" axis.

Precipitation technique is used to separate labeled antigen-antibody complex (Ag^{+}-Ab) and the radioactivity of ^{131}I present in labeled antigen-antibody complex (Ag^{+}-Ab). It is determined by the usual radioactivity method.

Applications:

1. Estimation of hormones and proteins that exhibit antigenic properties.
2. Several substances elicit specific antibody responses by making it as antigenic with the use of haptens (non-antigenic small molecules such as dinitrophenol). Hence, RIA can be used for the estimation of a wide variety of compounds like peptides, steroid hormones, vitamins, drugs, antibiotics, nucleic acids, structural proteins, and hormone receptor proteins.
3. RIA is used for the diagnosis of hormonal disorder.
4. It is also used for the diagnosis of cancer.
5. It also plays a role in therapeutic drug monitoring (TDM).
6. It is also very useful in biomedical research.

Enzyme Linked Immunosorbant Assay (ELISA)

This is a non-isotopic immune assay because no isotopes are used here. In place of radioactive isotopes employed in radioimmunoassay (RIA), enzymes are used as labels in the enzyme linked immunosorbant assay (ELISA). There are two advantages to ELISA compared to RIA. The first one is the more sensitivity issue (ELISA is as or even more sensitive than RIA). The second one is no risk (Risk of radiation hazards in RIA). Diagrammatically ELISA is represented in Figure 11.11.

Principle:

The basic principle involved in ELISA is the reaction between antigen and antibody to form antigen-antibody complex.

$$\underset{\textbf{(Antigen)}}{\text{Ag}} + \underset{\textbf{(Antibody)}}{\text{Ab}} \longrightarrow \underset{\textbf{(Antigen-antibody complex)}}{\text{Ag-Ab}}$$

The following are the various steps involved in ELISA.

1. Initially, to an inert solid like polystyrene, the antibody (Ab) against the protein to be determined is fixed.
2. Then, to the antibody-coated surface, the biological samples containing protein (antigen; Ag) to be estimated are applied. This results in the formation of the protein antibody complex (Ag-Ab).
3. Later, the second antibody (protein specific) covalently linked enzyme is added to react with the protein antibody complex (Ag-Ab). This results in the formation of an enzyme-bound second antibody complex. In general, the enzymes used in this method are easily assayable and preferably produce colored products. The most commonly used enzymes in ELISA are *peroxidase, amylase,* and *alkaline phosphatase*.
4. Then, the unbound second antibody linked enzymes are washed and the enzyme bound to the second antibody complex is assayed.
5. Finally, the activity of the enzyme is estimated. This estimation is based on the ability of the enzyme to form colored products when it reacts with the substrate. This is related to the concentration of protein being estimated.

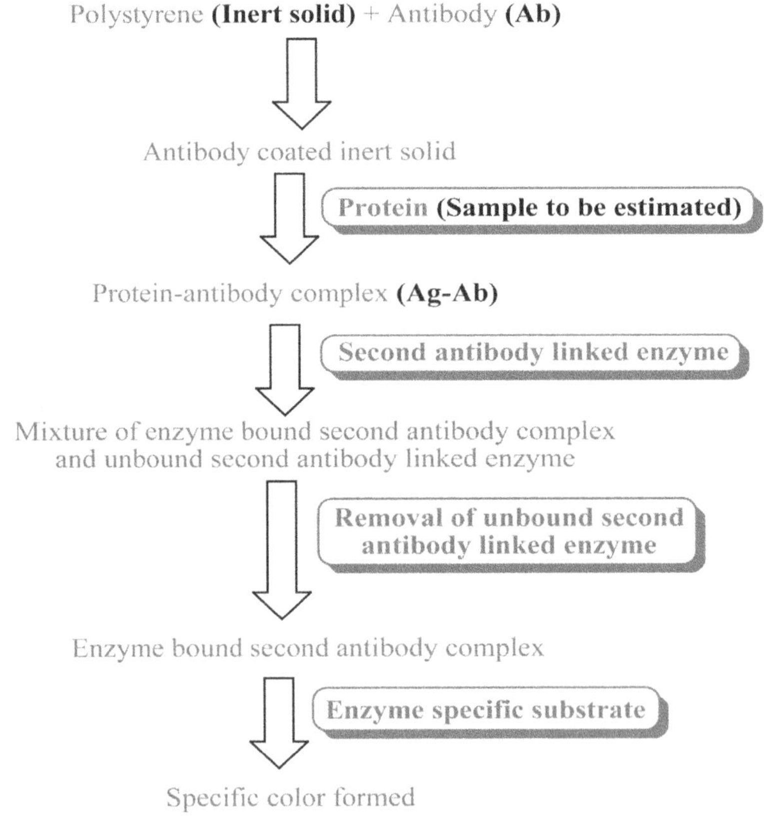

6. For example, *peroxidase* acts on substrate hydrogen peroxide and produces a water molecule and a nascent oxygen atom. This nascent oxygen atom reacts with colorless reduced diaminobenzidine and produces a brown colored oxidized diaminobenzidine. This is the primary principle involved in the use of *peroxidase* in ELISA.

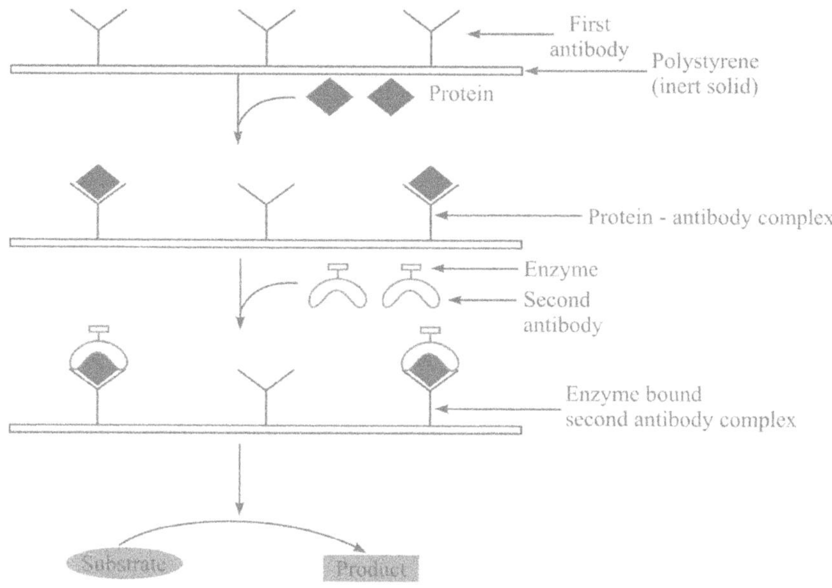

Figure 11.11 ELISA (Diagrammatic representation).

Applications:

1. ELISA is used for the estimation of small quantities of proteins like hormones, antigens, and antibodies.
2. It is also used for the estimation of small quantities of other biological substances.
3. ELISA is used for the diagnosis of acute immune deficiency syndrome (AIDS).
4. It is the basis behind the most commonly used pregnancy tests for the detection of human chorionic gonadotropin (HCG) in the urine.

PROBABLE QUESTIONS

PART – A: Multiple Choice Questions

1. What is the concentration of hormones present in the 1 ml of circulating blood?
   (a) Picogram to nanogram (b) Nanogram to microgram
   (c) Microgram to Milligram (d) Milligram to gram
2. One picogram is equal to how many grams?
   (a) 10^{-3} (b) 10^{-6}
   (c) 10^{-9} (d) 10^{-12}
3. One nanogram is equal to how many grams?
   (a) 10^{-3} (b) 10^{-6}
   (c) 10^{-9} (d) 10^{-12}
4. Which is foreign substances when introduced into an animal can stimulate a specific immune response in the form of production of antibodies and specific reactive T-lymphocytes?
   (a) Monoclonal antibody (b) Polyclonal antibody
   (c) Epitope (d) Antigen
5. Which are glycoproteins that bind specifically to the antigen that induced their formation?
   (a) Antigen (b) Antibody
   (c) Epitope (d) Prostaglandin

6. Which of the following one is also known as the antigenic determinant?
   (a) Epitope (b) Monoclonal antibody
   (c) Polyclonal antibody (d) Antigen
7. ____________ is the part of an antigen that is recognized by the immune system, specifically by antibodies, B-cells, or T-cells?
   (a) Antigen (b) Polyclonal antibody
   (c) Epitope (d) Monoclonal antibody
8. Which of the following statement is wrong with respect to characteristics of the immunochemical technique?
   (a) Simple, rapid, and robust
   (b) Low sensitive
   (c) Easily automated
   (d) Useful for both qualitative and quantitative measurements
9. Which of the following statement is wrong with respect to application of the immunochemical technique?
   (a) Used for identifying the function of the newly identified or novel proteins
   (b) Used to identify the importance of uncharacterized proteins in their natural environment
   (c) Used for the determination of species or tissues in which the protein or residues is expressed
   (d) Not useful for the diagnosis and treatment of a particular disease
10. ____________ is the region of an antigen binding to an antibody.
   (a) Epitope (b) Eicosanoid
   (c) Fab (d) Prostaglandin
11. Which statement is wrong?
   (a) Antibodies are immunoglobins (b) Antibodies contain four polypeptide units
   (c) Antibodies contain two polypeptide units (d) Antibodies are Y-shaped molecules
12. ____________ is the domain of antibodies site where it binds to an antigen.
   (a) Fab (b) Epitope
   (c) Prostaglandin (d) Eicosanoid
13. ____________ heavy chains and ____________ light chains are present in antibody.
   (a) One & one (b) Two & one
   (c) One & two (d) Two & two
14. Which technique is used for the measurement of the antibody-antigen complex?
   (a) Quantitative precipitin curve (b) Qualitative precipitin curve
   (c) Both a & b (d) None of the above
15. Which zone is present in quantitative precipitin curve?
   (a) Antibody excess zone (b) Equivalence zone
   (c) Antigen excess zone (d) All the above
16. Which immunochemical technique is not a particle method technique?
   (a) Agglutination (b) Immunoprecipitation
   (c) Immunoassay (d) Immunoelectrophoresis
17. Which immunochemical technique is not a particle method technique?
   (a) Immunostaining (b) Immunonephelometry
   (c) Immunoturbidimetry (d) Immunofixation

18. Which of the following technique is a label method immunochemical technique?
    (a) Immunoprecipitation (b) Immunoassay
    (c) Immunoblotting (d) Immunodetection
19. Which of the following technique is not a particle & label method immunochemical technique?
    (a) Immunofixation (b) Immunoassay
    (c) Immunoblotting (d) Immunoturbidimetry
20. In which process, an antibody reacts with a particulate antigen producing clumping of cells.
    (a) Agglutination (b) Precipitation
    (c) Fixation (d) Electrophoresis
21. Determination of the blood group (ABO type) comes under which type of agglutination?
    (a) Direct agglutination (b) Indirect agglutination
    (c) Agglutination inhibition (d) Hemagglutination
22. Widal test used for the diagnosis of *Salmonella typhi* is example for ____________.
    (a) Direct agglutination (b) Indirect agglutination
    (c) Agglutination inhibition (d) Hemagglutination
23. Pregnancy test using human chorionic gonadotropin is based on ______________.
    (a) Hemagglutination (b) Agglutination inhibition
    (c) Indirect agglutination (d) Direct agglutination
24. Which type of agglutination is involved in the diagnosis of rheumatoid arthritis?
    (a) Hemagglutination (b) Agglutination inhibition
    (c) Indirect agglutination (d) Direct agglutination
25. Diseases and other viruses, blood typing, etc. are detected using red blood cells involving reactions are example for ______________.
    (a) Agglutination inhibition (b) Direct agglutination
    (c) Hemagglutination (d) Indirect agglutination
26. The concentration of soluble antigen in the sample is determined by the competitive binding of an antigen comes under which type of agglutination?
    (a) Indirect agglutination (b) Agglutination inhibition
    (c) Direct agglutination (d) Hemagglutination
27. Which type of agglutination is also known as reverse agglutination?
    (a) Direct agglutination (b) Hemagglutination
    (c) Agglutination inhibition (d) Indirect agglutination
28. Immunoelectrophoresis is combination of which two technique?
    (a) Gel electrophoresis & immunodiffusion (b) Gel electrophoresis & immunofixation
    (c) Gel electrophoresis & immunoassay (d) Gel electrophoresis & immunoturbidimetry
29. The rocket immunoelectrophoresis is a ______________ technique.
    (a) Qualitative (b) Quantitative
    (c) Both a & b (d) None of the above
30. In which of the following technique, the intensity of the scattered light from the sample is measured directly?
    (a) Immunoelectrophoresis (b) Immunonephelometry
    (c) Immunoturbidimetry (d) Immunofixation

31. In which of the following technique, intensity or the amount of light that passes through the sample is measured?
    (a) Immunoturbidimetry (b) Immunofixation
    (c) Immunonephelometry (d) Immunoelectrophoresis
32. Which of the following is used as label in immunoassay?
    (a) Enzyme (b) Radio isotope
    (c) DNA reporters (d) All the above
33. Which of the following is used as label in immunoassay?
    (a) Fluorogenic reporters (b) DNA reporters
    (c) Electroluminescent tags (d) All the above
34. What is the basic principle involved in the immunoassay technique?
    (a) Competitive binding (b) Non-competitive binding
    (c) Both a & b (d) None of the above
35. Which is the most commonly used label in immunoassays?
    (a) DNA reporters (b) Enzyme
    (c) Radio isotope (d) Fluorogenic reporters
36. The enzyme labeled immunoassays is known as ____________________.
    (a) Enzyme-linked immunosorbent assay (b) Enzyme immunoassay
    (c) Both a & b (d) Radioimmunoassay
37. Which of the following is most frequently used enzyme for labeling in immunoassay?
    (a) *Horse radish peroxidase* (b) *Alkaline phosphatase*
    (c) *Glucose oxidase* (d) All the above
38. Radioactive isotopes labeled immunoassays are known as ____________.
    (a) Enzyme-linked immunosorbent assay (b) Enzyme immunoassay
    (c) Both a & b (d) Radioimmunoassay
39. In the real-time immuno quantitative *polymerase* chain reaction which label is used?
    (a) Enzyme (b) Radioactive isotope
    (c) DNA reporter (d) Fluorogenic reporter
40. Which label is used in protein microarray?
    (a) Fluorogenic reporter (b) DNA reporter
    (c) Radioactive isotope (d) Enzyme
41. RIA is a combination of which two techniques?
    (a) Radioactivity & immunological reactions (b) Radioactivity & turbidimetry
    (c) Radioactivity & nephelometry (d) Radioactivity & electrophoresis
42. In RIA, the substance to be determined is called as ____________________.
    (a) Labeled antigen (b) Unlabeled antigen
    (c) Both a & b (d) None of the above
43. In RIA, the substance to be determined is specifically labeled or treated with radioactive isotopes such as ^{131}I, with known radioactivity is called as _____________.
    (a) Labeled antigen (b) Unlabeled antigen
    (c) Both a & b (d) None of the above

44. In RIA, when the concentration of the unlabeled antigens is increased, what happened to the concentration of the labeled antigen-antibody complex?
    (a) Increased (b) Decreased
    (c) Neither increased nor decreased (d) Initially increased followed by decreased
45. Which is correct with respect to RIA application?
    (a) Estimation of hormones (b) Diagnosis of cancer
    (c) Useful in biomedical research (d) All the above
46. Which of the following statement is wrong with respect to ELISA?
    (a) Non-isotopic immune assay (b) Enzymes are used as label
    (c) More sensitivity (d) High risk
47. Which is correct with respect to ELISA application?
    (a) Estimation of small quantities of proteins (b) Diagnosis of AIDS
    (c) Basis behind the detection of HCG in urine (d) All the above
48. Which is the first phase of quantitative precipitin curve?
    (a) Antigen excess zone (b) Antibody excess zone
    (c) Equivalence zone (d) Antigen-antibody excess zone
49. Fewer antigens are present in which zone of quantitative precipitin curve?
    (a) Antibody excess zone (b) Antigen-antibody excess zone
    (c) Antigen excess zone (d) Equivalence zone
50. No free antibody or antigen is present in which zone of quantitative precipitin curve?
    (a) Antigen excess zone (b) Antibody excess zone
    (c) Equivalence zone (d) All the above

Key for Multiple Choice Questions

1. (a)	2. (d)	3. (c)	4. (d)	5. (b)
6. (a)	7. (c)	8. (b)	9. (d)	10. (a)
11. (c)	12. (a)	13. (d)	14. (a)	15. (d)
16. (c)	17. (a)	18. (b)	19. (c)	20. (a)
21. (a)	22. (a)	23. (c)	24. (c)	25. (c)
26. (b)	27. (d)	28. (a)	29. (b)	30. (b)
31. (a)	32. (d)	33. (d)	34. (a)	35. (b)
36. (c)	37. (d)	38. (d)	39. (c)	40. (a)
41. (a)	42. (b)	43. (a)	44. (b)	45. (d)
46. (d)	47. (d)	48. (b)	49. (a)	50. (c)

PART – B: Short Answers

1. What is immunochemistry?
2. What are immunochemical techniques?
3. Define antigen & epitope.

4. Define and classify antibodies.
5. What is the difference between monoclonal and polyclonal antibodies?
6. List out the important characteristics of the immunochemical techniques.
7. Write a note on applications of immunochemical techniques.
8. Write a short note on antigen-antibody reaction.
9. What is quantitative precipitin curve?
10. Define and classify immunochemical techniques.
11. Explain the term agglutination.
12. Write a note on immunoprecipitation.
13. What is immunoelectrophoresis?
14. Explain immunofixation.
15. What is immunoturbidimetry and immunonephelometry?
16. How immunoturbidimetry is differ from immunonephelometry?
17. Explain the term "immunoassay".
18. Write a note on labels used in immunoassay technique.
19. Define and classify immunoassays.
20. What is RIA? Write any two applications of the same.
21. What is ELISA? Write any two applications of the same.
22. Explain IgM.
23. What is the basic principle involved in radioimmunoassay?
24. What is the basic principle involved in enzyme linked immunosorbent assay?
25. Compare RIA with ELISA.

PART – C: Long Answers

1. Write a detailed note on immunochemical techniques.
2. Define various terms used in immunochemical techniques. Add a note on important characteristics and applications of immunochemical techniques.
3. Define and classify immunochemical techniques with suitable example. Add a note on principle involved in the immunochemical techniques.
4. Define and classify immunochemical techniques. Explain any one technique in detail.
5. Explain particle methods of immunochemical techniques.
6. Write a detailed note on label methods of immunochemical techniques.
7. Explain immunoassay in detail.
8. Define and classify immunoassay. Explain any one assay in datail.
9. Describe the principle and diagnostic applications of RIA.
10. What is ELISA? Explain the principle and techniques involved in various types with the applications.
11. Write about different types of immunoglobulins. Add a note on principle and applications of ELISA.

12

Water, Electrolytes and Acid-Base Balance

To survive against the odds and maintain homeostasis, the organisms possess a tremendous capacity. Water, electrolyte, and acid-base status are true examples of this. These three are interrelated and the kidney actively participates in their regulation .

Water

Functions of water:

The solvent of life is water. In life, compared to any other single compound, water is undoubtedly more important. The following are the major biological functions of water:

1. The aqueous medium is more important for biochemical reactions in the organisms. This is provided by water.
2. In several metabolic reactions, water directly participates as a reactant.
3. For the transport of solutes, water serves as a vehicle.
4. Water is closely linked with the regulation of body temperature.

Distribution of water:

Water is the major body constituent. In a normal healthy adult, about 60 % of the body weight is composed of water. For men, it is 55 to 70 % and for women, it is 45 to 60 %. In women and obese persons, high amount of fat is stored in anhydrous form. Hence, they have relatively less water content.

In general, the amount of water present in a normal healthy adult weighing 70 kg is 42 liters. Out of these 42 liters, 28 liters of water is distributed in the intracellular (inside the cells) compartment, and the remaining 14 liters of water is distributed in the extracellular (outside the cell) compartment. The intracellular compartment water is known as intracellular fluid or simply ICF, and the extracellular compartment water is known as extracellular fluid or simply ECF. The extracellular fluid is further sub-divided into two compartments as intestinal fluid (contains 10.5 liters of water) and plasma (contains 3.5 liters of water). In humans, the distribution of water in various compartments is presented in the Table 12.1 and Figure 12.1.

Table12.1 Distribution of water in various compartments (Adult man weighing 70 kg).

S. No.	Compartment name	% Body weight	Volume (in liters)
1	Total	60	42
2	Intracellular fluid or ICF	40	28
3	Extracellular fluid or ECF	20	14
4	Intestinal fluid	15	10.5
5	Plasma	5	3.5

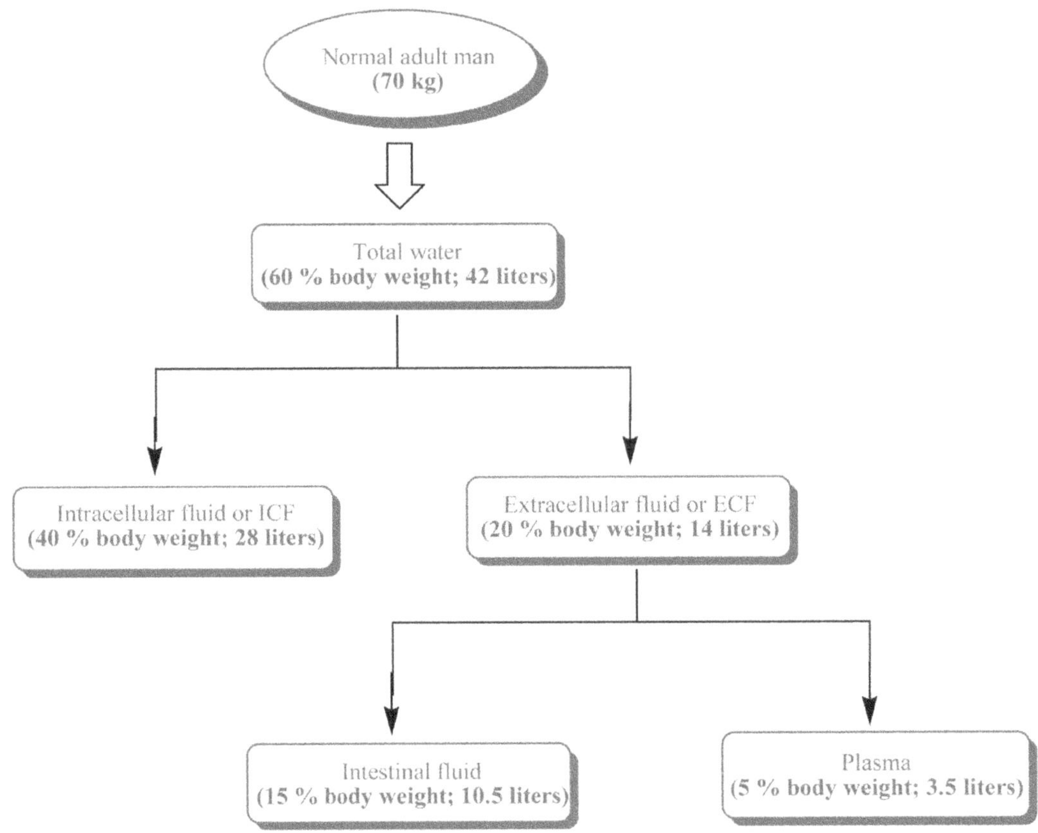

Figure 12.1 Water compartments in adult human.

Water Turnover and Balance

To regulate the water content, the body possesses a tremendous capacity. Daily water intake and water output balance are used to regulate the water content in a healthy individual.

Water intake:

The sources which supply water to the body are broadly classified into two major classes as exogenous and endogenous sources and the corresponding supplied water is known as exogenous and endogenous water, respectively.

Exogenous water: The sources for exogenous water are ingested water, and the water content of solid foods, and beverages. Intake of water may vary from 0.5 to 5 liters/day and it mainly depends on the social habits and climate. The thirst center located in the hypothalamus generally controls the ingestion of water. People who live in a hot climate drink more water in general. The thirst center is stimulated when the osmolality of plasma increased leads to an increased water intake.

Endogenous water: The sources for endogenous water are metabolic water produced in the body. The oxidation of food generally produces 300 to 350 ml of water/day. It is determined that 0.6 ml, 0.4 ml, and 1.1 ml of water are yielded for 1 g carbohydrate, protein, and fat, respectively. On average, for the consumption of 1000 cal by the body, 125 ml of water is generated.

Water output:

Water losses are variable in the body. The water from the body is eliminated by four distinct routes like urine, skin, lungs and feces.

Urine: From the body, water is mainly lost by this route only. The urine output in a healthy individual is varying from 1 to 2 liters/day. The loss of water from the kidney is highly variable and generally, the body demands to regulate it to either get rid of water or retain it. In a man, the urine production cannot be stopped completely despite there being any water intake. This happens because some amount of water is essential (500 ml/day) for the body to eliminate the waste products.

Everyday, around 180 liters of water are filtered by glomeruli in the renal tubules. However, only 1 to 2 liters of water is excreted as urine per day because most of the water is reabsorbed in the kidney. Vasopressin is the antidiuretic hormone (ADH) secreted by the posterior pituitary gland that tightly controls the water excretion by the kidney. The osmotic pressure of the plasma regulates the secretion of ADH. The increased osmolality of plasma stimulates the secretion of ADH leading to increased water reabsorption from the renal tubule (Urine output is less). On the other hand, decreased osmolality of plasma suppresses the secretion of ADH leading to decreased water reabsorption from the renal tubule (Urine output is more). The concentration of sodium in plasma plays a major role in the osmolality of plasma. Hence, the amount of water in the body is indirectly controlled by sodium. The deficiency of ADH produces a disorder called diabetes insipidus in which loss of water from the body is increased.

Skin: Perspiration is a process by which the body surface losses water (450 ml/day). This elimination process mainly depends on the atmospheric temperature and humidity. The body generally does not regulate this process. In a hot climate, the loss of water is more. In fever, water loss through the skin is increased. About 15 % increased water loss is observed through the skin for every 1 °C rise in the body temperature.

Lungs: Some amount of water (400 ml/day) is lost through the expired air during respiration. Air is saturated with water and expelled from the body. The water lost through the lung is increased during hot climates and /or fever. Insensible water loss is the collective loss of water by perspiration and respiration via skin and lungs, respectively.

Feces: Intestine reabsorbs most of the water and it enters the GIT. In a healthy individual, about 150 ml of water is lost through feces per day. In diarrhea, the fecal loss of water is tremendously increased.

In the body, the water balance is predominantly maintained by controlling the urine output. This happens after an obligatory water loss via skin, lungs and feces. A summary of water balance in the body is depicted in the Figure 12.2.

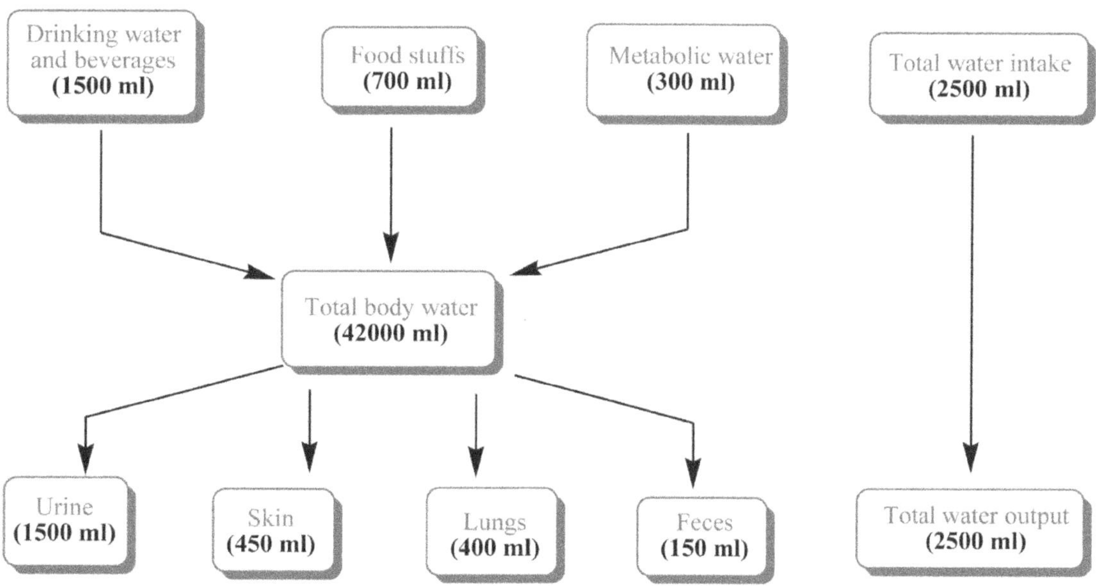

Figure 12.2 Summary of water balance in body.

Electrolyte Balance

An electrolyte is defined as a compound which readily dissociates in a solution and exists as ions i.e., positively and negatively charged particles (**Example:** NaCl (sodium chloride) exists as Na^+ (sodium cation) and Cl^- (chloride anion) and not as such.

The concentrations of electrolytes is expressed in mill equivalents (mEq/l) instead of milligrams (mg). A gram equivalent weight of the compound is defined as its weight in grams that can combine or displace 1 g of hydrogen. 1000 mill equivalents are equals to one-gram equivalent. The conversion of mg/l to mEq/l is generally calculated by using the following formula.

$$\frac{mEq}{l} = \frac{mg\ per\ litre \times Valency}{Atomic\ weight}$$

Body fluids electrolyte composition:

The osmotic equilibrium and water balance are maintained in the body fluid by well distribution of electrolytes. In each body compartment (ECF or ICF), the total concentrations of cations and anions are equal to maintain the electrical neutrality. A marked difference is present in the total concentration of electrolytes present between the ICF and ECF. For the survival of the cell, this concentration difference is essential and is maintained by sodium-potassium (Na^+-K^+) pump. The principle extracellular cation is sodium cation (Na+) and the intracellular cation is potassium cation (K^+). In ECF, the most predominant anion is chloride anion (Cl^-) and bicarbonate anion (HCO_3^-), while in ICF, it is phosphate anion (PO_4^{2-}), proteins, and organic acids. The compositions of electrolytes in the body fluids are summarized in the table 12.2.

Electrolyte distribution:

Electrolytes are the compounds which readily dissociate in solution and exist as ions i.e., positively and negatively charged particles. The distribution of electrolytes in the body may vary from one to another. The following are the various electrolytes present and their respective distribution in the body.

1. **Calcium:** It is the most abundant mineral in the body. About 1 to 1.5 kg of calcium is present in a normal adult. Out of this, about 99 % is present in the bones and teeth. The remaining small fraction i.e., 1 % calcium is present outside the skeletal tissue and performs a wide variety of functions. The normal plasma calcium level is 4.5 to 5.5 mEq/l.
2. **Sodium:** It is the chief cation of the ECF. About 50 % of sodium is present in the bones, 40 % in the ECF and the remaining 10 % is in the soft tissues. The normal plasma sodium level is 135 to 145 mEq/l.
3. **Potassium:** It is the chief cation of the ICF. About 98 % of potassium is present inside the cell i.e., ICF and the remaining 2 % in the plasma i.e., ECF. More than 95 % of total potassium is exchangeable. The normal plasma potassium level is 3.4 to 5 mEq/l.

Table12.2 The compositions of electrolytes in the body fluids.

Electrolytes concentration (in mEq/l)							
Extracellular fluid / ECF (Plasma)				Intracellular fluid / ICF (Muscle)			
Cations		Anions		Cations		Anions	
Sodium cation (Na^+)	142	Chloride anion (Cl^-)	103	Sodium cation (Na^+)	10	Chloride anion (Cl^-)	2
Potassium cation (K^+)	5	Bicarbonate anion (HCO_3^-)	27	Potassium cation (K^+)	150	Bicarbonate anion (HCO_3^-)	10
Calcium cation (Ca^{2+})	5	Proteins	16	Calcium cation (Ca^{2+})	2	Proteins	40
Magnesium cation (Mg^{2+})	3	Organic acids	6	Magnesium cation (Mg^{2+})	40	Organic acids	5
		Phosphate anion (HPO_4^{2-})	2			Phosphate anion (HPO_4^{2-})	140
		Sulphate anion (SO_4^{2-})	1			Sulphate anion (SO_4^{2-})	5
	155		**155**		**202**		**202**

4. **Magnesium:** About 20 g of magnesium is present in a normal healthy adult body. About 70 % of magnesium is present in the bones in combination with calcium and phosphorous and the remaining 30 % is in the soft tissues and body fluids. The normal plasma magnesium level is 2 to 3 mg/dl.
5. **Chloride:** It is an inorganic anionic halogen that is exclusively distributed within the ECF which comprises the blood or plasma compartment and intestinal fluid compartment. About 115 g of chloride is present in a normal healthy adult. About 90 % of chloride is present in the ECF and it contributes for 70 % of the total anionic charge of ECF. The remaining 10 % is present in the other parts. Chlorine is a constituent of sodium chloride. Hence, the metabolism of chlorine and sodium are related to each other. The normal plasma chlorine level is 95 to 105 mEq/l.
6. **Bicarbonate:** It is difficult to estimate how much bicarbonate is present in the body because it is constantly dissociated into carbondioxide and water. Water is abundantly present in the body and carbondioxide is massively volatile. Hence, the total body bicarbonate is mainly dependent on total body carbondioxide. About 70 % carbondioxide is converted into carbonic acid of which bicarbonate ion is the conjugate base. About 42 g or 700 mmol free bicarbonate ion is present in a normal healthy adult. About 60 % is present in ECF and the remaining 40 % is present in ICF.
7. **Phosphate:** It is the most abundant intracellular anion. In a normal healthy adult, about 700 g or 22.5 moles of phosphorus are present. About 85 % of phosphorus is present in the matrix of the bone in bound form with hydroxy apatite and the rest of 15 % is dissolved and exists largely as the phosphate ion. In that 15 %, about 14.99 % (3.4 moles) of phosphate ions are present in ICF, and the remaining 0.01 % are present in ECF.
8. **Sulphate:** The concentration of inorganic sulfate is maintained at high levels (~ 0.3–0.5 mM) as the fourth abundant anion in the plasma. Sulfate homeostasis in the body depends on the intestinal absorption of dietary sulfate, metabolism of sulfur-containing molecules, and renal reabsorption of the inorganic sulfate.

Osmotic pressure:

Osmosis is defined as a process by which molecules of a solvent tend to pass through a semi-permeable membrane from a less concentrated solution into a more concentrated one. The osmotic pressure is defined as the pressure that would have to be applied to a pure solvent to prevent it from passing into a given solution by osmosis, often used to express the concentration of the solution. There are two ways of expressing the concentration of molecules with regard to osmotic pressure.

1. **Osmolarity:** It is defined as the number of moles or millimoles per liter of solution.
2. **Osmolality:** It is defined as the number of moles or millimoles per kilogram (Kg) of solvent.

There is almost no difference between the osmolarity and osmolality if the solvent is pure water. The osmolality is more commonly used in biological fluids containing molecules such as proteins to express their concentration because it is about 6 % greater than osmolarity.

Osmolality of plasma:

The solute particles present in the fluid medium are measured by osmolality. The normal osmolality of plasma varies from 285 to 295 milliosmoles/Kg. The osmolality is measured by using an osmometer. The osmolality of plasma is largely (~ 90 %) contributed by sodium and its associated anions. Practically, plasma osmolality is calculated from the concentrations (in mmol/l) of a sodium cation (Na^+), potassium cation (K^+), urea and glucose as follows,

$$\text{Plasma osmolality}\left(in\frac{mmol}{l}\right) = 2Na^+ + 2K^+ + Urea + Glucose$$

For the account of associated anion, the concentration factor 2 is used for sodium cation (Na^+) and potassium cation (K^+), assuming complete ionization of the molecules. For osmolality of plasma, sodium cation (Na^+) is the most predominant contributor, hence, the above formula is simplified as follows,

$$\text{Plasma osmolality}\left(in\frac{mmol}{kg}\right) = 2 \times Plasma\ Na^+\left(in\frac{mmol}{l}\right)$$

If glucose and urea are present in the normal range then the above formula works well. In severe hyperproteinemia and lipemia, this formula will not be valid. The distribution of constituents in plasma osmolality is depicted in Table 12.3.

Table 12.3 Distribution of constituents in plasma osmolality.

S. No.	Constituents (Solute)	Osmolality (in mosm/Kg)
1	Sodium cation (Na^+)	135.0
2	Associated anions of Na^+	135.0
3	Potassium cation (K^+)	3.5
4	Associated anions of K^+	3.5
5	Calcium cation (Ca^{2+})	1.5
6	Associated anions of Ca^{2+}	1.5
7	Magnesium cation (Mg^{2+})	1.0
8	Associated anions of Mg^{2+}	1.0
9	Urea	5.0
10	Glucose	5.0
11	Protein	1.0
	Total	293.0

Osmolality of ECF and ICF:

The osmotic pressure difference between the ICF and ECF is responsible for the movement of water across the biological membrane. In a healthy individual, the osmotic pressure of ICF mainly due to potassium cations (K^+) is equal to the osmotic pressure of ECF mainly due to sodium cations (Na^+). Due to this osmotic equilibrium as such, there is no passage of water molecules in or out of the cells.

Osmotic pressure of ICF (due to K^+) = Osmotic pressure of ECF (due to Na^+)

Regulation of electrolyte balance:

The kidney plays a major role in the regulation of water and electrolyte balance together. Hormones such as aldosterone, antidiuretic hormone (ADH), and renin-angiotensin system are used to achieve this regulation.

Aldosterone: It is secreted by the adrenal cortex and is a mineralocorticoid. At the expense of potassium cation (K^+) and hydrogen cation (H^+), aldosterone increases the reabsorption of sodium cation (Na^+) by the renal tubules. The net effect of aldosterone is the retention of the sodium cation (Na^+) in the body.

Antidiuretic hormone (ADH): Hypothalamus is stimulated to release antidiuretic hormone (ADH) when the plasma osmolality is increased mostly due to sodium cation (Na^+). ADH effectively increases the water reabsorption by renal tubules.

Renin-angiotensin system: Renin-angiotensin system controls the secretion of aldosterone. Renin is secreted by juxtaglomerular apparatus by sense when the blood pressure is decreased due to a fall in ECF volume. Later, angiotensin-I is produced from angiotensinogen when the rennin acts on angiotensinogen. Further, angiotensin-I is converted to angiotensin-II which stimulates the release of aldosterone.

To maintain the normal fluid and electrolyte balance, aldosterone and antidiuretic hormone (ADH) coordinate with each other. In the regulation of sodium cation (Na^+) balance, the relationship between rennin, angiotensin, and aldosterone is presented in the Figure 12.3.

Atrial natriuretic factor (ANF) or atriopeptin: It is a peptide containing 28 amino acids. Increased blood volume, elevated blood pressure, and high salt intake stimulate the atrium of the heart to produce ANF or atriopeptin. GFR, sodium excretion, and the urine output is increased when ANF or atriopeptin acts on the kidney. ANF or atriopeptin produces opposite effects of renin and aldosterone which generally increases salt retention and blood pressure.

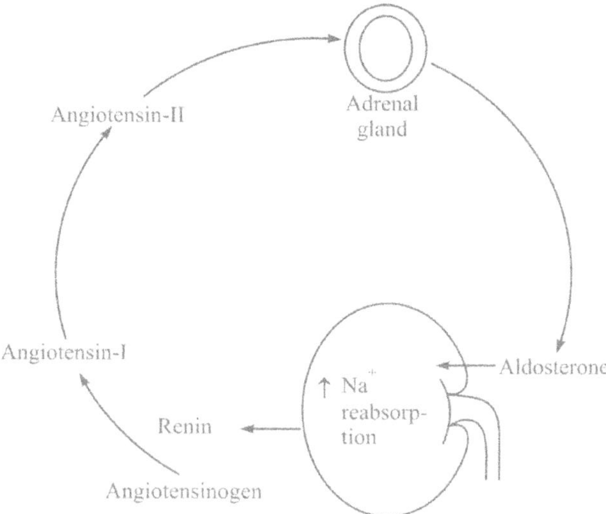

Figure 12.3 Relationship between rennin, angiotensin, and aldosterone in regulation of electrolyte balance.

Sodium cation (Na^+) concentration and ECF: It is important to know that sodium cation (Na^+) and its anions (mainly chloride anion i.e., Cl^-) are confined to the extracellular fluid. The osmotic effect of these anions and cation is responsible for the retention of water in ECF. Hence, the volume of ECF is ultimately determined by the amount of sodium cation (Na^+).

Dietary intake and electrolyte balance: The electrolyte requirement of the body is generally supplied by the consumption of a well-balanced diet. Salt hunger and water hunger cannot be differentiated by humans. Electrolyte intake is also regulated by thirst. The loss of electrolytes in a hot climate is usually higher. Sometimes, it is necessary to supplement drinking water with electrolytes.

Dehydration:

The depletion of water in the body is one of the most important characterizations of dehydration. Excessive water loss or insufficient intake or both may be the reason for dehydration. Based on the reason, dehydration is broadly classified into two major types as follows,

1. Dehydration due to loss of water alone.
2. Dehydration due to deprivation of water and electrolytes.

Causes: Dehydration may occur due to several causes such as a) diarrhea, b) vomiting, c) excessive sweating, d) fluid loss in burns, e) dysfunction of ADH, f) kidney disease like renal insufficiency, g) deficiency of ADH, etc.

Characteristic features: The severity of dehydration may be represented in three degrees as mild, moderate and severe. The following are the various salient features of dehydration:

1. Elevated pulse rate, decreased blood pressure, sunken eyeballs, decreased skin turgor, lethargy, confusion, and coma are the most important clinical symptoms of severe dehydration.
2. Osmotic pressure and electrolyte concentrations are concomitantly increased when the volume of ECF (**Example:** Plasma) is decreased.
3. Increased blood urea and plasma protein concentration.
4. Cells are shrunken and disturbed metabolism (**Example:** Increased protein breakdown) are due to drawing of water from ICF.
5. From the body, water depletion is often accompanied by loss of electrolytes like Na^+, K^+, etc.
6. Increased ADH secretion causes increased water retention in the body that leads to a very low urine volume.

Treatment: Intake of plenty of water is the choice of treatment for dehydration. Water should be administered intravenously in an isotonic solution (usually 5 % glucose) for the subjects who cannot take it orally. If the loss of electrolytes takes place along with dehydration, then the same should be administered either by oral or intravenous routes. This can be achieved by careful monitoring of the status of water and electrolytes.

Osmotic imbalance and dehydration in cholera: *Vibrio cholera* is the causative organism for cholera which is transmitted through contaminated water and foods. Into the intestinal lumen, various ions (Na^+, K^+, Cl^-, HCO_3^-, etc.) are secreted as a result of toxin produced by bacterium through stimulation of intestinal cells. The osmotic pressure is increased and water is sucked into the lumen by these ions resulting in diarrhea with heavy loss of water (5 to 10 liters/day). Due to the loss of dissolved salts and dehydration, the victims of cholera will die if not treated in time. In many developing countries, cholera and other forms of severe diarrhea are the major reasons for the death of young children. In general, cholera and other diarrheal disease are commonly treated using oral rehydration therapy (ORT).

Overhydration or water intoxication:

Excessive retention of the water in the body causes overhydration or water intoxication. The various reasons behind the overhydration are excessive intake of large volumes of salt-free fluids, renal failure, overproduction of ADH, etc. In general, after major surgery or trauma, lung infection, etc. overhydration is observed. The osmolality of ECF and ICF is decreased and both ECF and ICF are diluted in overhydration. Headache, lethargy and convulsions are the symptoms of overhydration. Stoppage of water intake and hypertonic saline administration are the treatment options for overhydration.

Water tank model: This model easily explains the distribution of body water in ICF and ECF, dehydration and overhydration. The water intake (mostly through oral) and water output (mostly urine) of the body are represented by the tank inlet and outlet, respectively. When the water output exceeds the water intake, it causes dehydration, and when the water intake exceeds the water output, it causes overhydration. The water tank model representing body fluid compartments are presented in the Figure 12.4.

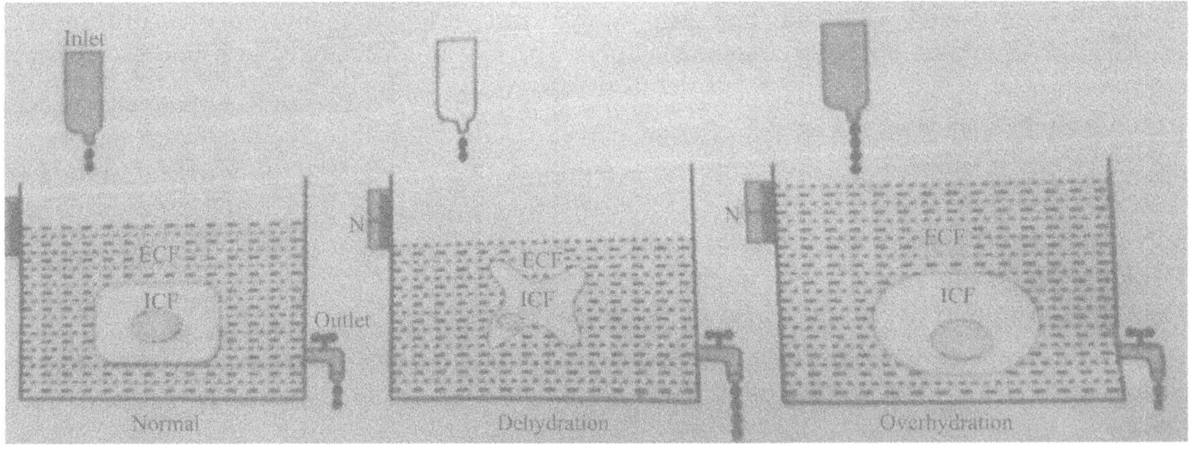

Figure 12.4 Water tank model (Body fluid comportments representation).

Diuretics: These are the drugs that increase the urine volume by stimulating water and sodium excretion. Bendrofluazide, frusemide, spironolactone and mannitol are the commonly used diuretics. Generally, diuretics are used in the treatment of edema, heart failure, and hypertension.

Determination of Sodium in Body Fluids (Colorimetric Method)

Sodium is the major cation of extracellular fluid. It plays a central role in the maintenance of the normal distribution of water and the osmotic pressure in the various fluid compartments. The main source of body sodium is the sodium chloride contained in ingested foods. Only about one-third of the total body sodium is present in the skeleton since most of it present in the extracellular body fluids.

Principle:

Sodium present in body fluids is estimated by several different methods such as flame photometry method, ion-selective electrodes method, and colorimetric method. The colorimetric estimation is old and the most popular method for determining sodium in body fluids. In this method, sodium present in body fluids is precipitated as the triple salt, sodium uranyl zinc acetate. In 1927, Kolthoff introduced this technique with subsequent utilization of the precipitate in several ways. One approach was a direct measurement of the solubilized residue itself by the colorimetric method. In another method, after precipitation color fade of the yellow supernatant liquid is monitored and measured.

In the present method, sodium present in body fluid is precipitated from a protein-free supernatant liquid as the triple salt, sodium uranyl zinc acetate by treating with uranyl acetate, zinc acetate and aqueous acetic acid-ethanol mixture. Sodium concentration present in body fluid is directly proportional to the resulting decrease in the absorbance of the supernatant-color reagent mixture.

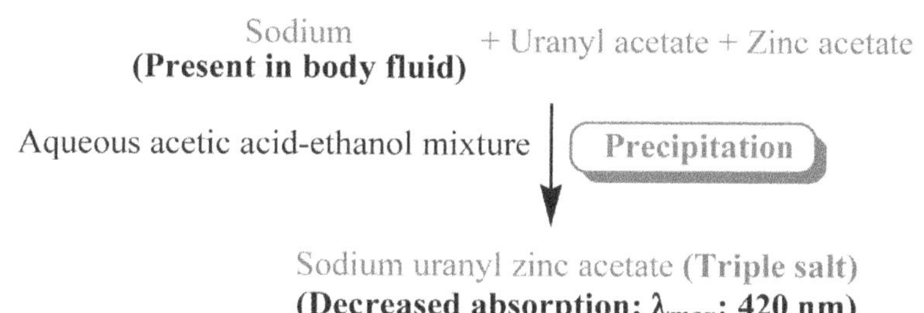

Concentration of sodium present α Decreased absorbance of mixture

Reagents:

1. **Sodium color reagent:** Solution of uranyl acetate (5.3 g/dl) and zinc acetate (15.4 g/dl), in aqueous acetic acid-ethanol mixture.
2. **Precipitating reagent:** Aqueous solution of trichloroacetic acid (10 g/dl).
3. **Standard sodium solution (140 mmol/l):** Sodium chloride (4.091 g/l) in aqueous trichloroacetic acid.

Collection and preparation of specimen:

1. **Serum:** Remove from clot promptly and carefully to prevent hemolysis.
2. **Plasma:** Use lithium heparinate, ammonium heparinate, or lithium oxalate as anticoagulant.
3. **Urine:** Use 24 hours collected; well mixed dilute portion of urine. Depends on the sodium content the dilution such as 1:10 (1 ml urine + 9 ml distilled water) or 1:5 (1 ml urine + 4 ml distilled water) or 1:2 (1 ml urine + 1 ml distilled water) may be required.
4. **Preparation of protein-free supernatant liquid:** Add 0.5 ml of serum plasma or diluted urine to a test tube. To this sample, add 0.5 ml of precipitating reagent dropwise with vigorous mixing. Allow the resulting mixture to stand for 5 minutes and centrifuge at high speed for 5-10 minutes.

Procedure:

Take three test tubes and label as standard, blank, and unknown. In the unknown test tube, take 0.5 ml of protein-free supernatant liquid and in the standard test tube, take 0.5 ml of standard sodium solution. In the blank test tube, take 0.5 ml of distilled water. Add 2.5 ml of sodium color reagent to all the three test tubes and mix well. Incubate all three tubes for 10 minutes at 15-30 °C and centrifuge at high speed for 5 minutes. Finally, transfer the supernatant liquid carefully and measure the color intensity. Measure the intensity of the color obtained in the standard, unknown, and blank against water at 420 nm within 30 minutes. Calculate the concentration of sodium present in the unknown sample using the following formula.

$$\textit{Concetration of sodium present in body fluid}\left(in\ \frac{mmol}{l}\right)=\frac{(E_b - E_u)}{(E_b - E_s)}\times C_s = \frac{(E_b - E_u)}{(E_b - E_s)}\times 140$$

Where, E_b = Optical density of the blank
E_u = Optical density of unknown body fluid
E_s = Optical density of standard sodium solution
C_s = Concentration of standard sodium solution

Take three test tubes and label as standard, blank, and unknown

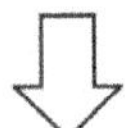

In the unknown test tube, take 0.5 ml of protein-free supernatant liquid and in the standard test tube, take 0.5 ml of standard sodium solution

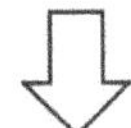

In the blank test tube, take 0.5 ml of distilled water

Add 2.5 ml of sodium color reagent to all the three test tubes and mix well

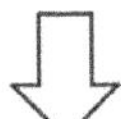

Incubate all three tubes for 10 minutes at 15-30 °C and centrifuge at high speed for 5 minutes

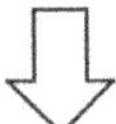

Transfer the supernatant liquid carefully and measure the color intensity of the color obtained in the standard, unknown, and blank against water at 420 nm within 30 minutes

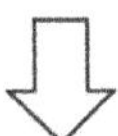

Calculate the concentration of sodium present in the unknown sample

Significance:

Hyponatremia (low serum sodium level) is found in a variety of clinical conditions such as severe polyuria, metabolic acidosis, Addison's disease, diarrhea, and renal tubular disease. Hypernatremia (increased serum sodium level) is found in the clinical conditions like hyperadrenalism, severe dehydration, diabetic coma after therapy with insulin, excess treatment with sodium salts.

Determination of Calcium in Body Fluids (Titrimetric Method)

Ionized calcium, calcium bound to protein, and calcium bound to other organic anions like citrate are the three different forms of calcium present in the serum. The ionized fractions of calcium perform most of the physiological functions but for routine work, the total calcium in the serum is estimated.

Principle:

This method is called as Clark and Collip method which is a titrimetric method of estimation. In this method, calcium present in biological fluid is treated with ammonium oxalate to precipitate calcium as calcium oxalate. Later, ammonia is used to wash the obtained precipitate to remove the excess oxalate. Calcium oxalate is treated with sulphuric acid results in formation of oxalic acid. The liberated oxalic acid is titrated with standard potassium permanganate.

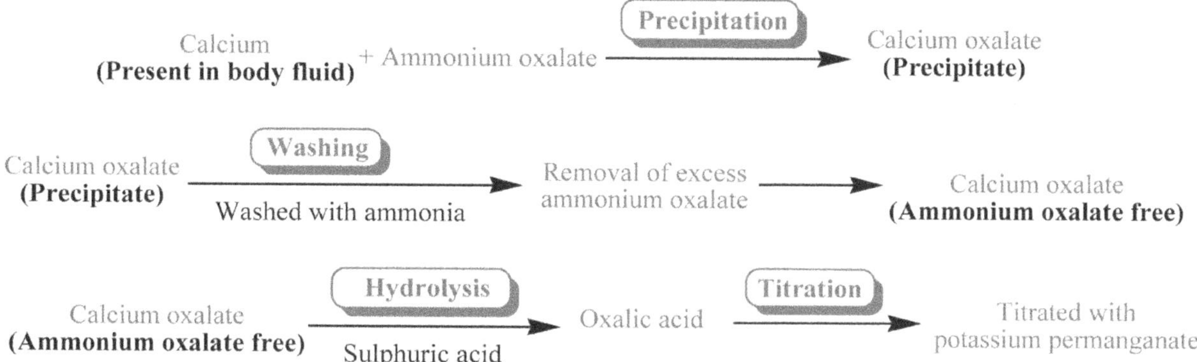

Reagents:

1. **4 % Ammonium oxalate solution:** Dissolve 4 g of ammonium oxalate in 50 ml of water and dilute to 100 ml with distilled water.
2. **2 % Ammonia solution:** Dilute 2 ml of concentrated ammonia to 100 ml with distilled water.
3. **1 N Sulphuric acid:** Dilute 28 ml of concentrated sulphuric acid to 1000 ml with distilled water.
4. **0.01 N Potassium permanganate solution:** Dissolve 3.158 g of potassium permanganate in 50 ml of water and dilute to 1000 ml with distilled water. Further, dilute 10 ml of above solution to 100 ml using distilled water. Standardize the prepared 0.01 N potassium permanganate solution using 0.01 N sodium oxalate. 1 ml of 0.01 N potassium permanganate is equivalent to 0.2 mg of calcium.
5. **0.01 N Sodium oxalate solution:** Dissolve 0.67 g of sodium oxalate in 50 ml of water and add 5 ml concentrated sulphuric acid. Then, dilute the solution to 1000 ml with distilled water. 1 ml of 0.01 N sodium oxalate is equivalent to 1 ml of 0.01 N potassium permanganate.

Procedure:

In a centrifuge tube, take 2 ml of serum, 2 ml of water and 1 ml of 4 % ammonium oxalate solution and mix well. Allow the centrifuge tube to stand for 30 minutes. Mix well the mixture and centrifuge at 1500 rpm for 15 minutes. Pour the supernatant liquid and drain the tube by keeping it inverted on a filter paper for a few minutes. Wipe the mouth of the tube dry with a filter paper. Further, add 3 ml of 2 % ammonia to the centrifuge tube, mix, centrifuge, and drain as before. In a conical flask, add 2 ml of 1 N sulphuric acid to the obtained precipitate and shake vigorously. Boil the conical flask in a water bath with frequent shaking until the precipitate dissolves completely. While the conical flask was still hot, titrate the content of the conical flask against 0.01 N potassium permanganate until a pink color develops and persists for at least one minute. Note the volume of 0.01 N potassium permanganate consumed as "X". Perform a blank experiment by avoiding body fluid in the same manner and note the volume of 0.01 N potassium permanganate consumed as "Y" (Blank: Titrate 2 ml of 1 N sulphuric acid with 0.01 N potassium permanganate exactly as before). Calculate the concentration of calcium present in body fluid using the following formula.

$$\textit{Concetration of calcium in 100 ml serum} = (X - Y) \times \frac{0.2}{2} \times 100\,mg$$

Where, X = Volume of 0.01 N potassium permanganate consumed in serum assay

Y = Volume of 0.01 N potassium permanganate consumed in the blank assay

Estimation of calcium in urine: Dilute the urine to 1:10 (1 ml urine + 9 ml distilled water) with water. Estimate the calcium present in the diluted urine by the above method and multiply the results with 10 (Dilution factor). Obtain better results by allowing the mixture of diluted urine, water and ammonium oxalate to stand for 24 h.

In a centrifuge tube, take 2 ml of serum, 2 ml of water and 1 ml of 4 % ammonium oxalate solution and mix well

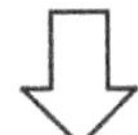

Allow the centrifuge tube to stand for 30 minutes

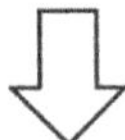

Mix well the mixture and centrifuge at 1500 rpm for 15 minutes

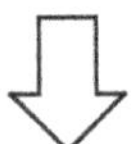

Pour the supernatant liquid and drain the tube by keeping it inverted on a filter paper for a few minutes

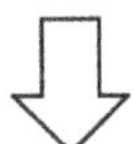

Wipe the mouth of the tube dry with a filter paper

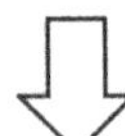

Further, add 3 ml of 2 % ammonia to the centrifuge tube, mix, centrifuge, and drain as before

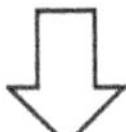

In a conical flask, add 2 ml of 1 N sulphuric acid to the obtained precipitate and shake vigorously

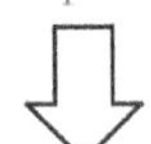

Boil the conical flask in a water bath with frequent shaking until the precipitate dissolves completely

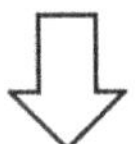

While the conical flask was still hot, titrate the content of the conical flask against 0.01 N potassium permanganate until a pink color develops and persists for at least one minute **(Note the volume of 0.01 N potassium permanganate consumed as "X")**

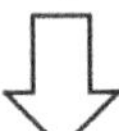

Perform a blank experiment by avoiding body fluid in the same manner **(Note the volume of 0.01 N potassium permanganate consumed as "Y")**

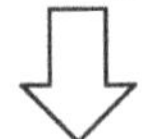

Calculate the concentration of calcium present in body fluid

Significance:

In healthy people, the serum calcium level may vary from 9 to 11 mg/100 ml. In adults, the product of serum calcium and serum inorganic phosphorous concentration is around 40 mg/100 ml and in case of children, it is around 50 mg/100 ml. In general, the concentration of serum calcium and serum inorganic phosphate are indirectly proportional to each other.

$$\text{Concetration of serum calcium } \alpha \frac{1}{\text{Concentration of serum inorganic phosphate}}$$

Serum calcium level is increased (hypercalcemia) in a variety of clinical conditions such as hyperparathyroidism, hypervitaminosis-D, multiple myeloma, extensive metastatic involvement of bones, sarcoidosis, idiopathic infantile hypercalcemia, milk-alkali syndrome, and polycythemia.

Determination of Serum Potassium (Turbidimetric Method)

In all body tissues, potassium is present and is required for normal cell function due to its role in maintaining intracellular fluid (ICF) volume and transmembrane electrochemical gradients.

Principle:

Serum potassium is estimated by the turbidimetric method. In this method, the potassium present in the serum is treated with sodium tetraphenylboron present in potassium turbid reagent that results in the formation of colloidal suspension. The turbidity of this formed colloidal solution is proportional to serum potassium concentration in the range of 2-7 mEq/l. The turbidity produced in the solution is measured photometrically at 620 nm.

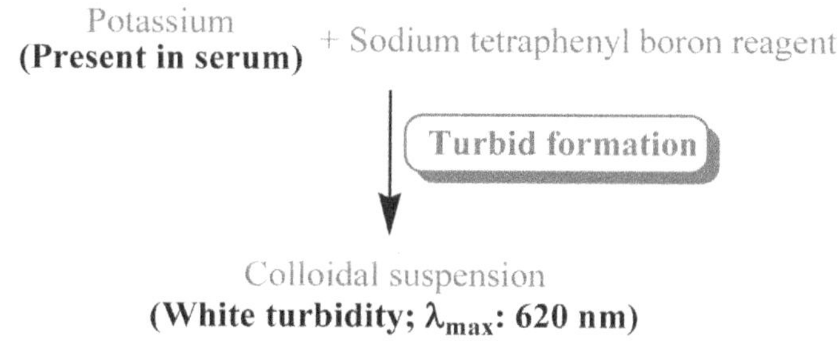

Reagents:

1. **Potassium turbid reagent:** Solution of sodiumtetraphenylboron.
2. **Standard potassium solution (140 mmol/l):** Solution of potassium chloride

Procedure:

Take three test tubes and label as standard, blank, and unknown. In the unknown test tube, take 0.05 ml of serum and in the standard test tube, take 0.05 ml of standard potassium solution. In the blank test tube, take 0.05 ml of distilled water. To all test tubes, add 1.0 ml of potassium turbid reagent and mix well. Incubate all three tubes for 5 minutes at room temperature. Measure the intensity of the turbidity in standard, unknown against the blank at 620 nm. Calculate the concentration of potassium present in the unknown sample using the following formula.

$$\text{Concetration of potassium present in serum}\left(in\ \frac{mmol}{l}\right)=\frac{E_u}{E_s}\times C_s=\frac{E_u}{E_s}\times 5$$

Where, E_u = Optical density of unknown serum sample

E_s = Optical density of standard potassium solution

C_s = Concentration of standard potassium solution

Significance:

Serum potassium level is increased (hyperkalemia) in a variety of clinical conditions such as renal failure, dehydration shock, or adrenal insufficiency. Serum potassium level is decreased (hypokalemia) in a variety of clinical conditions such as malnutrition, negative nitrogen balance, gastrointestinal fluid losses, and hyperactivity of the adrenal cortex.

Take three test tubes and label as standard, blank, and unknown

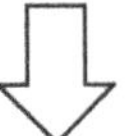

In the unknown test tube, take 0.05 ml of serum and in the standard test tube, take 0.05 ml of standard potassium solution

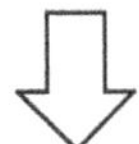

In the blank test tube, take 0.05 ml of distilled water

To all test tubes, add 1.0 ml of potassium turbid reagent and mix well

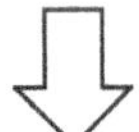

Incubate all three tubes for 5 minutes at room temperature

Measure the intensity of the turbidity in standard, unknown against the blank at 620 nm

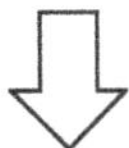

Calculate the concentration of potassium present in the unknown sample

Determination of Chloride in Body Fluids (Colorimetric Method)

The principal serum anions are chloride and bicarbonate; whereas the principal serum cations are sodium and potassium. These ions are involved in maintaining normal anion-cation balance, osmotic pressure, and proper water distribution between ICF and ECF. Several methods are available for the estimation of chloride such as the colorimetric method, titrimetric method, amperometric method, and use of chloride meter. Out of these methods, the colorimetric method is the most preferable due to its simplicity and rapidity. The present method is based on the modified Schoenfeld & Lewellen colorimetric method.

Principle:

In this method, chloride anions present in the biological fluid are estimated by the colorimetric method. Initially, the chloride anions present in a biological fluid is reacted with mercuric thiocyanate to produce mercuric chloride with a release of thiocyanate ions. Later, the released thiocyanate ions are reacted with ferric ions to produce a red-colored complex of ferric thiocyanate. The intensity of the red color complex formed is measured at 510 nm. The absorbance of the red-colored complex is directly proportional to the chloride concentration.

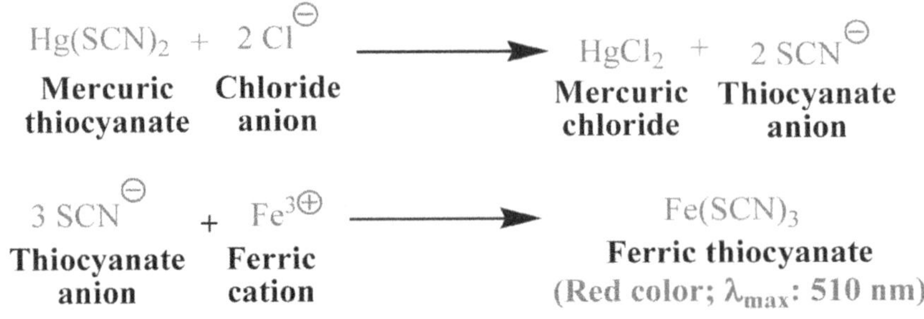

Reagents:

1. **Chloride reagent:** A mixture of buffer (50 mmol/l), mercuric thiocyanate (1.8 mmol/l), ferric nitrate (20 mmol/l), surfactants and anti-oxidants.
2. **Standard chloride solution (100 mmol/l):** Solution of potassium chloride.

Procedure:

Take three test tubes and label as standard, blank, and unknown. In the unknown test tube, take 0.01 ml of body fluid and in the standard test tube, take 0.01 ml of standard chloride solution. In the blank test tube, take 0.01 ml of distilled water. To all test tubes, add 1.0 ml of chloride reagent and mix well. Incubate all three tubes for 5 minutes at room temperature. Measure the intensity of the red color formed in the standard and unknown against the blank at 510 nm. Calculate the concentration of chloride present in the unknown sample using the following formula.

$$\textit{Concetration of chloride present in body fluid}\left(in\,\frac{mmol}{l}\right)=\frac{E_u}{E_s}\times C_s=\frac{E_u}{E_s}\times 100$$

Where, E_u = Optical density of unknown body fluid sample

E_s = Optical density of standard chloride solution

C_s = Concentration of standard chloride solution

Take three test tubes and label as standard, blank, and unknown

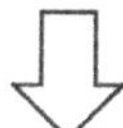

In the unknown test tube, take 0.01 ml of body fluid and in the standard test tube, take 0.01 ml of standard chloride solution

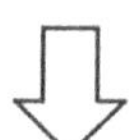

In the blank test tube, take 0.01 ml of distilled water

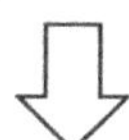

To all test tubes, add 1.0 ml of chloride reagent and mix well. Incubate all three tubes for 5 minutes at room temperature

Measure the intensity of the red color formed in the standard and unknown against the blank at 510 nm

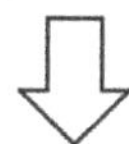

Calculate the concentration of chloride present in the unknown sample

Significance:

The normal serum chloride level is 98 to 109 mmol/l, urine chloride level is 170 to 250 mmol/24 hours and CSF chloride level are 118 to 132 mmol/l. In clinical conditions like dehydration and in conditions causing decreased renal blood flow such as congestive heart failure, increased serum chloride level (hyperchloridemia) is observed. In clinical conditions such as salt-losing nephritis, metabolic acidosis, and vomiting, decreased serum chloride levels (hypochloridemia) may be seen. In a normal person, when plasma chloride level falls below the lower limit of the normal range, urinary chloride excretion ceases. However, due to adrenal cortical insufficiency in Addison's disease in spite of its low plasma level, the excretion of chloride continues. In meningitis, especially untreated tuberculous meningitis, CSF chloride values may be decreased.

Determination of Bicarbonate in Body Fluids (Enzymatic Method)

Many potentially serious disorders associated with changes in the body, acid-base balance is diagnosed and treated with the help of bicarbonate estimation. The acid-base status is evaluated by bicarbonate estimation in conjunction with other clinical and laboratory information.

Principle:

Generally, bicarbonates present in the body fluids are estimated by the enzymatic method developed by Forrester *et al.* In this method, initially, the bicarbonate (HCO_3^-) present in the body fluid reacts with phosphoenolpyruvate in the presence of *phosphoenolpyruvate carboxylase* to produce oxaloacetate and inorganic phosphate ion ($H_2PO_4^-$). Later, the formed oxaloacetate is reduced by NADH + H^+ to malate in the presence of *malate dehydrogenase* with the concomitant oxidation of NADH + H^+ to NAD^+. In addition, the oxidation of NADH affects the reaction equilibrium of carbonic acid formation (reaction of carbondioxide and water) and their degradation (into hydrogen and bicarbonate ion). Hence, the total concentration of carbondioxide is also measured. This oxidation of NADH results in a decreased absorbance of the reaction mixture which is measured dichromatically at 405 or 415 nm. The absorbance of the reaction mixture is proportional to the bicarbonate content of the sample or total carbondioxide present in the sample.

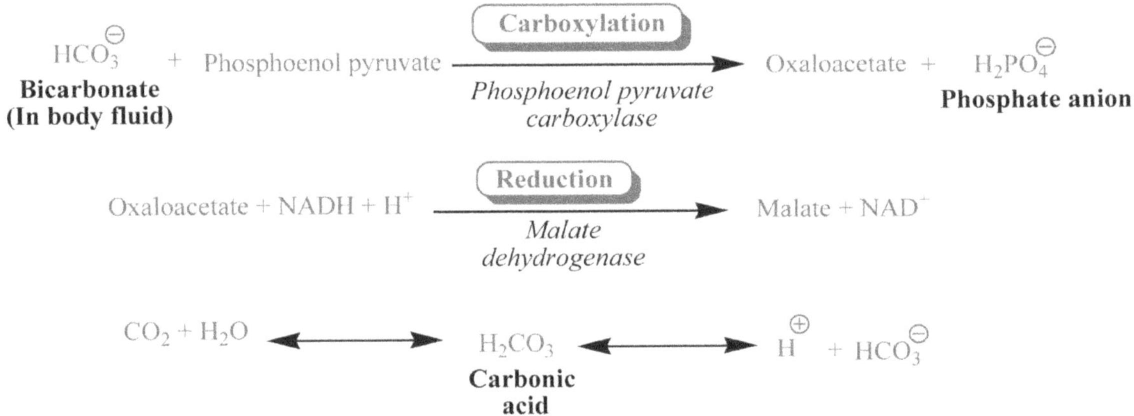

Reagents:

1. **Bicarbonate reagent:** A mixture of buffer (pH 7.5), phosphoenolpyruvate (12.5 mmol/l), *phosphoenolpyruvate carboxylase* (> 400 U/l), *malate dehydrogenase* (> 4100 U/l and NADH analog (0.6 mmol/l).
2. **Standard bicarbonate solution (30 mmol/l):** Solution of sodiumbicarbonate.

Procedure:

Take three test tubes and label as standard, blank and unknown. Take 10 µl of body fluid, 10 µl of standard bicarbonate solution, and 10 µl of distilled water in the unknown test tube, standard test tube, and blank test tube, respectively. To all test tubes, add 1000 µl of bicarbonate reagent and mix well. Incubate all three tubes at room temperature. Measure the intensity of the color formed in the standard and unknown against the blank at 405 nm after 2 minutes exactly and at 415 nm after 10 minutes exactly. Calculate the concentration of bicarbonate present in the unknown sample using the following formula.

$$\text{Concetration of bicarbonate present in body fluid}\left(in\,\frac{mmol}{l}\right)=\frac{\Delta E_u}{\Delta E_s}\times C_s=\frac{\Delta E_u}{\Delta E_s}\times 30$$

Where $\Delta E_u = E_u$ at 415 nm after 10 minutes – E_u at 405 nm after 2 minutes

$\Delta E_s = E_s$ at 415 nm after 10 minutes – E_s at 405 nm after 2 minutes

E_u = Optical density of unknown body fluid sample

E_s = Optical density of standard bicarbonate solution

C_s = Concentration of standard bicarbonate solution.

Take three test tubes and label as standard, blank and unknown

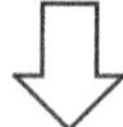

Take 10 µl of body fluid, 10 µl of standard bicarbonate solution, and 10 µl of distilled water in the unknown test tube, standard test tube, and blank test tube, respectively

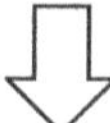

To all test tubes, add 1000 µl of bicarbonate reagent and mix well

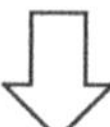

Incubate all three tubes at room temperature

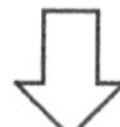

Measure the intensity of the color formed in the standard and unknown against the blank at 405 nm after 2 minutes exactly and at 415 nm after 10 minutes exactly

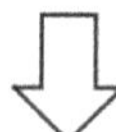

Calculate the concentration of bicarbonate present in the unknown sample

Significance:

In clinical conditions like compensated respiratory acidosis and metabolic alkalosis, increased bicarbonate levels may be observed. On the other hand, in clinical conditions such as compensated respiratory alkalosis and metabolic acidosis decreased bicarbonate levels may be observed. The differentiation between metabolic and respiratory conditions is identified using additional laboratory determinations.

Acid-base Balance

Normally, the pH of the blood is slightly alkaline i.e., 7.35 to 7.45. The intracellular fluid (ICF) pH is rather variable. For example, pH of erythrocyte is 7.2 and the pH of skeletal muscle is as low as 6.0. The important homeostatic mechanism of the body is the maintenance of the blood pH. Generally, the pH of the blood varies very little in normal circumstances due to effective regulation. A change in the blood pH affects the pH of the intracellular fluid (ICF) leading to a metabolism influence such as distortion in enzyme activity, protein structure, etc. For a compatible life, the pH of blood must be between 6.8 and 7.8.

According to Lowry and Bronsted, an acid is a proton (H^+) donor and a base is a proton (H^+) acceptor. pH is defined as the negative logarithm of hydrogen ion (H^+) concentration. Buffers are defined as the solutions which resist change in pH by the addition of small amounts of acids or bases.

Production of acids by the body: Generally, normal metabolism of the body is accompanied by the overall production of acids including volatile acids (**Example:** Carbonic acid; the most predominant; about 20000 mEq/day) and non-volatile acids (about 80 mEq/day) such as sulphuric acid, lactic acid, phosphoric acid, etc. From the metabolic product carbondioxide, carbonic acid is formed; in anaerobic metabolism lactic acid is produced; from sulphur containing amino acid, sulphuric acid is generated; from organic phosphates like phospholipids, phosphoric acid is derived. All the above acids add up hydrogen ion (H^+) to the blood. More acid is produced in the body while consuming a diet rich in animal protein which ultimately increases the acidic nature of the urine.

Production of bases by the body: Only a negligible amount of basic compounds are produced in the body under normal circumstances. From organic acids such as citrate and lactate, a small amount of bicarbonate is produced. A vegetarian diet has a tendency for the net production of bases. The reason behind this is the utilization of hydrogen ion (H^+) produced in the body by the salts of organic acids such as sodium lactate produced by vegetarian diet. Hence, the alkalizing effect produced by the vegetarian diet results in excretion of neutral or slightly alkaline urine by these subjects.

Maintenance of Blood pH

Regulation of the body's acid-base balance and maintenance of the blood pH (around 7.4) in the biological system is performed by three different defense mechanisms such as,

1. Blood buffers
2. Respiratory mechanism
3. Renal mechanism

1. **Blood buffers:**

A solution of a weak acid (HA) and its salt (BA) with a strong base is called buffer and it resists the change in pH by the addition of acid or alkali. Absolute concentrations of salt and acid are responsible for the buffering capacity of buffers. The protons (H^+ ions) cannot be removed from the body by buffer. Temporarily, it reduces the concentration of protons (H^+ ions) by acting as a shock absorbent. Ultimately, by the renal mechanism, the protons (H^+ ions) have to be eliminated. Three buffer systems are present in blood. They are, a) bicarbonate buffer, b) phosphate buffer, c) protein buffer.

(a) **Bicarbonate buffer system:** The predominant buffer system of the extracellular fluid (ECF) particularly plasma is sodiumbicarbonate and carbonic acid ($NaHCO_3$-H_2CO_3). Generally, carbonic acid is dissociated into hydrogen cation (H^+) and bicarbonate anion (HCO_3^-).

$$\underset{\textbf{Carbonic acid}}{H_2CO_3} \rightleftharpoons \underset{\textbf{Hydrogen cation}}{H^+} + \underset{\textbf{Bicarbonate anion}}{HCO_3^-}$$

At equilibrium by the law of mass action,

$$K_a = \frac{[H^+][HCO_3^-]}{[H_2CO_3]} \quad .....(1)$$

Where, K_a is the dissociation constant of H_2CO_3. The equation (1) can be written as follows,

$$[H^+] = K_a \frac{[H_2CO_3]}{[HCO_3^-]} \quad .....(2)$$

Taking logarithms on both side of equation (2),

$$\log [H^+] = \log K_a + \log \frac{[H_2CO_3]}{[HCO_3^-]} \quad .....(3)$$

Reciprocal of equation (3),

$$\log \frac{1}{[H^+]} = \log \frac{1}{Ka} + \log \frac{[HCO_3^-]}{[H_2CO_3]} \quad .....(4)$$

We know that, $pH = \log \frac{1}{[H^+]}$ and $pK_a = \log \frac{1}{K_a}$; substituting this in the equation (4),

$$pH = pK_a + \log \frac{[HCO_3^-]}{[H_2CO_3]} \quad .....(5)$$

For any buffer equation (5) is valid and the general equation for any buffer i.e., Henderson-Hassselbach equation can be written as,

$$pH = pK_a + log\frac{[Base]}{[Acid]} \quad .....(6)$$

From equation (6) it is evident that pH is dependent on the ratio of the concentration of the base to acid (HCO_3^- and H_2CO_3) in equation (5).

Blood pH and the ratio of HCO_3^- and H_2CO_3: 24 mmol/l (range: 22 to 26 mmol/l) is the normal bicarbonate (HCO_3^-) concentration in plasma. The solution of carbondioxide in water is carbonic acid (H_2CO_3) & the concentration of carbonic acid is given by the product of p^{co_2} (For carbondioxide, arterial partial pressure is 40 mmHg and the solubility constant is 0.03). Therefore,

Concentration of carbonic acid $= p^{co_2}$

= Arterial partial pressure of carbondioxide × Solubility constant of carbondioxide

= 40 × 0.03 = 1.2 mmol/l

The pH of the blood is 7.4; the pK_a for carbonic acid (H_2CO_3) is 6.1; concentration of bicarbonate (HCO_3^-) is 24 mmol/l and the concentration of carbonic acid (H_2CO_3) is 1.2 mmol/l. Substituting these values in Henderson-Hassselbalch equation for bicarbonate buffer i.e., equation (5),

$$pH = pK_a + log\frac{[HCO_3^-]}{[H_2CO_3]} \quad .....(7)$$

$$7.4 = 6.1 + log\frac{24}{1.2} = 6.1 + \log 20 = 6.1 + 1.3 = 7.4$$

It is evident that the blood pH is 7.4 and the ratio of bicarbonate to carbonic acid is 20:1. Thus, in the blood, the concentration of bicarbonate is 20 times higher than the carbonic acid concentration. This is responsible for the effective buffering of hydrogen cation (H^+) generated in the body and referred to as alkali reserve. Normally, the pH of the blood is determined by the concentration of bicarbonate and carbonic acid. In addition, the bicarbonate buffer system serves as an index to understand the disturbances in the acid-base balance of the body.

(b) **Phosphate buffer system:** The phosphate buffer system is mostly intracellular (ICF) buffer and is constituted by sodium dihydrogen phosphate and disodium hydrogen phosphate ($NaHPO_4$-Na_2HPO_4). In plasma, due to its low concentration, it is of less importance. It would have been more effective, had it been present in a high concentration due to its pK_a (6.8 which is close to blood pH 7.4). It is estimated that in phosphate buffer, the ratio of base to acid is 4, compared to 20 in bicarbonate buffer.

(c) **Protein buffer system:** In blood, the protein and hemoglobin together constitute this protein buffer system. pK_a of the ionizable group of the amino acid is responsible for the buffering capacity of the proteins. For protein buffer, the most effective contributor is the imidazole group of histidine (pK_a: 6.7). In the total buffering capacity of the plasma, only 2 % is accounted for the plasma proteins.

Another important buffer is the hemoglobin of RBC and it is mainly involved in the transport of gases such as oxygen and carbondioxide. Hemoglobin mainly buffers the fixed acids. The details of the hemoglobin buffer for the regulation of pH are discussed under respiratory mechanism.

2. **Respiratory mechanism:**

The acid-base balance is maintained by a rapid mechanism provided by the respiratory system through regulation of carbonic acid (H_2CO_3) concentration in blood i.e., the denominator in the bicarbonate buffer system. The carbondioxide is transported from peripheral tissues to lungs with the help of hemoglobin.

Under normal circumstances, all the carbondioxide produced by the cellular metabolic activity is eliminated from the body via the lungs in the expired air. The respiratory center located in the medulla of the brain controls the rate of the removal of carbondioxide or the rate of respiration. This center is highly sensitive to changes in blood pH. Hyperventilation causes to blow off carbondioxide when any decrease in the blood pH takes place. Hence, carbonic acid (H_2CO_3) concentration is decreased with the simultaneous elimination of hydrogen cation (H^+) as water. This mechanism is rapid but only for a short term because hyperventilation cannot be produced for long.

Hemoglobin as a buffer: The hemoglobin acts as a buffer. At the tissue level, it binds to hydrogen cation (H^+) and helps to transport carbondioxide as bicarbonate (HCO_3^-) with a minimum change in pH (termed as isohydric transport). It is estimated that for every 2 protons bound to hemoglobin, four oxygen molecules are released and the details are presented in the figure 12.5.

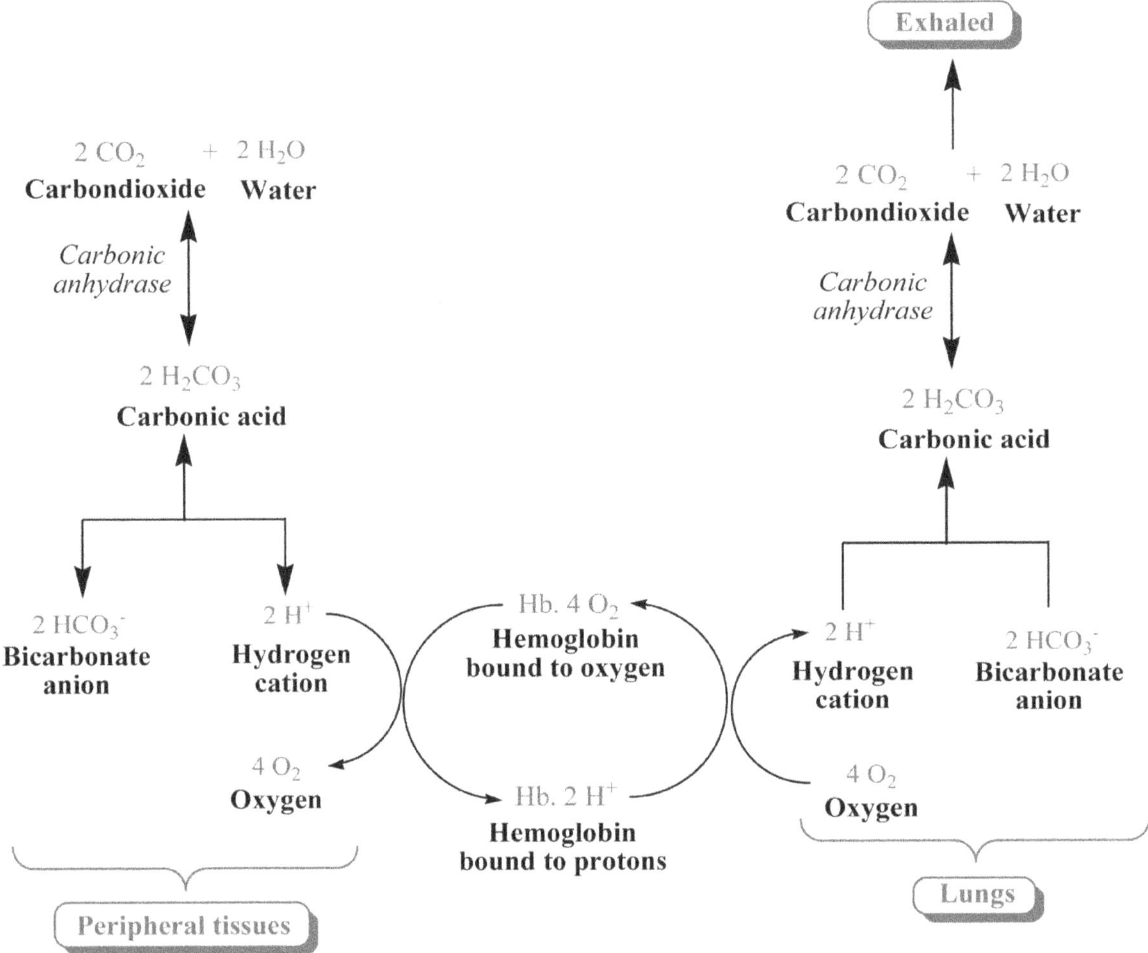

Figure 12.5 Transport of carbondioxide through the mediation of hemoglobin.

Production of bicarbonate (HCO_3^-) by RBC: RBC produce only a small amount of carbondioxide due to the lack of aerobic metabolic pathways. Along the concentration gradient, the plasma carbondioxide is diffused into the RBC. Later, it combines with water and produces carbonic acid (H_2CO_3) which dissociates into hydrogen cation (H^+) and bicarbonate anion (HCO_3^-). The hydrogen cation (H^+) is trapped by the hemoglobin for buffering action and the bicarbonate anion (HCO_3^-) is diffused into the plasma along the concentration gradient by the exchange of chloride ion (Cl^-) to maintain electrical neutrality. This process is referred as chloride shift for the generation of bicarbonate anion (HCO_3^-). Generation of bicarbonates in erythrocytes is presented in Figure 12.6.

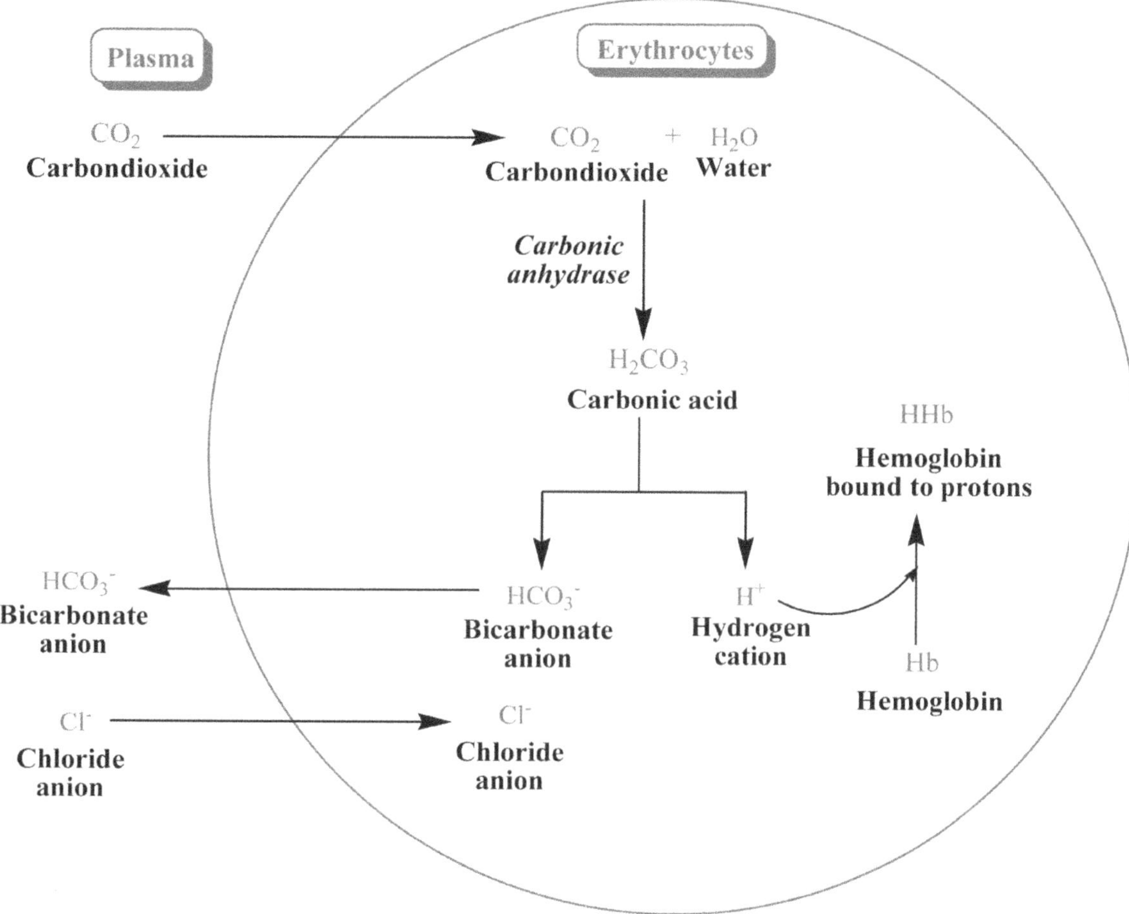

Figure 12.6 Generation of bicarbonate by the erythrocytes.

3. **Renal mechanism:**

Kidneys play a highly significant role in the maintenance of the acid-base balance of the body (blood pH). To an acid-base disturbance, a permanent solution is provided by a renal mechanism where a buffer system is temporary and the respiratory mechanism is only for a short term. Depending on the situation, along with the excretion and reabsorption of acidic or basic substances, the kidney maintains the alkali reserve for the regulation of blood pH.

Normally, the pH of the urine is acidic (6.0) compared to the slightly alkaline pH of blood plasma (7.4) because the kidney eliminates the hydrogen cation (H^+) generated under normal circumstances by the body. Depending on the concentration of hydrogen cation (H^+), the pH of the urine may vary from 4.5 to 9.5. *Carbonic anhydrase* is the central molecule involved in the regulation of blood pH by the following mechanisms.

(a) Excretion of hydrogen cation (H^+)
(b) Reabsorption of bicarbonate anion (HCO_3^-)
(c) Excretion of titratable acid
(d) Excretion of ammonium ions

(a) Excretion of hydrogen cation (H^+): From the body, the hydrogen cation (H^+) can excrete only through the kidneys and it occurs in proximal convoluted tubules (renal tubular cells) with the regeneration of bicarbonate anion (HCO_3^-). The hydrogen cation (H^+) produced form the carbonic acid (H_2CO_3) in renal tubular cell is secreted in the tubular lumen in exchange for a sodium cation (Na^+). This sodium in association with the bicarbonate anion (HCO_3^-) is reabsorbed into the blood. The secreted hydrogen cation (H^+) in the tubular lumen is combined with non-carbonate base and excreted in the urine. This is an effective mechanism for the excretion of hydrogen cation (H^+) with the simultaneous generation of bicarbonate anion (HCO_3^-). This bicarbonate anion (HCO_3^-) adds up to the alkali reserve of the body. The details of the excretion of hydrogen cation (H^+) mechanism is depicted in the Figure 12.7.

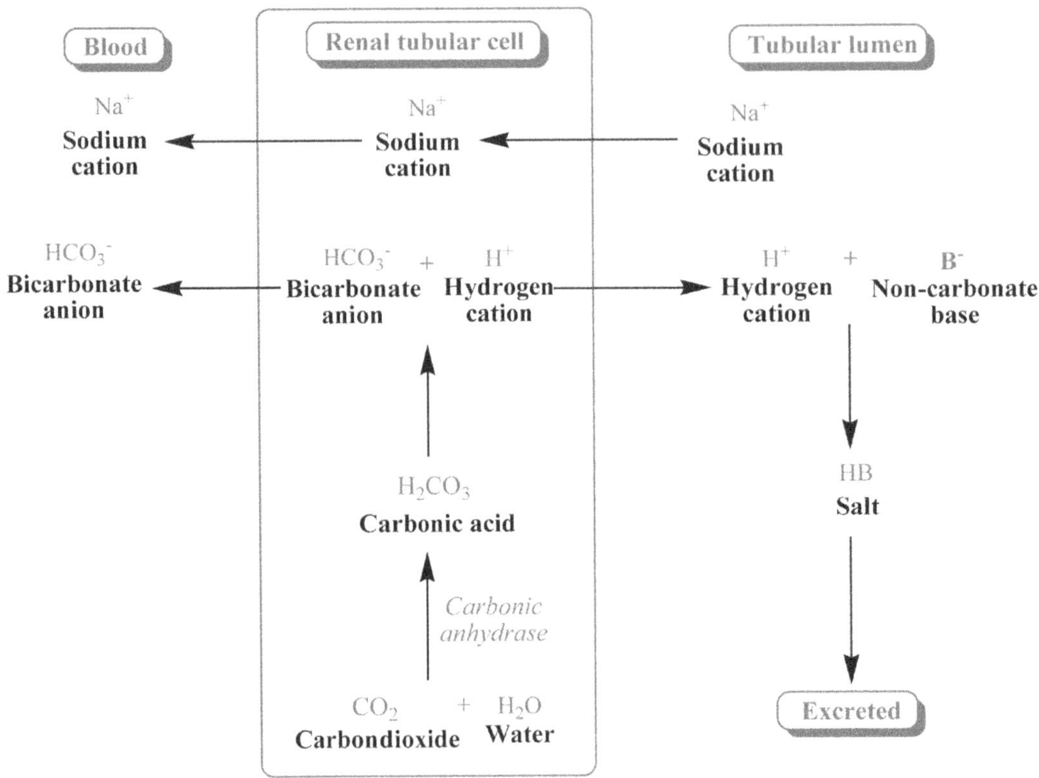

Figure12.7 Renal mechanism for blood pH regulation (Excretion of hydrogen cation (H^+)).

(b) **Reabsorption of bicarbonate anion (HCO_3^-):** The normal urine is almost free from bicarbonate anion (HCO_3^-) and this mechanism is primarily responsible to conserve the blood bicarbonate anion (HCO_3^-) with simultaneous excretion of hydrogen cation (H^+). This mechanism is helpful for maintaining the steady-state and will not be effective for the elimination of hydrogen cation (H^+) or the generation of bicarbonate anion (HCO_3^-) and the details are presented in the Figure 12.8.

(c) **Excretion of titratable acid:** The estimation of acid excreted by the kidney in urine is called titratable acidity. The urine is back titrated to the normal pH of the blood i.e., 7.4. Titratable acidity is defined as the number of ml of 0.1 N sodium hydroxide required to titrate 1 liter of urine to pH 7.4. It reflects the hydrogen cation (H^+) excreted into the urine which results in a fall of pH from 7.4 (that of blood). The phosphate buffer is used to buffer the actually excreted hydrogen cation (H^+) in the urine. The base disodium hydrogen phosphate (Na_2HPO_4) is dissociated into a sodium cation (Na^+) and a sodium hydrogen phosphate anion ($NaHPO_4^-$). Now, the sodium cation (Na^+) is exchanged for the secretion of hydrogen cation (H^+) in the tubular lumen; whereas the sodium hydrogen phosphate anion ($NaHPO_4^-$) is combined with the hydrogen cation (H^+) and produces sodium dihydrogen phosphate (NaH_2PO_4). The major quantity of titratable acid in urine is present in this form. More and more hydrogen cations (H^+) are added when the tubular fluid moves down the renal tubules resulting in the acidification of urine as low as 4.5. The depletion of the sodium cation (Na^+) takes place as a result of any further fall in the pH of urine. Excretion of titratable acid by phosphate buffer system is schematically presented in Figure 12.9.

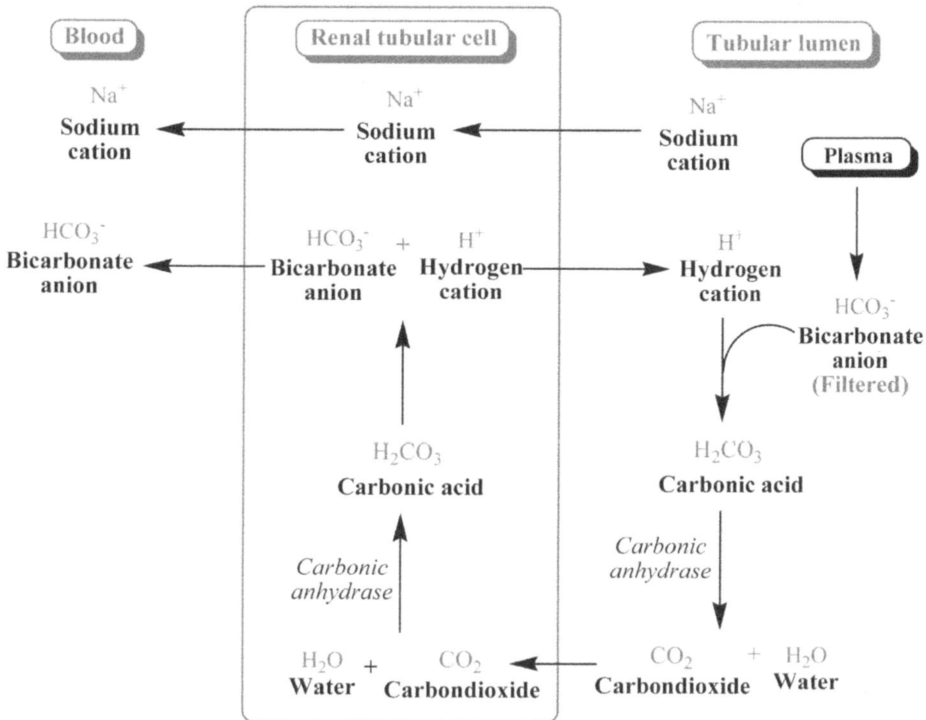

Figure 12.8 Renal mechanism for blood pH regulation (Reabsorption of bicarbonate anion (HCO_3^-)).

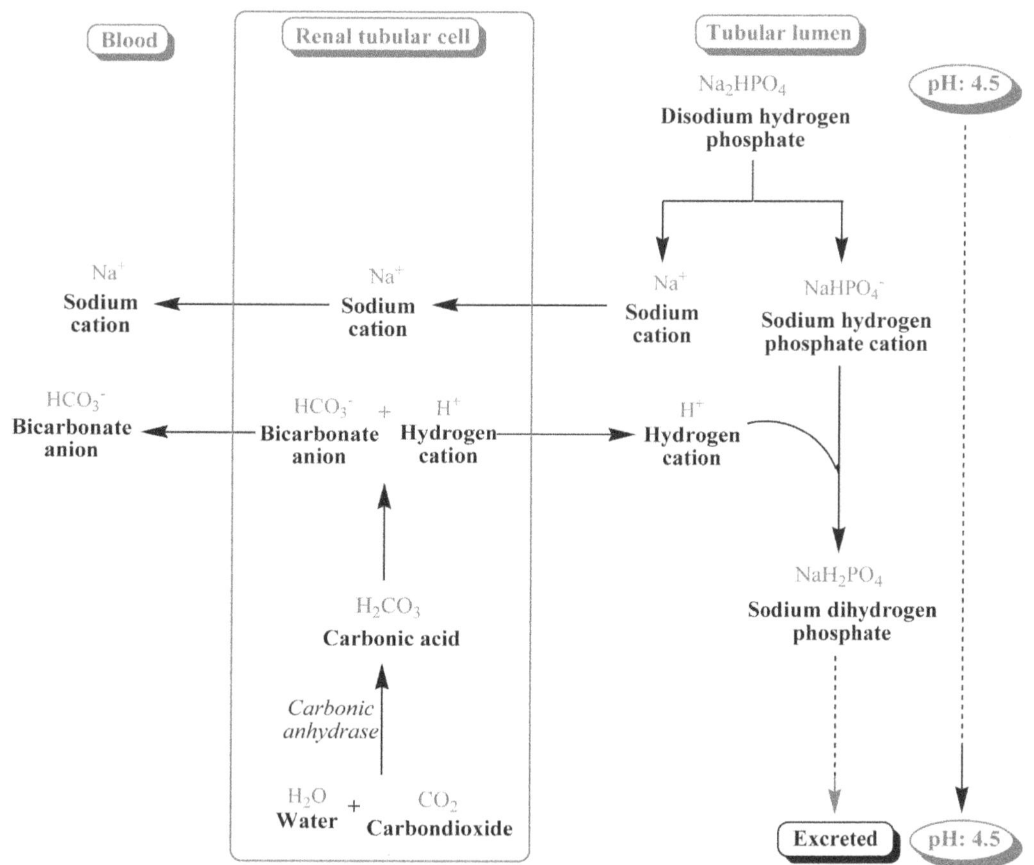

Figure 12.9 Renal mechanism for blood pH regulation (Excretion of titratable acid by phosphate buffer system).

(d) **Excretion of ammonium ions:** In this renal mechanism, the hydrogen cation (H^+) secreted in the tubular lumen is buffered with ammonia (obtained from the deamidation of glutamine to glutamate in presence of *glutaminase* in renal tubular cell and diffused into the tubular lumen) to produce ammonium cation (NH_4^+). This ammonium cation (NH_4^+) is excreted in the urine and not diffused back into the renal tubular cells. The major urine acid is ammonium cation (NH_4^+) and in this ammonium cation (NH_4^+) form, only about half to two-thirds of the body acid load is eliminated. Hence, this mechanism is very effective to eliminate large quantities of acid produced in the body and it becomes predominant, particularly in acidosis. Excretion of ammonium cation (NH_4^+) mechanism is presented in Figure 12.10.

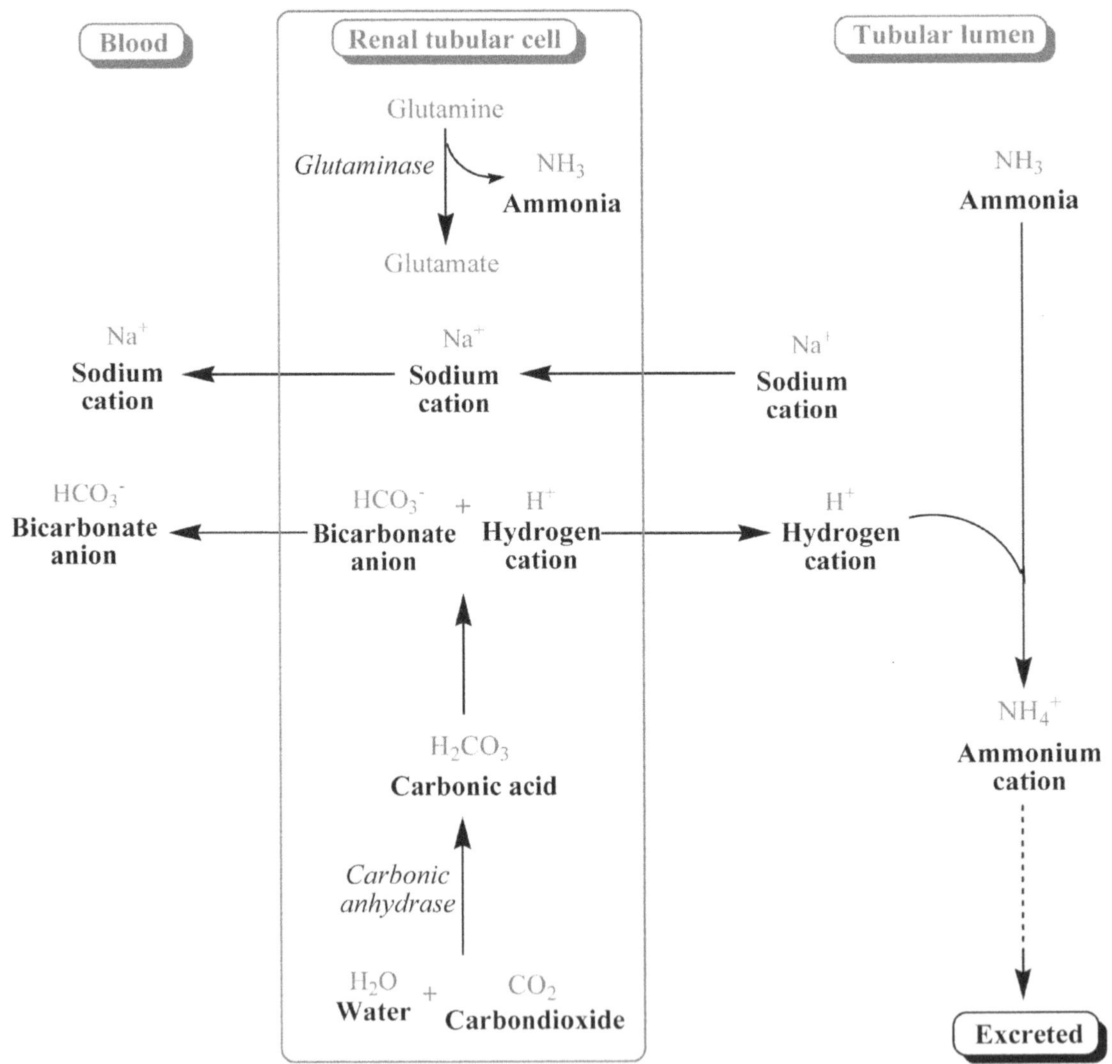

Figure 12.10 Renal mechanism for blood pH regulation (Excretion of ammonium cation (NH_4^+)).

Carbondioxide - The central molecule of pH regulation:

In the acid-base balance of the body, carbondioxide is the central molecule. Carbondioxide (CO_2) has the ability to combine with water and produce carbonic acid (H_2CO_3) which can dissociate into hydrogen cation (H^+) and bicarbonate anion (HCO_3^-). To maintain the pH of blood, handling of carbondioxide (CO_2) between the lungs, erythrocytes, and kidneys are summarized in the Figure 12.11. In aerobic metabolism, the produced carbondioxide (CO_2) may be exhaled via lungs or converted to bicarbonate anion (HCO_3^-) by erythrocytes and kidneys to add to the alkali reserve of the body.

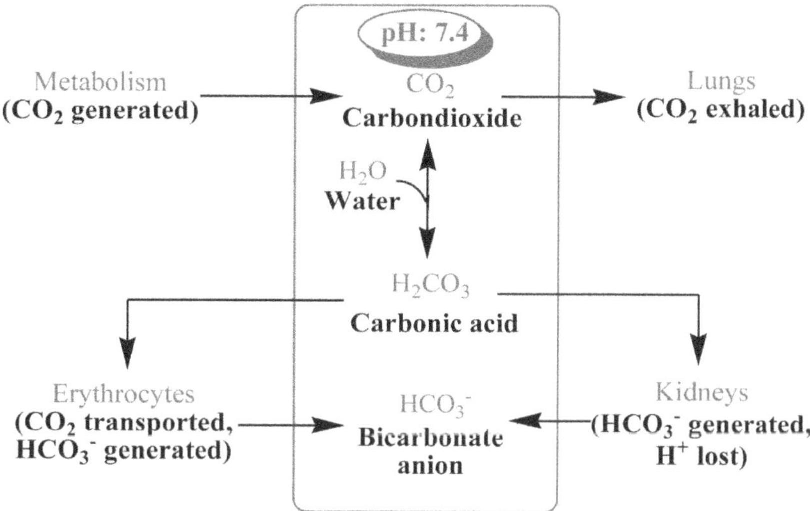

Figure 12.11 Carbondioxide – The central molecule of blood pH regulation.

Buffers of intracellular fluids (ICF):

Like extracellular fluids (ECF), the regulation of pH within the cell (ICF) is also important. The hydrogen cation (H^+) produced in the cells is exchanged for sodium cation (Na^+) and potassium cation (K^+) which reduces the potential accumulation of hydrogen cation (H^+) in the cells. Particularly, it is observed in the skeletal muscle.

Disorders of Acid-base Balance

The compatible blood pH for the existence of life is 6.8 to 7.8 and life cannot exist beyond that pH. The Henderson-Hassselbalch equation is used for a better understanding of the acid-base balance disorders.

$$pH = pK_a + log\frac{[HCO_3^-]}{[H_2CO_3]}$$ .....(Henderson-Hassselbalch equation)

From the above equation, it is evident that the pH of blood (concentration of hydrogen cation (H^+)) depends on the relative concentration of bicarbonate anion (HCO_3^-) and carbonic acid (H_2CO_3).

Classification:

Theoretically, there are two major classes of acid-base disorders and each class is further divided into two sub-classes as follows,

1. Acidosis (pH of blood decreased)
   (a) Metabolic acidosis (Due to decreased bicarbonate anion (HCO_3^-))
   (b) Respiratory acidosis (Due to increased carbonic acid (H_2CO_3))
2. Alkalosis (pH of blood increased)
   (a) Metabolic alkalosis (Due to increased bicarbonate anion (HCO_3^-))
   (b) Respiratory alkalosis (Due to decreased carbonic acid (H_2CO_3))

The metabolic acid-base disorder is due to direct changes in the concentration of bicarbonate anion (HCO_3^-) and the respiratory acid-base disorder is due to direct changes in the concentration of carbonic acid (H_2CO_3). But clinically mixed types of disorders are common. An increase or decrease in the concentration of hydrogen cation (H^+) in the blood is termed as acidemia and alkalemia respectively. But these terms are not commonly used.

Compensation of acid-base disorders: The body gears up its homeostatic mechanism to counter the acid-base disturbances and makes every attempt to restore the pH to a normal level. This process is termed as compensation, which may be partial or full. Sometimes, it may be uncompensated also. Acute metabolic disorders are compensated by the respiratory compensation through regulating the concentration of carbonic acid (H_2CO_3) by hyperventilation or hypoventilation. In the case of acute respiratory disorders, it is compensated renal compensation through regulating the concentration of bicarbonate anion (HCO_3^-) by increasing or decreasing its excretion. The primary change and the compensatory mechanism for various acid-base disorders are summarized in the Table 12.4.

Table 12.4 The primary change and the compensatory mechanism for various acid-base disorders.

S. No.	Disorder name	Primary change	Compensatory mechanism	Timescale for compensation
1	Metabolic acidosis	Plasma bicarbonate anion (HCO_3^-) decreased	Hyperventilation (increased elimination of carbondioxide)	Minutes to hours
2	Respiratory acidosis	Plasma carbondioxide increased	Plasma bicarbonate anion (HCO_3^-) and renal absorption of bicarbonate anion (HCO_3^-) is increased	Days
3	Metabolic alkalosis	Plasma bicarbonate anion (HCO_3^-) increased	Hypoventilation (decreased elimination of carbondioxide)	Minutes to hours
4	Respiratory alkalosis	Plasma carbondioxide decreased	Plasma bicarbonate anion (HCO_3^-) and renal absorption of bicarbonate anion (HCO_3^-) is decreased	Days

Anion gap: To maintain the electrical neutrality in the body fluids, the total concentration of the cations and anions is equal. The anion gap is defined as the difference between the total measured concentration of cations (sodium cation (Na^+) and potassium cation (K^+)) and that of the total measured concentration of anions (chloride anion (Cl^-) and bicarbonate anion (HCO_3^-)). In fact, unmeasured anions in the plasma are represented by anion gap (A^-) and the following formula is used to calculate the anion gap.

$$\text{Anion gap } (A^-) = \text{Concentration of cations} - \text{Concentration of anions}$$

$$= [Na^+ + K^+] - [Cl^- + HCO_3^-] = [136 + 4] - [100 + 25] = 140 - 125 = 15 \text{ mEq/l}$$

In a healthy individual, the anion gap is 15 mEq/l (In the range of 8 to 18 mEq/l). The anion gap is altered generally in acid-base disorders.

Metabolic acidosis: In this disorder, the blood pH is decreased due to reduced concentration of bicarbonate anion (HCO_3^-). The reasons behind the decreased concentration of the bicarbonate anion (HCO_3^-) are- a) utilization in buffering hydrogen cation (H^+), b) loss in urine, or gastrointestinal tract (GIT), c) failure to be regenerated. The most important one is the over production of organic acid which combines with sodium bicarbonate ($NaHCO_3$) and depletes the alkali reserve of the body by converting into corresponding sodium salt with the production of carbondioxide and water.

$$\underset{\textbf{Sodium bicarbonate}}{NaHCO_3} + \text{Organic acid} \longrightarrow \text{Sodium salt of organic acid} + CO_2 + H_2O$$

Metabolic acidosis occurs in clinical conditions such as diabetes mellitus (ketoacidosis), lactic acidosis, renal failure, etc. The anion gap is increased in metabolic acidosis due to the increased production and accumulation of organic acids. In general, metabolic acidosis is compensated by the hyperventilation of lungs by increased elimination of carbondioxide (decreased carbonic acid (H_2CO_3)) from the body.

Respiratory acidosis: In this disorder, the blood pH is decreased due to the retention of carbondioxide resulting in increased concentration of carbonic acid (H_2CO_3). The major reasons for respiratory acidosis is depression of respiratory center (overdose of drugs), pulmonary disorder (bronchopneumonia), and breathing air with a high concentration of carbondioxide. Respiratory acidosis occurs in clinical conditions like severe asthma and cardiac arrest. In general, respiratory acidosis is compensated by a renal mechanism in which more bicarbonate anion (HCO_3^-) is generated and retained by the kidney which adds up to the alkali reserve of the body. In urine, titratable acidity and ammonium cation (NH_4^+) is increased.

Metabolic alkalosis: In this disorder, the blood pH is increased due to an increased concentration of bicarbonate anion (HCO_3^-). Metabolic alkalosis occurs in clinical conditions such as vomiting (results in loss of hydrogen cation (H^+)) and hypokalemia. In general, metabolic alkalosis is compensated by the hypoventilation of lungs by decreased elimination of carbondioxide (increased carbonic acid (H_2CO_3)) from the body. This is slowly taken over by renal mechanism which exerts more bicarbonate anion (HCO_3^-) and retains hydrogen cation (H^+).

Respiratory alkalosis: In this disorder, blood pH is increased due to the decreased concentration of carbonic acid (H_2CO_3). The major reasons for the respiratory alkalosis are prolonged hyperventilation results in increased exhalation of carbondioxide by the lungs. Respiratory alkalosis occurs in clinical conditions like hyperventilation (hysteria, hypoxia, increased intracranial pressure, excessive artificial ventilation, and the action of some drugs which stimulate respiratory center, to produce hyperventilation) and severe anemia. In general, respiratory alkalosis is compensated by a renal mechanism in which the plasma bicarbonate anion (HCO_3^-) and the renal absorption of the bicarbonate anion (HCO_3^-) are decreased.

Mixed acid-base disorders: Simultaneously, when two or more acid-base disturbances occur, the concentration of both bicarbonate anion (HCO_3^-) and carbonic acid (H_2CO_3) are altered. Many times, mixed acid-base disorders occur as a result of a compensatory mechanism.

Acid-base disorders & plasma potassium: The normal plasma potassium concentration is 3.5 to 5.0 mEq/l and it affects the contraction of the heart. Hence, it is very important. Both hypokalemia (decreased plasma K^+) and hyperkalemia (increased plasma K^+) are life-threatening. In metabolic acidosis, particularly diabetic ketoacidosis is associated with hypokalemia (decreased plasma K^+) and the patient is treated with potassium supplement along with insulin. Metabolic alkalosis is associated with increased renal excretion of potassium cation (K^+). Hence, in acid-base disorders, it is necessary to measure the plasma potassium cation (K^+) concentration. Incase if the disorder is associated with hypokalemia, careful monitoring of plasma potassium cation (K^+) and potassium supplementation must be considered.

BLOOD GAS MEASUREMENT

Blood gas measurement is an important investigation associated with respiratory failure and/or acid-base disorders. In general, from the radial artery of the forearm or femoral artery of the leg, arterial blood is collected for blood gas analysis. The plasma concentration of oxygen, cabondioxide, and pH is measured and the bicarbonate concentration is calculated using the Henderson-Hassselbalch equation. The normal blood gas analysis values for different parameters are as follows,

1. **Hydrogen cation (H^+):** 35 - 43 mmol/l
2. **pH:** 7.35 - 7.45
3. **Plasma carbondioxide:** 4.5 to 6.0 kPa
4. **Plasma oxygen:** 10.5 to 13.5 kPa
5. **Bicarbonate:** 24 to 30 mmol/l.

PROBABLE QUESTIONS

PART – A: Multiple Choice Questions

1. What are functions of water?
   (a) In several metabolic reactions, water directly participates as a reactant
   (b) For the transport of solutes, water serves as a vehicle
   (c) Water is closely linked with the regulation of body temperature
   (d) All the above

2. In a normal healthy adult, how much body weight is composed of water?
   (a) 60 % (b) 70 %
   (c) 85 % (d) 90 %
3. Intake of water may vary from ________ liters/day and it mainly depends on the social habits and climate.
   (a) 0.4 to 4 (b) 0.5 to 5
   (c) 0.6 to 6 (d) 0.7 to 7
4. How much amount of water is produced per day by the oxidation of food stuffs?
   (a) 300 to 350 ml (b) 400 to 450 ml
   (c) 500 to 550 ml (d) 600 to 650 ml
5. Which of the following one route is not a distinct route for elimination of water from the body?
   (a) Urine (b) Skin
   (c) Lungs (d) Blood
6. Which gland secretes vasopressin (The antidiuretic hormone)?
   (a) Anterior pituitary (b) Posterior pituitary
   (c) Thyroid (d) Adrenal
7. Where the kidney is exactly located?
   (a) Between the peritoneum and posterior wall of the abdomen
   (b) Between the peritoneum and posterior wall of the liver
   (c) Between the peritoneum and anterior wall of the abdomen
   (d) Between the peritoneum and anterior wall of the liver
8. Body surface losses how much water per day by perspiration process?
   (a) 400 ml/day (b) 450 ml/day
   (c) 500 ml/day (d) 550 ml/day
9. About 15 % increased water loss is observed through the skin for every ________ °C rise in the body temperature?
   (a) 1 (b) 4
   (c) 6 (d) 8
10. Which is the most abundant mineral in the body?
    (a) Sodium (b) Potassium
    (c) Calcium (d) Magnesium
11. Which is the chief cation of the ECF?
    (a) Potassium (b) Magnesium
    (c) Sodium (d) Calcium
12. Which is the chief cation of the ICF?
    (a) Calcium (b) Sodium
    (c) Magnesium (d) Potassium
13. Which is the most abundant anion of the ECF?
    (a) Chloride (b) Phosphate
    (c) Sulphate (d) Bicarbonate
14. Which is the most abundant anion of the ICF?
    (a) Bicarbonate (b) Chloride
    (c) Phosphate (d) Sulphate

15. What is the normal plasma magnesium level?
    (a) 0 to 1 mg/dl
    (b) 2 to 3 mg/dl
    (c) 4 to 5 mg/dl
    (d) 6 to 7 mg/dl.
16. What is the normal plasma chlorine level?
    (a) 95 to 105 mEq/l
    (b) 100 to 105 mEq/l
    (c) 105 to 110 mEq/l
    (d) 125 to 150 mEq/l
17. Osmosis is defined as a process by which molecules of a solvent tend to pass through a semi-permeable membrane from a __________ concentrated solution into a ______________ concentrated one.
    (a) More, more
    (b) More, less
    (c) Less, more
    (d) Less, less
18. The number of moles or millimoles per liter of solution is commonly known as ______________.
    (a) Osmolality
    (b) Osmolarity
    (c) Molarity
    (d) Molality
19. The number of moles or millimoles per kilogram of solvent is ______________.
    (a) Molarity
    (b) Molality
    (c) Osmolality
    (d) Osmolarity
20. The normal osmolality of plasma varies from ___________ milliosmoles/Kg.
    (a) 255-265
    (b) 265-275
    (c) 275-285
    (d) 285-295
21. Which instrument is used to measure the osmolality?
    (a) Osmometer
    (b) Colorimeter
    (c) pH meter
    (d) Refractometer
22. Which of the following statement is wrong with respect to aldosterone?
    (a) Secreted by the thyroid gland
    (b) It is a mineralocorticoid
    (c) It increases the reabsorption of sodium cation by the renal tubules
    (d) Secreted by the adrenal cortex
23. Hypothalamus is stimulated to release antidiuretic hormone when the plasma osmolality is ______________ mostly due to ______________.
    (a) Increased & calcium cation
    (b) Increased & sodium cation
    (c) Decreased & calcium cation
    (d) Decreased & sodium cation
24. Atrial natriuretic factor or atriopeptin is a peptide containing how many amino acids?
    (a) 38
    (b) 28
    (c) 18
    (d) 8
25. Which of the following stimulate the atrium of the heart to produce ANF or atriopeptin?
    (a) Increased blood volume
    (b) Elevated blood pressure
    (c) High salt intake
    (d) All the above
26. What happened when ANF or atriopeptin acts on the kidney?
    (a) Increased GFR
    (b) Increased sodium retention
    (c) Increased urine output
    (d) All the above
27. Which of the following causes dehydration?
    (a) Diarrhea & vomiting
    (b) Fluid loss in burns
    (c) Kidney disease like renal insufficiency
    (d) All the above

28. Which of the following statement is wrong with respect to characteristic of dehydration?
    (a) Elevated pulse rate
    (b) Increased blood pressure
    (c) Sunken eyeballs
    (d) Decreased skin turgor
29. Which of the following statement is wrong with respect to diuretics?
    (a) Stimulates water and sodium excretion
    (b) Used in the treatment of edema
    (c) Used in the treatment of hypotension
    (d) Used in the treatment of heart failure
30. Which of the following method is used for estimation of sodium in body fluids?
    (a) Flame photometry method
    (b) Ion-selective electrodes method
    (c) Colorimetric method
    (d) All the above
31. In colorimetric method, sodium present in body fluids is precipitated as the ________ salt.
    (a) Single
    (b) Double
    (c) Triple
    (d) Tetra
32. Which substance is act as a precipitating agent in the estimation of sodium by colorimetric method?
    (a) Trichloroacetic acid
    (b) Uranyl acetate
    (c) Zinc acetate
    (d) Acetic acid-ethanol mixture
33. Low serum sodium level is known as ________________.
    (a) Hypernatremia
    (b) Hyperkalemia
    (c) Hyponatremia
    (d) Hypokalemia
34. Hypernatremia is found in which clinical conditions?
    (a) Metabolic acidosis
    (b) Hyperadrenalism
    (c) Addison's disease
    (d) Renal tubular disease
35. In Clark and Collip titrimetric method estimation of calcium which one is used as titrant?
    (a) Sodium hydroxide
    (b) Perchloric acid
    (c) Hydrochloric acid
    (d) Potassium permanganate
36. Which of the following compound is used as precipitating agent in Clark and Collip titrimetric method estimation of calcium?
    (a) Ammonium oxalate
    (b) Zinc acetate
    (c) Barium chloride
    (d) Potassium nitrate
37. What is the relationship between the concentration of serum calcium and serum inorganic phosphate?
    (a) Directly proportional
    (b) Indirectly proportional
    (c) Both a & b
    (d) None of the above
38. In which clinical conditions serum calcium level is not increased?
    (a) Hyperparathyroidism
    (b) Multiple myeloma
    (c) Hypovitaminosis-D
    (d) Sarcoidosis
39. Which compound is present in potassium turbid reagent?
    (a) Sodium tetraphenyl boron
    (b) Sodium triphenyl boron
    (c) Magnesium tetraphenyl boron
    (d) Magnesium triphenyl boron
40. What is hyperkalemia?
    (a) Decreased serum calcium level
    (b) Increased serum calcium level
    (c) Decreased serum potassium level
    (d) Increased serum potassium level

41. Serum potassium level is decreased in which clinical conditions?
    (a) Renal failure
    (b) Negative nitrogen balance
    (c) Dehydration shock
    (d) Adrenal insufficiency
42. Serum potassium level is increased in which clinical conditions?
    (a) Dehydration shock
    (b) Malnutrition
    (c) Gastrointestinal fluid loss
    (d) Hyperactivity of the adrenal cortex
43. Which method is available for the estimation of chloride?
    (a) Colorimetric method
    (b) Titrimetric method, and amperometric method
    (c) Use of chloride meter
    (d) All the above
44. Mercuric thiocyanate is used in estimation of which electrolyte?
    (a) Bicarbonate
    (b) Calcium
    (c) Chloride
    (d) Potassium
45. Hypochloridemia is observed in which clinical condition?
    (a) Metabolic acidosis
    (b) Dehydration
    (c) Congestive heart failure
    (d) Conditions causing decreased renal blood flow
46. Hyperchloridemia is observed in which clinical condition?
    (a) Salt-losing nephritis
    (b) Metabolic acidosis
    (c) Vomiting
    (d) Dehydration
47. Which of the following enzymes are useful for the estimation of bicarbonate?
    (a) *Phosphoenolpyruvate carboxylase & lactate dehydrogenase*
    (b) *Phosphoenolpyruvate carboxylase & malate dehydrogenase*
    (c) *Phosphoenolpyruvate carboxy kinase & lactate dehydrogenase*
    (d) *Phosphoenolpyruvate carboxy kinase & malate dehydrogenase*
48. What is the normal pH of the blood?
    (a) Strongly acidic
    (b) Strongly basic
    (c) Slightly acidic
    (d) Slightly basic
49. What is buffer?
    (a) Solution of a strong acid and its salt with a strong base
    (b) Solution of a weak acid and its salt with a strong base
    (c) Solution of a strong acid and its salt with a weak base
    (d) Solution of a weak acid and its salt with a weak base
50. Which one is the predominant buffer system of the extracellular fluid particularly plasma?
    (a) Bicarbonate buffer system
    (b) Phosphate buffer system
    (c) Protein buffer system
    (d) Oxalate buffer system

Key for Multiple Choice Questions

1 (d)	2 (a)	3 (b)	4 (a)	5 (d)
6 (b)	7 (a)	8 (b)	9 (a)	10 (c)
11 (c)	12 (d)	13 (a)	14 (c)	15 (b)

16 (a)	17 (c)	18 (b)	19 (c)	20 (d)
21 (a)	22 (a)	23 (b)	24 (c)	25 (d)
26 (d)	27 (d)	28 (b)	29 (c)	30 (d)
31 (c)	32 (a)	33 (c)	34 (b)	35 (d)
36 (a)	37 (b)	38 (c)	39 (a)	40 (d)
41 (b)	42 (a)	43 (d)	44 (c)	45 (a)
46 (d)	47 (b)	48 (d)	49 (b)	50 (a)

PART – B: Short Answers

1. Write a short note on functions of water.
2. How water is distributed in human biological system?
3. What is ICF and ECF?
4. Explain the term "water turnover".
5. What is exogenous and endogenous water?
6. What are four distinct routes of water excretion from the body?
7. Write the electrolyte composition of intracellular fluid.
8. Write the electrolyte composition of extracellular fluid.
9. Define osmolarity and osmolality.
10. Write a note on plasma osmolality.
11. How electrolyte balance is regulated?
12. What is atriopeptin?
13. Write a note on dehydration.
14. What is overhydration?
15. Explain distribution of body water using water tank model.
16. Write the principle involved in the estimation of sodium in body fluids by colorimetric method.
17. What is hyponatremia and hypernatremia?
18. Write the principle involved in the estimation of calcium in body fluids by titrimetric method.
19. Write the significance of serum potassium level.
20. Write the principle involved in the estimation of chloride in body fluids by colorimetric method.
21. Explain the principle involved in the estimation of bicarbonate in body fluids by enzymatic method.
22. How acid and bases are produced in the body?
23. What are blood buffers?
24. What is metabolic acidosis and respiratory acidosis?
25. What is an anion gap?

PART – C: Long Answers

1. What are all the functions of water? How water is distributed in biological system?
2. Write a detailed note on water turnover and water balance.
3. What is the importance of electrolyte balance in body fluids? How it is regulated?
4. Write about electrolyte composition of body fluids. Comment on its diagnostic applications.
5. Explain about water balance and its regulation in the body.
6. List out various electrolyte present in body and explain their respective distribution in detail.
7. How electrolyte balance is regulated in the body fluids?
8. Explain dehydration and overhydration in detail with treatment option.

9. Explain the methods for determination of sodium in body fluids.
10. Write the principle and procedure involved in the estimation of calcium in body fluids. Add a note on significance of calcium.
11. Write a note on estimation of serum potassium by turbidimetric method.
12. How presence of chloride in body fluids are estimated by colorimetric method.
13. Write the principle and procedure involved in the estimation of bicarbonate in body fluids. Add a note on significance of bicarbonate.
14. Explain calcium and phosphate homeostasis in the body.
15. Write the mechanism involved in regulation of body's acid base balance and maintenance of blood pH.
16. Write notes on blood buffers and explain disorders of acid-base balance.
17. Explain how pH of blood is maintained.
18. Explain respiratory and renal mechanism of blood pH maintenance.
19. Discuss disorders of acid–base balance in detail.

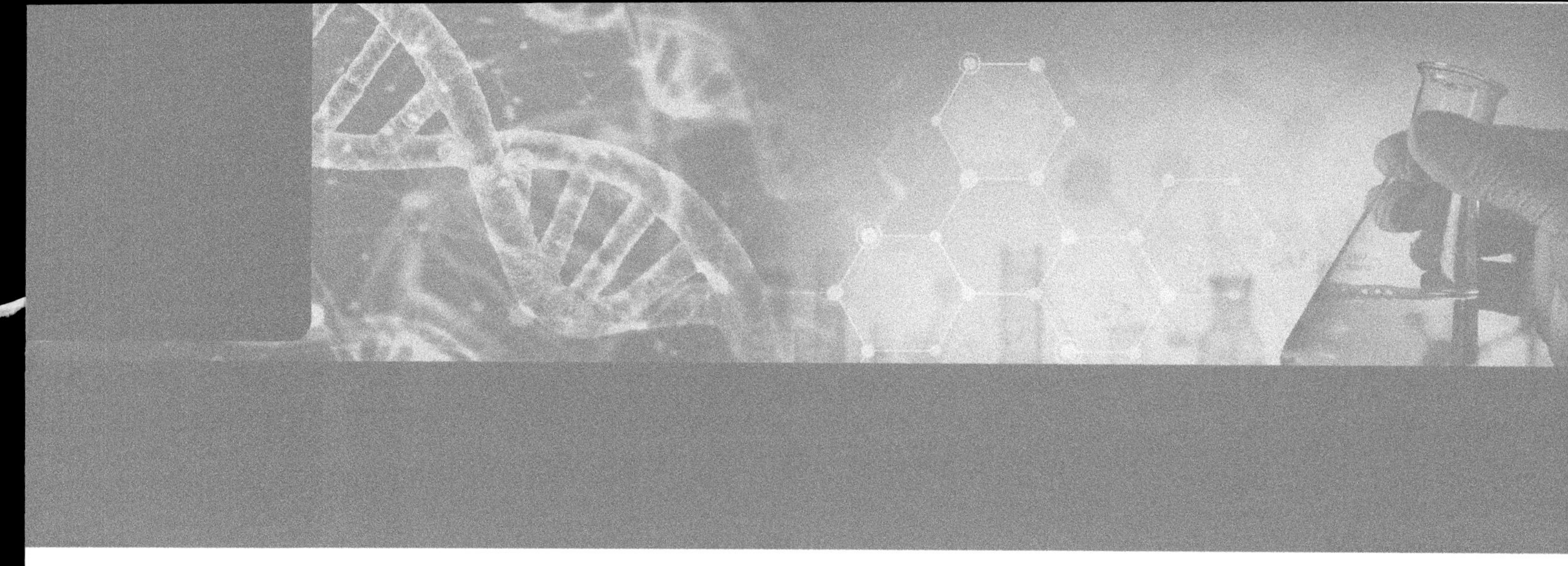

SYMBOLS

A

B

C

D

E

F

G

H

I

J

K

L

M

N

O

P

Q

R

S

T

U

V

W

X

Z

www.ingramcontent.com/pod-product-compliance
Ingram Content Group UK Ltd.
Pitfield, Milton Keynes, MK11 3LW, UK
UKHW061536190726
13845UKWH00005B/122